This book is due for return on or before the last date shown below.

- 2 DEC 2014		

GASTROINTESTINAL IMAGING CASES

The McGraw-Hill Radiology Series

This innovative series offers indispensable workstation reference material for the practicing radiologist. Within this series is a full range of practical, clinically relevant works divided into three categories:

- **Patterns:** Organized by modality, these books provide a pattern-based approach to constructing practical differential diagnoses.
- **Variants:** Structured by modality as well as anatomy, these graphic volumes aid the radiologist in reducing false positive rates.
- **Cases:** Classic case presentations with an emphasis on differential diagnoses and clinical context.

GASTROINTESTINAL IMAGING CASES

Stephan W. Anderson, MD
Associate Professor of Radiology
Boston University School of Medicine
Section Chief, Abdominal Imaging, Department of Radiology
Boston Medical Center
Boston, Massachusetts

Christine Menias, MD
Professor of Radiology
Mallinckrodt Institute of Radiology
Washington University
St. Louis, Missouri

Jorge A. Soto, MD
Professor of Radiology
Boston University School of Medicine
Vice Chairman, Department of Radiology
Boston Medical Center
Boston, Massachusetts

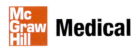 **Medical**

New York   Chicago   San Francisco   Lisbon   London   Madrid   Mexico City
New Delhi   San Juan   Seoul   Singapore   Sydney   Toronto

ISBN 978-0-07-163659-9
MHID 0-07-163659-5

Notice

Medicine is an ever-changing science. As new research and clinical experience broaden our knowledge, changes in treatment and drug therapy are required. The authors and the publisher of this work have checked with sources believed to be reliable in their efforts to provide information that is complete and generally in accord with the standards accepted at the time of publication. However, in view of the possibility of human error or changes in medical sciences, neither the authors nor the publisher nor any other party who has been involved in the preparation or publication of this work warrants that the information contained herein is in every respect accurate or complete, and they disclaim all responsibility for any errors or omissions or for the results obtained from use of the information contained in this work. Readers are encouraged to confirm the information contained herein with other sources. For example and in particular, readers are advised to check the product information sheet included in the package of each drug they plan to administer to be certain that the information contained in this work is accurate and that changes have not been made in the recommended dose or in the contraindications for administration. This recommendation is of particular importance in connection with new or infrequently used drugs.

This book was set in TradeGothic by Cenveo Publisher Services.
The editors were Michael Weitz and Brian Kearns.
The production supervisor was Catherine Saggese.
Project management was provided by Anupriya Tyagi, Cenveo Publisher Services.
The designer was Eve Siegel.
China Translation & Printing Services, Ltd. was printer and binder.

Library of Congress Cataloging-in-Publication Data

Anderson, Stephan, 1975
  Gastrointestinal imaging: cases/Stephan Anderson, Christine Menias, Jorge Soto.
      p. ; cm.
  ISBN 978-0-07-163659-9 (alk. paper)—ISBN 0-07-163659-5 (alk. paper)
I. Menias, Christine, 1968 II. Soto, Jorge A. III. Title. [DNLM: 1. Digestive System
  Diseases—radiography—Case Reports. 2. Diagnosis, Differential—Case Reports.
  3. Diagnostic Imaging—methods—Case Reports. WI 141]
616.3′30754—dc23   2012038223

To my wife and sons.
Stephan W. Anderson, MD

I would like to thank all of the Mallinckrodt family of residents, fellows, and faculty who have and continue to teach me. It's been a great privilege. The contributions to the "Cooky Jar" all these years is the reason that this review can be made.
Christine Menias, MD

I dedicate this book to my parents, wife, and children.
Jorge A. Soto, MD

CONTENTS

CONTRIBUTORS

Rahul Arya, MD
Department of Radiology
Boston University Medical Center
Boston, Massachusetts

Tharakeswara Kumar Bathala, MD
Department of Radiology
University of Texas MD
Anderson Cancer Center Houston, Texas

German Castrillon, MD
Staff Radiologist
Universidad de Antioquia
Medellin, Colombia

David Hindson, MD
Department of Radiology
Boston University Medical Center
Boston, Massachusetts

Steven Kussman, MD
Department of Radiology
Boston University Medical Center
Boston, Massachusetts

Vijay Ramalingam, MD
Department of Radiology
Boston University Medical Center
Boston, Massachusetts

Emilio Sanin, MD
Staff Radiologist
Hospital Pablo Tobon Uribe
Medellin, Colombia

Jennifer Uyeda, MD
Department of Radiology
Boston University Medical Center
Boston, Massachusetts

PREFACE

While many radiologists attain a fair degree of comfort with gastrointestinal (GI) imaging, this book aims both to reinforce the more common knowledge and expand the breadth of familiarity of radiologists with GI pathologies and disease entities. This includes the presentation of clinically relevant subtleties and nuances of common conditions, increasing the added values of the radiologists in these common GI diagnoses. In addition, we present the less common GI conditions and diseases which, while not encountered on a daily basis, may have significant clinical impact in a given patient's care.

This book, entitled *Gastrointestinal Imaging Cases* aims to familiarize the reader with a wide range of entities encountered in GI image practice. Included herein are diseases and conditions ranging from those which are commonly encountered to those which, while less common, remain clinically relevant. Importantly, common variants and benign conditions are presented to allow the reader to confidently detect malignant and other life-threatening conditions. Naturally, the images provided are paramount to gaining a complete understanding of the various imaging presentations of a particular condition, along with useful imaging features which allow for confident diagnoses. In addition, included in the body of each case, a *Presentation* section highlights common or classic clinical signs and symptoms related to the condition at hand. Subsequently, the *Findings* section presents a brief overview of the salient points of the imaging features of the case. The *Differential Diagnosis* lists other conditions which may be entertained given a similarity in clinical presentation or imaging features. The *Comments* section provides a detailed description of each case, including pertinent background information, clinical presentation, pathophysiology, and imaging findings on modalities typically employed in a particular case. Finally, the *Pearls* section lists several salient take-home points for each case, from the clinical presentation to the imaging findings. Ultrasound, computed tomography (CT), and magnetic resonance imaging (MRI) are the predominant modalities employed throughout this text, a reflection of appropriate clinical practice. In addition, where relevant, plain radiography, fluoroscopy, and positron emission tomography (PET) are presented.

This book is intended to be a good resource for the practicing radiologist but is also felt to be highly appropriate for the radiologist in training, from those interested in more advanced training in GI imaging to those in dedicated GI imaging fellowships. The intent of this work is not to provide an encyclopedic presentation of all aspects of GI imaging, but to present those conditions which are felt to be relevant in the clinical practice of GI radiology.

CHAPTER 1

LIVER

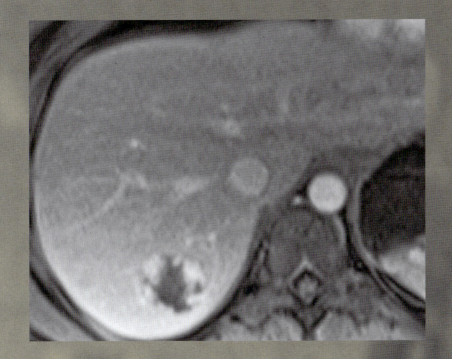

BENIGN LIVER LESIONS

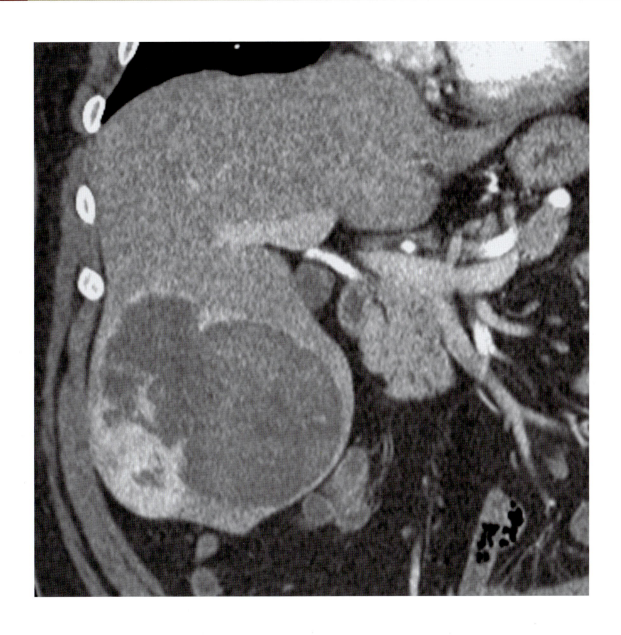

PRESENTATION

Hemangiomas are usually asymptomatic unless extremely large. These are incidental findings that frequently have typical imaging characteristics that, when present, allow a confident diagnosis without need for biopsy or follow-up.

FINDINGS

Well-circumscribed, homogenous, hyperechoic masses with posterior acoustic enhancement on ultrasound (US) imaging, hypoattenuating on unenhanced, and on magnetic resonance (MR) T1 hypointense and T2 hyperintense on MR. After contrast injection, globular, peripheral, discontinuous enhancement, which progresses to uniform, centripetal filling, and contrast retention on portal, equilibrium, and delayed phases. Atypical appearances are common.

DIFFERENTIAL DIAGNOSIS

- Hepatocellular carcinoma
- Focal nodular hyperplasia
- Liver metastasis

COMMENTS

Cavernous hemangiomas are the most common liver tumor, present in 1% to 20% of the population. They are benign lesions that arise from the endothelial cells that line the blood vessels and consist of multiple, large vascular channels lined by a single layer of endothelial cells. Hemangiomas are less frequent in cirrhotic livers, thought to regress secondary to the fibrotic process. Most have typical imaging characteristics, but some atypical variants have also been described.

Typical cavernous hemangiomas will be well-circumscribed, homogenous, hyperechoic masses with posterior acoustic enhancement on US imaging. On unenhanced CT they will be hypoattenuating, and on MR they will be T1 hypointense and T2 hyperintense. After contrast injection, arterial phase imaging will demonstrate a globular, peripheral, discontinuous enhancement, which will progress to uniform, centripetal filling, and contrast retention on portal, equilibrium, and delayed phases. These lesions do not demonstrate diffusion restriction, although the T2 shine-through phenomenon can be expected. Atypical hemangiomas include those that are flash-filling (completely fill in the arterial phase), giant hemangiomas (larger than 12 cm, without complete filling in delayed imaging, and central cystic-necrotic degeneration), hyalinized hemangiomas (slightly T2 hyperintense, nonenhancing; require biopsy for diagnosis), and calcified hemangiomas. In the presence of hepatic steatosis or cirrhosis, the imaging appearance of

cavernous hemangiomas is variable. Cavernous hemangiomas are uncommon in patients with advanced cirrhosis. It is believed that hemangiomas may undergo thrombosis and subsequently involute as the hepatic fibrosis progresses.

PEARLS

- Cavernous hemangiomas are benign lesions that arise from the endothelial cells that line the blood vessels and consist of multiple, large vascular channels lined by a single layer of endothelial cells.

- Typical cavernous hemangiomas are well-circumscribed, homogenous, hyperechoic masses with posterior acoustic enhancement on US imaging.

- After contrast injection, arterial phase CT or MR images demonstrate a globular, peripheral, discontinuous enhancement, which progresses to uniform, centripetal filling, and contrast retention on the portal, equilibrium, and delayed phases.

- Atypical presentations of hemangiomas on imaging are common and depend on the status of the background liver parenchyma (such as steatosis and cirrhosis).

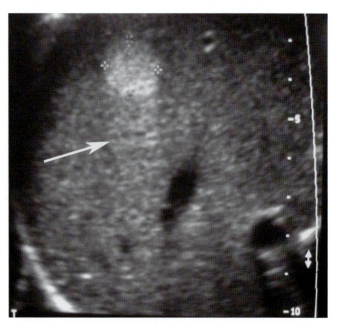

1. US image demonstrates a well-circumscribed, hyperechoic mass with posterior acoustic enhancement (arrow). The appearance is characteristic of a cavernous hemangioma.

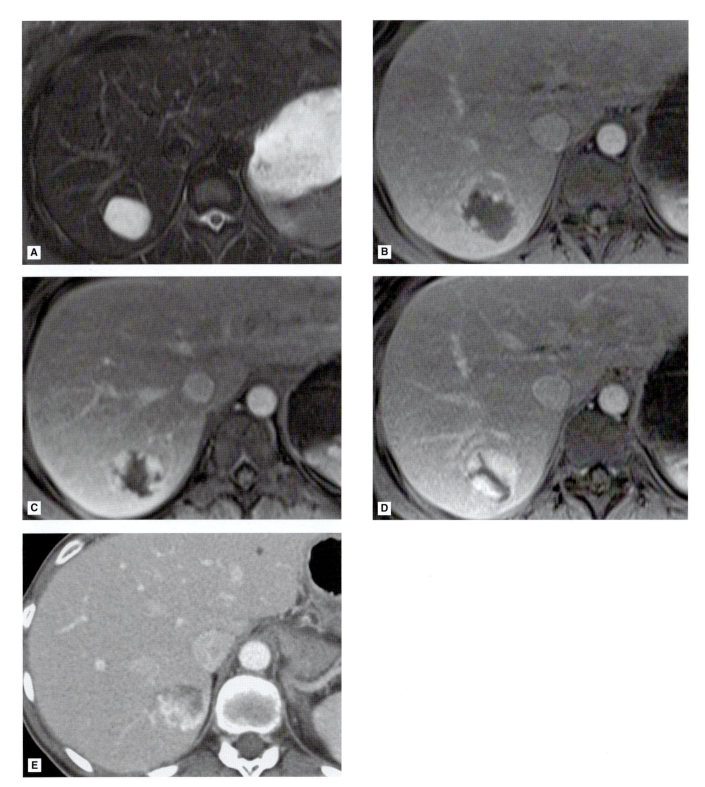

2. A. Axial T2-weighted image reveals a rounded, homogeneous, markedly hyperintense lesion. On the postcontrast images obtained in the arterial (**B**), portal venous (**C**), and delayed (**D**) phases the lesion demonstrates globular, peripheral, discontinuous enhancement that progresses centripetally over time. This enhancement pattern is characteristic of a cavernous hemangioma. **E.** Axial contrast-enhanced CT image acquired in the portal venous phase reveals a similar contrast enhancement behavior.

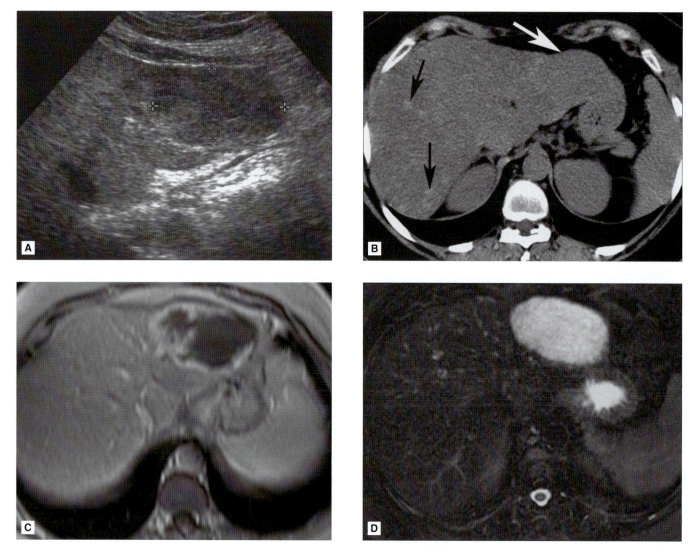

3. Atypical appearance of cavernous hemangioma on US and CT. Transverse US image (**A**) demonstrates a large, predominantly hypoechoic lesion in the left hepatic lobe (borders marked with calipers). Noncontrast CT image (**B**) shows the lesion (white arrow) as being nearly isoattenuating with the fatty-infiltrated liver parenchyma. Note multiple hyperattenuating (siderotic) nodules (black arrows). On the contrast-enhanced (**C**) and fat-suppressed T2-weighted (**D**) MR images, the appearance of the lesion is typical of a cavernous hemangioma.

PRESENTATION

- Often incidental finding
- If large enough, palpable mass and/or compression of adjacent structures
- Rupture: Pain, hemorrhagic shock

FINDINGS

The appearance on US is nonspecific. On unenhanced computed tomography (CT), they are typically iso-hypoattenuating. On MR, these lesions are iso- to hyperintense on T1W images and slightly hyperintense on T2W images. After contrast injection, enhancement is moderate. Hepatobiliary-specific MR contrast agents allow a more confident diagnosis. Intralesional fat is common and can be detected with US, CT, or MR.

DIFFERENTIAL DIAGNOSIS

- Hepatocellular carcinoma
- Focal nodular hyperplasia
- Hypervascular liver metastases
- Liver abscess

COMMENTS

Hepatic adenoma is a rare, benign tumor of the liver. At histopathologic analysis, adenomas contain normal-appearing hepatocytes with absent bile ducts and portal triads, and most do not contain Kupffer cells. They are usually solitary and have a male-female ratio of 1:9. Predisposing factors have been identified: oral contraceptive use, anabolic steroids, and glycogen storage disease. Currently, most surgeons advocate resection of any presumed hepatic adenoma, regardless of the size, mainly because of the risk of rupture and hemorrhagic shock and, second, because of the known possibility of malignant transformation to hepatocellular carcinoma.

Patients with hepatic adenoma are usually asymptomatic, in which case the lesion is discovered during laparoscopy, laparotomy, or imaging carried out for other conditions. Occasionally, an adenoma may be large enough to cause a palpable right upper quadrant mass or symptoms derived from compression of adjacent structures. Large adenomas may rupture and bleed into the peritoneal cavity, presenting with pain and even hemorrhagic shock.

The ultrasonographic appearance of adenomas is highly nonspecific. They may appear iso-, hypo-, or hyperechoic and are usually heterogeneous with fat and liquid components from prior hemorrhage or necrosis. They are

well-circumscribed, generally lobulated lesions. On unenhanced CT, adenomas are typically iso-hypoattenuating relative to the surrounding parenchyma. On MR, these lesions are iso- to hyperintense on T1W images and slightly hyperintense on T2W images. After contrast injection, they demonstrate moderate enhancement during the arterial phase and show washout and enhancement similar to the rest of the liver in the venous and delayed phases. The contrast agents Gadobenate Dimeglumine (Gd-BOPTA), and more recently, gadoxetate disodium, have been effectively used to characterize adenomas, which are intensely hypointense relative to the surrounding parenchyma on delayed images due to the lack of normally functioning hepatocytes. A ruptured adenoma will demonstrate perihepatic fluid and greater internal heterogeneity.

PEARLS

- Adenomas are usually solitary lesions, much more common in women than men and associated with use of oral contraceptives or anabolic steroids and glycogen storage disease.

- Large adenomas may rupture and bleed into the peritoneal cavity, presenting with pain and even hemorrhagic shock.

- Imaging appearance is not specific, but they may contain internal fat.

- Surgical resection of adenomas is advocated, regardless of the size, mainly because of the risk of rupture and hemorrhagic shock and because of the known possibility of malignant transformation to hepatocellular carcinoma.

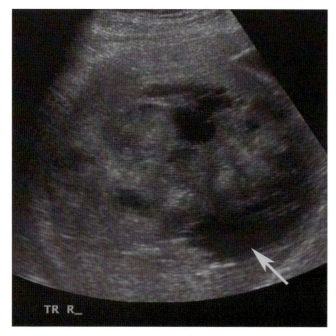

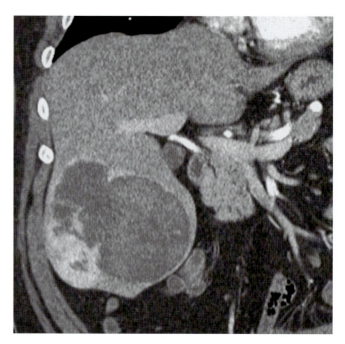

1. Transverse US image of the right lobe of the liver reveals a heterogeneous lesion with an anechoic component (arrow), due to probable hemorrhage and necrosis.

2. Coronal reformation of an arterial-phase abdominal CT shows a circumscribed lesion in the right hepatic lobe with moderate peripheral enhancement and central hypoattenuating, probably necrotic, component.

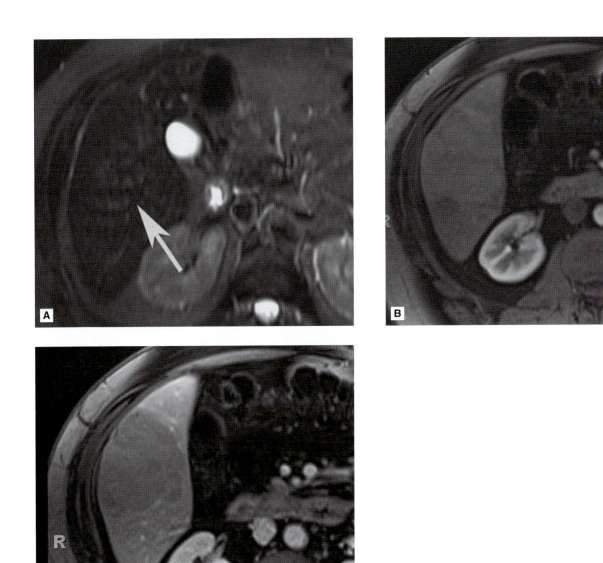

3. A. Axial T2-weighted FS image of the liver demonstrates a slightly hyperintense lesion in segment 5 of the liver (arrow). In the axial T1-weighted image after administration of intravenous gadolinium contrast in the arterial phase (**B**), the lesion presents moderate, homogeneous enhancement (arrow), with washout relative to the adjacent liver in the equilibrium phase (**C**).

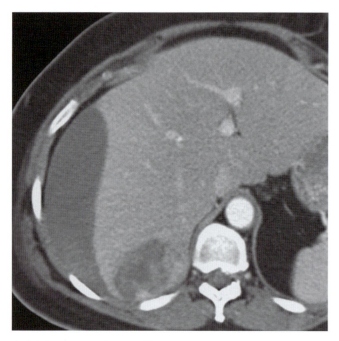

4. Axial contrast-enhanced CT image demonstrates signs of a ruptured liver lesion (white arrow), with a subcapsular hematoma (black arrow); the lesion was resected and found to be an adenoma.

PRESENTATION

Focal Nodular Hyperplasia (FNH) is typically an incidental finding in a patient imaged for unrelated symptoms. Occasionally, symptoms may arise secondary to the size of the lesion and capsular distention or compression of adjacent structures.

FINDINGS

Focal mass is homogeneous and may appear similar to the background liver on US and on noncontrast CT and MR. With contrast, the lesion enhances avidly on the arterial postcontrast phase and becomes isodense to the liver parenchyma on portal and delayed phases. The central scar displays delayed enhancement and is usually T1 hypointense and T2 hyperintense on MR.

DIFFERENTIAL DIAGNOSIS

- Hemangioma
- Hepatic adenoma
- Hepatocellular carcinoma (HCC)
- Cholangiocarcinoma
- Hypervascular liver metastases

COMMENTS

FNH is the second benign liver tumor in frequency, surpassed only by hepatic hemangioma. It has a male-to-female ratio of 1:8 and occurs in otherwise healthy, young individuals. It is composed of abnormally arranged, normal hepatic constituents. It is thought to be derived from hyperplasia secondary to an underlying congenital arteriovenous malformation. On pathology, multiple spherical nodules of hepatocytes are found, held together by a network of fibrous tissue, many times with a dominant central scar that contains multiple malformed vessels, which ultimately connect to a main, malformed feeding artery. Accurately differentiating FNH from adenoma and HCC is important, since the former requires no further workup or intervention, avoiding unnecessary biopsies or surgery.

On US, the lesion is usually a homogeneous mass that may appear iso-, hypo-, or hyperechoic. The central scar is infrequently recognized, as is the enlarged feeding artery, which could be better evaluated using Doppler ultrasound. The lesion is iso- or hypoattenuating on unenhanced CT, avidly enhances on the arterial postcontrast phase, and becomes isodense to the liver parenchyma on portal and delayed phases. The central scar, if present, is hypoattenuating in the arterial phase and displays delayed enhancement. The lesion has well-defined margins and does not invade adjacent structures. The main feeding artery can be seen in the arterial phase in many studies. On MRI, the lesion is typically T1 hypo- to isointense and T2 iso- to mildly hyperintense. The scar is usually T1 hypointense and T2 hyperintense. The behavior of the lesion and of the central scar after gadolinium injection is similar to what is found on CT. Because the lesion contains normally functioning hepatocytes, the biliary excreted contrast agent gadoxetate disodium can be administered to differentiate FNH from adenomas at delayed imaging, where they will appear hyperintense while the latter will be markedly hypointense.

PEARLS

- Focal nodular hyperplasia is the second benign liver tumor in frequency and is much more common in women than men.

- The lesion often has a dominant central scar that contains multiple malformed vessels, which ultimately connect to a main malformed feeding artery.

- The lesion is iso- or hypoattenuating on unenhanced CT, avidly enhances on the arterial postcontrast phase and becomes isodense to the liver parenchyma on portal and delayed phases. The central scar, if present, may display delayed enhancement.

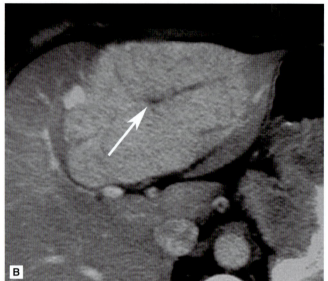

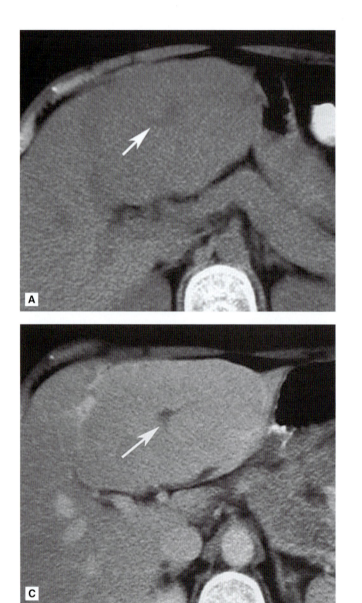

1. Noncontrast (**A**), arterial phase (**B**), and portal venous (**C**) CT images demonstrate typical features of FNH. The lesion is nearly isoattenuating with the liver parenchyma on the unenhanced (**A**) and portal venous phase (**C**) images. Enhancement is intense, diffuse, and homogeneous on the arterial-phase image (**B**). The low-attenuation central scar is well seen on all three images (arrows).

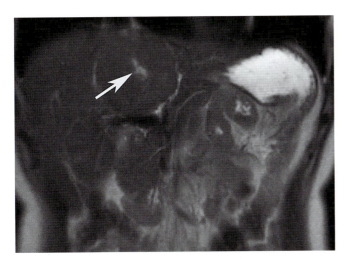

2. Coronal T2-weighted image demonstrates a rounded, well-circumscribed lesion in the left hepatic lobe, which is nearly isointense with the liver parenchyma with a hyperintense central scar (arrow) and surrounding pseudocapsule. The rest of the liver is otherwise normal.

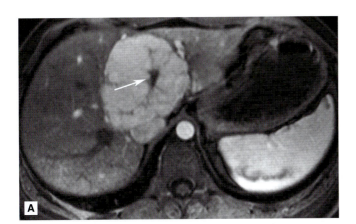

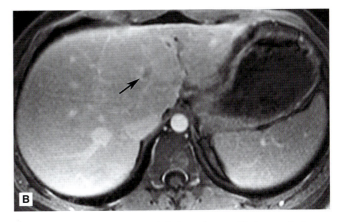

3. Axial T1-weighted fat suppressed images obtained after administration of intravenous contrast. Arterial phase image (**A**) demonstrates avid homogeneous enhancement of the lesion, except in the central scar (arrow). On the portal venous phase image (not shown), the lesion was isointense to the hepatic parenchyma. On the delayed phase image (**B**), acquired 1 hour post administration of intravenous contrast, the lesion shows relative hyperenhancement of the central scar (arrow), while the lesion itself remains isointense to the liver parenchyma.

PRESENTATION

- Usually asymptomatic
- Dull right upper quadrant pain or early satiety when large
- Occasionally palpable abdominal mass
- Jaundice (if causing bile duct obstruction)

FINDINGS

On US, simple hepatic cysts are anechoic with posterior acoustic enhancement, while on CT they are homogeneous and of low attenuation (0-15 HU). Signal intensity is homogenously on T1-weighted MR images and high on T2-weighted images. Simple cysts do not enhance with intravenous contrast.

DIFFERENTIAL DIAGNOSIS

- Hepatic abscess
- Hydatid cyst
- Cystadenoma/cystadenocarcinoma
- Cystic metastases

COMMENTS

The term hepatic cyst refers to solitary nonparasitic cysts of the liver, also known as simple cysts. Simple hepatic cysts are lined by epithelium and can be sporadic or, rarely, associated with systemic multiorgan diseases. Given the benign nature of simple hepatic cysts, once the diagnosis is established, no further imaging or workup is necessary. However, several other (more aggressive) cystic lesions must be distinguished from true simple cysts: parasitic (usually hydatid/echinococcal) cysts, cystic tumors, and abscesses. Multiple simple cysts can occur in the setting of polycystic liver disease. These conditions can usually be distinguished on the basis of the patient's symptoms and the imaging appearance. Peribiliary cysts, choledochal cysts, and Caroli disease arise from or originate from the bile ducts and are reviewed in the chapter devoted to biliary duct pathology.

The vast majority of simple hepatic cysts do not cause symptoms and are usually discovered as incidental findings on imaging or at laparotomy. They have been estimated to occur in 5% of the population, and prevalence increases progressively with age. The cause of simple liver cysts is not known, but they may be congenital in origin. The cysts are lined by biliary-type epithelium and the fluid contained within has a composition that mimics plasma. Simple cysts can occur in the setting of adult polycystic liver disease, a congenital disorder that is usually associated with autosomal-dominant polycystic kidney disease, and in these patients the kidney cysts usually precede the liver cysts. Occasionally, polycystic liver disease may be seen in the absence of significant cystic disease in the kidneys. Patients with polycystic disease often develop renal failure, whereas liver cysts only rarely are associated with hepatic fibrosis and liver failure.

On ultrasound, simple hepatic cysts are anechoic with posterior acoustic enhancement, while on CT they are homogeneous and of lower attenuation than the normal liver parenchyma. Measured internal attenuation typically varies between 0 and 15 Hounsfield units (consistent with simple fluid). Signal intensity is homogenously low signal intensity on T1-weighted MR images and high on T2-weighted images. An increase in the echo time (TE), ie, heavily T2-weighted images, leads to a progressive increase in the signal intensity, which is useful in discriminating cysts from metastatic deposits. Simple hepatic cysts have no discernible wall and do not enhance following the administration of iodinated contrast or gadolinium. Rim calcification is rare but occurs occasionally. Complications of simple hepatic cysts include infection, rupture, and hemorrhage. These complications may alter the imaging appearance of normal cysts. For example, intracystic hemorrhage causes hyperintensity on T1-weighted MR images and hyperattenuation on CT images. Cysts may be solitary or multiple; the possibility of polycystic disease should be considered if the number of cysts exceeds 10.

PEARLS

- Simple hepatic cysts are lined by epithelium and can be sporadic or, rarely, associated with systemic multiorgan diseases.

- On ultrasound, simple hepatic cysts are anechoic with posterior acoustic enhancement, while on CT they are homogeneous and of lower attenuation than the normal liver parenchyma.

- Signal intensity is homogenously low signal intensity on T1-weighted MR images and high on T2-weighted images.

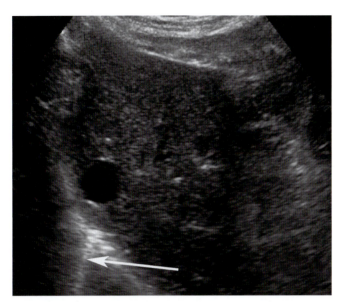

1. Transverse US image shows an anechoic lesion in the right hepatic lobe, which has imperceptible walls and increased through transmission (arrow).

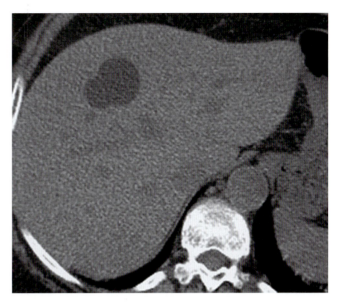

2. Noncontrast CT image demonstrates a lobulated, homogeneous low attenuation lesion in the left hepatic lobe. The wall of the lesion is not discernible. Measured internal attenuation was 9 Hounsfield units.

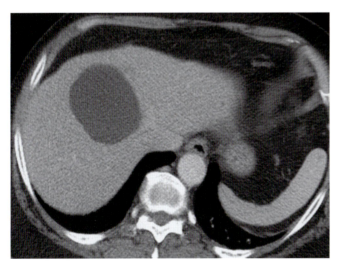

3. Contrast-enhanced CT image shows a large low attenuation lesion (12 Hounsfield units) without any wall or internal enhancement elements. This appearance is characteristic of a simple hepatic cyst.

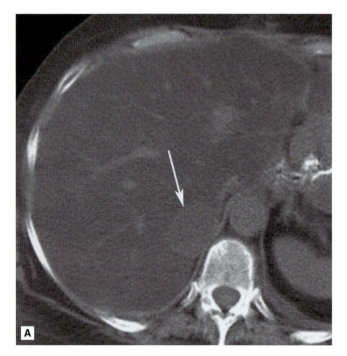

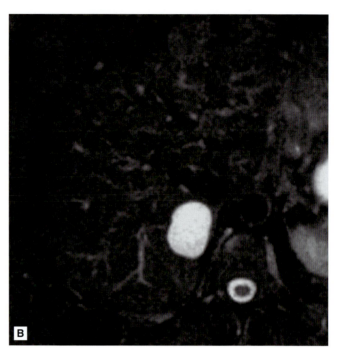

4. A. Noncontrast CT image shows a marked diffuse decrease in the attenuation of the hepatic parenchyma, indicative of hepatic steatosis. There is a homogeneous lesion with smooth margins in the posterior aspect of the right hepatic lobe (arrow). The internal attenuation measured 7 Hounsfield units, higher than the hepatic parenchymal attenuation measured −5 Hounsfield units. **B.** Fat-suppressed T2-weighted MR image confirms the cystic nature of the lesion, which is markedly hyperintense and no discernible wall.

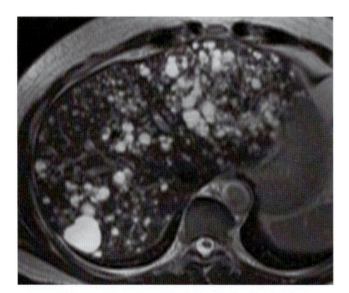

5. Axial T2-weighted MR image shows innumerable high-signal intensity lesions throughout the liver parenchyma. Multiple similar lesions were present in the kidneys as well (not shown). These findings are characteristic of polycystic disease.

PRESENTATION

- Usually found in the setting of a patient with tuberous sclerosis.
- Can be sporadic and discovered incidentally.
- Usually asymptomatic.
- Criteria for resection given the risk of rupture are the same as those for renal lesions.

FINDINGS

Imaging focuses on the detection of intralesional macroscopic fat. Larger lesions may demonstrate large vessels visible on arterial and portal venous phases of CT or MR.

DIFFERENTIAL DIAGNOSIS

- Intrahepatic lipoma
- Adenoma
- Hepatocellular carcinoma (HCC)
- Cavernous hemangioma
- Focal fatty infiltration

COMMENTS

Angiomyolipomas (AML) are benign neoplastic lesions that are composed of smooth muscle cells, fat, and proliferating, thick blood vessels. Diagnosis is made upon identification of intratumoral fat at imaging or biopsy in the absence of other findings suggestive of malignancy. These lesions may be sporadic or be associated with the tuberous sclerosis complex (TSC). They are usually asymptomatic, unless large or ruptured. Given the different tissue components, imaging characteristics depend on the amount of each of the tissues present in the lesion. Fat attenuating and hyper-enhancing components are seen on contrast enhanced CT. Larger lesions, more often seen in sporadic cases, may even demonstrate large vessels visible on arterial and portal venous phases. On the other hand, AMLs associated with TSC are usually more numerous and smaller, many times fat-deficient and therefore difficult to accurately characterize. AMLs are identified as markedly hyperechoic masses on US and can be confused for cavernous hemangiomas; the presence of sound attenuation can help in differentiating these lesions. Magnetic resonance imaging will demonstrate T1 hyperintense foci of fat with a significant drop in signal intensity on fat-suppressed sequences. Enhancement of the soft tissue component in the lesion is usually later in the arterial phase than for HCCs and mild enhancement of the fatty component may be identified, while the fat in fat-containing HCCs will not enhance. Even so, differentiation from HCC is difficult and sometimes impossible on imaging requiring biopsy. Surgical management is not required unless ruptured and many surgeons advocate preventive resection once an AML reaches 4 cm, as in renal lesions.

PEARLS

- Angiomyolipomas are benign neoplastic lesions that are composed of smooth muscle cells, fat and proliferating, thick blood vessels.

- Diagnosis is made upon identification of intratumoral fat at imaging or biopsy in the absence of findings suggestive of malignancy.

- Angiomyolipomas can occur sporadically or in the setting of tuberous sclerosis, in which case they are associated with renal angiomyolipomas.

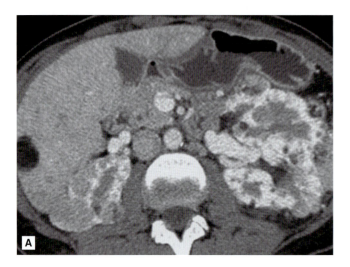
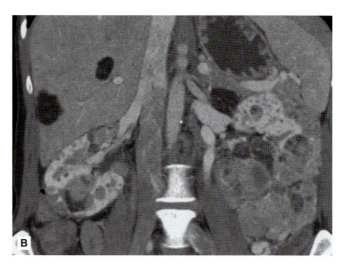

1. Axial (**A**) and coronal reformat (**B**) contrast enhanced images of the abdomen in a patient with history of known tuberous sclerosis. Multiple fat density lesions are noted in the kidneys and liver, consistent with angiomyolipomas.

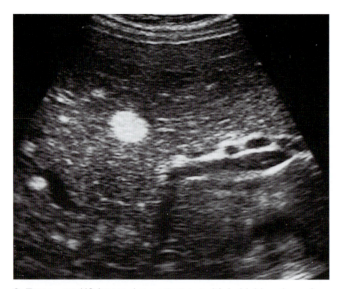

2. Transverse US image demonstrates multiple highly echogenic focal lesions in the liver, representing angiomyolipomas in a patient with tuberous sclerosis.

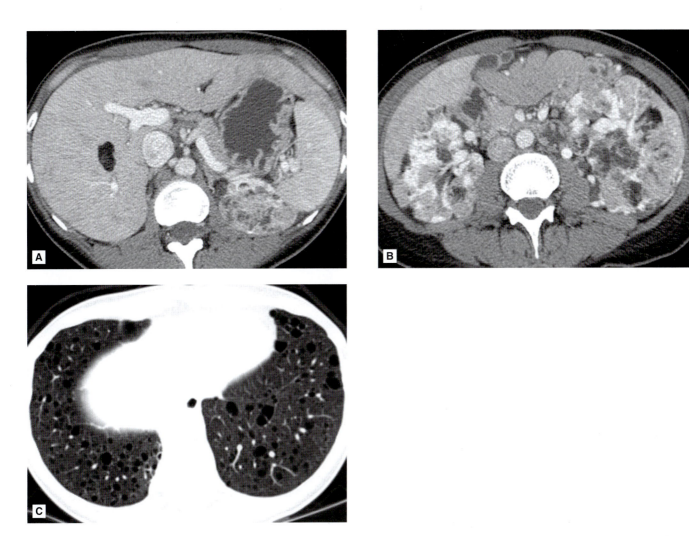

3. Computed tomography images show multiple fat-containing lesions in both kidneys (**B**), with loss of the normal renal architecture. The hepatic angiomyolipoma (**A**) has very low internal attenuation, similar to that of subcutaneous fat. **C.** CT image of the lower chest shows multiple thin-wall cystic lesions replacing the lung parenchyma. Final diagnosis was multiple renal and hepatic angiomyolipomas and lymphangioleiomyomatosis of the lungs in a patient with tuberous sclerosis complex.

PRESENTATION

Dysplastic nodules present in patients with cirrhosis of the liver. Symptoms arise from this condition rather than from the dysplastic nodule itself.

FINDINGS

Indistinguishable from typical regenerating nodules on CT. On T2-weighted MR images, they are usually iso- to hypointense, but high-grade lesions can have higher intensity. They are iso- or hyperintense on T1-weighted images. Enhancement pattern after contrast administration is variable.

DIFFERENTIAL DIAGNOSIS

• Hepatocellular carcinoma

• Regenerative nodule

• Metastasis

• Thrombosed hemangioma

COMMENTS

Dysplastic nodules are composed of hepatocytes that show histologic characteristics of abnormal growth caused by a genetic alteration. These characteristics include cytoplasmic changes and varying degrees of nuclear atypia. They typically occur in cirrhotic livers, should be over 1 mm in diameter, and lack criteria definitive of malignancy. They can be divided into low and high grade, the latter nearer to HCC in the disease continuum. In the process of transformation of regenerative nodules to dysplastic nodules to HCC, neoangiogenesis takes place, allowing characterization with imaging. While a completely satisfactory definition of the imaging characteristics of a dysplastic nodule have not been reached, and the clinical relevance of diagnosing such a lesion is unclear, mistaking one for an HCC and vice versa could result in important changes in a patient's management and prognosis.

Because of their variable histologic characteristics, dysplastic nodules have varying imaging features. On CT, dysplastic nodules are indistinguishable from typical regenerating nodules. On T2-weighted imaging, low-grade lesions tend to be iso- to hypointense while high-grade lesions tend to have a higher intensity. Both low- and high-grade lesions may be hypo-, iso-, or hyperintense on T1-weighted images, but high-grade lesions are typically more hyperintense, probably due to a greater amount of copper or fatty degeneration. After contrast injection, the behavior is also variable. Low-grade lesions may be indistinguishable from the liver parenchyma while high-grade lesions may behave exactly like an HCC, but most frequently will present arterial phase enhancement and no washout. Although characteristics of high-grade dysplastic nodules resemble those of an HCC, usually all of the criteria are not met, allowing for differentiation, case in which a closer follow-up will be necessary. Small lesions and ambiguous imaging characteristics may require biopsy to ruleout malignancy.

PEARLS

• **Dysplastic nodules occur in cirrhotic livers and are composed of hepatocytes that show histologic characteristics of abnormal growth but lack criteria definitive of malignancy.**

• **On CT, dysplastic nodules are indistinguishable from typical regenerating nodules.**

• **High-grade lesions tend to be hyperintense on T2-weighted images and relatively hyperintense on T1-weighted images.**

• **Low-grade lesions are more often iso- to hypointense on T2-weighted images and hypo- to isointense on T1-weighted images.**

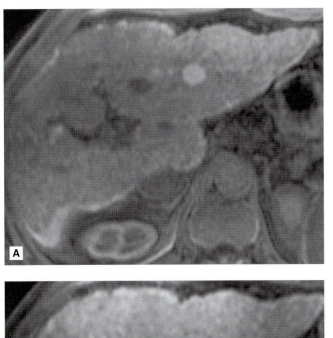

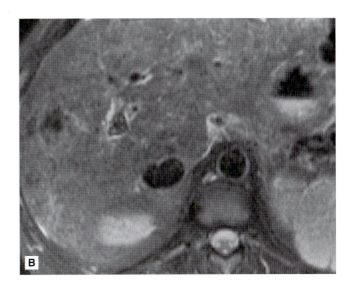

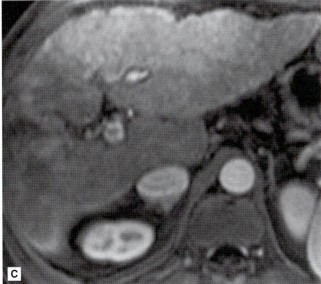

1. A. Noncontrast, fat-suppressed, T1-weighted axial image demonstrates a high-signal intensity nodule in the left hepatic lobe (arrow). Note also signs of advanced cirrhosis. On the axial T2-weighted image (**B**), the nodule exhibits low-signal intensity (arrow). After administration of intravenous contrast (**C**, arterial phase image), the nodule demonstrates mild enhancement.

PRESENTATION

Biliary hamartomas are almost always discovered incidentally in patients in whom imaging is done for unrelated symptoms.

FINDINGS

On US, bright foci with a comet-tail artifact. Noncontrast CT demonstrates multiple small, hypodense, cystic-appearing lesions and variable enhancement. Magnetic resonance imaging shows T1 hypointense and T2 hyperintense lesions.

DIFFERENTIAL DIAGNOSIS

• Simple hepatic cysts

• Adult poly-cystic kidney (hepatic) disease

• Caroli disease

• Primary sclerosing cholangitis

• Peribiliary cysts

• Liver metastasis

COMMENTS

Biliary hamartomas, also called von Meyenburg complexes are benign liver malformations that arise from the ductal plates and small interlobular bile ducts. They are typically 2 to 15 mm in diameter, of uniform size, and scattered throughout the liver mainly in the subcapsular region. These lesions are seen in up to 3% of autopsy specimens. Microscopically, biliary hamartomas consist of multiple dilated, tortuous, or branching bile ducts, lined by a single layer of cuboidal cells, embedded in a fibrocollagenous stroma, and are not connected to the normal biliary tree. Since this is typically an incidental finding, the importance lies in the possibility of a misdiagnosis of a different entity, altering the patients' clinical care.

On US, multiple bright foci with a comet-tail artifact may be seen and larger cysts will be anechoic with posterior echo enhancement. Noncontrast CT demonstrates multiple small, hypodense, cystic-appearing lesions with a distribution pattern as previously described. Although enhancement of the lesions to the point where they are difficult to discern on portal phase imaging has been described, most biliary hamartomas will be unenhancing. Magnetic resonance imaging will reveal T1 hypointense and T2 hyperintense lesions, frequently better demonstrated on MRCP, where a normal intra- and extrahepatic biliary tree will also help in the correct identification of this condition.

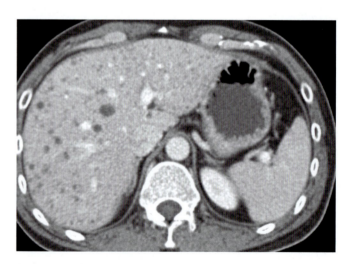

1. Contrast-enhanced CT image acquired in the portal venous phase demonstrates innumerable small, hypodense, nonenhancing, cystic lesions scattered throughout the liver parenchyma.

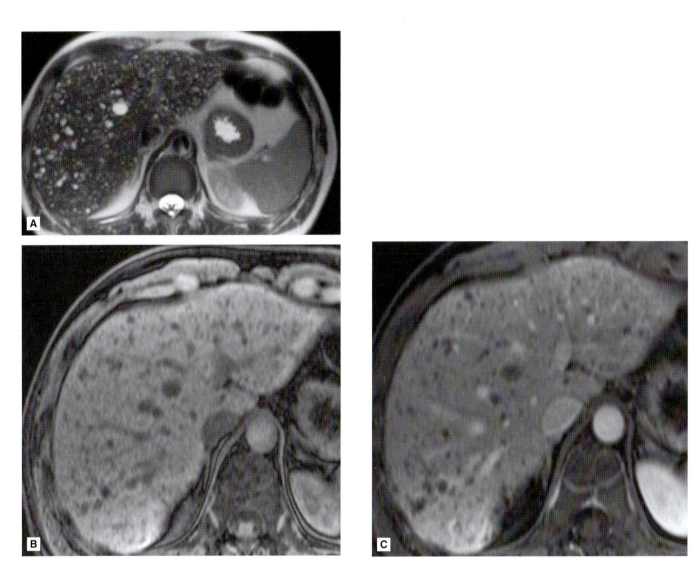

2. Axial T2-weighted (**A**) of the same patient as Figure **1** demonstrates innumerable small hyperintense lesions in the liver. T1-weighted MR images obtained before (**B**) and after (**C**) administration of intravenous contrast show the same lesions as hypointense and essentially nonenhancing cystic lesions. The liver parenchyma is otherwise unremarkable.

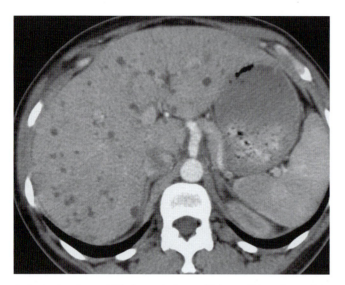

3. Contrast-enhanced CT demonstrates multiple small low-attenuation lesions in the liver, uniform in size, in an asymptomatic patient. The appearance is characteristic of biliary hamartomas.

PRESENTATION

- Usually asymptomatic
- Can reach considerable size and produce compression of adjacent structures
- Pain
- Jaundice
- Palpable mass

FINDINGS

Multiloculated cystic lesions with internal septa and nodularity. On US, the internal echogenicity depends on the contents. On CT, lesions are well circumscribed, hypoattenuating, with septa and nodularity that may enhance and thin calcifications may also be seen in the cyst walls. On MRI, signal intensity is variable.

DIFFERENTIAL DIAGNOSIS

- Simple liver cyst
- Biliary cystadenocarcinoma
- Hydatid cyst
- Cystic liver metastases
- Cystic hepatocellular carcinoma

COMMENTS

Biliary cystadenomas and cystadenocarcinomas are rare, cystic neoplasms that arise from the biliary ducts covered by mucin-secreting epithelium. Biliary cystadenomas, although histologically benign, are premalignant potential with potential to degenerate to cystadenocarcinoma. They may be uni- or multiloculated, the former being difficult to differentiate from a simple liver cyst on imaging. These neoplasms grow slowly, are more frequent in middle-aged individuals, and have a women-to-men ratio of 4:1. Cystadenomas and cystadenocarcinomas are difficult to distinguish because clinical and imaging characteristics overlap greatly, which is one of the reasons why resection is usually recommended.

At imaging, cystadenomas are seen as uni- or, more frequently, multiloculated cystic lesions, and internal septa and nodularity may be seen. On US, septa are easily recognized and the internal echogenicity depends on the contents, usually mucin, but also hemorrhagic, serous, and bilious contents have been described. On CT, these lesions are well circumscribed, hypoattenuating, with septa and nodularity that may enhance. Both cystadenomas and cystadenocarcinomas may have internal septa and nodularity, but the lack of them is suggestive of the former. Thin calcifications may also be seen in the cyst walls. The signal intensity of the lesion is variable at MRI depending on its contents, usually T1W hypointense and T2W hyperintense. After contrast injection, cystadenomas usually do not enhance or faint enhancement of septations and mural nodules may be seen, given their lack of pericystic edema. Cystadenocarcinomas more commonly have thick septations, internal or peripheral nodules and satellite lesions. Extrahepatic spread of tumor to the peritoneum or regional lymph nodes is also confirmatory of malignant histology.

PEARLS

- These primary cystic neoplasms of the bile duct epithelium grow slowly and are more frequent in middle-aged individuals, with a women-to-men ratio of 4:1.

- At imaging, cystadenomas are seen as uni- or, more frequently, multiloculated cystic lesions, and internal septa and nodularity may be seen.

- Differentiating between cystadenoma and cystadeno-carcinoma is difficult, but cystadenocarcinomas more commonly have thick septations, internal or peripheral nodules, and satellite lesions.

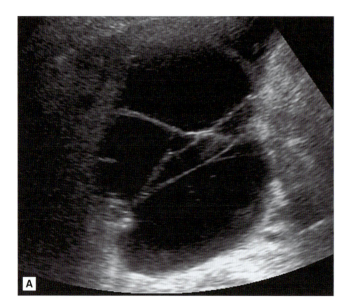

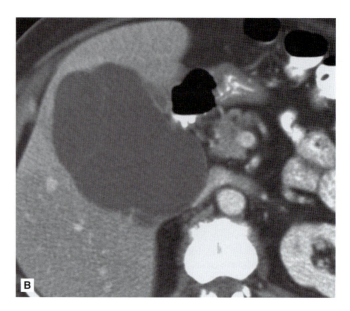

1. A. US image of the right lobe of the liver in a patient with right upper quadrant abdominal pain shows a cystic, multiseptated lesion, with no evidence of calcifications or mural nodules. **B.** Axial contrast-enhanced CT demonstrates a well-circumscribed, hypodense -cystic-lesion, with fine internal septations, no calcifications. The rest of the liver parenchyma shows no evidence of disease.

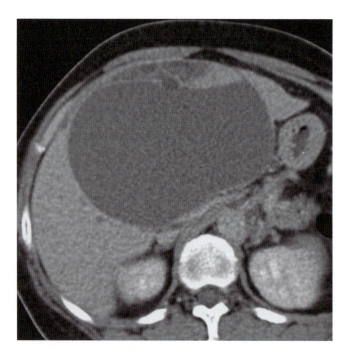

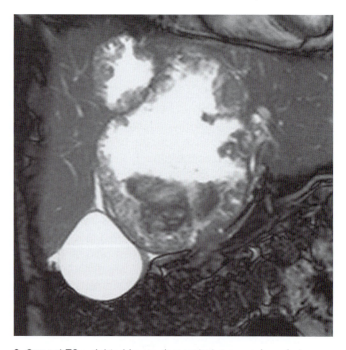

2. Contrast-enhanced CT image shows a large, cystic lesion with a solid component anteriorly. The lesion was proven to be a cystadenocarcinoma.

3. Coronal T2-weighted image demonstrates a very large heterogeneous mass with a dominant central cystic component, thick solid walls, and a satellite lesion superiorly. The appearance is characteristic of a biliary cystadenocarcinoma.

PRESENTATION

- Right upper quadrant pain
- Weight loss
- Often incidental finding
- Hepatomegaly, palpable mass
- Occasionally jaundice or liver failure

FINDINGS

On US, typically appears as a hypoechoic mass. On CT, they are mostly peripheral and hypoattenuating lesions with a rim of intense peripheral enhancement. Capsular retraction and calcifications may also be seen. On MR, the enhancement pattern is similar to that seen on CT.

DIFFERENTIAL DIAGNOSIS

- Cholangiocarcinoma
- Hepatocellular carcinoma
- Confluent fibrosis in cirrhosis

COMMENTS

Epithelioid hemangioendothelioma is a solid tumor of vascular origin that is composed primarily of epithelioid-appearing endothelial cells. Epithelioid hemangioendothelioma of the liver usually occurs in young adults and is slightly more common in women than men. However, because of the prolonged course and nonspecific clinical manifestations, the age of the patient at the time of diagnosis by biopsy or imaging studies varies widely. The clinical course is variable, but the aggressiveness generally is between that of benign endothelial tumors (cavernous hemangiomas) and malignant angiosarcomas. Most patients survive 5 to 10 years after diagnosis. Metastases occur in approximately 30% of patients and are seen most commonly in the lungs, abdominal lymph nodes, omentum, mesentery, and peritoneum. More familiarity with the pathologic findings and better access to advanced imaging techniques may allow discovery of this tumor at earlier ages. Tumor marker levels, such as alfa-fetoprotein and cancer antigen 19-9 levels, are almost always normal.

Macroscopically, the tumor is composed of firm nodules with a hyperemic periphery and dense fibrous center. Tumor infiltration and occlusion of hepatic sinusoids and small vessels cause a narrow avascular zone between the tumor nodules and liver parenchyma. The imaging findings correlate well with the pathologic findings. The typical sonographic appearance of epithelioid hemangioendothelioma is a hypoechoic mass with occasional foci of central increased echogenicity. On CT, the lesions are mostly peripheral and hypoattenuating, are readily visible on unenhanced scans, and commonly have a rim of intense peripheral enhancement and/or an outer hypodense halo. Hypertrophy of unaffected liver regions is seen in advanced cases. Capsular retraction is also common finding in epithelioid hemangioendothelioma. After contrast administration on CT or MR, the periphery of the lesions is hypervascular, whereas the central portions of the tumor nodules remain relatively hypoattenuating (hypointense on MR images). Some lesions demonstrate a peripheral halo or a target-type enhancement pattern after administration of contrast material. With progression of this disease, the nodules often coalesce in the periphery of the liver. Calcifications have been described both histologically and on CT.

PEARLS

- Hepatic epithelioid hemangioendothelioma is a solid tumor of vascular origin that is composed primarily of epithelioid-appearing endothelial cells and usually occurs in young adults (slightly more common in females).

- The clinical course is variable, but the aggressiveness generally is between that of benign endothelial tumors (cavernous hemangiomas) and malignant angiosarcomas.

- On CT, epithelioid hemangioendotheliomas are mostly peripheral and hypoattenuating, are readily visible on unenhanced scans, and commonly have a rim of intense peripheral enhancement and/or an outer hypodense halo.

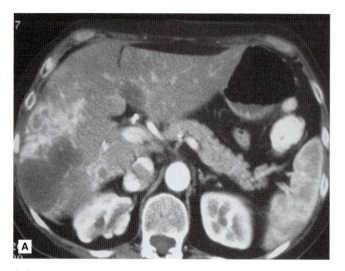

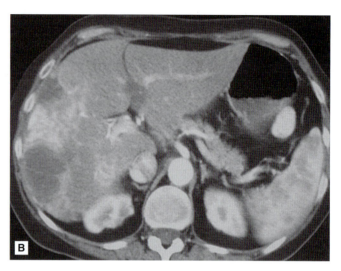

1. Contrast-enhanced CT images acquired in the hepatic arterial (**A**) and portal venous (**B**) phases of enhancement demonstrate multiple peripheral hypoattenuating masses with an intensely enhancing rim. Histological diagnosis was hepatic epithelioid hemangioendothelioma.

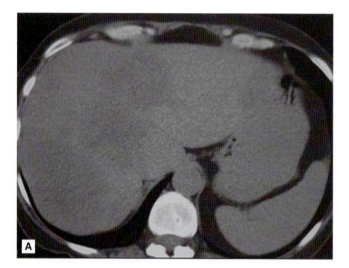

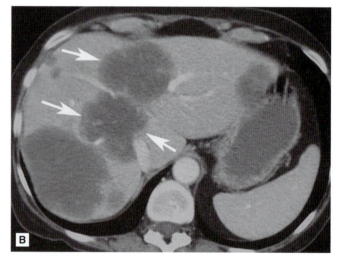

2. Noncontrast (**A**) and contrast-enhanced (**B**) CT images demonstrate multiple low attenuation lesions with heterogeneous enhancement. Note the peripheral halo of enhancement (**B**, arrows).

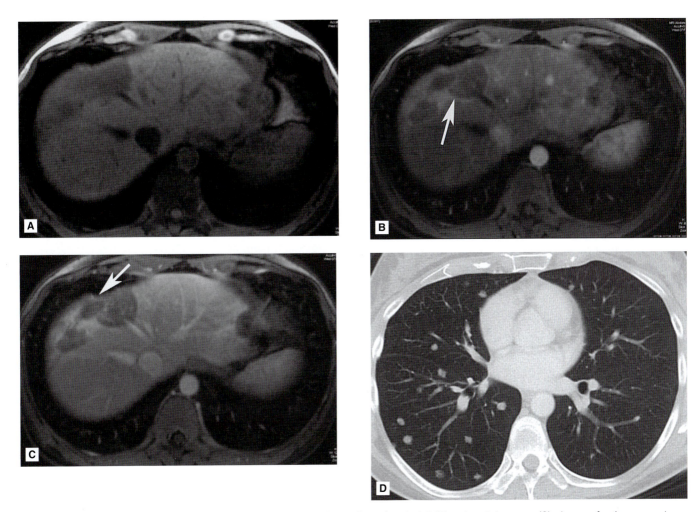

3. Noncontrast (**A**) and contrast-enhanced MR images obtained in the hepatic arterial (**B**) and portal venous (**C**) phases of enhancement. There are multiple hypointense lesions in the periphery of the liver, with perilesional hypervascularity (**B**, arrow). Note also a small indentation on the surface of the liver, due to capsular retraction (**C**, arrow). **D.** CT image of the chest demonstrates multiple pulmonary metastases.

PRESENTATION

- Most frequently described in patients with portal hypertension, usually from cirrhosis
- Less frequently in patients with inflammatory liver conditions
- Worsening jaundice has been attributed to extrinsic compression of the biliary ducts

FINDINGS

Peribiliary cysts are distributed along the portal triad and/or the hepatic hilum. Ultrasound reveals small anechoic lesions that follow this distribution. On CT, the cysts are hypoattenuating and do not enhance with contrast. Magnetic resonance imaging will demonstrate small lesions that follow the portal triad. The cysts do not fill with contrast injected during Endoscopic Retrograde Cholangiopancreatography (ERCP).

DIFFERENTIAL DIAGNOSIS

- Simple liver cysts
- Primary sclerosing cholangitis
- Caroli disease
- Recurrent cholangitis
- Choledochal cysts
- Dilated bile ducts
- Biliary hamartomas

COMMENTS

Peribiliary glands are located in the periductal connective tissue and are distributed in a linear fashion along both sides of the biliary ducts, following the portal triad or in the hepatic hilum. Peribiliary cysts are essentially retention cysts, without communication with the liver parenchyma or the bile ducts. On histological examination, the cyst wall is lined by a single layer of cuboidal epithelium and a dense fibrous band with inflammation. They are round or ovoid, measure from 0.2 to 15 mm and do not contain bile. The most common cause of peribiliary cysts is thought to be portal hypertension, although they have been found in specimens of livers affected by infectious processes like ascending cholangitis.

On imaging, peribiliary cysts have the same appearance of any other cystic lesion. It is their distribution along the portal triad and/or the hepatic hilum that is most characteristic, allowing for a probable diagnosis. Ultrasound will reveal small, round, anechoic lesions that follow the above mentioned distribution. On CT they will be hypoattenuating and will not enhance after contrast injection. Magnetic resonance imaging will demonstrate multiple T1 hypointense and T2 hyperintense, rounded, small, cystic lesions that follow the portal triad. On MRCP, distortion of the adjacent bile ducts may be seen, as well as on ERCP. The cysts should never fill up with the contrast injected during ERCP or after utilization of cholangiographic gadolinium-based agents.

PEARLS

- Peribiliary cysts are essentially retention cysts, without communication with the liver parenchyma or the bile ducts.

- The most common cause of peribiliary cysts is thought to be portal hypertension, although they have been found in specimens of livers affected by infectious processes like ascending cholangitis.

- On imaging, the distribution along the portal triad and/or the hepatic hilum is most characteristic, allowing for a probable diagnosis.

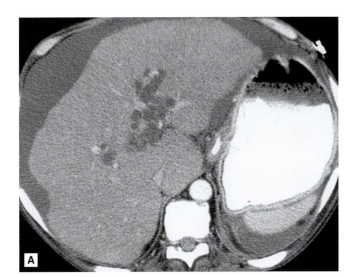

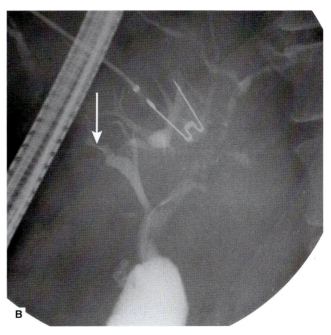

1. A. Axial, contrast-enhanced, CT image demonstrate changes consistent with cirrhosis in the liver, with associated portal hypertension. Multiple, rounded, periportal cystic spaces are noted. ERCP (**B**) was performed due to suspected biliary ductal dilatation on CT. However, ERCP demonstrates that there is no biliary dilatation. There are multiple areas of extrinsic compression of the bile ducts, with scalloping (arrow). The combination of findings is characteristic of peribiliary cysts.

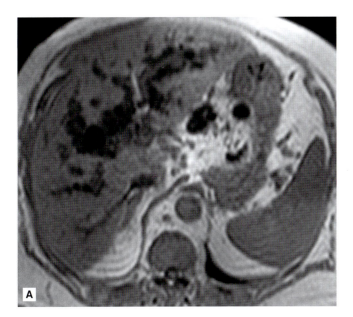

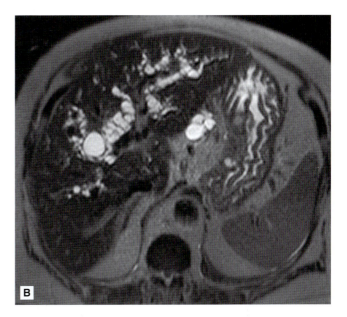

2. T1-weighted (**A**) and T2-weighted (**B**) axial images demonstrate multiple T1-low signal and T2-high signal intensity lesions in the distribution of the intrahepatic bile ducts. This appearance is characteristic of peribiliary cysts.

MALIGNANT LIVER LESIONS

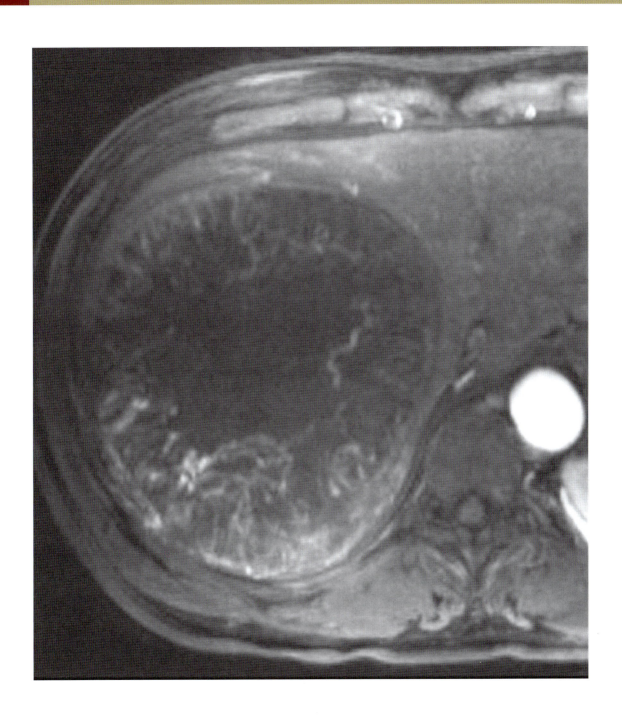

PRESENTATION

- Pruritus, jaundice

- Splenomegaly, variceal bleeding

- Cachexia

- Increasing abdominal girth (portal vein occlusion by thrombus with rapid development of ascites)

- Right upper quadrant pain

- Hepatomegaly

FINDINGS

Hepatocellular carcinoma (HCC) is typically hypervascular on the arterial phase and washes out on the portal venous phase. Appearance on MR is usually a lesion that is isointense, hypointense, or hyperintense relative to the liver on T1-weighted images and hyperintense on T2-weighted images. Diffusion-weighted MR images demonstrate restricted diffusion in HCC. On US, the lesion most commonly appear as hypoechoic nodules or masses, but hyperechogenicity is not rare.

DIFFERENTIAL DIAGNOSIS

- Cholangiocarcinoma

- Cirrhosis with dysplastic nodules

- Hepatocellular adenoma

- Fibrous nodular hyperplasia

- Metastatic disease

COMMENTS

Hepatocellular carcinoma is an aggressive primary malignancy of the hepatocyte that usually arises as a complication of long-standing chronic liver disease and cirrhosis (most commonly from hepatitis B and C infection and alcohol), often appearing 20 to 30 years following the initial insult to the liver. Other, less common, associations include primary biliary cirrhosis, androgenic steroids, primary sclerosing cholangitis, 1-antitrypsin deficiency, and hemochromatosis. Obesity and diabetes have also been implicated as risk factors for HCC, most likely through the development of non-alcoholic steatohepatitis. Hepatocellular carcinoma is more common in men than women and average age at diagnosis is approximately 65 years. The extent of hepatic dysfunction limits treatment options, and as many patients die of liver failure as from tumor progression. Currently, HCC is one of

the most common worldwide causes of cancer death. However, the incidence of HCC should decrease in the coming years through successful vaccination strategies for hepatitis B virus infection and screening and treatment of hepatitis C virus infection. Tumors are multifocal in the liver 75% of the time. Late in the disease, metastases may develop in the lung, portal vein, periportal nodes, bone, or brain.

Liver function tests are typically abnormal, to the extent that liver damage and dysfunction has developed. Total bilirubin, aspartate aminotransferase, alkaline phosphatase, albumin, and prothrombin show results that are consistent with cirrhosis.

Alpha-fetoprotein is elevated in 75% of cases and the level of elevation correlates inversely with prognosis. Liver imaging using US, CT, or MRI is required to make the diagnosis. Sensitivity of each test varies between approximately 60% and 85% for a solitary lesion; sensitivity is higher with multiple tumors and with larger lesions. Ultrasonography is the least expensive choice for screening, but it is highly operator-dependent. An advantage is that Doppler imaging can be performed at the same time to determine the patency of the portal vein.

Computed tomography, especially with multi-detector technology and a triphasic technique (noncontrast, arterial, and portal venous phases) has a higher sensitivity than US. The addition of the arterial phase to conventional CT scanning increases the number of tumor nodules detected, since HCC is typically hypervascular on the arterial phase and washes out on the portal venous phase. The CT appearance of HCC varies depending on tumor size and the phase of image acquisition. The most common attenuation pattern is iso-, hyper-, and isoattenuating on precontrast, arterial phase, and portal venous phase images, respectively; however, this pattern can also be seen in other hepatocellular nodules, including regenerative and dysplastic nodules. Computed tomography scanning has the added benefit of detecting extrahepatic disease, especially lymphadenopathy and peritoneal carcinomatosis.

Magnetic resonance imaging may detect smaller lesions than triphasic CT scanning. Magnetic resonance imaging is particularly advantageous in patients with nodular cirrhotic livers. The appearance of HCC on MRI depends on various factors, such as presence of fat, hemorrhage, fibrosis, degree of cellular differentiation, and necrosis. On T1-weighted images, HCC may be isointense, hypointense, or hyperintense relative to the liver. On T2-weighted images, HCC is generally hyperintense. Magnetic resonance imaging can help differentiate between the different types of nodules in the setting of cirrhosis: If the lesion is bright on T2-weighted images, it is HCC until proven otherwise; if the mass is dark on T1- and T2-weighted images, it is an iron-containing (siderotic) regenerative nodule or siderotic dysplastic nodule;

if the mass is bright on T1-weighted images and dark or isointense on T2-weighted images, it is usually a dysplastic nodule or low-grade HCC. Gadolinium-enhanced MRI typically demonstrates that HCC nodules enhance intensely, usually in the arterial phase and particularly if they are small. A lesion showing arterial enhancement is most likely HCC; however, dysplastic nodules and, less likely, regenerative nodules can show similar enhancement. Malignant nodules usually become isointense in the portal venous phase ("washout").

Biopsy is often required in order to make a definitive diagnosis. Core biopsy is preferred over fine needle biopsy since larger amounts of tissue can be obtained and, at the same time, the surrounding liver parenchyma can be sampled if indicated. A careful analysis of potential risks and complications should be weighed against the expected benefits before performing a biopsy. Biopsy may be omitted in the patient with a growing lesion greater than 2 cm diagnosed on two different imaging techniques with one of the techniques showing contrast enhancement and washout. Likewise, a growing mass in a cirrhotic liver on one imaging modality with an associated Alpha Fetal protein (AFP) level greater than 500 to 1000 ng/mL is sufficient evidence to make the presumptive diagnosis of hepatocellular carcinoma.

Surgical resection and liver transplantation are the best definitive therapeutic options to achieve a cure of the disease.

Accurate determination of the size and number of tumor nodules is critical in order to determine the best means for therapy. Extensive multifocal disease, tumors larger than 4 or 5 cm and evidence of main portal vein invasion, or extrahepatic spread preclude resection or transplantation.

PEARLS

- Hepatocellular carcinoma is an aggressive primary malignancy of the hepatocyte that usually arises as a complication of long-standing chronic liver disease and cirrhosis (most commonly from hepatitis B and C infection and alcohol).

- Although currently HCC is one of the most common worldwide causes of cancer death, the incidence of HCC should decrease in the coming years through successful vaccination strategies for hepatitis B virus infection and screening and treatment of hepatitis C virus infection.

- Magnetic resonance imaging may detect smaller lesions than triphasic CT scanning and is particularly advantageous in patients with nodular cirrhotic livers.

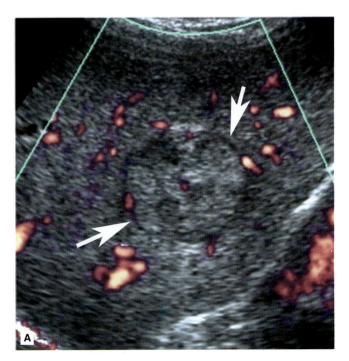

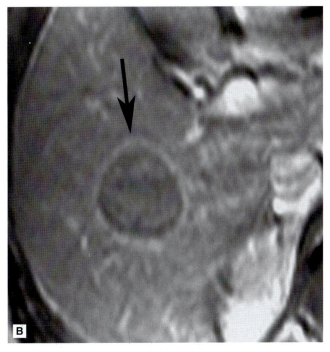

1. A. Power Doppler US image in the transverse plain demonstrates a focal solid lesion with heterogeneous echogenicity and a subtle hypoechoic halo representing a capsule (arrows). **B.** Contrast-enhanced MR image acquired in the portal venous phase demonstrates the well-circumscribed low signal lesion with a hyperenhancing pseudocapsule (arrow).

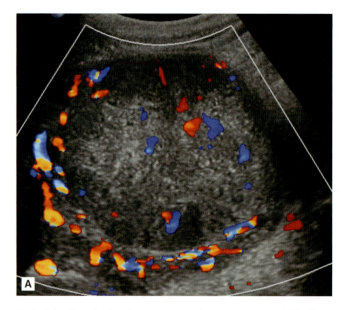

2. A. Color Doppler US image shows a heterogeneous solid lesion with internal vascularity. The central area of the lesion is echogenic.
B. Contrast-enhanced CT demonstrates the lesion as hypervascular with a stellate, hypoattenuating, central scar.

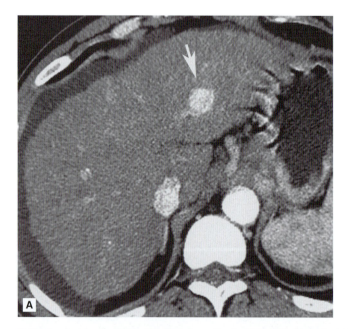

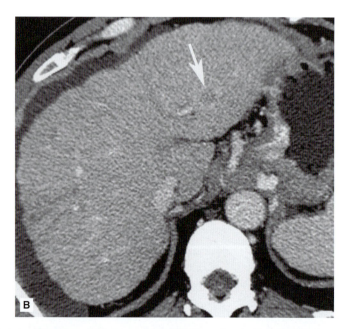

3. Contrast-enhanced CT of a cirrhotic patient obtained in the arterial phase (**A**) and portal venous phase (**B**). There is a hypervascular lesion in the left hepatic lobe (**A**) that "washes out" in the portal venous phase (**B**). This appearance is characteristic of hepatocellular carcinoma.

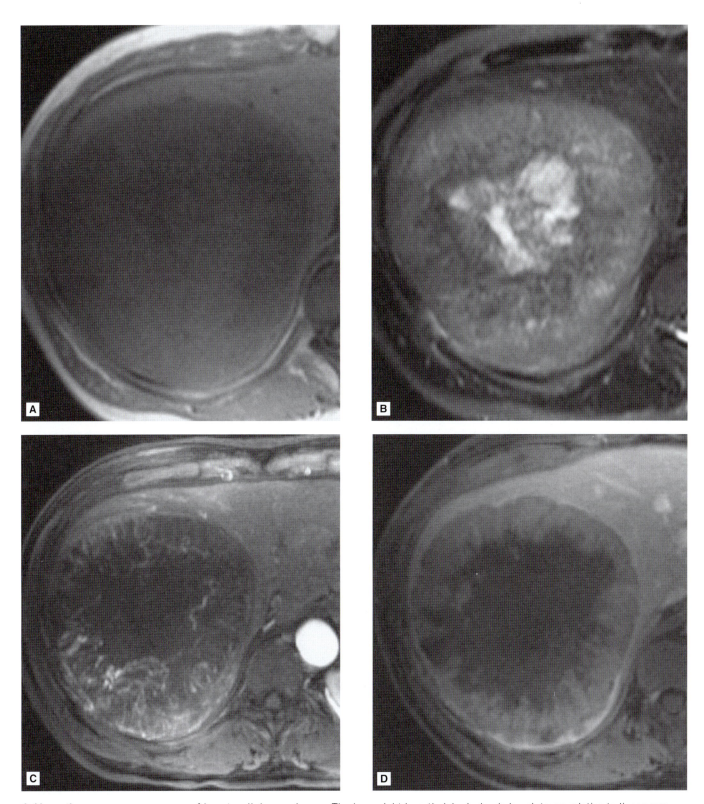

4. Magnetic resonance appearance of hepatocellular carcinoma. The large right hepatic lobe lesion is hypointense relative to liver parenchyma on the T1-weighted image (**A**) and slightly hyperintense on the T2-weighted image (**B**). On the arterial phase image of the dynamic contrast-enhanced sequence (**C**), the lesion demonstrates heterogeneous enhancement. The enhancing areas of the lesion are hypointense relative to the liver parenchyma on the portal venous phase image (**D**).

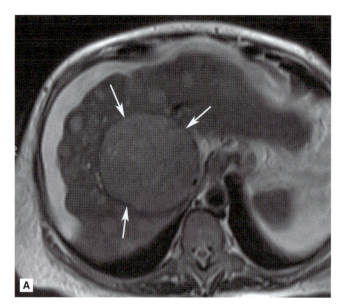

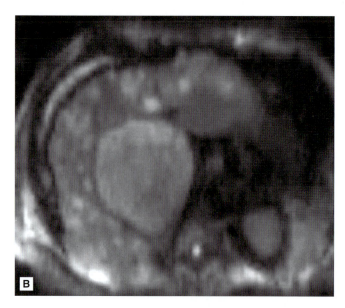

5. A. T2-weighted MR image shows findings of multifocal hepatocellular carcinoma in a cirrhotic patient. The larger dominant lesion has a hypointense pseudocapsule (arrows). **B.** Diffusion-weighted image acquired at the same level as **A** shows demonstrates hyperintensity (indicating restricted diffusion) in the multifocal liver lesions.

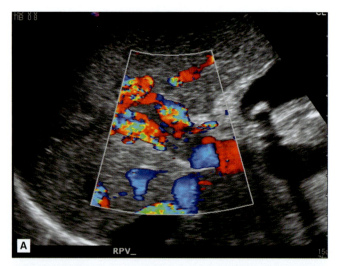

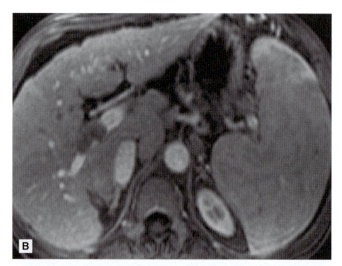

6. Color Doppler US (**A**) and contrast-enhanced MR image in the portal venous phase (**B**) of a cirrhotic patient demonstrate echogenic (**A**) and low intensity (**B**) thrombus in the main portal vein. The thrombus demonstrates internal vascularity confirming the malignant nature of the thrombus.

PRESENTATION

- Abdominal pain
- Weight loss
- Malaise
- Migratory thrombophlebitis (Trousseau syndrome)
- Fever
- Obstructive jaundice
- Gynecomastia

FINDINGS

On CT, typically appears as a large, solitary, hypoattenuating mass with well-circumscribed and lobulated margins and heterogeneous enhancement. A central scar is present in 60% to 70% of cases and calcifications in 35% to 60%. On T1-weighted MR images, the tumor is homogeneous and hypointense relative to the liver, and on T2-weighted MR images the tumor is most often hyperintense. The central scar usually appears hypointense on all images obtained with all sequences.

DIFFERENTIAL DIAGNOSIS

- Cavernous hemangiomas
- Hepatocellular carcinoma
- Hepatocellular adenoma
- Focal nodular hyperplasia
- Peripheral (intrahepatic cholangiocarcinoma)
- Hepatic metastasis

COMMENTS

Fibrolamellar hepatocellular carcinoma is an uncommon malignant neoplasm of the liver with characteristic clinical, epidemiologic, histologic, and imaging features that distinguish it from the more common hepatocellular carcinoma (HCC). Fibrolamellar carcinoma is a distinct clinical entity. The tumor occurs in a younger population than does HCC and usually occurs in the setting of a normal liver parenchyma, while typical hepatocellular carcinoma occurs in the setting of a cirrhotic liver at least 80% of the time. Fibrolamellar carcinoma is not associated with elevated levels of alpha-fetoprotein in serum. Also, the prognosis of fibrolamellar carcinoma is better than HCC. Survival of patients with fibrolamellar carcinoma is 73% at 1 year and 32% at 5 years, whereas survival of patients

with hepatocellular carcinoma is 26% at 1 year and 7% at 5 years.

On noncontrast CT images, the typical fibrolamellar tumor appears as a large, solitary, hypoattenuating mass with well-circumscribed and lobulated margins. During the arterial phase, the tumor enhances heterogeneously and usually becomes hyperattenuating relative to the surrounding hepatic parenchyma. The tumor becomes more isoattenuating on the portal venous and delayed phases. A central scar is present in 60% to 70% of fibrolamellar carcinomas and appears on CT scans as a stellate hypoattenuating and hypoenhancing area in the center of the mass. Calcifications occur in 35% to 60% of fibrolamellar carcinomas.

Metastatic lymphadenopathy (most commonly in the porta hepatis) is common. On T1-weighted MR images, the tumor is homogeneous and hypointense relative to the liver, and on T2-weighted MR images the tumor is most often hyperintense. The central scar usually appears hypointense on all images obtained with all sequences. The appearance of the scar on MR images can be useful in differentiating fibrolamellar carcinomas from FNH, because scars in FNH tend to be hyperintense on T2-weighted images. Fibrolamellar carcinomas typically do not contain intracellular fat; therefore, the demonstration of intralesional fat with fat-saturated or in-phase and out-of-phase MR images are more consistent with HCC or adenoma. On gadolinium-enhanced MR images, the enhancement patterns seen in fibrolamellar carcinomas are very similar to those found on contrast-enhanced CT. Early heterogeneous enhancement occurs during the arterial phase and progresses to more homogeneous enhancement during delayed phases. The central scar does not enhance during the arterial phase, but it may demonstrate mild enhancement in the later portal or equilibrium phases. On ultrasonography, the characteristic appearance is a solitary, well-defined hepatic mass with heterogeneous echogenicity. When present, the central scar may be seen as a hyperechoic area.

PEARLS

- Fibrolamellar hepatocellular carcinoma occurs in a younger population than does HCC and usually occurs in the setting of a normal liver parenchyma.

- The tumor is usually large and heterogeneous on imaging studies and demonstrates heterogeneous enhancement with intravenous contrast.

- A central scar is present in 60%-70% of fibrolamellar carcinomas and calcifications occur in 35%-60% of cases.

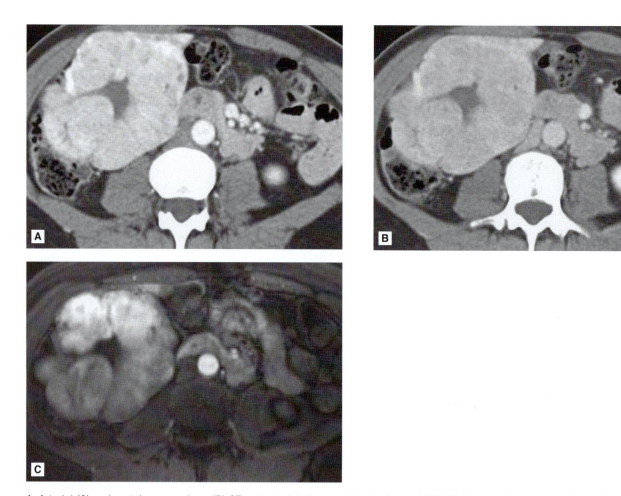

1. Arterial (**A**) and portal venous phase (**B**) CT and arterial phase contrast-enhanced MR (**C**) images demonstrate a large, lobulated, but well-circumscribed mass with a hypoattenuating/hypointense central scar. Enhancement is heterogeneous initially (**A** and **C**), but then becomes more homogeneous (**B**).

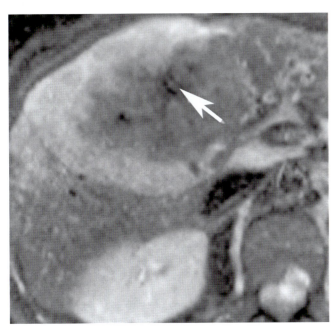

2. T2-weighted MR image of a large fibrolamellar hepatocellular carcinoma. The tumor mass is slightly hyperintense relative to the liver parenchyma. However, the central scar (arrow) is hypointense.

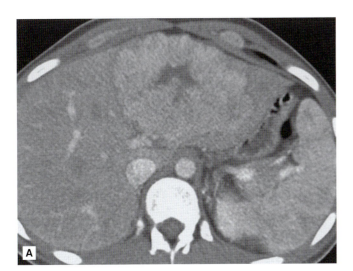

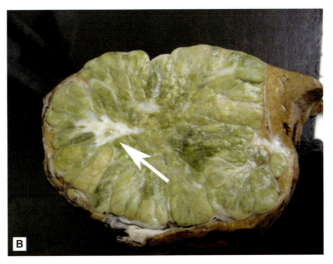

3. Arterial phase image of a contrast-enhanced CT scan (**A**) demonstrates a large mass in the left lobe of the liver with heterogeneous early enhancement and a hypoattenuating central scar. This appearance is characteristic of fibrolamellar hepatocellular carcinoma. **B.** The resected tumor specimen shows the tumor lesion with a fibrotic scar (arrow).

PRESENTATION

- Abdominal pain, upper abdominal discomfort

- Hepatomegaly, sometimes with nodularity of the liver edge

- Ascites

- Elevated liver function tests, especially increased levels of alkaline phosphatase

FINDINGS

The appearance of liver metastases on the various imaging studies varies widely. They vary in size, shape, vascularity, growth pattern, and presence of fibrosis and calcifications. The majority of metastases are hypovascular, but some are characteristically hypervascular metastases. The most common pattern on US is the "bull's eye" or "target" appearance. On diffusion-weighted images, metastases exhibit restricted diffusion.

DIFFERENTIAL DIAGNOSIS

- Biliary cystadenoma/cystadenocarcinoma

- Hepatocellular carcinoma

- Cavernous hemangioma

- Cholangiocarcinoma

- Focal nodular hyperplasia

- Hepatic adenoma

- Granulomatous diseases (tuberculosis, sarcoidosis)

COMMENTS

The liver is a common site for metastases from malignancies of multiple sources because of its dual blood supply with extensive microvasculature and also because of various humoral factors that facilitate cell growth. In fact, the liver is the parenchymal organ, most commonly involved with metastatic disease. In most Western countries, a malignant focal liver lesion is more likely to represent a metastasis than a primary tumor. Metastases to the liver may arise from virtually any malignant neoplasm, but the most common sources are tumors of the colon, stomach, pancreas, lung, and breast. In children, liver metastases are most commonly from neuroblastoma and Wilms tumor. In the majority of cases, liver metastases are multiple and both lobes are involved. Only in approximately 10% of patients is a metastasis solitary. Size of liver metastases is typically very variable, perhaps indicating that seeding occurs in episodes. Factors that influence the incidence and pattern of liver metastases include the patient's gender and age, the primary site, the histologic type, and the duration of the tumor. Most patients diagnosed with metastatic disease to the liver are treated with systemic therapy, as it is assumed that other organs are involved as well. However, in some specific circumstances (such as colorectal carcinoma), some metastases may be surgically resectable or treated with ablation techniques, such as radiofrequency. Studies have shown a 20% to 40% 5-year survival rate after hepatic resection in select patients. Thus, the confirmation of a liver lesion as a metastatic focus has a significant impact on the patient's treatment and prognosis.

The appearance of liver metastases on the various imaging studies varies with histological and morphological characteristics. Metastases may be expansive or infiltrative. They vary in size, shape, vascularity, growth pattern, and presence of fibrosis and calcifications. Large metastases often outgrow their blood supply, causing hypoxia and necrosis at the center of the lesion. The majority of metastases are hypovascular, but some primary tumors characteristically have hypervascular metastases. These include metastases from carcinoid, sarcomas, neuroendocrine tumors, renal carcinoma, thyroid carcinomas, choriocarcinomas, and some breast carcinomas.

Ultrasonography is widely used in the investigation of suspected liver metastases. Metastases can appear hypoechoic, isoechoic, or hyperechoic on US. A common pattern of metastases on US is the "bull's eye" or "target" appearance, where a halo (representing a compressed normal hepatic parenchyma and/or a zone of proliferation of cancer cells) is observed. This halo usually suggests an aggressive behavior. The accuracy of transabdominal US is approximately 80%. Where available, contrast-enhanced US in the liver-specific phase of contrast enhancement improves the detection of hepatic metastases, relative to unenhanced conventional US. Computed tomography is widely available and reproducible and it is the preferred imaging examination as it is highly sensitive for detecting liver metastases and simultaneously permits a comprehensive evaluation of the involvement of extrahepatic tissues, including the bones, bowel, lymph nodes, and mesentery. The appearance of metastases on CT is variable. The majority of liver metastases are hypoattenuating relative to the surrounding contrast-enhanced liver parenchyma on portal venous phase images. Nonenhanced scans are not routinely obtained in the evaluation of liver metastases but are useful for the detection of calcified metastases, such as those arising from mucinous primary tumors of the colon, ovary, and breast. When hypervascular metastases are suspected, an arterial phase (20-30 seconds) is added to the imaging protocol. These hypervascular metastases exhibit homogeneous enhancement in the arterial phase and often become isoattenuating to normal liver in the portal phase. Other CT techniques, such as delayed (4-6 hours) images and CT portography are now rarely used.

There is also ample evidence supporting the use of MRI in the evaluation of liver metastases, although this modality is usually reserved for problem solving, when characterization of a lesion detected with US or CT is necessary. Most liver metastases appear as hypointense lesions on T1-weighted images and as hyperintense lesions on T2-weighted images. Use of dynamic gadolinium-enhanced MR sequences improves the detection of metastases and helps in the differentiation of benign lesions from malignant lesions with high accuracy. Metastases typically enhance heterogeneously and may show central nonenhancing areas as a result of tumor necrosis. Hypervascular metastases enhance more than the surrounding liver in the arterial phase of the dynamic study, whereas hypovascular metastases enhance less than the surrounding liver. On diffusion weighted-images, metastases are characteristically hyperintense, secondary to the hypercellularity, and restricted diffusion.

The sensitivity and specificity of MR can be improved even further with the administration of hepatobiliary specific contrast agents. Unfortunately, the imaging appearance of liver metastases is often nonspecific, and biopsy specimens are required for tissue diagnosis.

PEARLS

- The liver is the parenchymal organ most commonly involved with metastatic disease.

- The most common primary sources of liver metastases are tumors of the colon, stomach, pancreas, lung, and breast.

- The appearance of liver metastases on the various imaging studies varies widely and depends on histological and morphological characteristics as well as on the status of the liver parenchyma.

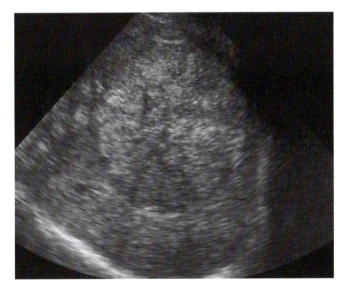

1. The transverse US image demonstrates a large hepatic colorectal cancer metastasis as a heterogeneous space-occupying lesion with areas of hypo- and hyperechogenicity.

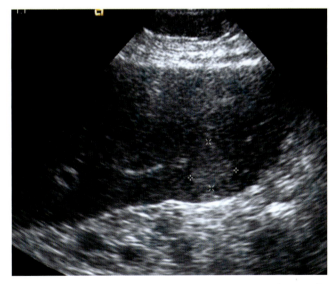

2. Small hyperechoic metastasis in the left hepatic lobe (calipers). The primary tumor was breast carcinoma.

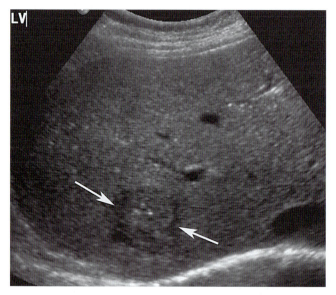

3. Metastatic lesion from colorectal carcinoma in the right hepatic lobe has a heterogeneous appearance on the transverse US image. Notice the surrounding hypoechoic halo (arrows), which is an indication of the aggressive nature of the lesion.

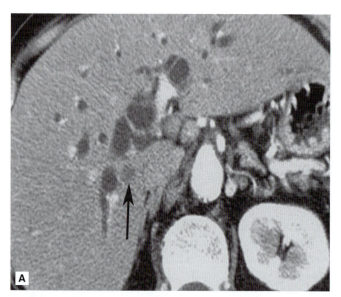

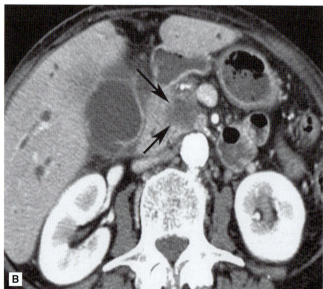

4. Axial portal-venous phase CT images of a patient with painless jaundice demonstrate severe biliary ductal dilatation, with a small hypoattenuating hepatic lesion (**A**, arrow), which was proven to be a metastasis from pancreatic ductal adenocarcinoma. The primary tumor in the head of the pancreas is well seen on **B** (arrows).

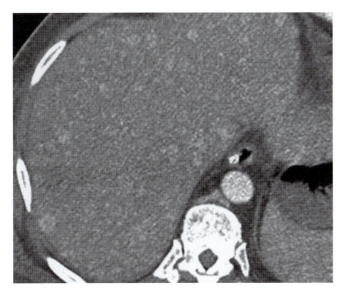

5. Diffuse hypervascular metastases from melanoma. The liver is enlarged and contains innumerable hypervascular lesions of variable size.

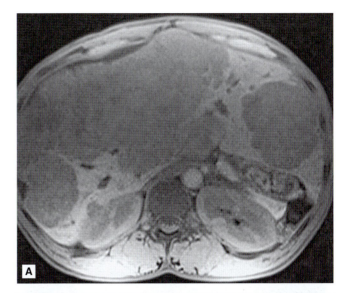

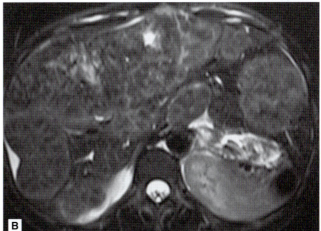

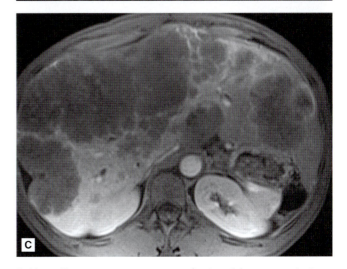

6. Magnetic resonance appearance of colorectal cancer metastases. The large tumor lesions are hypointense on the T1-weighted image (**A**), slightly hyperintense on the T2-weighted image (**B**), and hypovascular on the portal venous phase of the dynamic contrast-enhanced sequence (**C**).

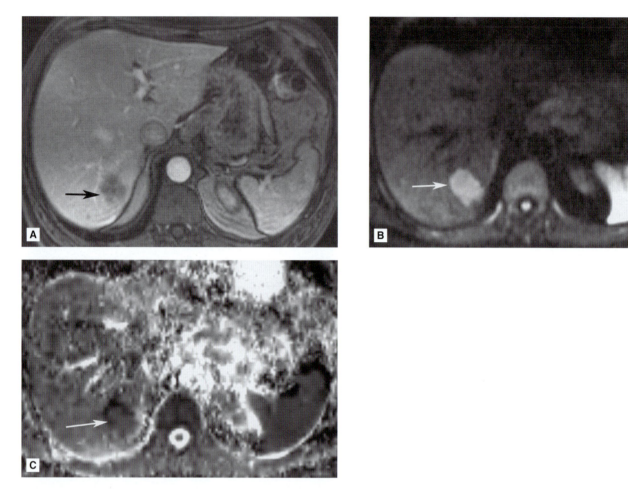

7. Colorectal cancer metastasis with restricted diffusion. On the contrast-enhanced image (**A**), the lesion (arrow) is hypovascular relative to the liver parenchyma. On the diffusion-weighted image (**B**) and corresponding ADC map (**C**) the lesion (arrows) exhibits high and low signal intensity, respectively.

PRESENTATION

- Abdominal pain
- Palpable masses
- Weight loss
- Painless jaundice

FINDINGS

Typically present as large tumors with heterogeneous echogenicity on US, irregular and hypoattenuating on CT, and hypointense on T1- and isointense to slightly hyperintense on T2-weighted MR images. There is a characteristic delayed enhancement with intravenous contrast. Segmental bile duct dilatation is also common.

DIFFERENTIAL DIAGNOSIS

- Hepatocellular carcinoma
- Hepatic adenoma
- Cavernous hemangioma
- Focal nodular hyperplasia
- Hepatic metastasis

COMMENTS

Intrahepatic (also commonly referred to as "peripheral") cholangiocarcinoma is a slow-growing malignant hepatic tumor (adenocarcinoma) arising from the epithelium of the bile duct. It is the second most common primary hepatic malignant tumor after hepatocellular carcinoma. Although the cause of peripheral cholangiocarcinoma is not clearly established, groups at higher risk for development of cholangiocarcinoma include patients with chronic parasitic infestation with Clonorchis sinensis, untreated choledochal cysts, chronic primary sclerosing cholangitis, alpha-1 antitrypsin deficiency, autosomal dominant polycystic kidney disease, and exposure to Thorotrast. In general, these tumors grow slowly, although they may be diffuse or multicentric. Surgical resection remains as the main therapeutic option, but prognosis is poor, with a median survival of approximately 25 months. Less than 20% of tumors are resectable at the time of diagnosis.

Solitary, well-demarcated, intrahepatic tumors are difficult to differentiate from primary hepatocellular carcinomas. Compared with other tumors, peripheral cholangiocarcinomas are less cellular and have relatively few well-differentiated

carcinoma cells in a dense connective tissue stroma. Intrahepatic tumors have a special predilection for perineural spread. Hematogenous spread to the liver, peritoneum, or lung is extremely rare. Lymphatic spread is common and occurs in the cystic and common bile duct nodes Infiltration of adjacent liver and peritoneal seeding are common.

The first-line investigation in a patient with jaundice or right upper quadrant pain is ultrasonography. Tumors may be very large (5-20 cm) at the time of presentation. The echogenicity of the tumor mass can be homogeneous or heterogeneous, but it usually appears at least partially hyperechoic. On CT, intrahepatic cholangiocarcinomas are predominantly hypoattenuating, with irregular margins, rounded or oval in shape. Segmental biliary ductal dilatation is common. Enhancement with intravenous contrast is variable initially, but there is a characteristic delayed enhancement with increasing attenuation in as many as 74% of patients. This pattern of enhancement differs from hepatocellular carcinoma, which more commonly shows an early peak with progressive washout. The overlying liver capsule may be retracted when the lesions are peripheral. A central scar is present in about 30% of patients. On MR, the intrahepatic mass is hypointense relative to normal liver on T1-weighted images and isointense to slightly hyperintense on T2-weighted images. The intravenous administration of gadolinium-based contrast material results in an enhancement pattern similar to that observed with CT.

PEARLS

- Intrahepatic (also commonly referred to as "peripheral") cholangiocarcinoma is a slow-growing malignant hepatic tumor (adenocarcinoma) arising from the epithelium of the bile duct and is the second most common primary hepatic malignant tumor after hepatocellular carcinoma.

- Peripheral cholangiocarcinomas are relatively hypocellular and have few well-differentiated carcinoma cells in a dense connective tissue stroma.

- On CT, intrahepatic cholangiocarcinomas are large, predominantly hypoattenuating, with irregular margins, rounded or oval in shape, may cause segmental biliary ductal dilatation and exhibit a characteristic delayed enhancement with increasing attenuation over time.

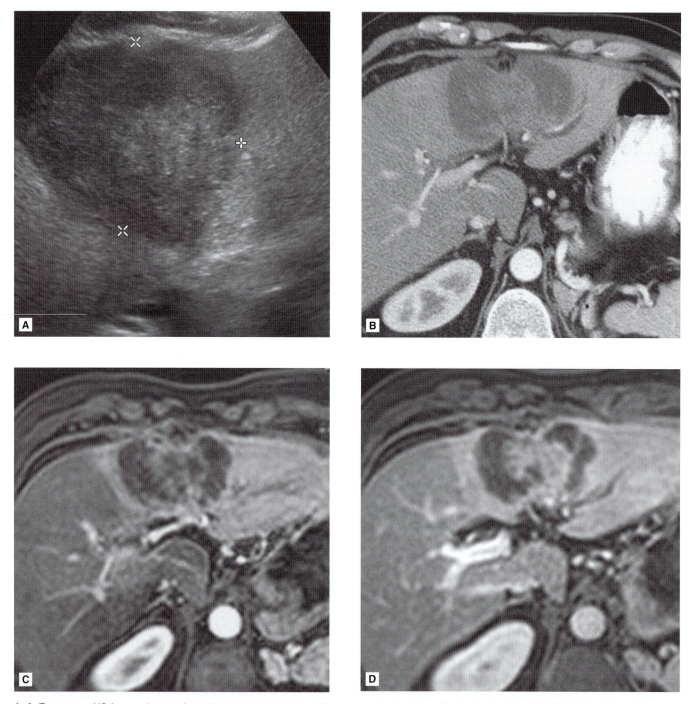

1. A. Transverse US image shows a large, heterogeneous mass with a hyperechoic center. **B.** Contrast-enhanced CT demonstrates the heterogeneous tumor lesion in the left lobe of the liver. The mass is causing capsular retraction. On the contrast-enhanced MR images obtained in the arterial (**C**) and equilibrium (**D**) phases the mass enhances with contrast initially in the periphery, with retention of contrast in the center on the delayed phase.

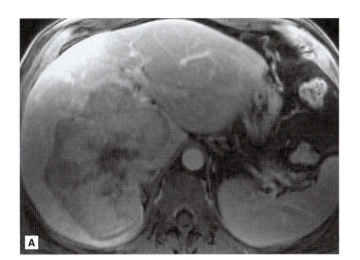

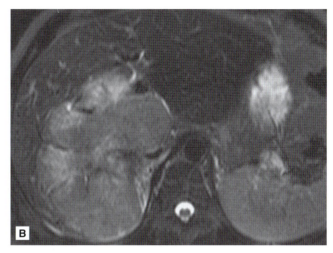

2. Delayed phase contrast-enhanced (**A**) and T2-weighted (**B**) MR images demonstrate a large mass in the right hepatic lobe. The tumor lesion retains contrast centrally in **A** and is predominantly hyperintense, with a hypointense center, in **B**.

INFECTIOUS/INFLAMMATORY

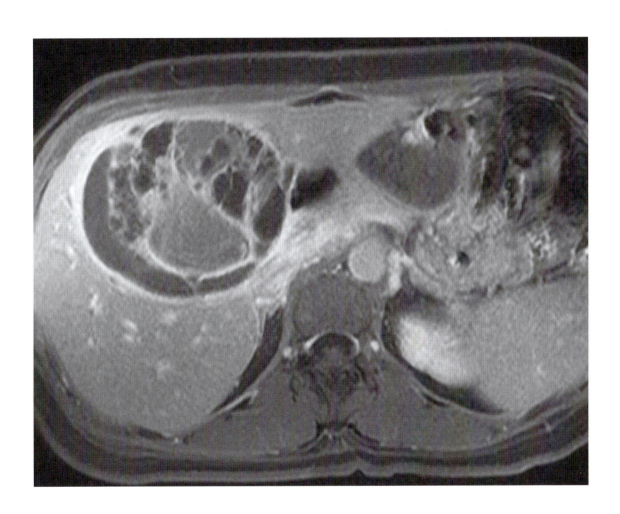

PRESENTATION

- High fever, chills, malaise
- Right upper quadrant pain
- Pleuritic or right shoulder pain
- Right upper quadrant tenderness
- Jaundice

FINDINGS

The appearance on US is variable and nonspecific. A round or oval anechoic or hypoechoic mass is consistent with a pyogenic abscess. Computed tomography shows low attenuation lesions with enhancing rim (or wall) and MR reveals T1-hypointense, T2-hyperintense lesions.

DIFFERENTIAL DIAGNOSIS

- Acute cholecystitis
- Acute complicated appendicitis
- Amebic liver abscess
- Acute pyelonephritis

COMMENTS

Pyogenic hepatic abscesses usually occur as a complication of an intra-abdominal inflammatory or infectious process, a remote infection with septicemia or secondary to biliary obstruction and infection (ascending cholangitis). Pyogenic abscesses of the liver are challenging from the diagnostic and therapeutic points of view. Most hepatic abscesses are polymicrobial in origin. *Escherichia coli* is the most common organism isolated in Western series, while *Klebsiella pneumoniae* is a common pathogen in other groups of patients. Coinfection with anaerobic organisms, such as *Bacteroides* species, is also common.

The clinical presentation of a hepatic abscess is variable: acute with high fever and sepsis or insidious with dull pain and low-grade fever. Symptoms are easily misdiagnosed as acute cholecystitis. The most common finding at physical examination is right upper quadrant tenderness, often with hepatomegaly. Leukocytosis with elevated band cells, anemia, high erythrocyte sedimentation rate, and abnormal liver function test results are common laboratory abnormalities seen in patients with pyogenic liver abscesses.

The chest radiograph is abnormal in approximately 50% of the patients. Nonspecific findings may include an elevated right hemidiaphragm, subdiaphragmatic air-fluid level, pneumonitis, consolidation, and pleural effusion. Ultrasonography is highly sensitive for detection of large abscesses, although their appearance is variable and nonspecific. A round or oval anechoic or hypoechoic mass is consistent with a pyogenic abscess. Increased through transmission suggests that the lesion is at least partially fluid-containing. Computed tomography usually reveals a low attenuation lesion with enhancing rim (or wall) and thick internal septations which may also enhance. However, the purulent material contained within the abscess cavity does not enhance. In multiphasic scans, a halo of hyperemia may be present on the early arterial phase images. Magnetic resonance is only used if the diagnosis is elusive on other imaging tests or as a problemsolving tool. Pyogenic abscesses appear as T1-hypointense, T2-hyperintense lesions with thick enhancing walls and internal septations.

PEARLS

- **Pyogenic hepatic abscesses usually occur as a complication of an intra-abdominal inflammatory or infectious process, a remote infection with septicemia or secondary to biliary obstruction and infection (ascending cholangitis).**

- **On US, a round or oval anechoic or hypoechoic mass is consistent with a pyogenic abscess.**

- **Computed tomography usually reveals a low attenuation lesion with an enhancing rim (or wall) and thick internal septations that may also enhance.**

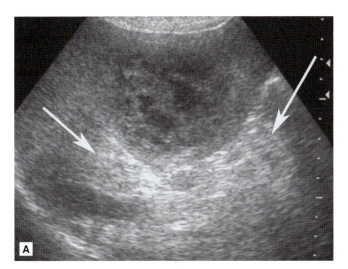

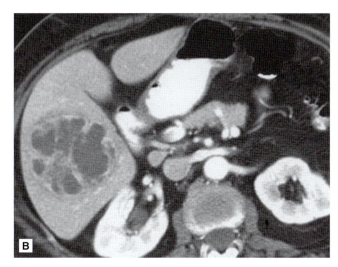

1. Patient who presented with intra-abdominal sepsis and persistent right upper quadrant pain. **A.** Longitudinal US image demonstrates a heterogeneous but predominantly hypoechoic lesion in the right hepatic lobe, with increased through transmission (arrows). **B.** The contrast-enhanced CT image shows the septated, thick-walled, fluid-containing lesion. This appearance is highly consistent with a pyogenic liver abscess.

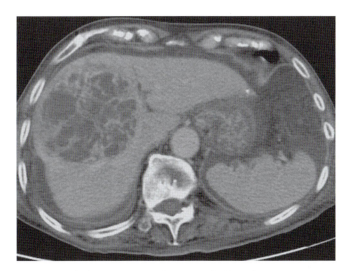

2. Characteristic appearance of a pyogenic liver abscess on contrast-enhanced CT. The fluid-containing lesion is multi-loculated, with a thick wall and multiple enhancing internal septations.

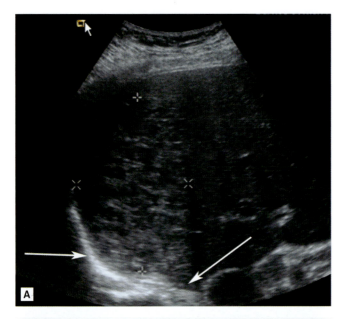

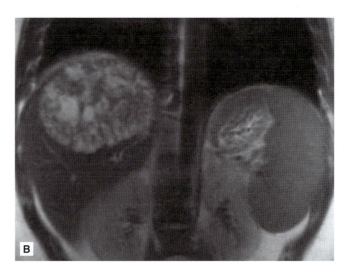

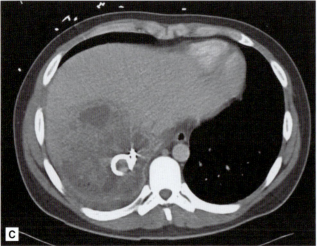

3. A. Transverse US image shows a complex (containing hypo- and hyperechoic areas) focal lesion in the right hepatic lobe with fine internal septations. The appearance is nonspecific, but increased through transmission (arrows) suggests fluid contents. **B.** The appearance of the lesion on the coronal T2-weighted MR image correlates well with the US; the fluid components are bright, whereas the linear septations are hypointense. The patient underwent percutaneous drainage of the pyogenic abscess. A post-drainage CT image (**C**) shows the pigtail catheter in good position, but the abscess remains grossly unchanged. This reflects the very complex nature of these abscess cavities.

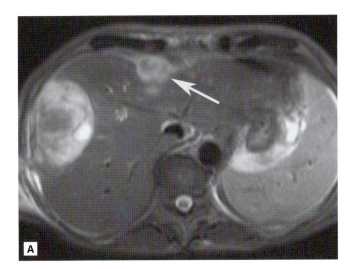

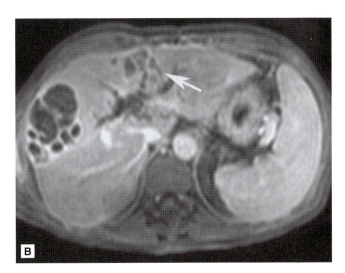

4. Magnetic resonance appearance of a large pyogenic abscess in the right hepatic lobe. The lesion is predominantly hyperintense on the T2-weighted image (**A**). After administration of intravenous contrast (**B**), there is enhancement in the wall and internal septations, but the majority of the lesion remains markedly hypointense. Note smaller abscess in the left lobe (**A** and **B**, arrows).

PRESENTATION

- Can be asymptomatic for years.

- Symptoms generally arise secondary to the large size of the cystic lesion and compression of adjacent structures (jaundice, biliary colic, liver mass) or peritonitis following cyst rupture.

FINDINGS

On US, a cyst with a split internal wall (a floating membrane or "water lily" sign) is pathognomonic. On CT, hydatid cysts are hypoattenuating with a discrete wall, with coarse calcifications in 50% of cases. On MR, the cyst is typically T1 hypointense, markedly T2 hyperintense, with a T1- and T2-hypodense fibrotic and calcified rim.

DIFFERENTIAL DIAGNOSIS

- Simple liver cyst

- Hepatic abscess

- Cystic liver metastases

- Undifferentiated embryonal sarcoma

- Biliary cystadenoma and cystadenocarcinoma

COMMENTS

Hepatic echinococcal disease is endemic to certain areas of the world, particularly in sheep-herding regions. It is caused by the ingestion of the eggs of the tapeworm *Echinococcus granulosus* in water or food contaminated with the feces of an infected dog. Dogs become infected by the ingestion of the viscera of infected sheep and other herbivores. Once in the intestine, the egg hatches and the larvae invade the intestinal mucosa and travel through the portal system to the liver, developing into a cystic structure made up of an endo- and ectocyst (the surrounding liver parenchyma). Daughter cysts are also detected in the periphery of the main cyst as a result of the invagination of the endocyst. Every organ in the body can be affected by the disease, but about 80% of patients have single-organ involvement, two-thirds affecting the liver.

Patients develop symptoms when the cyst reaches considerable size and compresses adjacent structures. Jaundice, biliary colic, right upper quadrant mass, and even thrombosis of the inferior vena cava or hepatic veins may ensue. The cyst may spontaneously, traumatically, or iatrogenically rupture into the peritoneal cavity with secondary spread of the disease and potential peritonitis. The disease is rarely fatal, with sporadic reports of anaphylactic shock secondary to cyst rupture or tamponade if ruptured into the heart. The diagnosis of hydatid cyst is made through imaging findings and confirmed by a positive serology in 90% of patients.

Ultrasound is the main imaging modality in this disease. Although some may have characteristics similar to a simple cyst, finding a split internal wall (a floating membrane or "water lily" sign) is pathognomonic. Septated cysts and daughter cysts are also indicative of echinococcal disease. Some may demonstrate a solid heterogeneous appearance, difficult to distinguish from a neoplasm, but calcifications should prompt ruling out this entity by other means. On CT, echinococcal cysts are typically seen as hypoattenuating lesions with a discrete wall, with coarse calcifications in 50% of cases. The daughter cysts can also be recognized. On MR, the main cyst is typically T1 hypointense, markedly T2 hyperintense, with a T1- and T2-hypodense fibrotic and calcified rim. Daughter cysts are usually less T2 hyperintense than the main lesion.

PEARLS

- Hepatic echinococcal disease is endemic to certain areas of the world, particularly in sheep-herding regions.

- The diagnosis of hydatid cyst is made through imaging findings and confirmed by a positive serology in 90% of patients.

- Although the appearance on US may be very similar to a simple cyst, the finding of a split internal wall (a floating membrane or "water lily" sign) is pathognomonic.

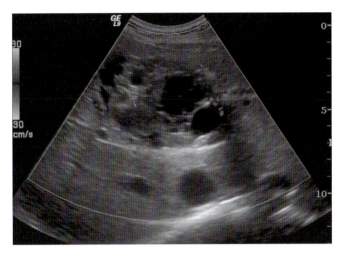

1. Ultrasound of the liver demonstrates a mainly hypoechoic, apparently cystic, complex lesion with areas of posterior acoustic shadowing due to calcifications and satellite daughter cysts.

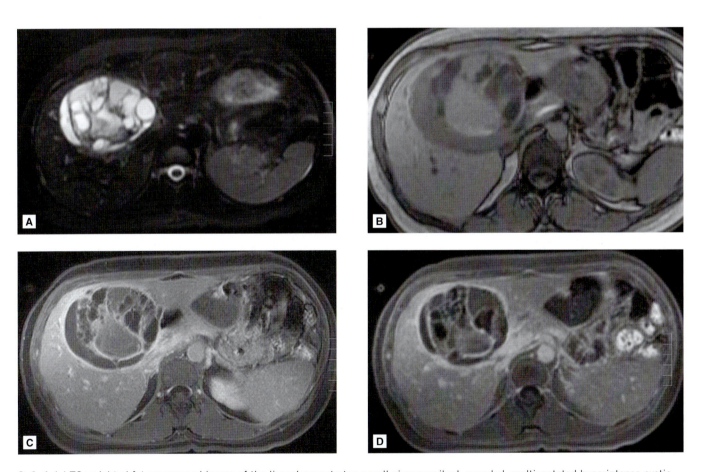

2. A. Axial T2-weighted fat-suppressed image of the liver demonstrates a well-circumscribed, rounded, multiseptated hyperintense cystic lesion, with other similarly appearing smaller and more hyperintense peripheral daughter cysts. Axial T1-weighted out of phase (**B**) and T1-weighted fat-suppressed postgadolinium (**C** and **D**) images of the liver. Hyper- and hypointense components to this complex cystic lesion can be appreciated. Marked peripheral ring-like enhancement of the lesion is noted, concerning for superimposed infection.

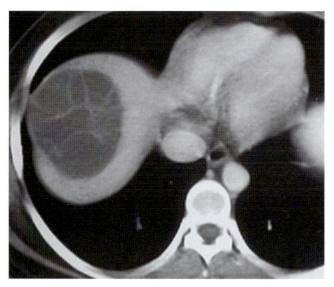

3. Axial contrast-enhanced computed tomography (CECT) of the abdomen of a different patient. Image demonstrates a multiseptated, hypoattenuating, well-circumscribed lesion, proven to be a hydatid cyst.

PRESENTATION

- Abdominal pain most common in the right upper quadrant, may radiate to the right shoulder or scapular area and usually constant and dull

- Constitutional symptoms: fever, rigors, nausea and vomiting, weight loss

- Diarrhea, occasionally bloody in nature

- Pulmonary symptoms: cough and chest pain

- Hepatomegaly and abdominal tenderness

- Jaundice (< 10% of cases) causes

FINDINGS

Ultrasonography shows a large lesion, round or oval in shape, with well-defined margins, and hypoechoic. On CT, the lesion is typically hypoattenuating, with a thick enhancing rim (capsule) and may contain internal septations.

DIFFERENTIAL DIAGNOSIS

- Hydatid cysts

- Cholecystitis

- Pyogenic liver abscess

- Malaria (in endemic regions)

- Hemangiomas, hepatocellular carcinoma and other liver tumors

- Hepatic cysts

- Hepatitis, typhoid fever

COMMENTS

Amebic liver abscess is the most frequent extraintestinal manifestation of infection by *Entamoeba histolytica*, which ascends into the liver via the portal venous system after penetrating the mucosal layer of the colon. Amebic liver abscess is rare and is currently seen almost exclusively in developing countries or, in the United States, in immigrants, or travelers. Prompt recognition and appropriate treatment of amebic liver abscess lead to improved morbidity and mortality rates. The right lobe of the liver is more commonly affected than the left lobe. This has been attributed to the fact that the right lobe portal laminar blood flow is supplied predominantly by the superior mesenteric vein, whereas the left lobe portal blood flow is supplied by the splenic vein.

Leukocytosis is common and anemia may be present as well. A small proportion of patients have associated jaundice. Levels of aspartate aminotransferase (AST) and alkaline phosphatase are commonly elevated. A combination of serologic and imaging tests are the most widely used methods for confirming the diagnosis of amebic liver abscess. The preferred serologic method is the enzyme-linked immunosorbent assay (ELISA) immunoassay, which detects antibodies specific for *E histolytica* in approximately 95% of patients with extraintestinal amebiasis, in 70% of patients with active intestinal infection, and in 10% of persons who are asymptomatic carriers. The role of microscopic stool examination is currently limited, since only a minority of patients have trophozoites in their stool.

Ultrasonography is the preferred initial imaging diagnostic test. It is rapid, inexpensive, widely available in areas where amebiasis is endemic and is reported to be only slightly less sensitive than CT scan (75%-80% sensitivity vs 88%-95% for CT scan). Ultrasonography simultaneously evaluates the gallbladder, which is always a focus of interest in the differential diagnosis. The lesions can be large and tend to be round or oval in shape, with well-defined margins, and hypoechoic. On CT, the lesion is typically hypoattenuating, with a thick enhancing rim (capsule) and may contain internal septations of variable thickness. The lesion may be lobulated. Although hepatic liver abscesses can be multiple, they are characteristically less numerous than pyogenic abscesses. Magnetic resonance imaging is only used when the diagnosis remains questionable after other tests have been performed. A chest radiograph may show elevation of the right diaphragm, basilar atelectasis, and right pleural effusion. Therapy is usually with administration of oral or intravenous antiprotozoal medications. However, since other lesions (such as pyogenic abscess or tumor can be difficult to differentiate from amebic abscess), image-guided aspiration or drainage is often required for confirmation of the diagnosis or as part of the therapy. The content retrieved has been classically described as resembling "anchovy paste."

PEARLS

- **The condition is rare and seen almost exclusively in developing countries or, in the United States, in immigrants or travelers.**

- **On US, the lesions are usually hypoechoic, large, and round or oval in shape, with well-defined margins.**

- **On CT, the lesion is typically hypoattenuating, with a thick enhancing rim (capsule) and may contain internal septations of variable thickness.**

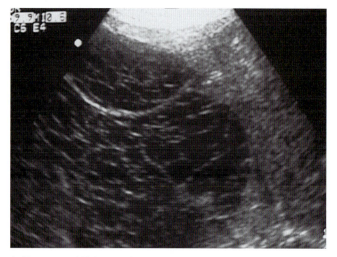

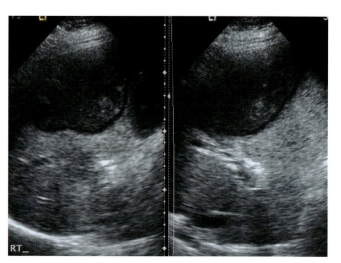

1. Transverse US image demonstrates a large hypoechoic lesion replacing most of the right hepatic lobe. The lesion contains fine internal septations giving it a "lacy" appearance, characteristic of amebic abscess.

2. Two transverse images on a different patient show a large, well-circumscribed, hypoechoic lesion with internal echoes representing debris.

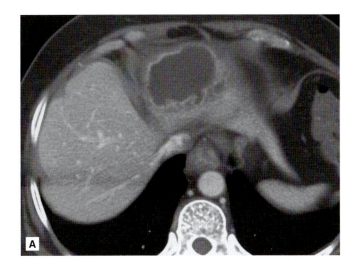

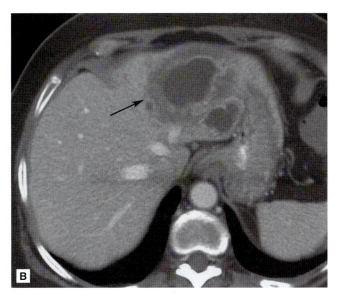

3. Two axial images (**A**, **B**) demonstrate a large dominant lesion with a smaller, "daughter" lesion in the left lobe of the liver. Both lesions have a homogeneous, low attenuation center and a thick enhancing wall (capsule, arrow on. **B**).

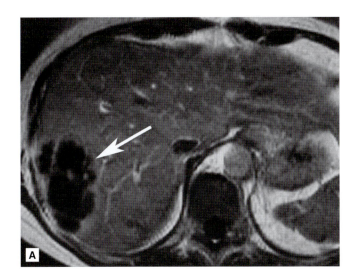

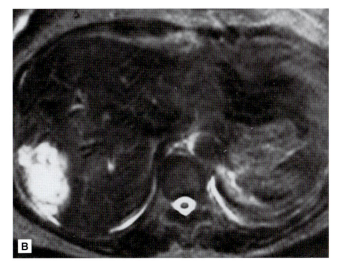

4. A. Axial contrast-enhanced T1-weighted MR image and (**B**) axial T2-weighted MR image show a T1-low, T2-bright signal intensity–lobulated lesion with enhancing walls (**A**, arrow).

PRESENTATION

- Pain in right side of upper abdomen in patient with pelvic inflammatory disease
- Signs and symptoms of peritonitis

FINDINGS

On cross-sectional images, there is thickening and abnormal enhancement of the anterior liver capsule, with varying degrees of loculated perihepatic ascites and peritoneal septations extending to the undersurface of the diaphragm. Imaging of the pelvis reveals signs of coexistent pelvic inflammatory disease.

DIFFERENTIAL DIAGNOSIS

- Acute cholecystitis
- Hepatic abscess
- Acute appendicitis
- Acute diverticulitis

COMMENTS

Curtis in 1930 and Fitz-Hugh in 1934 described a syndrome characterized clinically by pain in the right side of the upper abdomen in women with concurrent pelvic inflammatory disease. The condition is now known as Fitz-Hugh-Curtis syndrome. At surgery, the classic finding is string-like adhesions between the anterior surface of the liver and the parietal peritoneum and that is the origin of the term "perihepatitis." Although the original cases of Fitz-Hugh-Curtis syndrome occurred from a complication of salpingitis caused by gonococcal infection, most cases today are caused by chlamydial infections.

Reports of cross-sectional imaging features (with US, CT, or MR) in Fitz-Hugh-Curtis syndrome have largely focused on the anterior liver surface, corresponding to the classic surgical findings. Such findings include thickening and abnormal enhancement of the anterior liver capsule, with varying degrees of loculated perihepatic ascites and peritoneal septations extending to the undersurface of the diaphragm. Both sonographic and CT findings of localized peritonitis have been described in this syndrome. Cross-sectional imaging findings of peritonitis in the right upper quadrant or right paracolic gutter, in the absence of findings to suggest acute appendicitis or acute diverticulitis should suggest the diagnosis. Involvement of the hepatorenal fossa (Morison pouch) is also commonly observed, given its more dependent location in the supine position. Gallbladder wall thickening and transient hepatic attenuation difference have also been reported in association with perihepatitis. Additionally, imaging of the pelvis often demonstrates typical signs of coexistent pelvic inflammatory disease (thickening and hyperenhancement of adnexal structures with free peritoneal fluid) and/or frank tubo-ovarian abscess.

PEARLS

- **Fitz-Hugh-Curtis syndrome (perihepatitis) is characterized clinically by pain in the right side of the upper abdomen in women with concurrent pelvic inflammatory disease.**

- **Most cases of Fitz-Hugh-Curtis syndrome today are caused by chlamydial infections.**

- **Cross-sectional imaging findings of localized right upper quadrant peritonitis associated with salpingitis should suggest the diagnosis.**

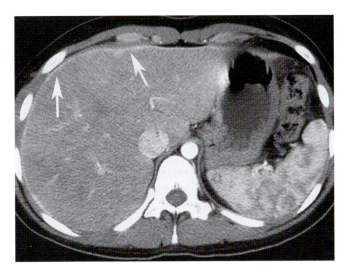

1. Contrast-enhanced CT image demonstrates marked hyperenhancement and thickening of the liver capsule. This appearance is characteristic of Fitz-Hugh-Curtis (perihepatitis).

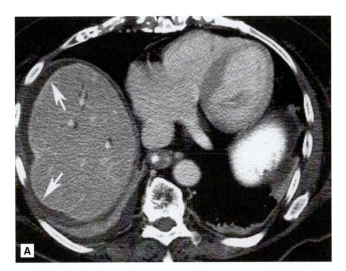

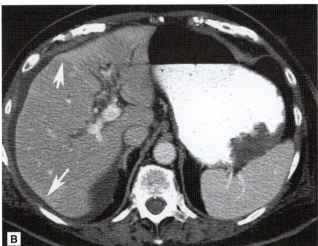

2. Contrast-enhanced CT images of a patient with Fitz-Hugh-Curtis syndrome show enhancement of the liver capsule (**A**, arrows) and of the subcapsular liver parenchyma (**B**, arrows). There is associated perihepatic fluid.

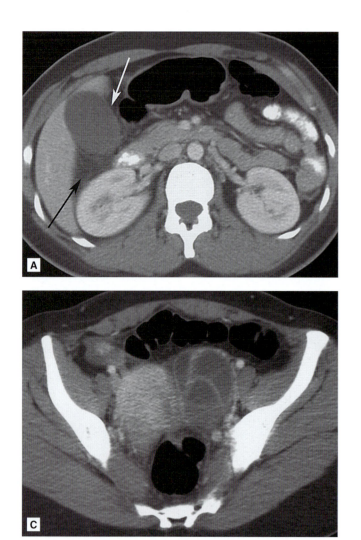

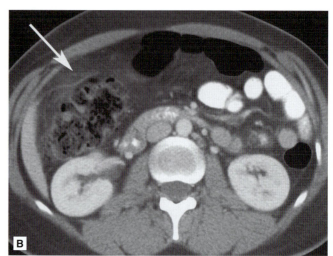

3. Contrast-enhanced CT images demonstrate mild gallbladder wall thickening and enhancement (**A**, white arrow), fluid in Morrison pouch (**A**, black arrow), thickening of the anterior peritoneum on the right side (**B**, arrow) and a large left tubo-ovarian abscess (**C**). This combination of findings is highly consistent with Fitz-Hugh-Curtis syndrome.

PRESENTATION

Fever or sepsis in an immunocompromised patient (neutropenia or undergoing chemotherapy)

FINDINGS

These are usually well-defined microabscesses distributed diffusely throughout the liver. The appearance on US is highly variable. CT reveals innumerable small (< 1 cm) hypoattenuating lesions which may enhance in the periphery. The lesions are hypointense on T1-weighted and hyperintense on T2-weighted MR images.

DIFFERENTIAL DIAGNOSIS

• Septicemia

• Infection with other opportunistic infections (mycobacteria, *Cryptosporidium*, *Pneumocystis carinii*)

• Sarcoidosis

• Ascending cholangitis

COMMENTS

Fungal infections of the liver and spleen occur primarily in the setting of prolonged or recurrent severe neutropenia, such as patients with acute leukemia, patients with lymphoproliferative disorders being treated with high-dose chemotherapy and in patients of post bone marrow transplantation. The most common causative organism is *Candida albicans*. Hepatic candidiasis is a common infection in immunocompromised patients and is caused by hematogenous spread and seeding of *Candida* strains from the intestine, mostly via the portal venous circulations. Complications occur when the microabscesses coalesce or rupture into the peritoneal cavity or into the biliary tract, causing cholangitis. Hepatosplenic candidiasis is associated with high morbidity and mortality.

Although a definitive diagnosis is made with microbiologic or histologic confirmation of presence of the organisms, the clinical status and comorbidities often preclude obtaining a tissue diagnosis. Thus, empiric antifungal therapy is often instituted in patients with high clinical suspicion and suspicious imaging findings. *Candida albicans* characteristically causes multiple rounded, well-defined microabscesses which are distributed diffusely throughout the hepatic parenchyma. Ultrasonography and CT have an important role in the diagnosis of hepatic and splenic fungal infection and in the follow-up of affected patients. Various morphologic patterns of US findings of liver candidiasis have been described in the literature. These include the "wheel within a wheel" and "wagon wheel" patterns which are found in early disease and the "bull's eye" pattern, which usually indicates more advanced disease. CT reveals innumerable small (< 1 cm) hypoattenuating lesions which may enhance in the periphery. The same lesions are hypointense on T1-weighted MR images, hyperintense on T2-weighted MR images, and show evidence of restricted diffusion in diffusion-weighted images. As the lesions heal, scattered calcifications may appear. Overall, CT is superior to US in depicting fungal liver microabscesses and dynamic contrast-enhanced MR imaging may even be superior to dynamic contrast-enhanced portal venous phase CT. As the lesions heal, scattered calcifications may appear.

PEARLS

• Fungal infections of the liver and spleen occur primarily in the setting of prolonged or recurrent severe neutropenia, such as patients with acute leukemia, patients with lymphoproliferative disorders being treated with high-dose chemotherapy and patients of post bone marrow transplantation.

• *Candida albicans* (the most common causative organism) characteristically causes multiple rounded, well-defined microabscesses which are distributed diffusely throughout the hepatic parenchyma.

• CT reveals innumerable small (< 1 cm) hypoattenuating lesions which may enhance in the periphery.

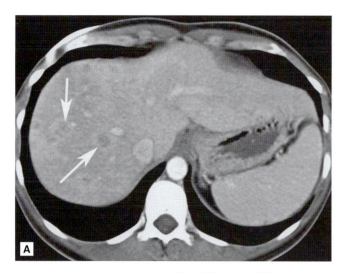

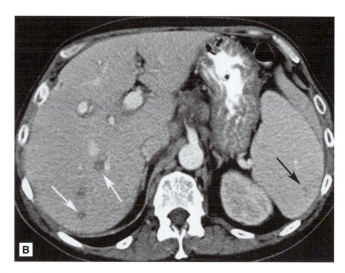

1. Contrast-enhanced CT images (**A** and **B**) of two different patients with confirmed hepatosplenic candidiasis. Both patients have multiple, discrete, small hypoattenuating lesions in the liver (**A** and **B**, white arrows). Note also splenomegaly and small hypoattenuating splenic lesion on **B** (black arrow).

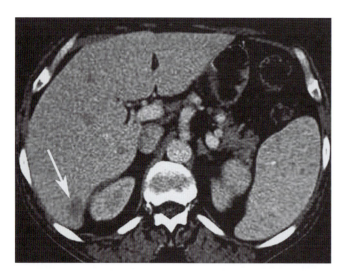

2. Contrast-enhanced CT image of a neutropenic patient with fever and proven hepatosplenic candidiasis. There are multiple ill-defined low-attenuation lesions in the liver and spleen (arrow).

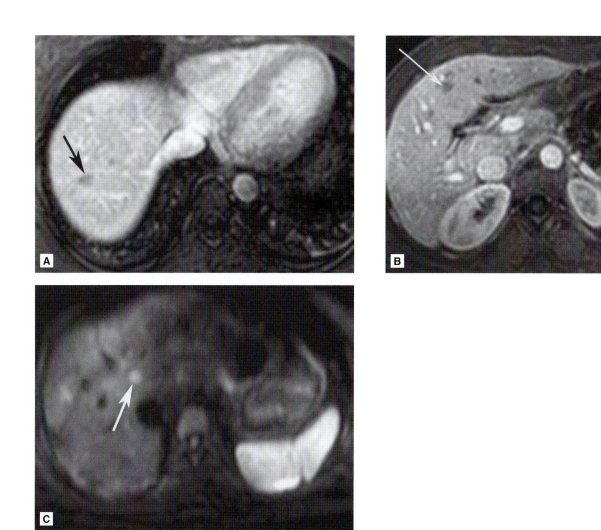

3. MR images of a patient with hepatosplenic candidiasis. Contrast-enhanced images demonstrate multiple small, low–signal intensity lesions in the liver (**A**, black arrow and **B**, white arrow). Lesions with a similar appearance are also present in the spleen (**B**, black arrow). The diffusion-weighted image (**C**) shows hyperintensity in the liver lesions, indicating presence of restricted diffusion (white arrow).

PRESENTATION

- Subclinical disease (asymptomatic).
- Malaise, fatigue.
- Anorexia, nausea, and vomiting.
- Markedly elevated liver enzymes in serum.
- Severe cases may cause hepatic encephalopathy.

FINDINGS

Hepatomegaly and diffuse parenchymal hypoechogenecity are seen on ultrasound producing the classic "starry sky" appearance. Heterogeneous liver on nonenhanced CT and heterogeneous enhancement with contrast are seen. On MR, hepatomegaly and regions of hyperintensity on T2-weighted images and heterogeneous enhancement on multiphase contrast-enhanced MR. The gallbladder has a characteristic appearance: collapsed lumen and a markedly thickened wall.

DIFFERENTIAL DIAGNOSIS

- Obstructive jaundice
- Acute cholecystitis
- Cirrhosis
- Hepatic abscess

COMMENTS

The term hepatitis refers to inflammation of the liver parenchyma and can result from multiple causes, such as viruses, alcohol, drugs, autoimmune diseases, and metabolic diseases. Viral infections (mainly hepatitis A, B, C, and E) cause more than 50% of the cases of acute hepatitis in the United States. At histology, hepatitis is characterized by periportal hepatocellular necrosis, Kupffer cell proliferation, and portal inflammation of plasma cells. The process may be self-limiting, with complete healing, or progress to segmental scarring or diffuse cirrhosis. Acute hepatitis lasts less than 6 months whereas the term chronic hepatitis describes hepatic parenchymal inflammation that does not regress in periods longer than 6 months. Approximately 20% of patients with chronic hepatitis B or hepatitis C develop cirrhosis.

The clinical presentation of acute hepatitis varies between subclinical disease and fulminant hepatic failure. Symptomatic acute hepatitis causes malaise, anorexia, fatigue, nausea, and vomiting. Liver enzymes are markedly elevated, with aminotransferase values often exceeding 1000 U/L and severe hyperbilirubinemia. The more severe cases of acute hepatitis may progress to acute hepatic failure, which is characterized by poor synthetic function (defined as a prothrombin time of at least 16 seconds or an international normalized ratio of 1.5). Fulminant hepatic failure is defined as acute liver failure that is complicated by hepatic encephalopathy with brain edema that may be potentially fatal. The specific cause of the hepatitis is determined based on clinical history, results of serum serology and, if necessary, liver biopsy.

Morphologically, acute hepatitis causes hepatomegaly and edema of the liver capsule with focal areas of necrosis that result in an irregular liver contour. In its fulminant variant, acute hepatitis causes extensive necrosis with significant loss of parenchymal volume. Ascites and splenomegaly can accompany severe hepatitis. On US, the liver is enlarged and the parenchymal echogenicity is decreased diffusely. This is caused by hepatocyte edema. The portal spaces appear relatively hyperechoic, causing a characteristic "starry night" appearance of the enlarged liver. CT images of acute and fulminant courses of hepatitis show generalized hepatomegaly combined with peripheral edema. Nonenhanced CT can show heterogeneous attenuation patterns. The overall hepatic parenchymal attenuation is usually equal to or less than that of the spleen. Contrast-enhanced CT can demonstrate irregular perfusion with heterogeneous regions of attenuation. MR also shows generalized hepatomegaly combined with edema of the liver capsule. In addition, regions of hyperintensity can be seen surrounding the portal venous branches on T2-weighted images. A heterogeneous enhancement pattern, similar to that seen at CT, can be seen on dynamic and multiphase contrast-enhanced MR images. The gallbladder has a characteristic appearance in patients with acute hepatitis: collapsed lumen with a markedly thickened wall. This is thought to be secondary to a combination of factors: decreased bile duct production and submucosal edema from direct inflammation, lymphatic obstruction and hypoalbuminemia.

PEARLS

- Clinical presentation of acute hepatitis varies between subclinical disease and fulminant hepatic failure.

- The "starry night" appearance is often seen on US: hepatomegaly with decreased parenchymal echogenicity and relatively hyperechoic portal spaces.

- The gallbladder has a characteristic appearance in patients with acute hepatitis: collapsed lumen with a markedly thickened wall.

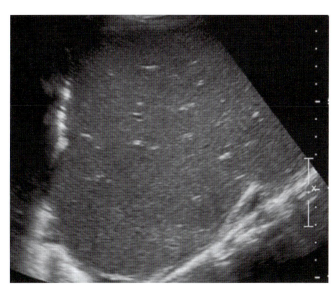

1. Patient with acute viral hepatitis. The transverse US image demonstrates an enlarged liver with hypoechoic parenchyma and relative hyperechogenicity of the portal spaces. This is the "starry night" appearance of the liver.

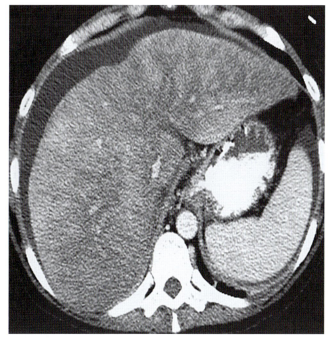

2. Contrast-enhanced CT image shows a markedly heterogeneous enhancement pattern of the liver parenchyma, irregular hepatic surface, and ascites. The patient was subsequently diagnosed with acute hepatitis.

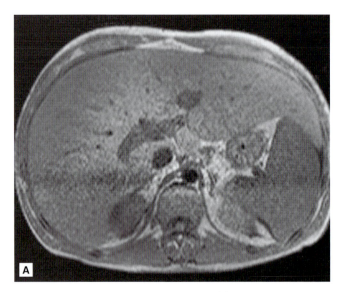

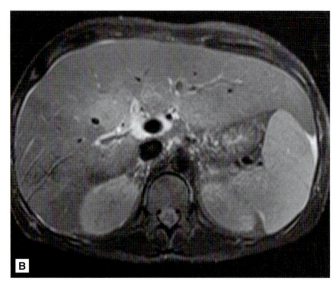

3. Axial T1-weighted (**A**) and T2-weighted (**B**) MR images demonstrate hepatomegaly and diffuse T1-low signal and T2-low signal intensity of the liver parenchyma. These findings are indicative of increased water content in the hepatocytes. The appearance is characteristic of acute hepatitis.

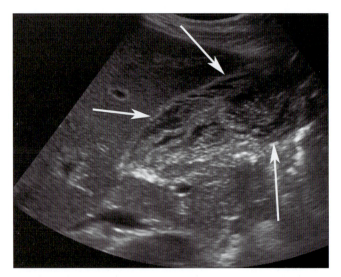

4. Transverse US image shows the typical appearance of the gallbladder in a patient with acute hepatitis. There is severe wall thickening with a multilayered appearance (arrows) and no discernible lumen.

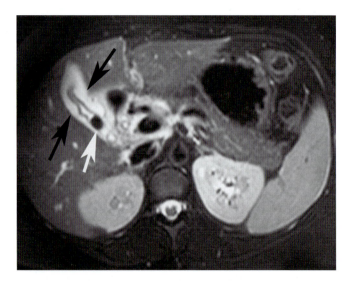

5. Axial T2-weighted MR image demonstrates a collapsed gallbladder with severe, diffuse, wall thickening with intramural hyperintensity (black arrows), indicating submucosal edema. Note also hypointense stone in the gallbladder neck (white arrow). Although the combination of wall thickening and gallstone may also be seen in acute cholecystitis, lack of luminal distention helps make the correct diagnosis.

PRESENTATION

- Fever, chills

- Right upper quadrant or epigastric pain

- Upper gastrointestinal tract symptoms (nausea, indigestion)

- Malaise, weight loss

FINDINGS

Inflammatory pseudotumor masses are typically solitary, with variable morphology, mostly hypoattenuating and with variable enhancement on CT and MR. Fibrous tissue components exhibit delayed enhancement.

DIFFERENTIAL DIAGNOSIS

- Hepatic abscess

- Metastasis

- Peripheral cholangiocarcinoma

- Hepatocellular carcinoma

COMMENTS

Hepatic inflammatory pseudotumor is a rare benign non-neoplastic lesion characterized by proliferating fibrous tissue and infiltration with polyclonal plasma cells and other inflammatory cells. The disease is usually acute or subacute and can develop anywhere in the body. The exact etiology of inflammatory pseudotumor remains unclear, but several mechanisms have been postulated for lesions occurring in the liver: infection, immune reaction, intraparenchymal hemorrhage and necrosis, occlusive phlebitis of intrahepatic veins, and secondary reaction to intrahepatic rupture of a biliary radical with cholangitis. In the liver, the disorder usually affects infants and young men and is more commonly located in the medial segments of the left lobe.

The majority of patients present with signs and laboratory evidence of an active inflammatory process. It is very difficult to make the specific diagnosis of inflammatory hepatic pseudotumor based on laboratory or imaging findings, because there is no specific serologic marker or radiographic appearance. Therefore, the vast majority of inflammatory pseudotumors of the liver require tissue diagnosis with image-guided biopsy or surgery. Once the diagnosis is confirmed, most patients respond adequately to therapy with antibiotics.

Inflammatory pseudotumor masses are typically solitary, with variable morphology. On CT, the mass appears mostly hypoattenuating, with variable degrees of enhancement with intravenous contrast. Areas of hyperattenuation correspond histologically with a greater concentration of fibrous tissue. Internal septations and delayed enhancement of fibrous areas are frequently observed. Only a few reports have described the MRI features of hepatic inflammatory pseudotumors. The lesion is predominantly hypointense lesion on T1-weighted images and isointense, with a hyperintense ring, on T2-weighted images. Nonspecific hyperintense areas on T1-weighted images may be present. Postcontrast sequences demonstrate early, intense, irregular enhancement and rapid washout. As with CT, delayed enhancement of fibrous tissue may be seen.

PEARLS

- Hepatic inflammatory pseudotumor is a rare benign non-neoplastic lesion characterized by proliferating fibrous tissue and infiltration with polyclonal plasma cells and other inflammatory cells.

- On CT, the mass appears mostly hypoattenuating, with variable degrees of enhancement with intravenous contrast.

- A specific diagnosis of inflammatory hepatic pseudotumor is rarely made on the basis of laboratory or imaging findings alone and, therefore, the vast majority of the lesions require tissue diagnosis with image-guided biopsy or surgery.

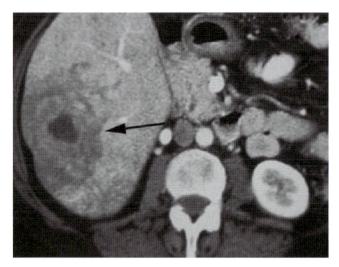

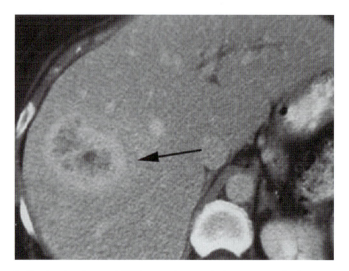

1. Contrast-enhanced CT image shows a large hypoattenuating lesion (arrow) with heterogeneous enhancement and a necrotic center in the right hepatic lobe.

2. Contrast-enhanced CT image shows a heterogeneous lesion with a thick enhancing wall and a low-attenuation center.

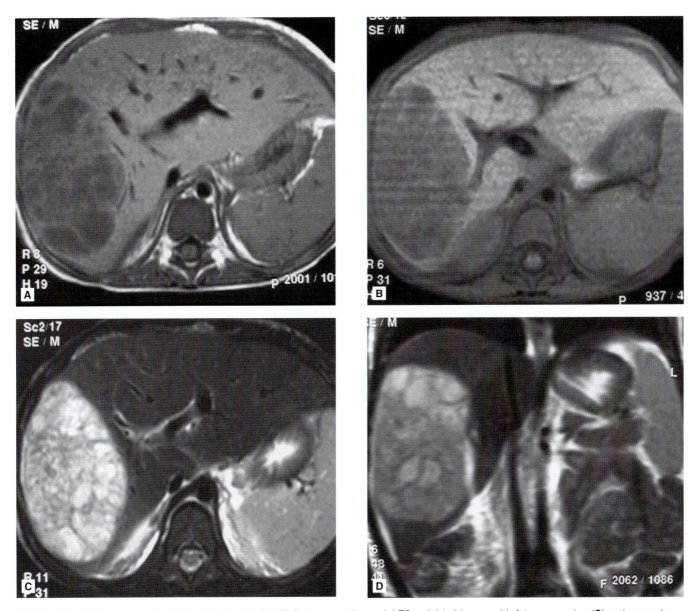

3. T1-weighted images acquired without (**A**) and with (**B**) fat suppression, axial T2-weighted image with fat suppression (**C**) and coronal T2-weighted image (**D**) demonstrate a large lesion in the right hepatic lobe. The lesion is predominantly hypointense on T1-weighted images and predominantly hyperintense on T2-weighted images.

PRESENTATION

- Dyspepsia
- Pain, weakness
- Abdominal distention
- Hepatosplenomegaly
- Hematemesis, and melena
- Rarely, signs and symptoms of liver failure

FINDINGS

US demonstrates echogenic thickening of the walls of the portal vein and branches, often extending to the porta hepatis, including the gallbladder. CT images demonstrate a peripheral, branching, pattern of linear calcifications along the hepatic surface and capsule. The liver mat assumes a characteristic "tortoise shell"–like appearance.

DIFFERENTIAL DIAGNOSIS

- *Salmonella* infection
- Gastroenteritis
- Hepatitis A, B, C

COMMENTS

Schistosomiasis is a parasitic disease caused by a type of blood fluke. Schistosomiasis is the third most devastating tropical disease in the world, after malaria and intestinal helminth infections. The disease is endemic in many African countries, where nearly 200 million people may be infected and coinfection with human immunodeficiency virus (HIV) is not uncommon. The disease is also common in some countries in the Caribbean, South America, and eastern Asia. All cases diagnosed in the United States are imported from foreign countries. Approximately 20 million people worldwide suffer the severe clinical form. Infection in endemic countries usually occurs during childhood; poor hygiene and playing in infested water and mud are contributing factors. The life cycle of these flatworms involves stages in the human and in the freshwater snail. The cercariae leave the snail and swim to a human or non-human animal, where they penetrate the skin. After penetrating the body, the cercariae travel to the heart and lungs, and reach the portal veins through the systemic circulation, and then develop into adult worms. The clinical form of the disease then results from immunological reactions to eggs trapped in tissues. Antigens released from the egg stimulate a granulomatous reaction that, in latter stages of the disease, causes collagen deposition and fibrosis.

The vast majority of gastrointestinal and hepatic schistosomiasis are caused by *Schistosoma mansoni* and *Schistosoma japonicum*. Most patients are asymptomatic or only mildly symptomatic and do not require medical attention. Only a small proportion of the endemic population develops clinically significant complications, such as periportal fibrosis, which leads to portal hypertension and gastrointestinal hemorrhage. Liver failure is uncommon.

Definitive diagnosis of schistosomiasis relies on detecting specific schistosome eggs in stool. Eosinophilia is prominent in acute schistosomiasis. Liver biopsy specimens may also demonstrate the eggs, confirming the diagnosis, as well as hepatic granulomas and findings of portal thrombophlebitis, with progressive deposition of fibrous tissue that ultimately compresses the hepatic venules. Hepatocyte damage and necrosis are rare. In chronic schistosomiasis, the main finding at US is echogenic thickening of the walls of the portal vein and branches, often extending to the porta hepatis, including the gallbladder. CT images demonstrate a peripheral, branching, pattern of linear calcifications along the hepatic surface and capsule. In the more advanced forms, the liver surface becomes distorted with large nodular formations of hepatic tissue separated by grooves and depressions, producing the characteristic "tortoise shell"–like appearance. As the disease progresses, evidence of portal hypertension appears on both US and CT.

PEARLS

- **Schistosomiasis is the third most devastating tropical disease in the world, after malaria and intestinal helminth infections.**

- **In chronic schistosomiasis, the main finding at US is echogenic thickening of the walls of the portal vein and branches, often extending to the porta hepatis, including the gallbladder.**

- **CT images demonstrate a peripheral, branching, pattern of linear calcifications along the hepatic surface and capsule and the liver surface becomes distorted with large nodular formations of hepatic tissue separated by grooves and depressions, producing the characteristic "tortoise shell"–like appearance.**

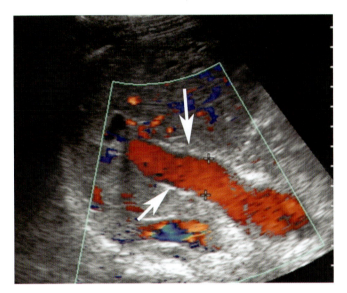

1. Transverse color Doppler US image demonstrates marked abnormal hepatic architecture and areas of parenchymal hyperechogenicity. The portal vein is dilated, a sign of portal hypertension. The wall of the portal vein is thickened as well (arrows).

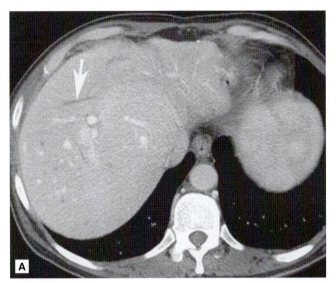

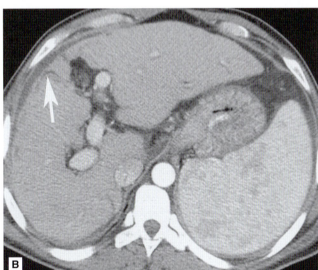

2. Contrast-enhanced CT images (**A**, **B**) demonstrate linear, branching, hypoattenuating areas in the periphery and subcapsular areas of the liver (arrows), characteristic of fibrosis in a patient with schistosomiasis and portal hypertension. Note the splenomegaly as well.

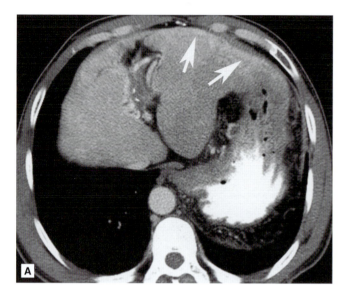

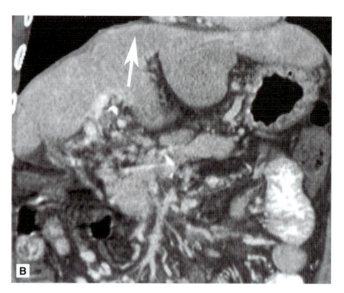

3. Axial contrast-enhanced CT image (**A**) and coronal reformation (**B**) demonstrate the markedly abnormal liver morphology and architectural distortion. Note also multiple small subcapsular hyperattenuating foci, representing calcifications.

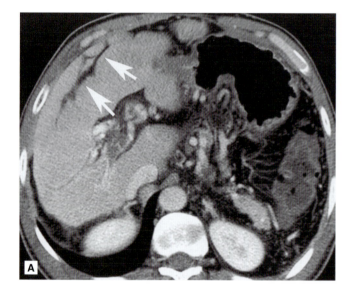

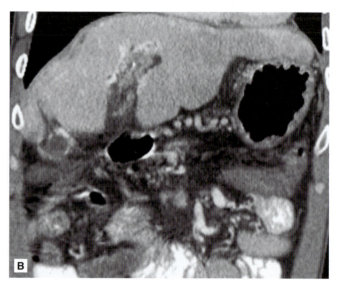

4. Contrast-enhanced axial (**A**) and coronal (**B**) CT images in a patient with advanced hepatic schistosomiasis demonstrates the lobulated liver surface with large nodular formations of hepatic tissue (arrows) separated by shallow grooves, producing the characteristic "tortoise shell"–like appearance.

DIFFUSE LIVER DISEASE

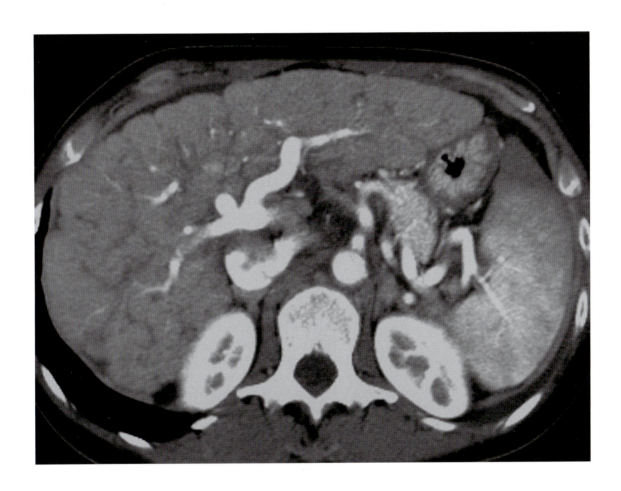

PRESENTATION

- Jaundice
- Muscle wasting
- Weight loss
- Marked ascites
- Variceal bleeding
- Hepatic encephalopathy
- Fatigue
- Gynecomastia
- Cutaneous manifestations: spider angiomata, skin telangiectasias, palmar erythema

FINDINGS

"Lumpy-bumpy" hepatic surface, enlargement of the left hepatic (especially the lateral segments) and caudate lobes, expanded gallbladder fossa, and expanded periportal space. Confluent hepatic fibrosis is common and appears as a wedge-shaped region with capsular retraction. Signs of portal hypertension include ascites, splenomegaly, and varices.

DIFFERENTIAL DIAGNOSIS

- Miliary infections
- Treated hepatic tumors (pseudocirrhosis)
- Sarcoidosis
- Diffuse metastases

COMMENTS

Cirrhosis represents the end-stage result of a wide variety of chronic liver diseases. Histologically, cirrhosis is a diffuse hepatic process in which the normal liver architecture is replaced by fibrosis and structurally abnormal nodules. Many causes of liver injury lead to fibrosis, which is defined as excessive extracellular matrix (especially collagen). Most of this increased collagen deposition occurs in the space of Disse (the space between hepatocytes and sinusoids). Fibrosis alone is potentially reversible. In contrast, in most patients, cirrhosis is not a reversible process. The progression of liver injury to cirrhosis may be fast (weeks) or slow (years). The correlation between the histologic severity of disease and the clinical findings is often poor.

Some patients are nearly asymptomatic while others have multiple symptoms of end-stage liver disease with limited survival. Signs and symptoms result from portal hypertension (variceal bleeding, ascites), poor synthetic function (coagulopathy), or decreased capability of the liver to detoxify the organism (hepatic encephalopathy).

Alcoholic liver disease was once the predominant cause of cirrhosis in the United States, but has been replaced by hepatitis C as the leading cause of chronic hepatitis and cirrhosis. Cryptogenic cirrhosis, a common cause in the past, is now considered to be secondary to nonalcoholic fatty liver disease (NAFLD) and nonalcoholic steatohepatitis (NASH) in many cases. Hepatic steatosis may regress in some patients as fibrosis progresses. Hepatitis B, often coincident with hepatitis D, is another common underlying etiology of cirrhosis. Other, less common, causes include autoimmune hepatitis, primary biliary cirrhosis, chronic biliary obstruction, primary sclerosing cholangitis, hemochromatosis, Wilson disease, alpha-1 antitrypsin deficiency, sarcoidosis, drug toxicity, and chronic right-sided heart failure.

The most common tool for gauging prognosis in cirrhosis is the Child-Turcotte-Pugh (CTP) system. Epidemiologic work shows that the CTP score may predict life expectancy in patients with advanced cirrhosis. A CTP score of 10 or greater is associated with a 50% chance of death within 1 year. Liver transplant programs in the United States have used the Model for End-Stage Liver Disease (MELD) scoring system to assess the relative severities of patients' liver diseases. Management of cirrhosis focuses on treating the underlying cause to stop or revert disease progression and treating complications as they arise.

Patients with cirrhosis should undergo periodic evaluation for early detection of complications, such as portal hypertension and hepatocellular carcinoma (HCC). Routine surveillance endoscopy is recommended to determine whether the patient has asymptomatic esophageal varices. Screening for interval development of HCC is also recommended, although the specific strategy is variable. Ultrasonography (see section on HCC) and alpha-fetoprotein are commonly obtained as part of a screening program, although the real utility is debatable. Increasingly, patients with clinical diagnosis of cirrhosis and confirmed or suspected HCC are monitored in the setting of liver transplant programs. Triple-phase CT and MRI are acquired in high-risk patients and in patients with suspected tumors based on results of screening tests.

Although cirrhosis is characterized by presence of innumerable regenerating nodules, the nodules themselves may not be readily apparent on imaging. The "lumpy-bumpy" appearance of the hepatic surface is usually visible when cirrhosis is moderate to severe and is more apparent in the presence of ascites. More subtle cases may only be evident with high-resolution US focused on the surface of the liver. In advanced cirrhosis, gross morphologic changes are easily recognized by the various imaging modalities. Enlargement of the left lobe (especially the lateral segments) and the caudate lobe, believed to be secondary to relative regeneration rather than fibrosis, is demonstrated by any cross-sectional technique. However, in autoimmune cirrhosis there is atrophy of the lateral segment of the left lobe and massive enlargement of the caudate lobe. Other morphologic findings of cirrhosis include the expanded gallbladder fossa and the expanded periportal space signs. In cirrhosis, portal venous flow is reduced and there is a compensatory increase in hepatic arterial flow and intrahepatic vascular shunts develop spontaneously. Multiphasic CT scanning can demonstrate these shunts as early opacification of the intrahepatic veins during the early arterial phase with associated, wedge-shaped perfusion abnormalities. Another imaging finding common in cirrhosis is confluent hepatic fibrosis, a region of atrophy that typically occurs in the anterior and medial segments. On CT, confluent hepatic fibrosis is seen as a wedge-shaped iso- or hypoattenuating region with capsular retraction. On MRI, focal confluent hepatic fibrosis is hypointense on T1-weighted images and usually hyperintense on T2-weighted images. Secondary manifestations of cirrhosis include findings of portal hypertension (ascites, splenomegaly, varices, recanalization of the paraumbilical vein), thickening and edema of the small and large bowel, and thickening of the gallbladder wall. Portal hypertension occurs once portal pressures reach 5 to 10 mm Hg above normal.

Continuous regeneration within the liver in cirrhosis may result in a variety of dysplastic lesions, which can range from premalignant to frankly malignant and invasive nodules. MR is the best method to differentiate between the various types of nodules. Regenerating nodules may contain high levels of iron (siderotic nodules), and be easily demonstrated on MR with gradient-echo sequences with a characteristic "blooming" artifact.

PEARLS

- Cirrhosis represents the end-stage result of a wide variety of chronic liver diseases in which, histologically, the normal liver architecture is replaced by fibrosis and abnormal nodules.

- Patients with cirrhosis should undergo periodic evaluation for early detection of complications, such as portal hypertension and HCC.

- The hepatic surface in cirrhosis is "lumpy-bumpy" due to the presence of multiple nodules. However this is seen only when cirrhosis is moderate to severe and is more apparent in the presence of ascites.

- Advanced cirrhosis causes gross morphologic changes: enlargement of the left lobe (especially the lateral segments) and the caudate lobe, relative atrophy of the right lobe, capsular retraction due to confluent fibrosis, and portal hypertension.

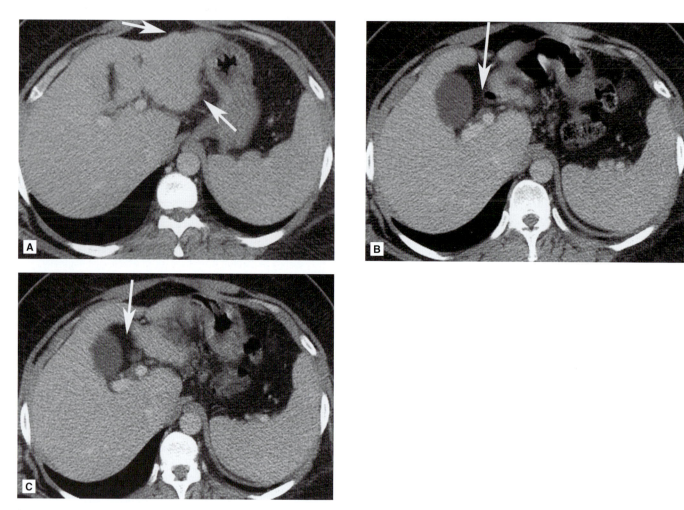

1. Axial CT images show findings characteristic of cirrhosis: surface nodularity (**A**, arrows), enlargement of the periportal space (**B**, arrow) and enlargement of the gallbladder fossa (**C**, arrow).

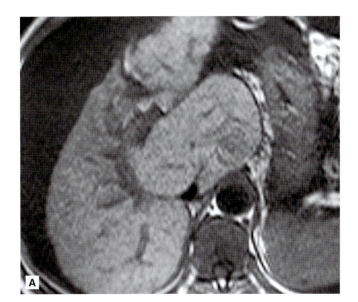

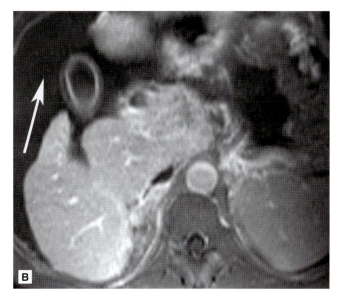

2. Precontrast (**A**), and contrast-enhanced (**B**) T1-weighted MR image demonstrates marked hypertrophy of the caudate lobe and atrophy of the right lobe. The gallbladder fossa is enlarged and there is abundant ascites.

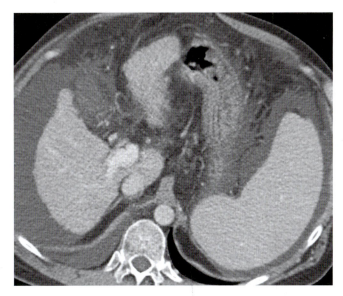

3. Contrast-enhanced CT image shows characteristic findings of cirrhosis and portal hypertension. There is surface nodularity, expansion of the gallbladder fossa, splenomegaly, and ascites.

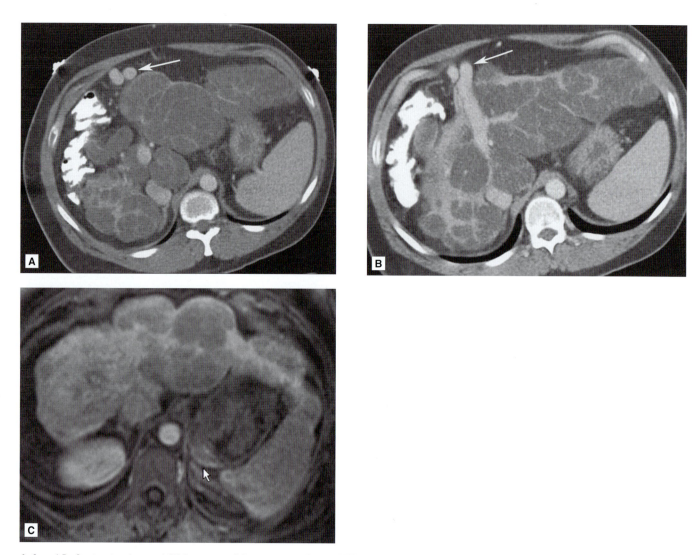

4. A and **B**. Contrast-enhanced CT images and **C**. contrast-enhanced T1-weighted MR image (**C**) show findings of advanced macronodular cirrhosis. The hepatic parenchyma is replaced with large nodules that cause severe architectural distortion. Note also the recanalized paraumbilical vein on **A** and **B** (arrows).

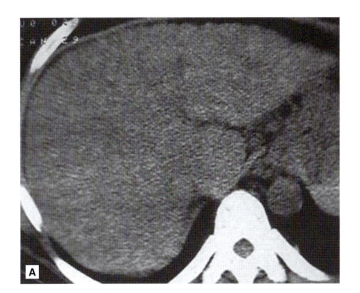

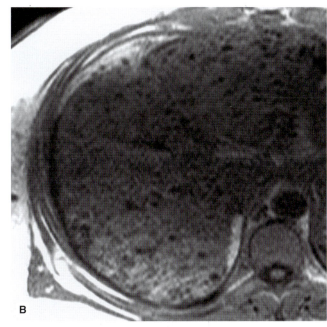

5. Noncontrast CT (**A**) and noncontrast T1-weighted MR image (**B**) of two different patients with siderotic (iron-containing) nodules. The siderotic nodules appear as multiple hyperattenuating foci on **A** and as hypointense nodules on **B**.

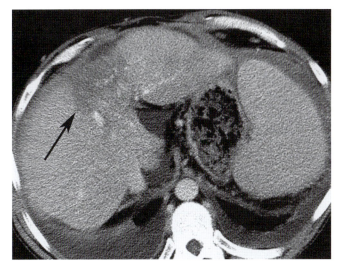

6. Contrast-enhanced CT image demonstrates characteristic findings of confluent hepatic fibrosis in cirrhosis. There is a wedge-shaped hypoattenuating area in the medial left hepatic lobe, with associated retraction of the capsule and surface.

PRESENTATION

- Symptoms and signs of liver metastases
- Symptoms and signs of portal hypertension
- Abnormal liver function tests

FINDINGS

Imaging findings include a lobulated liver surface with focal areas of volume loss, hypertrophy of the caudate lobe and, eventually, features of portal hypertension. Confluent areas of low attenuation extending to the liver capsule are commonly present.

DIFFERENTIAL DIAGNOSIS

- Cirrhosis
- Metastatic disease
- Sarcoidosis
- Diffuse infections

COMMENTS

Patients with liver metastases from various primary tumors (particularly breast carcinoma) who undergo treatment with systemic chemotherapy may develop areas of scarring that extend to the hepatic surface of the liver, with intervening regenerative hepatic parenchyma. This usually results from shrinkage of the metastatic nodules and retraction of the liver capsule, with a lobular margin. Between the areas of scarring, the liver parenchyma is regenerative. The result is a morphologic appearance that resembles macronodular cirrhosis and, thus, thisentity is referred to as "pseudocirrhosis." These changes can be observed within a few weeks or months after initiation of therapy. The pathogenesis is not completely understood, but it may result from the hepatoxic effects of systemic chemotherapy and/or hepatic infiltration by the metastatic tumor itself. There are also reports in the literature of a cirrhosis-like appearance of the liver in patients with metastases from breast carcinoma who had not previously undergone chemotherapy.

The imaging findings in patients with pseudocirrhosis include a lobulated liver surface with focal areas of volume loss, hypertrophy of the caudate lobe and, eventually, features of portal hypertension. Confluent areas of low attenuation extending to the liver capsule are commonly present as well. At pathology, the characteristic findings include elements of nodular regenerative hyperplasia without bridging fibrosis of the portal spaces (as seen in cirrhosis). The low-attenuation areas represent bands of fibrotic tissue, often with fatty infiltration as well. Frequently, foci of residual viable tumor are present, but they are difficult to detect given the advanced morphologic abnormalities.

PEARLS

- **Patients with liver metastases (particularly from breast carcinoma) who undergo treatment with systemic chemotherapy may develop areas of scarring that extend to the hepatic surface of the liver, with intervening regenerative hepatic parenchyma.**

- **The imaging findings in patients with pseudocirrhosis include a lobulated liver surface with focal areas of volume loss, hypertrophy of the caudate lobe and, eventually, features of portal hypertension.**

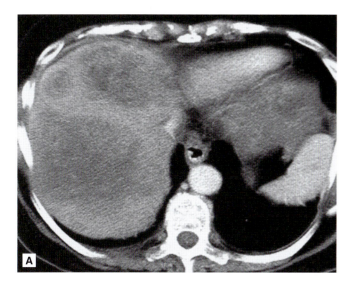

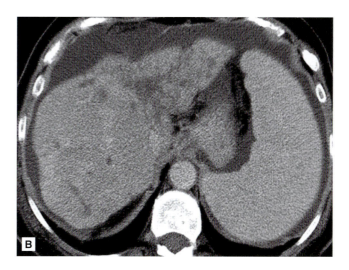

1. A. Contrast-enhanced CT image of a patient with breast cancer demonstrates multiple large, irregular, low-attenuation metastases in the liver. **B.** Contrast-enhanced CT image acquired 6 months after **A**, after 3 cycles of chemotherapy. The metastases have diminished considerably in size and the liver surface is irregular, with multiple bands of low attenuation that extend to the capsule. This appearance is characteristic of pseudocirrhosis. There are signs of portal hypertension as well (splenomegaly and ascites).

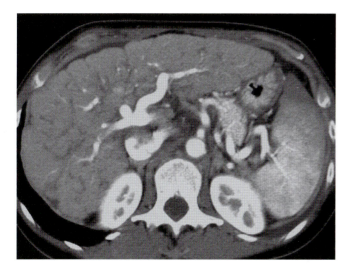

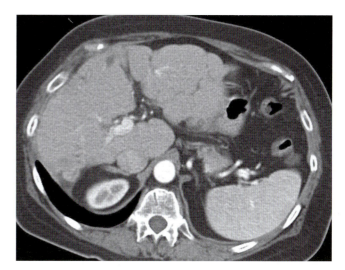

2. Contrast-enhanced CT image shows signs of pseudocirrhosis in a patient with treated liver metastases from breast carcinoma. There are multiple low-attenuation bands perpendicular to the hepatic capsule and extending to the liver surface, creating a lobulated appearance.

3. Contrast-enhanced CT image demonstrates multiple lobulations in the surface of the liver and small, low-attenuation bands that extend to the capsule.

PRESENTATION

- Most patients are asymptomatic.

- Fatigue, malaise, or upper abdominal discomfort.

- Ascites, edema, and jaundice in patients with cirrhosis due to progressive nonalcoholic steatohepatitis (NASH).

- Hepatomegaly is common.

FINDINGS

On US, the liver is characteristically hyperechogenic (bright). At unenhanced CT, fatty infiltration causes a lowering of the normal attenuation of the liver parenchyma. On opposed-phase MR images, areas of steatosis appear as regions of decreased signal intensity compared with the in-phase signal intensity.

DIFFERENTIAL DIAGNOSIS

- Acute hepatitis

- Hepatotoxicity from medications

- Cirrhosis

COMMENTS

Fatty change in the liver results from excessive accumulation of triglycerides and other lipids within the hepatocytes. Fatty liver disease is now the most common cause for elevated liver function tests in the United States, and this is mainly due to the ongoing obesity epidemic. Other risk factors include diabetes and high triglyceride levels. Steatosis affects approximately 25% to 35% of the general population. Fatty liver disease can range from fatty liver alone (steatosis) to fatty liver associated with inflammation (steatohepatitis). This condition can occur with the use of alcohol (alcohol-related fatty liver) or in the absence of alcohol (nonalcoholic fatty liver disease). If steatohepatitis is present but a history of alcohol use is not, the condition is termed NASH. Simple fatty liver is believed to be benign, but NASH can progress to fibrosis and cirrhosis and can be associated with hepatocellular carcinoma.

Fibrosis or cirrhosis in the liver is present in 15% to 50% of patients with NASH.

The most common associations with fatty liver disease are alcohol and the metabolic syndrome (type II diabetes, obesity, and hypertriglyceridemia). Other associations include drugs (steroids, tamoxifen, methotrexate), metabolic abnormalities (galactosemia, glycogen storage diseases, homocystinuria, tyrosinemia), total parenteral nutrition, and starvation. Mild-to-moderate elevation of the hepatic enzymes and hyperlipidemia are common. Importantly, viral markers should be tested and viral infection excluded, as the differential diagnosis always includes viral hepatitis.

On US, the liver is characteristically hyperechogenic (bright). However, steatosis is detected on US only when substantial (30% or more) fatty change is present.

At unenhanced CT, fatty infiltration causes a lowering of the normal attenuation of the liver parenchyma. In healthy adults, the attenuation value of the liver parenchyma is higher than that of the spleen. Mild degrees of diffuse fatty infiltration can be diagnosed when the attenuation value of the liver parenchyma is slightly less than that of the spleen; more severe involvement leads to attenuation levels lower than that of the intrahepatic blood vessels. Contrast-enhanced images are less reliable and less specific for detecting steatosis. Focal fatty infiltration, perivascular fat distributions, and residual foci of unaffected liver parenchyma surrounded by fatty infiltration may all be confused with neoplastic lesions at CT. Therefore, the identification of differentiating imaging characteristics becomes crucial, especially in patients being evaluated for possible liver metastases: Focal fatty infiltration commonly has a segmental or lobar distribution and often has a geographic shape that extends to the liver capsule. Common locations for fatty infiltration are in the anterior part of segment IV, adjacent to the falciform ligament and the fissure for the ligamentum teres. Vessels are seen coursing through the area of abnormal attenuation without any displacement. MR is highly sensitive for detecting diffuse or focal fatty infiltration. Gradient-echo phase shift images have been proved to be an excellent tool to detect fatty parenchyma. On opposed-phase images, focal fatty infiltration appears as a region of decreased signal intensity compared with the in-phase signal intensity. Noninvasive studies, such as US, CT, and MRI, are very useful to identify the presence of a fatty liver. However, these imaging techniques cannot distinguish between benign steatosis and steatohepatitis and biopsy is often necessary in these circumstances. Benign steatosis may be focal or diffuse, whereas steatohepatitis is usually diffuse. New techniques, such as diffusion-weighted MR imaging and elastography, are undergoing active investigation for this purpose.

PEARLS

- Fatty liver disease is now the most common cause for elevated liver function tests in the United States, and this is mainly due to the ongoing obesity epidemic.

- Fatty liver disease can range from fatty liver alone (steatosis) to fatty liver associated with inflammation (steatohepatitis).

- Noninvasive studies, such as US, CT, and MRI, are very useful to identify the presence of a fatty liver but cannot distinguish between benign steatosis and steatohepatitis; biopsy is often necessary in these circumstances.

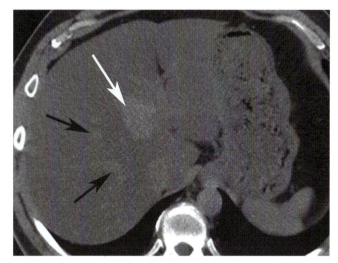

1. Axial noncontrast CT image demonstrates diffuse decreased attenuation of the liver parenchyma, consistent with steatosis. The attenuation of the intrahepatic vessels (black arrows) and spleen is higher than that of the liver. There is a focal area of sparing (relatively normal hepatic parenchyma) in the medial left lobe (white arrow).

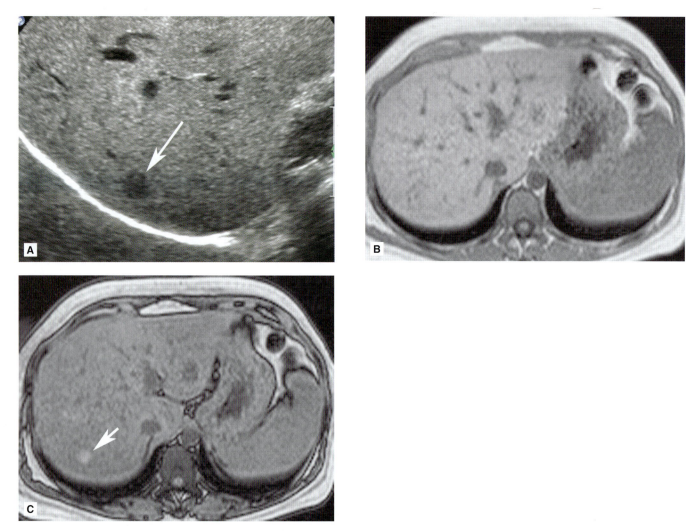

2. A. Transverse US image shows diffuse increased echogenicity of the hepatic parenchyma, indicative of fatty infiltration, and a nonspecific, rounded hypoechoic area in the posterior right lobe (arrow). **B.** In-phase MR image shows a normal appearance of the liver and spleen. **C.** On the opposed-phase MR image obtained at the same level as **B.** The signal intensity of the hepatic parenchyma has dropped, and is similar to that of the spleen and paraspinal muscles. The rounded area in the posterior right lobe (arrow) has relatively normal signal intensity, consistent with a focal area of normal liver (focal fatty sparing).

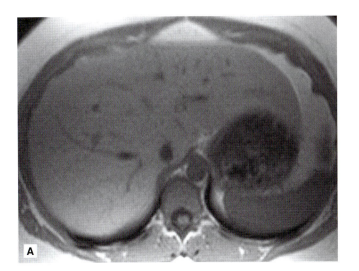

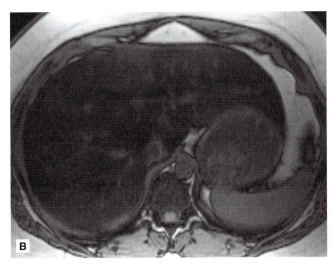

3. Severe diffuse fatty infiltration in an obese patient demonstrated with in-phase (**A**) and opposed-phase (**B**) images. The signal intensity of the hepatic parenchyma is markedly less on **B** as compared to **A**.

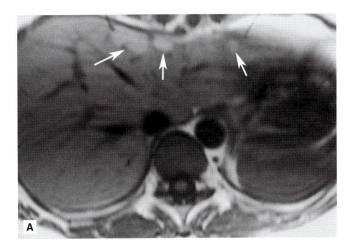

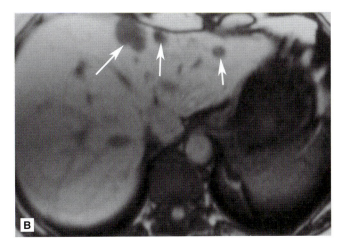

4. In-phase (**A**) and opposed-phase (**B**) images demonstrate characteristic findings of focal fatty infiltration in the left hepatic lobe. There are 3 peripheral hyperintense areas on **A** (arrows) which demonstrated marked signal loss on **B** (arrows).

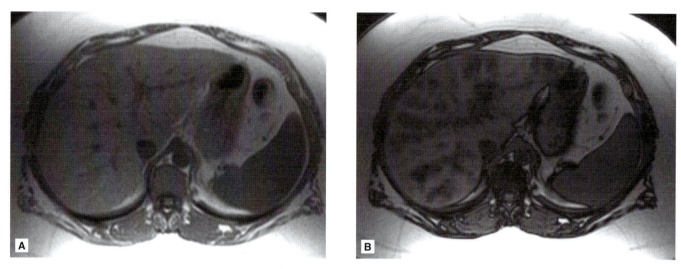

5. Obese patient with perivascular fatty infiltration demonstrated on in-phase (**A**) and opposed-phase (**B**) images. There are multiple areas of low signal intensity surrounding the branching portal venous system on **B**, which are not apparent on **A**.

PRESENTATION

- Symptoms and signs of liver disease
- Skin pigmentation
- Diabetes mellitus
- Arthropathy
- Impotence in males
- Cardiac enlargement, with or without heart failure or conduction defects

FINDINGS

On noncontrast CT, excessive hepatic iron causes increased attenuation of the liver parenchyma, usually greater than 75 Hounsfield units (HU). On MR, iron causes decreased signal intensity on MRI images. Iron content can be accurately quantified with MR techniques.

DIFFERENTIAL DIAGNOSIS

- Other causes of cirrhosis

COMMENTS

Hemochromatosis is the abnormal accumulation of iron in parenchymal organs, leading to organ dysfunction and failure. It is the most common inherited liver disease in whites and the most common autosomal recessive genetic disorder. Hereditary hemochromatosis is an adult-onset disorder characterized by inappropriately high iron absorption resulting in progressive iron overload. The organs involved are the liver, heart, pancreas, pituitary, joints, and skin. Excess iron is hazardous because it produces free radical formation which can produce deoxyribonucleic acid (DNA) cleavage that eventually leads to cell injury and fibrosis. Clinical manifestations include liver cirrhosis, heart failure, diabetes mellitus, impotence, and arthritis. If untreated, hemochromatosis may lead to death from cirrhosis, diabetes, hepatocellular carcinoma. The disease usually becomes apparent after age 40 in men and age 50 in women. Secondary hemochromatosis can be the result of a variety of disorders, most commonly chronic hemolytic anemias. Iron deposition in primary hemochromatosis occurs in the parenchymal cells of the liver (hepatocytes), whereas in secondary hemochromatosis the abnormal accumulation occurs in the reticuloendothelial system (Kupffer cells and spleen).

On CT, patients with abnormal accumulation of hepatic iron demonstrate hepatomegaly and diffuse increased attenuation of the liver parenchyma, usually greater than 75 HU on the noncontrast examination. The liver vasculature appears particularly prominent because of the increased contrast between the vessels and the high-attenuation liver. Other abnormalities that can cause increased attenuation of the liver on CT scans include amiodarone toxicity, Thorotrast, glycogen storage diseases, gold therapy, and Wilson disease. Increased iron in the liver can be detected and quantified by MRI. Iron causes magnetic susceptibility artifact, which leads to spin dephasing (T2*-related signal loss). This dephasing results in decreased signal intensity on MRI images.

T2-weighted gradient-echo images are most sensitive to magnetic susceptibility artifact and thus are the best sequences to detect increased iron in the liver. T2-weighted gradient-echo images can be performed as breath-hold images on most scanners. On a 1.5-T scanner, an echo time (TE) of at least 10 ms and a flip angle of less than 30 degrees should be used. In determining whether the signal intensity of the liver is abnormally low, skeletal muscle can be used as a control. If the liver demonstrates signal intensity equal to or lower than that of skeletal muscle, such as the paraspinal muscles, on either T2-weighted gradient echo, or T2-weighted spin-echo images, increased iron accumulation in the liver can be diagnosed. Iron deposits in the liver per se usually do not alter liver echogenicity. If ultrasonographic liver abnormalities are present, they are usually secondary to cirrhosis.

PEARLS

- **Hereditary hemochromatosis is an adult-onset disorder characterized by inappropriately high iron absorption resulting in progressive iron overload leading to dysfunction of the liver, heart, pancreas, pituitary, joints, and skin.**

- **On CT, patients with hemochromatosis demonstrate hepatomegaly and diffuse increased attenuation of the liver parenchyma, usually greater than 75 HU units on the noncontrast examination.**

- **Iron causes marked signal intensity loss on T2-weighted MR images, especially gradient-echo sequences (T2*-related signal loss). Increased iron in the liver can be detected and quantified with MRI.**

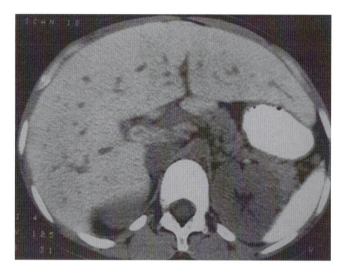

1. Noncontrast CT image of a patient with excessive iron deposition in the liver secondary to sickle cell disease and multiple transfusions. The attenuation of the liver parenchyma is increased diffusely (~ 90 HU) and the intrahepatic vessels are prominent. The spleen is diffusely calcified (autoinfarction).

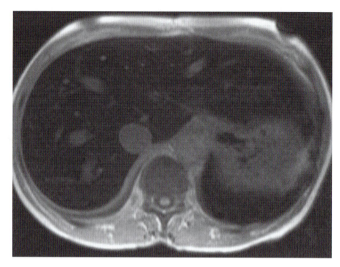

2. Axial gradient-echo MR image of a patient with hemochromatosis demonstrates diffuse hypointensity of the liver parenchyma. The excess iron causes susceptibility artifact and spin dephasing. The signal intensity is lower than that of the skeletal muscle, such as the paraspinal muscles.

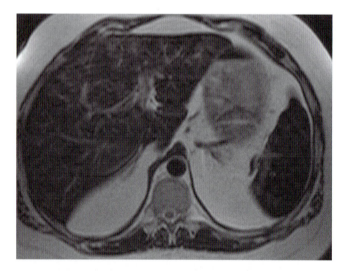

3. Axial T2-weighted fast spin-echo MR image demonstrates diffuse hypointensity of the liver parenchyma, consistent with abnormal iron deposition, in a patient with hemochromatosis.

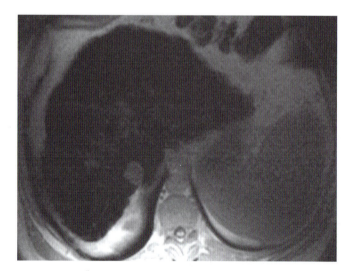

4. Axial gradient-echo MR image of a patient with hemochromatosis demonstrates abnormal low signal intensity of the liver parenchyma, secondary to iron deposition, and morphologic changes consistent with cirrhosis (abnormal hepatic architecture and nodular surface).

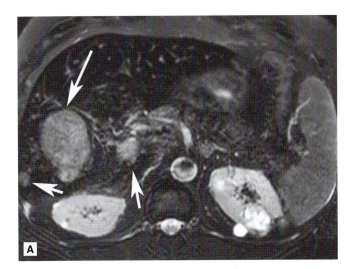
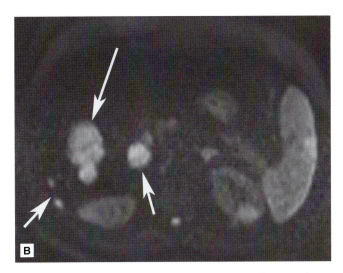

5. Axial T2-weighted (**A**) and diffusion-weighted (**B**) MR images obtained on a patient with hemochromatosis demonstrate diffuse hypointensity of the liver parenchyma and multiple high–signal intensity masses with restricted diffusion (**A** and **B**, arrows). The findings are characteristic of hemochromatosis with multifocal hepatocellular carcinoma.

PRESENTATION

- Usually incidental finding in a patient with known thoracic sarcoidosis

- Systemic symptoms (fatigue, weight loss, fever)

- Shortness of breath and cough (secondary to pulmonary involvement)

FINDINGS

Granulomas are seen as multiple hypoattenuating lesions on CT which are more conspicuous with intravenous contrast. On MR, these noncaseating granulomas are hypointense on T1-weighted images and hyperintense on T2-weighted images. On US, the nodules are hypoechoic relative to the background liver, although hyperechoic nodules have also been described.

DIFFERENTIAL DIAGNOSIS

- Lymphoma

- Metastatic disease

- Systemic infection

COMMENTS

Sarcoidosis is a generalized granulomatous disease that most commonly affects the pulmonary parenchyma and mediastinal and hilar lymph nodes. Although involvement of abdominal organs in patients with sarcoidosis is frequent, the abdominal manifestations are usually documented after the initial diagnosis has been made on the basis of thoracic findings. Noncaseating epithelioid granulomas scattered diffusely throughout the liver are the most common hepatic manifestation of multisystem sarcoidosis. Granulomas can be found in the spleen in 25% to 50% and in the liver in 25% to 75% of unselected patients with sarcoidosis.

Sarcoidosis frequently produces no symptoms. When present, symptoms associated with sarcoidosis are either systemic (fever and fatigue) or specific to the organ involved (such as dyspnea or cough in patients with pulmonary disease). Dysfunction of the liver and spleen is rare and, thus, most patients with hepatosplenic sarcoidosis are asymptomatic from the abdominal point of view. Serum levels of the angiotensin-converting enzyme (ACE) are often elevated in patients with sarcoidosis. This is helpful in the differential diagnosis of patients who have abdominal adenopathy and multiple small lesions in the liver and/or spleen. Specifically, patients with lymphoma do not usually have elevated ACE levels. Symptomatic patients usually respond well to therapy with steroids.

Hepatic noncaseating epithelioid granulomas manifest without specific multidetector CT or MR imaging features and range from submillimeter size of 1 to 2 cm. Larger granulomas are surrounded by fibrotic hepatic parenchyma, an indication of a more vigorous immunologic response. These granulomas are seen on noncontrast CT images as multiple intrahepatic and intrasplenic hypoattenuating lesions, usually in the setting of associated hepatosplenomegaly and intra-abdominal adenopathy. After administration of intravenous contrast material, these low-attenuation focal lesions are more conspicuous, but become rapidly isoattenuating to liver parenchyma on equilibrium and delayed phases. On MR images, these noncaseating granulomas are seen as multiple intrahepatic and intrasplenic nodules that are hypointense on T1-weighted images and hyperintense on T2-weighted images. On ultrasonography, sarcoidosis nodules are more commonly hypoechoic relative to the background liver, although hyperechoic nodules have also been described. The appearance may depend on the echogenicity of the liver.

PEARLS

- **Non-caseating granulomas are found in the spleen in 25% to 50% and in the liver in 25% to 75% of patients with sarcoidosis.**

- **Serum levels of the angiotensin-converting enzyme (ACE) are often elevated in patients with sarcoidosis.**

- **Sarcoid granulomas do not have specific multi-detector CT or MR imaging features and range in size from submillimeter to 1 to 2 cm.**

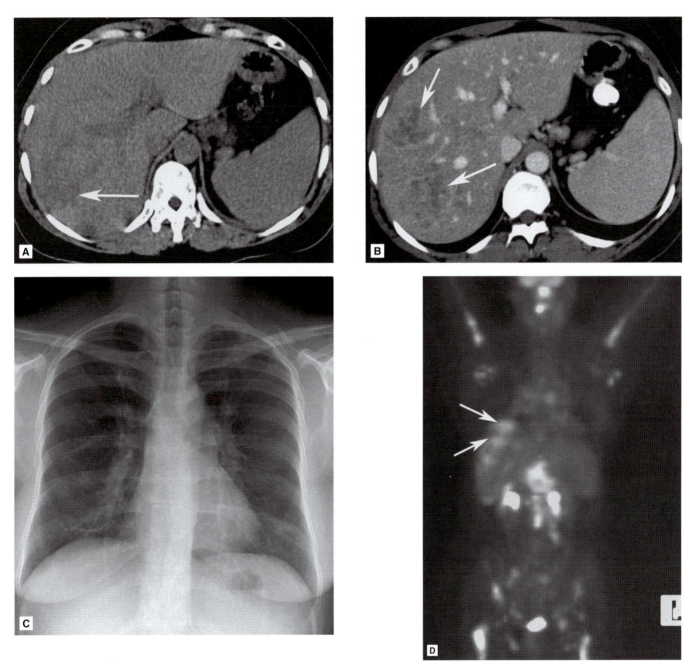

1. Noncontrast (**A**) and contrast-enhanced (**B**) CT images in a patient with known sarcoidosis show a cluster of poorly defined low-attenuation lesions in the liver (**A** and **B**, arrows). The posteroanterior radiograph of the chest (**C**) demonstrates bilateral hilar prominence, secondary to presence of enlarged lymph nodes. Whole body fluorodeoxyglucose positron emission tomography (FDG-PET) scan (**D**) shows multiple hypermetabolic lymph nodes and foci of hypermetabolism in the right lobe of the liver (arrows).

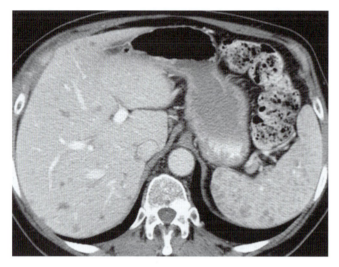

2. Contrast-enhanced CT image demonstrates multiple poorly defined low-attenuation lesions in the liver and spleen. The spleen is slightly enlarged as well.

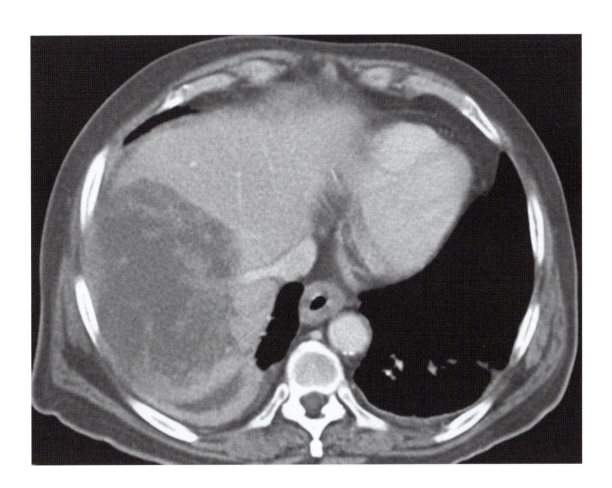

PRESENTATION

- Usually develops slowly and silently

- May present with gastrointestinal bleeding

- Abdominal pain in acute thrombosis

- Splenomegaly, ascites

FINDINGS

On US, echogenic material is seen in the lumen of the vein. Contrast-enhanced CT and MR demonstrate clot filling or expanding the portal vein. Cavernous transformation is characterized on imaging by a tangle of fine or markedly enlarged serpiginous vessels seen in place of the portal vein.

DIFFERENTIAL DIAGNOSIS

- Portal hypertension

COMMENTS

Portal vein thrombosis is caused by hepatic parenchymal disease with secondary reduced portal venous flow, acute intra-abdominal inflammation or sepsis (such as acute appendicitis or pancreatitis), hypercoagulable syndromes, trauma, or tumors. Segmental or global portal vein thrombosis occurs in up to 30% of patients with hepatocellular carcinoma and in 5% to 8% of patients with cirrhosis and portal hypertension. Portal vein thrombosis may remain clinically silent and not discovered until gastrointestinal hemorrhage develops, unless it is found incidentally during routine surveillance for an underlying process (such as cirrhosis). Acute thrombosis may lead to hypersplenism. Associated thrombosis of the mesenteric veins can also occur, causing intestinal ischemia and abdominal pain.

On ultrasonography, echogenic material (representing clot) is seen in the lumen of the vein. Overall, the clot usually has moderate echogenicity, but may be hypoechoic in cases of hyperacute thrombosis. Pulsed or color Doppler images show absence of the typical hepatopetal venous flow signal in the lumen of the portal vein, although partial thrombus may be surrounded by residual flow. Incomplete occlusion is particularly common in cases of neoplastic invasion of the portal vein. Contrast-enhanced CT images depict the low-attenuation material filling or expanding the portal vein, surrounded by peripheral enhancement. Arterial portography, which requires indirect opacification of the portal venous system with injection of contrast material into the splenic artery or superior mesenteric artery, is rarely performed for diagnosis. MR demonstrates abnormal intravascular intermediate-to-high–signal intensity clot replacing the usual flow voids seen in patent vessels.

Cavernous transformation (ie, the development of multiple periportal collateral vessels within the wall or surrounding the portal vein) occurs with long-standing portal vein thrombosis. The appearance on imaging studies is characteristic: A tangle of fine or markedly enlarged serpiginous vessels is seen in place of the portal vein, which is not identified. The application of color and/or pulsed Doppler imaging shows blood flow in these periportal collaterals that form around the thrombosed portal vein or that replace the vein. In cases of malignant thrombosis, the portal vein is expanded by soft tissue with internal vascularity, which can be demonstrated directly with Doppler US or as areas of enhancement on contrast-enhanced CT or MR.

PEARLS

- **Portal vein thrombosis is caused by hepatic parenchymal disease with secondary reduced portal venous flow, acute intra-abdominal inflammation or sepsis (such as acute appendicitis or pancreatitis), hypercoagulable syndromes, trauma, or tumors.**

- **On US, echogenic clot in the lumen of the vein, whereas pulsed or color Doppler images show absence of the typical hepatopetal venous flow signal.**

- **Cavernous transformation (ie, the development of multiple periportal collateral vessels within the wall or surrounding the portal vein) occurs with long-standing portal vein thrombosis and has a characteristic appearance on imaging studies: A tangle of fine or markedly enlarged serpiginous vessels is seen in place of the portal vein, which is not identified.**

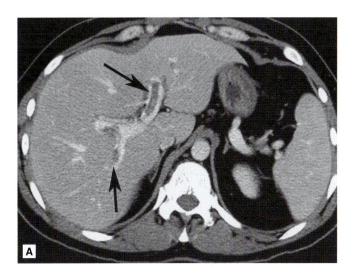

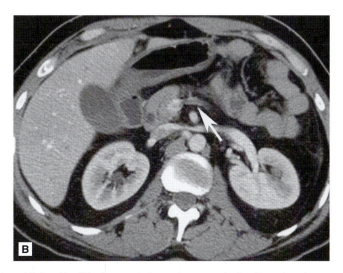

1. Contrast-enhanced CT images of a patient with complicated acute sigmoid diverticulitis demonstrate acute nonocclusive thrombus in the right and left portal veins (**A**, arrows) and in the inferior mesenteric vein (**B**, arrow).

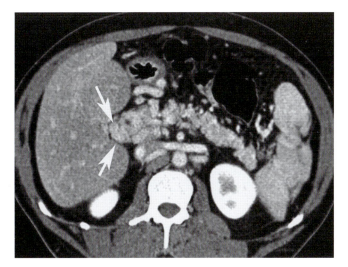

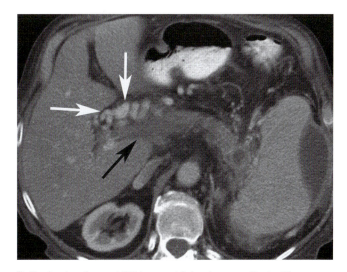

2. Contrast-enhanced CT image of a patient with chronic thrombosis of the portal vein and cavernous transformation. There is a tangle of fine tortuous, serpiginous vessels in the porta hepatis (arrows), replacing the portal vein.

3. Contrast-enhanced CT image obtained on a patient with subacute pancreatitis demonstrates thrombosis of the portal vein (black arrow) and cavernous transformation (white arrows). Notice also fluid collections in the tail of the pancreas and subcapsular aspect of the spleen.

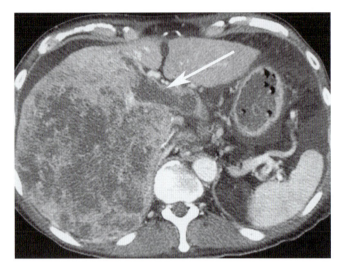

4. Tumor thrombus in the main portal vein demonstrated on a contrast-enhanced CT image. There is hypoattenuating tissue in the lumen of the portal vein, which also appears expanded (arrow). The right lobe of the liver is replaced with an irregular, heterogeneous mass, characteristic of hepatocellular carcinoma.

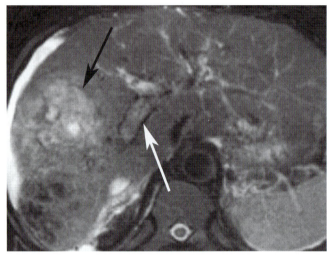

5. Axial fat-suppressed T2-weighted image demonstrates a heterogeneous, but predominantly high–signal intensity, mass in the right hepatic lobe (black arrow) with invasion of the right portal vein (white arrow). Percutaneous biopsy confirmed hepatocellular carcinoma.

PRESENTATION

- Painful hepatomegaly
- Ascites refractory to treatment
- Portal hypertension with variceal bleeding
- Jaundice
- Splenomegaly
- Vomiting

FINDINGS

On CT and MR, hepatic veins do not enhance and the inferior vena cava (IVC) is compressed by the enlarged caudate lobe. Ascites and splenomegaly are usually present. Over time, multiple regenerative nodules develop and the caudate lobe hypertrophies.

DIFFERENTIAL DIAGNOSIS

- Right-sided heart failure
- Hepatic veno-occlusive disease
- Cirrhosis with portal hypertension
- Constrictive pericarditis

COMMENTS

Budd-Chiari syndrome (BCS) is a manifestation of hepatic venous outflow obstruction that may occur at the level of the IVC, the hepatic veins, or at the venule level. The causes of BCS are numerous. Two types are generally recognized: acute and chronic. The acute form results from acute thrombosis of the main hepatic veins or the IVC. The chronic form results from fibrosis of the intrahepatic veins, presumably caused inflammation. Both the acute form and the chronic form of BCS result in severe centrilobular congestion and hepatocellular necrosis and atrophy. This in turn causes delay or reversal of portal venous blood flow and morphologic changes in the liver (resulting in abnormal liver function test results). The classic presentation is with ascites, hepatomegaly, and abdominal pain. BCS has been classified into a primary form, associated with congenital webs of the IVC and a secondary form, associated with numerous conditions: tumor, venous thrombosis caused by hematological (polycythemia rubra vera, antiphospholipid syndrome, pregnancy and the postpartum state, use of oral contraceptives, sickle cell disease, thrombocytosis, paroxysmal nocturnal hemoglobinuria) or autoimmune diseases (systemic lupus erythematosus, Behcet syndrome), use of immunosuppressive drugs, and trauma.

In most patients with BCS, hepatic venous outflow obstruction is not complete, with residual patent accessory veins such as the caudate veins, which drain into the IVC inferior to the major hepatic veins. Alternative pathways for drainage also develop via the azygos vein, the intercostal vessels, and the paravertebral veins. The parts of the liver that have preserved venous drainage undergo hypertrophy.

Although a definitive diagnosis requires a liver biopsy, imaging studies are very useful in the evaluation and to help rule out many of the differential considerations. The thrombosed hepatic veins are hypoattenuating, and the IVC is compressed by the enlarged caudate lobe. Ascites and splenomegaly are usually present as well. In subacute or chronic BCS, the morphologic changes become apparent, with hypertrophy of the areas with preserved drainage, and portosystemic and intrahepatic collateral vessels. Chronic BCS is also characterized by the development of multiple regenerative nodules, which are usually hypervascular on arterial phase images and remain slightly hyperattenuating on portal venous phase images. Venography of the IVC or hepatic veins shows a spiderweb pattern of collateral vessels, pathognomonic of BCS.

PEARLS

- **BCS is a manifestation of hepatic venous outflow obstruction that may occur at the level of the IVC, the hepatic veins, or at the venule level.**

- **Conventional US shows enlargement of the caudate lobe, ascites, splenomegaly, and narrowing or lack of visualization and thrombosis of the hepatic veins while color Doppler studies show absent or flat flow in the hepatic veins.**

- **In acute BCS, CT and MR images demonstrate patchy enhancement of the liver, with decreased peripheral enhancement and more intense enhancement of the central portion of the liver.**

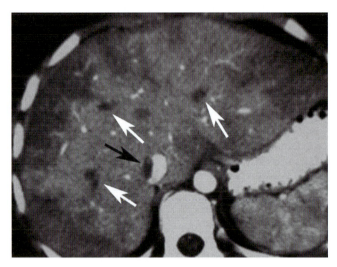

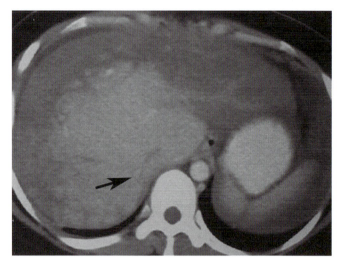

1. Contrast-enhanced CT image shows characteristic findings of acute BCS. There is eccentric low-attenuation clot in the IVC (black arrow) and nonfilling of the hepatic veins, which are completely filled with clot (white arrows). There is patchy enhancement of the liver parenchyma, with multiple foci of poor enhancement in the periphery.

2. Contrast-enhanced CT of chronic BCS. The central areas of the liver, especially the caudate lobe, are hypertrophied and there is atrophy of the peripheral areas. The IVC (arrow) is small and compressed. Note also perisplenic and perihepatic ascites.

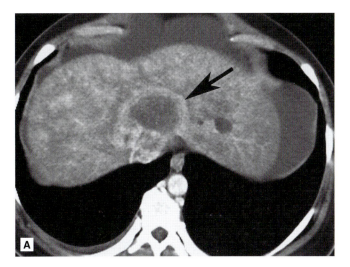

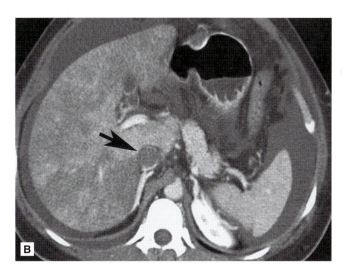

3. Peripheral cholangiocarcinoma causing BCS. Contrast-enhanced CT images demonstrate a large, heterogeneous, mass (**A**, arrow) which is invading the IVC with tumor thrombus (**B**, arrow). Enhancement of the hepatic parenchyma is heterogeneous, secondary to the obstructed venous outflow.

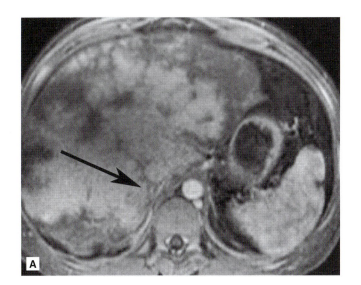

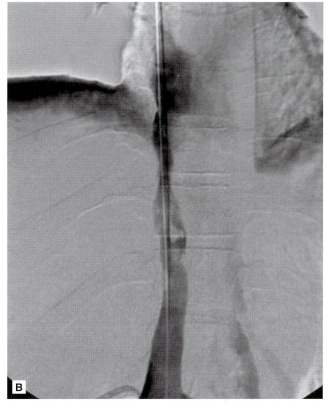

4. A. Contrast-enhanced MR image shows a patchy, heterogeneous enhancement of the liver parenchyma. The IVC is slit-like (arrow). **B.** Venography of the same patient shows marked narrowing of the IVC; the hepatic veins could not be canalized, indicating chronic thrombosis.

PRESENTATION

- Peliosis hepatis is often asymptomatic.

- Ascites, hepatomegaly.

- Hepatic failure.

- Acute abdominal pain and hypotension in cases of rupture.

FINDINGS

At US, peliosis hepatis lesions typically are hyperechoic lesion. On noncontrast CT, they are commonly hypoattenuating, often with areas of hemorrhage. After administration of intravenous contrast, early globular enhancement is observed with centripetal progression although brisk, homogeneous, enhancement is also possible. MR images also demonstrate the hemorrhagic components.

DIFFERENTIAL DIAGNOSIS

- Adenoma

- Cavernous hemangioma

- Focal nodular hyperplasia

- Hypervascular metastasis

- Hepatocellular carcinoma

COMMENTS

Peliosis hepatis is a rare benign vascular lesion characterized by sinusoidal dilatation and blood-filled spaces. Multiple causes of peliosis hepatis have been described, including toxins (such as arsenic and polyvinyl chloride), drugs (such as oral contraceptives, anabolic steroids, and corticosteroids), infectious agents in AIDS (such as *Bartonella* or "bacillary angiomatosis") and malignancies (mostly hepatocellular carcinoma). However, peliosis hepatis is idiopathic in 30% to 50% of patients.

Peliosis hepatis is often asymptomatic. In symptomatic patients, common finding include portal hypertension with ascites, hepatomegaly, cholestasis, and, ultimately, hepatic failure. Rupture of peliosis lesions and intraperitoneal hemorrhage cause acute abdominal pain and shock. Peliosis hepatis usually regresses after the causative factor is corrected, such as removing a drug, terminating steroid therapy, or successful therapy of any associated

infectious disease. However, if not treated, the disease may be rapidly fatal.

At gross pathology, peliosis hepatis is characterized by multiple irregular cavities, filled with blood, in the hepatic parenchyma. These lesions typically involve the entire liver, but cases of focal disease have been described. Imaging findings match these pathological findings. At US, peliosis hepatis lesions demonstrate variable echogenicity relative to the surrounding normal liver parenchyma and may have internal vascularity when evaluated with color Doppler. The more typical appearance is a focal hyperechoic lesion in patients with normal background liver; however, it may appear hypoechoic in patients with increased echogenicity of the liver parenchyma, such as in steatosis. Noncontrast CT images commonly show a focal hypoattenuating area; however, areas of hemorrhage may be hyperattenuating. After administration of intravenous contrast, early globular enhancement is observed, with a centripetal progression in more delayed phase. A brisk, homogeneous, enhancement may also be seen. Other findings include central areas of thrombosis or foci of calcification. On delayed phase images, peliosis hepatis is characteristically hyperattenuating relative to surrounding liver parenchyma. On MR, the signal intensity of peliosis hepatis lesions depends on the age of the hemorrhagic component. On T2-weighted images, peliotic lesions are usually hyperintense, whereas on T1-weighted images the lesions are usually hypointense although isointense and hyperintense areas may also be present. Enhancement after contrast administration is similar to that described for CT. On direct angiography, lesions are seen as vascular nodules in the arterial phase.

PEARLS

- **Peliosis hepatis is a rare benign vascular lesion characterized by sinusoidal dilatation and blood-filled spaces.**

- **Although multiple causes of peliosis hepatis have been described, the condition is often caused by infection with *Bartonella* species in patients with AIDS ("bacillary angiomatosis").**

- **After administration of intravenous contrast, early globular enhancement is observed, with a centripetal progression in more delayed phase.**

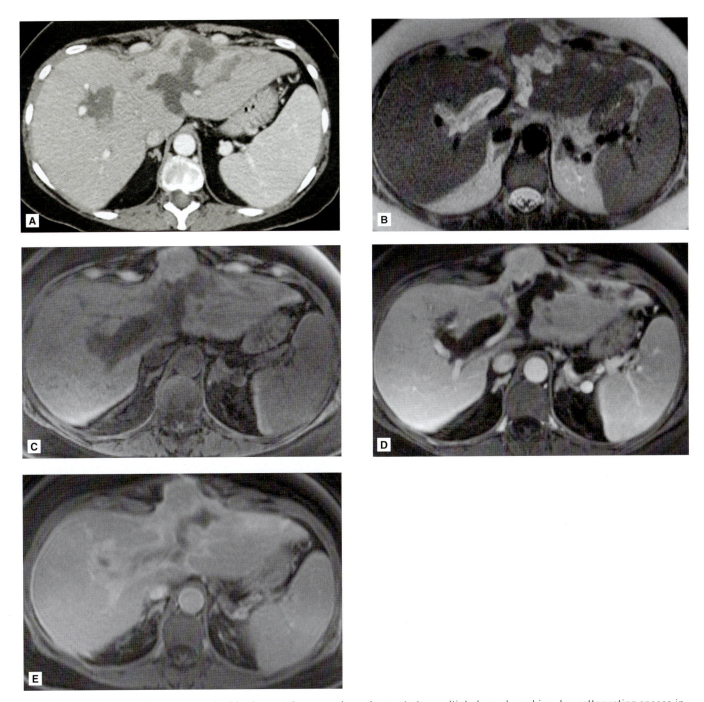

1. A. Contrast-enhanced CT image acquired in the portal venous phase demonstrates multiple large, branching, hypoattenuating spaces in the liver. The branching areas are markedly hyperintense on the axial T2-weighted image (**B**) and hypointense on the T1-weighted image (**C**). After intravenous contrast administration, the areas remain hypointense on the portal venous phase image (**D**) but demonstrate delayed enhancement on the equilibrium phase image (**E**).

PRESENTATION

- Asymptomatic liver enzyme elevation
- Jaundice
- Right upper quadrant discomfort
- Fatigue

FINDINGS

US, CT, and MR demonstrate ascites, hepatomegaly and enlarged inferior vena cava (IVC), hepatic veins, and coronary sinus. Intravenous contrast injected through an upper extremity vein may flow directly into the IVC and the hepatic veins. The enhanced liver commonly has a heterogeneous, mottled, reticulated appearance ("nutmeg" liver).

DIFFERENTIAL DIAGNOSIS

- Hemochromatosis
- Hepatic veno-occlusive disease
- Ischemic hepatitis

COMMENTS

Right-sided heart failure causes a variety of morphologic and functional abnormalities of the liver, broadly termed "congestive hepatopathy." The severity of liver involvement varies from hepatomegaly with congestive heart failure and passive congestion to liver fibrosis and cardiac cirrhosis. The most simple explanation of the cause is decompensated right ventricular (or biventricular) failure which allows direct transmission of elevated right atrial pressures to the hepatic parenchyma through the hepatic veins and IVC. At histologic examination, there is venous congestion with sinusoidal stasis and, ultimately, parenchymal necrosis, atrophy, collagen deposition, and fibrosis. Fortunately, the number of new cases with true cardiac cirrhosis has decreased considerably over the past several decades, as a result of lower rates of untreated rheumatic valvular disease and chronic constrictive pericarditis.

Clinically, the most common and important symptoms are those of right-sided congestive heart failure (pedal edema, weight gain, increased abdominal girth, right upper quadrant abdominal pain). The symptoms typically progress insidiously but may also appear suddenly, especially in cases of constrictive pericarditis or acute right ventricular decompensation. On physical examination, the liver is enlarged, firm, and pulsatile. The jugular venous pressure is elevated. Characteristically, the bilirubin levels are slightly elevated. Abdominal US usually demonstrates ascites, hepatomegaly, lack of normal respiratory variation in the caliber of the IVC and IVC diameter greater than or equal to 2.3 cm. Subcostal Doppler examination of the hepatic vein shows reversal of flow during systole, a finding that is highly specific for tricuspid regurgitation, a common finding in patients with passive congestion. CT and MR demonstrate hepatomegaly, hepatic congestion, enlargement of the IVC, hepatic veins and coronary sinus, and splenomegaly. The elevated central venous pressure in the right atrium may cause the intravenous contrast injected through an upper extremity vein to flow directly into the IVC and the hepatic veins. This finding is typically associated with tricuspid regurgitation. The enhanced liver also commonly has a heterogeneous, mottled, reticulated appearance ("nutmeg" liver).

PEARLS

- **The severity of liver involvement in right heart failure varies from hepatomegaly with congestive heart failure and passive congestion to liver fibrosis and cardiac cirrhosis.**

- **Abdominal US usually demonstrates ascites, hepatomegaly, lack of normal respiratory variation in the caliber of the IVC and IVC diameter greater than or equal to 2.3 cm.**

- **The enhanced liver on CT or MR commonly has a heterogeneous, mottled, reticulated appearance ("nutmeg" liver).**

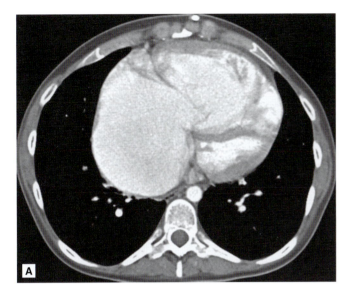
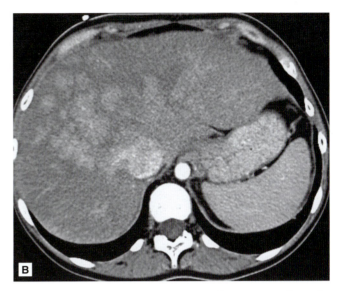

1. Contrast-enhanced CT images demonstrate a markedly enlarged right atrium (**A**) and a mottled, heterogeneous enhancement pattern of the hepatic parenchyma (**B**), characteristic of passive congestion.

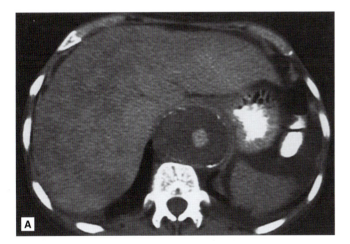
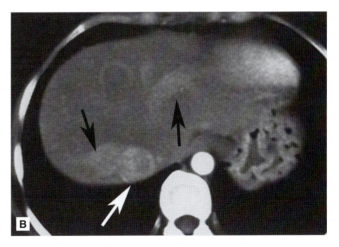

2. Contrast-enhanced CT images show the distended IVC (**B**, white arrow) and hepatic veins (**B**, black arrows); there is a reflux of contrast-enhanced blood from the right atrium into the IVC and hepatic veins. These are signs of increased right atrial pressures and tricuspid regurgitation. The liver has a mottled appearance (**A**). Note also large abdominal aortic aneurysm.

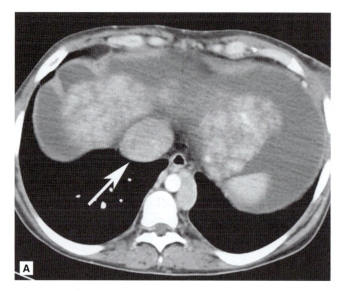
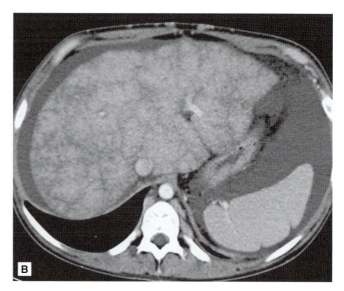

3. The contrast-enhanced CT images (**A**, **B**) demonstrate characteristic findings of chronic hepatic passive congestion. The IVC is distended (**A**, arrow), the hepatic parenchyma has a reticulated ("nutmeg") appearance (**B**), and there is massive ascites. The lobulated contours of the liver suggest development of cirrhosis as well.

PRESENTATION

- Abdominal pain

- Elevated liver enzymes, especially the low-dose heparin (LDH), in a patient at risk

- Abnormal liver function

FINDINGS

On CT, infarctions characteristically appear as sharply defined, wedge-shaped low-attenuation lesions without significant mass effect, extending to the liver surface. At MR imaging, lesions are typically hypointense on T1-weighted images and hyperintense on T2-weighted images. Gas may be seen in hepatic infarctions.

DIFFERENTIAL DIAGNOSIS

- Liver metastases

- Multiple abscesses

- Budd-Chiari syndrome

COMMENTS

Infarction of the hepatic parenchyma is rare, largely because of the dual blood supply provided by the hepatic arteries and the portal veins. The hepatic artery carries arterial blood, whereas the portal vein drains venous blood from the gastrointestinal tract and other parts of the splanchnic area, including the spleen and pancreas. Just over 70% of hepatic blood flow is supplied by the portal vein, but venous blood is only 80% saturated with oxygen. Thus, the portal venous blood supplies only 50% to 60% of the hepatic oxygen requirement. The remaining oxygen is supplied by hepatic arterial blood, which accounts for 25% of the flow. Therefore, clinically apparent infarcts require that both sources of hepatic blood supply are substantially compromised, as occurs in hypercoagulability disorders, acute shock, vascular complications following liver transplantation and pre-eclampsia or hemolytic anemia, elevated liver enzymes, low platelets (HELLP) syndrome. With the progressively increased use of liver transplantation for definitive therapy of end-stage liver disease there has been a noticeable increase in the incidence of liver infarctions that manifest clinically. In the setting of liver transplantation, the majority of hepatic infarctions occur secondary to arterial occlusion.

On US, hepatic infarctions are not easily detectable. Hepatomegaly and nonspecific changes in parenchymal echogenicity may be all that is present. However, evaluation with color or pulsed Doppler demonstrates absence of flow in the hepatic artery. The appearance of hepatic infarctions on CT is variable. The most characteristic presentation is as sharply defined, wedge-shaped low-attenuation lesions without significant mass effect, extending to the liver surface. However, they can also appear as rounded or oval in shape and centrally located. At MR imaging, lesions are typically hypointense on T1-weighted images but hyperintense on T2-weighted images. Although in the proper clinical setting the diagnosis of liver infarction is made easily in most cases, differential diagnosis should be made with focal fatty infiltration, abscess, or even a tumor. Gas may be seen in hepatic infarctions and, when present, differentiation from hepatic abscess is difficult. Aspiration may be necessary to confirm whether the area is sterile or infected. Segments IV and VIII are more commonly involved with hepatic abscess than other locations in the liver.

PEARLS

- **Infarction of the hepatic parenchyma is rare, largely because of the dual blood supply provided by the hepatic arteries and the portal veins.**

- **Causes of hepatic infarction include hypercoagulability disorders, acute shock, vascular complications following liver transplantation and pre-eclampsia or HELLP syndrome.**

- **The characteristic presentation at CT is as sharply defined, wedge-shaped low-attenuation lesions without significant mass effect, extending to the liver surface.**

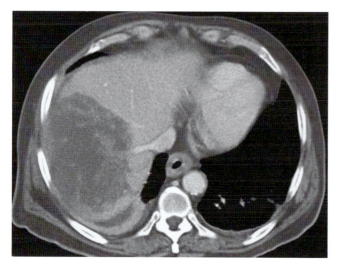

1. Hepatic infarction caused by iatrogenic ligation of the right hepatic artery during laparoscopic cholecystectomy. There is a large, peripheral, wedge-shaped area of low attenuation affecting most of the right hepatic lobe. Despite the large size of the lesion, there is no significant mass effect.

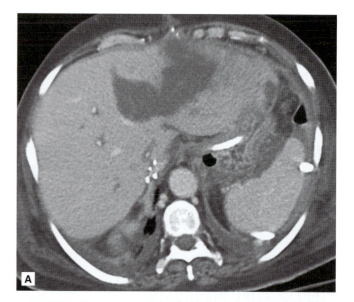

A

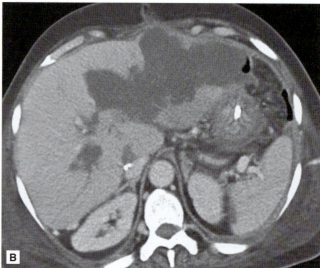

B

2. Contrast-enhanced CT images (**A**, **B**) of a patient with a large hepatic infarction that occurred as a complication of an orthotopic liver transplantation. There are large geographic areas of low attenuation extending to the surface of the left hepatic lobe, without significant mass effect, with a characteristic appearance of hepatic infarctions.

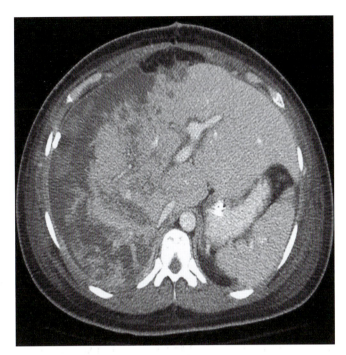

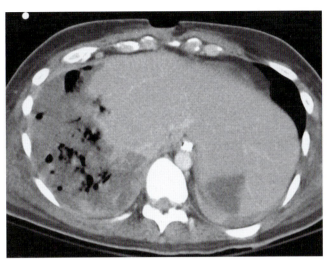

4. Hepatic infarction caused by a complication of blunt hepatic trauma. The patient underwent emergent laparotomy and ligation of the right hepatic artery. The entire right hepatic lobe is affected, with lack of enhancement and multiple intraparenchymal gas collections.

3. Contrast-enhanced CT image demonstrating infarctions of the periphery of the right hepatic lobe in a patient with HELLP syndrome. Note the characteristic subcapsular location and the lack of significant mass effect.

CHAPTER 2

GALLBLADDER AND BILIARY SYSTEM

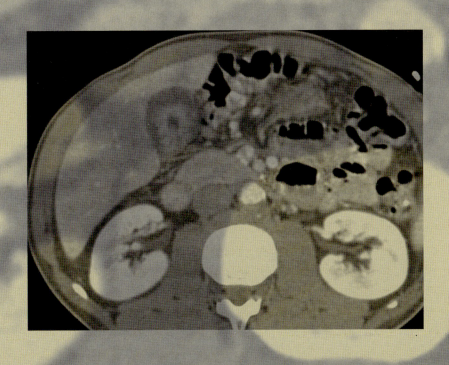

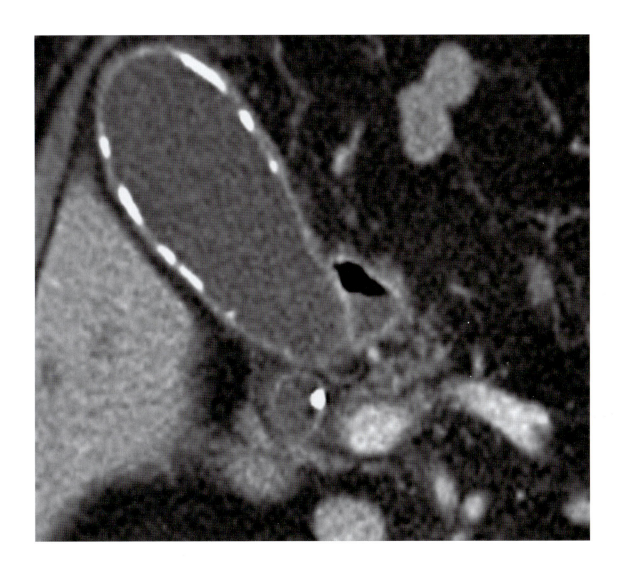

PRESENTATION

- Charcot triad with fever, jaundice, and right upper quadrant pain
- Elderly patients: atypical presentation with sepsis and mental status change

FINDINGS

Imaging tests demonstrate ductal dilatation, pneumobilia, and, possibly, stones in the common bile duct. Computed tomography (CT) and magnetic resonance (MR) show bile duct wall thickening and hyperenhancement, and periductal fat stranding. Contrast-enhanced CT and MR examinations may also demonstrate early, transient, hyperenhancement of the periductal hepatic parenchyma.

DIFFERENTIAL DIAGNOSIS

- Biliary colic and acute cholecystitis
- Acute pancreatitis
- Liver abscess
- Acute pyelonephritis
- Acute appendicitis
- Right-side diverticulitis

COMMENTS

Ascending cholangitis occurs when the obstructed and dilated biliary tree becomes secondarily infected with bacteria. The obstruction is most often caused by a stone, but it may also be associated with a neoplasm or benign stricture. Ascending cholangitis can occur as a complication of endoscopic retrograde cholangiopancreatography (ERCP), when contrast material is injected forcefully into the dilated proximal bile ducts of a patient with distal mechanical obstruction and poor drainage. Bacteria reach the biliary tree directly from the duodenum or from the portal venous system. An unobstructed biliary system that is colonized by bacteria typically does not result in acute cholangitis. However, with obstruction, progressively increasing intraductal biliary pressures push the infection proximally into the intra-hepatic ducts, hepatic veins, and perihepatic lymphatics, eventually leading to bacteremia and sepsis. Pyogenic liver

abscesses of various sizes, originating in the infected bile ducts, are commonly seen in ascending cholangitis.

The clinical presentation is variable, with the spectrum ranging from mild and nonspecific symptoms to rapidly progressive and otherwise unexplained sepsis. Charcot triad (right upper quadrant pain, fever, and jaundice) occurs in 20% to 25% of patients. The Reynolds pentad adds mental status changes and sepsis to the triad. In the past, mortality approached 100%, but increased awareness and timely interventions, such as therapeutic ERCP with sphincterotomy, stone extraction, and biliary stent or nasobiliary drain placement, have decreased this mortality rate from 5% to 10%.

On imaging studies, features of biliary obstruction and acute infection/inflammation are observed. Intraductal biliary gas (pneumobilia) is a common finding, since many of these patients have a history of recurrent biliary disease and prior retrograde interventions. Ultrasonography (US) examinations demonstrate ductal dilatation, pneumobilia, and, possibly, stones in the common bile duct. CT and MR show signs of bile duct inflammation, such as wall thickening and hyperenhancement, and periductal fat stranding. When a stone is suspected as the underlying etiology of acute obstruction, MR with magnetic resonance cholangiopancreatography (MRCP) has definite advantages in sensitivity over US and CT. Contrast-enhanced, multiphasic CT and MR examinations may also demonstrate a characteristic sign of ascending cholangitis: early, transient, hyperenhancement of the periductal hepatic parenchyma in the arterial phase. This sign is an indication of peribiliary hyperemia and rapidly disappears with appropriate therapy. ERCP, usually performed as an emergent therapeutic procedure, may show saccular abscesses and microabscesses communicating with the dilated intrahepatic ducts.

PEARLS

- **Most common underlying cause is an obstructive bile duct stone.**
- **Charcot triad (right upper quadrant pain, fever, and jaundice) is characteristic clinical presentation, but only present in 25% of patients.**
- **Emergent ERCP with stone extraction and biliary drainage are therapeutic interventions of choice.**

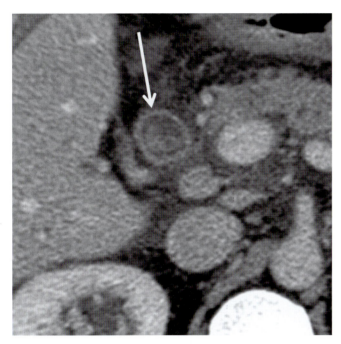

1. Contrast-enhanced CT image demonstrates a dilated common bile duct (arrow) with thickened and enhancing walls and multiple intraductal stones. There are inflammatory changes in the surrounding fat as well. These findings are characteristic of choledocholithiasis with complicating ascending cholangitis and pancreatitis.

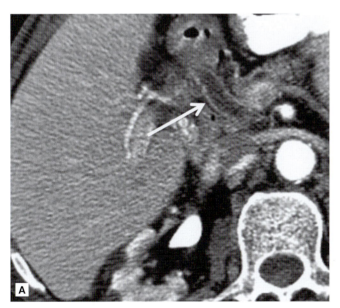

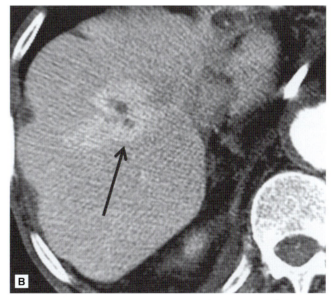

2. Two images of a contrast-enhanced CT examination demonstrate findings of ascending cholangitis. The common bile duct is slightly dilated, with thick and enhancing walls (**A**, arrow). There are small abscesses in the liver, with a hyperenhancing rim (**B**, arrow).

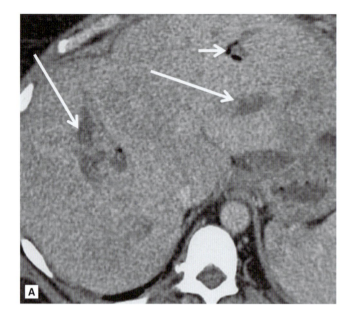

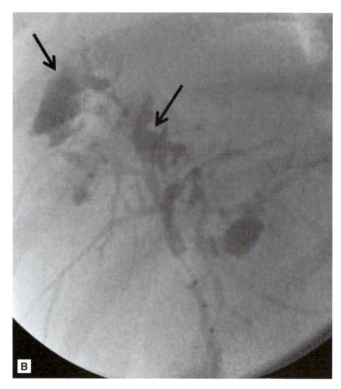

3. A. Contrast-enhanced CT image demonstrates dilated intrahepatic ducts and irregular low-attenuation lesions in the liver (long arrows). There is also pneumobilia in the left hepatic ducts (short arrow) from prior biliary instrumentations. **B.** ERCP image of the same patient shows the dilated, irregular, intrahepatic ducts, and filling of cavities (arrows) representing biliary necrosis and abscesses.

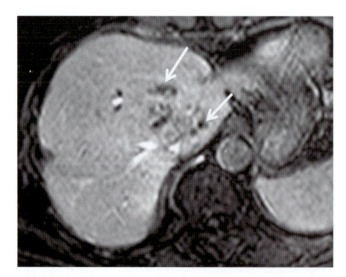

4. Contrast-enhanced MR image shows multiple small low–signal intensity lesions in the hepatic parenchyma, representing dilated bile ducts and microabscesses (arrows) from ascending cholangitis.

PRESENTATION

- Often asymptomatic

- Right upper quadrant and epigastric pain

- Diarrhea

- Fever and jaundice less common (10%-20% of patients)

FINDINGS

Imaging tests reveal dilated intrahepatic and extrahepatic bile ducts with associated bile duct wall thickening. The gallbladder demonstrates marked wall thickening and distention. Cholangiography (ERCP or MRCP) shows tapering of the distal common bile duct, extrahepatic bile duct dilation, and irregular focal beading of the intrahepatic ducts.

DIFFERENTIAL DIAGNOSIS

- Primary sclerosing cholangitis

- Papillary stenosis

COMMENTS

AIDS cholangiopathy is a syndrome of biliary obstruction resulting from infection-related strictures of the biliary. AIDS cholangiopathy occurred in as many as 26% of AIDS patients prior to the advent of highly active antiretroviral therapy; the current incidence of cholangiopathy is not well known, but has decreased in the era of potent antiretroviral therapy. It has been suggested that human immunodeficiency virus (HIV) cholangiopathy occurs more frequently in those patients with AIDS who are homosexual men. AIDS cholangiopathy is usually seen in patients with a cluster of differentiation 4 (CD4) count well below 100/mm^3 and may be their presenting manifestation. The organism most closely associated with AIDS cholangiopathy is *Cryptosporidium parvum*; other pathogens that have been identified include *Microsporidium*, cytomegalovirus (CMV), *Mycobacterium avium intracellulare*, *Candida albicans*, and *Cyclospora cayetanensis*. Involvement of the large intrahepatic ducts is usually associated with *C parvum* and CMV infection. In many cases, an organism cannot be recovered. The diagnostic yield is increased when bile is sampled in addition to obtaining biopsy specimens of the papilla and duodenum at endoscopy.

Many patients with HIV cholangiopathy are asymptomatic, presenting with only liver enzyme abnormalities. Symptomatic patients typically complain of right upper quadrant and

epigastric pain and diarrhea; pruritus, fever, and jaundice are less common. The severity of the abdominal pain varies with the biliary tract lesion. Severe abdominal pain is indicative of papillary stenosis, while milder abdominal pain is usually associated with intrahepatic and extrahepatic sclerosing cholangitis without papillary stenosis. The diarrhea in AIDS cholangiopathy is due to small bowel involvement with the infectious agent and may be the initial presenting feature. Approximately 20% of patients with symptomatic small bowel infection by *Cryptosporidium* subsequently developed biliary tract disease.

Abdominal US often reveals dilatation of the intrahepatic and extrahepatic bile ducts (70%-75% of cases) with associated bile duct wall thickening. The gallbladder demonstrates marked wall thickening and distention in approximately 50% of patients. Isolated involvement of the papilla may be seen as a hyperechoic "nodule" on US. Cholangiography (ERCP or MRCP) is the most important technique for the assessment of biliary ductal morphology and strictures. ERCP has the added value of allowing collection of specimens and performance of therapeutic sphincterotomy in selected patients. Findings at cholangiography may include tapering of the distal common bile duct, extrahepatic bile duct dilation, irregular focal beading of the intrahepatic ducts, and intraductal filling defects representing debris. The cholangiographic pattern differs from primary sclerosing cholangitis in that the intrahepatic bile ducts in HIV cholangiopathy are more often dilated and irregular as opposed to narrowed but there is considerable overlap. A cholangiographic pattern consistent with both papillary stenosis and sclerosing cholangitis is highly suggestive of HIV cholangiopathy.

Medical therapy for HIV cholangiopathy is usually not successful, and most patients require endoscopic interventions for relief of symptoms. HIV cholangiopathy is an infrequent cause of death, with most patients dying of other AIDS-related complications.

PEARLS

- **Cholangiographic pattern consistent with both papillary stenosis and sclerosing cholangitis is highly suggestive of HIV cholangiopathy.**

- **Symptoms, when present, include right upper quadrant and epigastric pain, diarrhea, pruritus, fever, and jaundice.**

- **Gallbladder usually involved.**

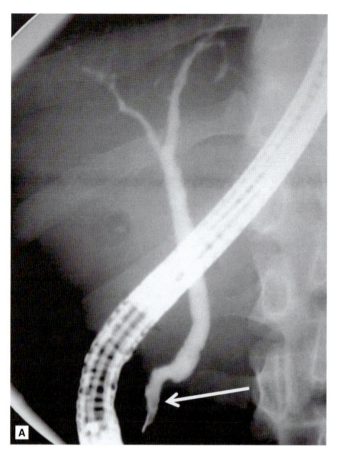
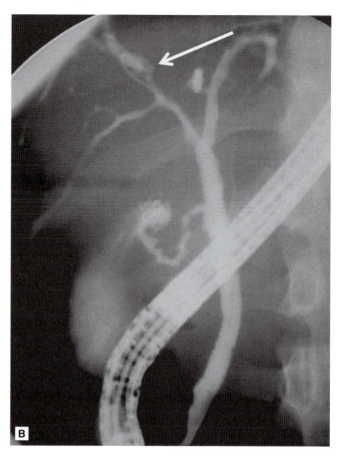

1. A and **B.** Two ERCP images demonstrate irregularity and a tapered stricture of the distal common bile duct (**A**, arrow) and stenotic segments with beading of the intrahepatic bile ducts (**A**, arrow).

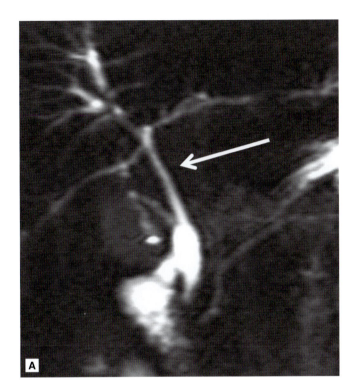

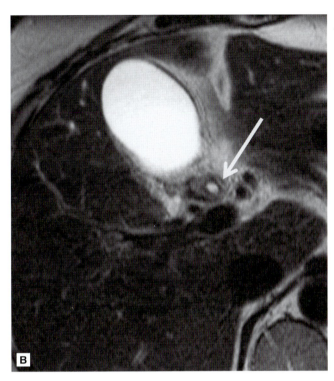

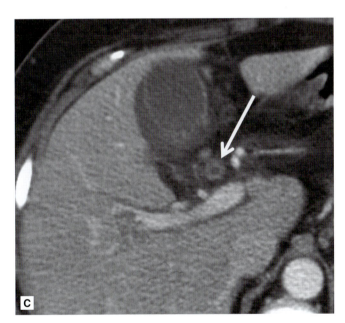

2. Thick-slab MRCP image (**A**), T2-weighted axial MR image (**B**) and contrast-enhanced CT image (**C**) demonstrate a long smooth stricture of the common bile duct (**A**, arrow), with wall thickening (**B** and **C**, arrows) and hyperenhancement (**C**) of the mid common bile duct.

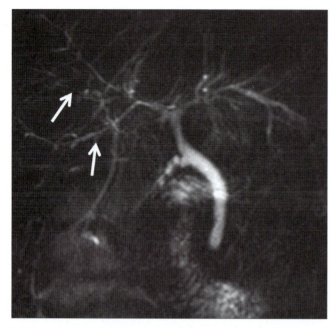

3. Thick-slab MRCP image show predominantly intrahepatic bile duct involvement, with multifocal strictures (arrows) in a patient with AIDS cholangiopathy.

PRESENTATION

- Pain and tenderness in the right upper abdomen or epigastrium
- Murphy sign: tenderness and inspiratory pause during palpation
- Signs of peritoneal irritation
- Nausea and vomiting
- Fever
- Jaundice (15% of cases)

FINDINGS

US demonstrates gallstones, distended gallbladder lumen, wall thickening, a positive ultrasonographic Murphy sign, pericholecystic fluid, and a hyperemic wall on evaluation with color Doppler. Additional findings on CT and MR include inflammation of the pericholecystic fat and hyper-enhancement in the gallbladder fossa.

DIFFERENTIAL DIAGNOSIS

- Acalculous cholecystitis
- Cholelithiasis
- Acute pancreatitis
- Ascending cholangitis
- Peptic ulcer perforation with perihepatitis

COMMENTS

Acute calculous cholecystitis occurs as a result of inflammation of the gallbladder wall, secondary to obstruction of the cystic duct by an impacted stone in the neck of the gallbladder or in the cystic duct. Acute cholecystitis occurs more commonly in women than men, reflecting the higher prevalence of gallstones in women as well. Acute acalculous cholecystitis represents inflammation of the gallbladder in the absence of calculi, and is discussed in a separate chapter of this book. If cystic duct patency is re-established, acute cholecystitis may resolve spontaneously within 5 to 7 days after onset of symptoms. However, this is not usually the case. Instead, if not treated in a timely fashion, inflammatory cell infiltration of the gallbladder wall in association with mural and mucosal hemorrhagic necrosis follows. Gangrenous cholecystitis occurs in as many as 20% of cases. Micro-organisms are identified in 80% of acute cholecystitis cases, although it is considered a secondary event and not an initiating one.

Most patients with acute cholecystitis describe a prior history of biliary pain. Frequently, the pain begins in the epigastric region and then localizes to the right upper quadrant. Although the pain may initially be described as colicky, it becomes constant in virtually all cases. In elderly and diabetic patients, the clinical presentation can be atypical or vague. Pain and fever may be absent, and localized tenderness may be the only presenting sign. Acute cholecystitis is differentiated from biliary colic by the persistence of constant severe pain for more than 6 hours. Palpation of the right subcostal area reveals tenderness which becomes worse with deep inspiration, leading to a sudden inspiratory arrest called the Murphy sign. The Murphy sign may be elicited with an ultrasound probe as well. In approximately 35% of patients, a distended, tender gallbladder may be palpable. Approximately 20% patients with acute cholecystitis have mild jaundice.

Ultrasonography is the preferred initial imaging examination for diagnosis of acute cholecystitis. The main features of acute calculous cholecystitis on US include, in addition to the presence of stones, distention of the gallbladder lumen, gallbladder wall thickening, a positive ultrasonographic Murphy sign, pericholecystic fluid, and a hyperemic wall on evaluation with color Doppler. All of these findings are suggestive but not diagnostic of acute cholecystitis. The sonographic Murphy sign is absent in as many as 70% of patients with acute cholecystitis. Inflammatory pericholecystic reaction in the gallbladder fossa is better depicted with CT than with US. CT is also useful in making the differential diagnosis when obesity or gaseous distention limits the use of ultrasonography. MR may demonstrate the same morphologic changes as CT, displaying inflammatory changes in the gallbladder wall and pericholecystic fat. Cholescintigraphy is a highly sensitive diagnostic modality for diagnosing acute cholecystitis, although the findings are nonspecific.

PEARLS

- **Right upper quadrant pain evolves from colicky to constant, usually lasting for more than 6 hours.**

- **US is test of choice and findings include stones, distention of the gallbladder lumen, wall thickening, a positive sonographic Murphy sign, pericholecystic fluid, and hyperemic wall.**

- **CT, MR, or nuclear medicine (hydroxy iminodiacetic acid [HIDA] scan) are useful in difficult or inconclusive US examinations.**

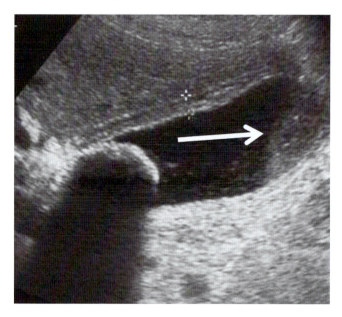

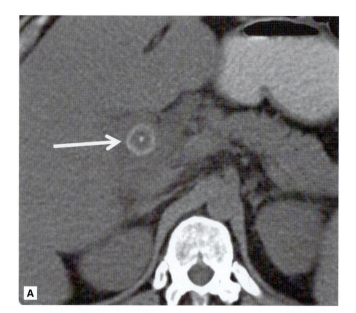

A

1. Longitudinal image of an ultrasonographic examination of the gallbladder demonstrates characteristic findings of acute cholecystitis. There is a large stone impacted in the gallbladder neck, with associated diffuse wall thickening (calipers) and sludge in the gallbladder (arrow). The patient also complained of exquisite pain in the region of the gallbladder (positive US Murphy sign).

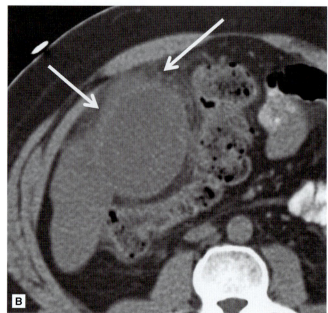

B

2. Two axial noncontrast CT images show a distended gallbladder with wall thickening and inflammatory changes in the pericholecystic fat (**B**, arrows). There is also a peripherally calcified stone impacted in the gallbladder neck (**A**, arrow).

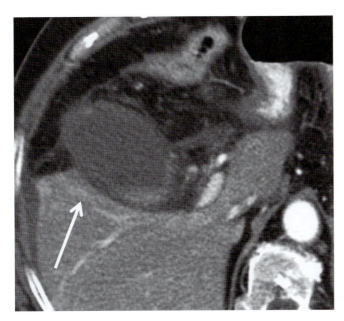

3. Hepatic arterial phase of a contrast-enhanced CT images demonstrate inflammatory changes in the gallbladder wall and pericholecystic fat. Note also a focal area of hyperenhancement in the liver parenchyma adjacent to the gallbladder (arrow). This transient hyperemia occurs secondary to the acute gallbladder inflammation.

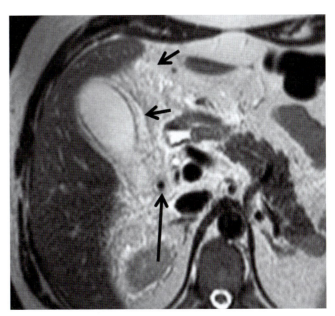

4. Axial T2-weighted image without fat suppression demonstrates findings of acute cholecystitis. The gallbladder is distended with wall thickening. There is also intramural and pericholecystic high signal (short arrows). Note also the hypointense stone impacted in the gallbladder neck (long arrow).

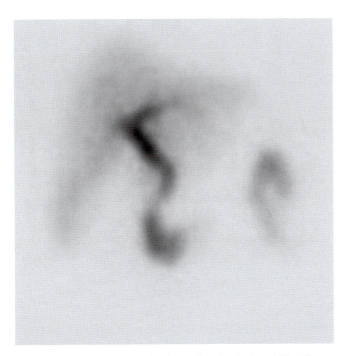

5. HIDA scan demonstrates findings of acute cholecystitis. The image was acquired 60 minutes after injection of the radiotracer. There is adequate filling of the bile ducts and passage of the tracer to the duodenum, but no filling of the gallbladder. In the proper clinical setting, these findings are highly consistent with acute cholecystitis.

PRESENTATION

- Abdominal or right upper quadrant pain
- Fever
- Elevated white blood cell count or sedimentation rate
- Unexplained sepsis

FINDINGS

US and CT demonstrate a distended gallbladder with thickened walls (> 3-4 mm), with or without pericholecystic fluid, often with intraluminal sludge but without stones.

DIFFERENTIAL DIAGNOSIS

- Ascending cholangitis
- Intra-abdominal abscess
- Sepsis
- Liver abscess

COMMENTS

Acalculous cholecystitis is a severe condition that most commonly occurs in hospitalized, debilitated patients with various types of underlying medical or surgical conditions. Acalculous cholecystitis causes approximately 5% to 10% of all cases of acute cholecystitis and the mortality rate (10%-50%) is considerably higher than that of calculous cholecystitis (1%-2%). It is most commonly observed in the setting of very ill patients (eg, patients in intensive care units on mechanical ventilation, uncontrolled diabetes, patients with sepsis or severe burn injuries and after severe trauma). In addition, compared to cholecystitis caused by stone disease, acalculous cholecystitis is associated with a higher incidence of complications such as gangrene, emphysema, and perforation.

The main cause of acalculous cholecystitis is thought to be long-standing bile stasis that leads to overdistention of the gallbladder. Critically ill patients are more prone because of prolonged fasting resulting in a decrease or absence of cholecystokinin-induced gallbladder contraction. In fact, acalculous cholecystitis is particularly common in patients on prolonged total parenteral nutrition. Over time, multiple factors lead to development of gallbladder wall ischemia and secondary infection. Dehydration and a slow flow state (such as heart failure) also play a role.

Routine laboratory tests usually demonstrate an elevated white blood cell count and altered liver function tests. However, these results are not specific in these very sick patients. Blood cultures may be positive but do not localize the focus of the infection either. US and CT are the imaging tests usually performed in these hospitalized patients with unexplained sepsis or elevated leucocytes. The usual finding is a distended gallbladder with thickened walls (> 3-4 mm), with or without pericholecystic fluid, often with intraluminal sludge but without stones. Unfortunately, these findings are not specific and can be mimicked by hepatitis, cirrhosis, and hypoalbuminemia. Nuclear medicine scans after injection of hydroxy iminodiacetic acid (HIDA) can be used to assess the patency of the cystic duct, but this test also has numerous potential pitfalls. Definitive therapy is achieved with cholecystectomy (open or laparoscopic). Nonsurgical candidates undergo percutaneous cholecystostomy under US guidance. This procedure also serves to confirm the diagnosis in complex or questionable cases. Because of concurrent antibiotic therapy, bile culture results are positive in only approximately 50% of patients with acalculous cholecystitis.

PEARLS

- Occurs most commonly in debilitated or hospitalized patients.
- Morbidity and mortality are higher than calculous cholecystitis.
- Difficult diagnosis, imaging findings often not specific.

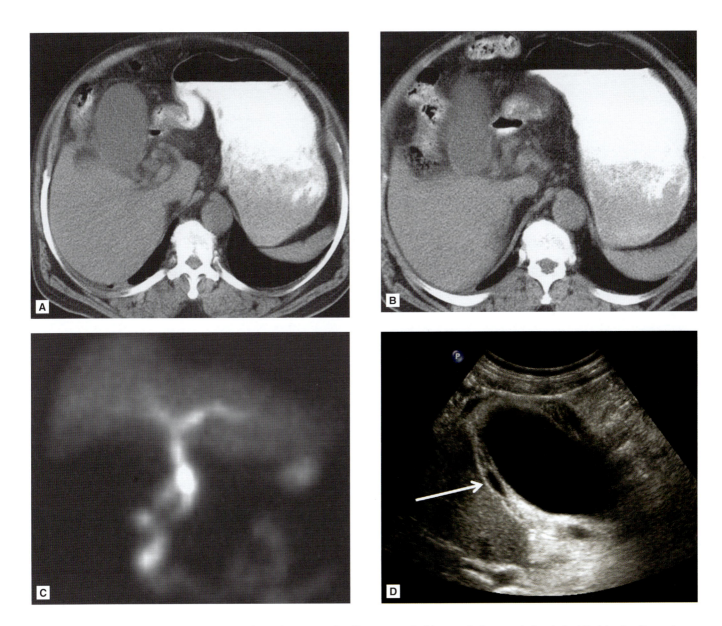

1. A 65-year-old male patient in the coronary intensive care unit with new onset of low-grade fever and elevated white blood cell count, 1 week after suffering a myocardial infarction. Nonintravenous contrast-enhanced CT images (**A** and **B**) demonstrate a markedly distended gallbladder with thickened wall and inflammatory changes in the pericholecystic fat. The HIDA scan static image obtained 60 minutes after injection of the radiotracer (**C**) shows patent bile ducts, but no filling of the gallbladder, confirming the clinical diagnosis of acute cholecystitis. The patient was not considered a good candidate for cholecystectomy and was treated with emergent percutaneous cholecystostomy tube placement under US guidance. Ultrasonography (**D**, **E**, and **F**) confirmed findings of acute cholecystitis (**D**), with thick wall and pericholecystic fluid (arrow), but no stone found. Figures **E** and **F** show the cholecystostomy tube in place (long white arrows). Figure **F**, obtained with color Doppler, also shows gallbladder wall hypervascularity (short white arrow).

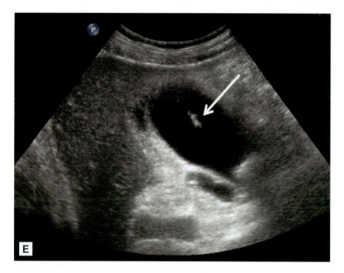

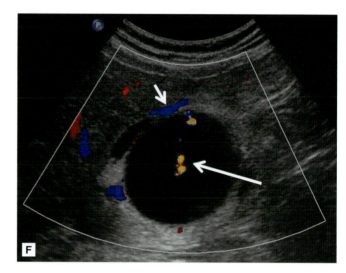

1. (*continued*)

PRESENTATION

- Persistent pain
- Worsening fever and leukocytosis
- More severe localized or generalized tenderness
- Systemic toxicity

FINDINGS

Complications include gallbladder empyema, mural hemorrhage, gangrenous cholecystitis, emphysematous cholecystitis, gallbladder perforation, and pericholecystic abscess. Imaging findings depend on the specific complication, and are present in the wall and the lumen of the gallbladder.

DIFFERENTIAL DIAGNOSIS

- Acute pancreatitis
- Perforated peptic ulcer
- Gonococcal perihepatitis (Fitz-Hugh-Curtis syndrome)
- Acute hepatitis
- Acute pyelonephritis

COMMENTS

Acute cholecystitis may be complicated by empyema, mural hemorrhage, gangrenous cholecystitis, emphysematous cholecystitis, gallbladder perforation, pericholecystic abscess, and bilioenteric fistula. All of these complications are more common in the elderly and in patients with significant comorbidities.

As the gallbladder wall inflammation progresses, bile becomes infected. In 85% of patients, disimpaction of the cystic duct occurs, and inflammation in the gallbladder settles. However, if the cystic duct remains obstructed, the process may progress to gallbladder empyema and eventually result wall gangrene or perforation.

Gangrenous cholecystitis is a surgical emergency. Patients are progressively toxic and may subsequently develop septicemia and shock. On US, gallbladder gangrene is typically seen as a thickened wall with a multilayered, striated appearance. Doppler US may demonstrate absent perfusion focally or diffusely. On contrast-enhanced CT or MR, the wall is indistinct, with absence of enhancement in the gangrenous areas.

In gallbladder perforation, the wall of the gallbladder is not well delineated on imaging tests and a localized defect in the wall may be noted at the site of perforation. Perforation may be localized and produce a pericholecystic abscess or free, resulting in peritonitis. An inflamed gallbladder may perforate into colon or duodenum because of the close proximity of the gallbladder to these structures. This may lead to gallstone ileus (impaction of a gallstone in the ileocecal valve with bowel obstruction) or, rarely, to Bouveret syndrome (impaction of a stone in the duodenum).

Emphysematous cholecystitis can complicate acute calculous or acalculous cholecystitis. In emphysematous cholecystitis, ischemia of the gallbladder wall is followed by infection with gas-forming organisms that produce gas in the gallbladder lumen, in the gallbladder wall, or both. In 30% to 50% of patients, diabetes mellitus is a predisposing condition. The mortality rate is 15%. Clinical symptoms can be deceptively mild.

PEARLS

- Complications of untreated acute cholecystitis include empyema, mural hemorrhage, gangrene, emphysematous cholecystitis, gallbladder perforation, and pericholecystic abscess.

- Complicated acute cholecystitis occurs primarily in elderly, diabetic and debilitated patients.

- Gangrenous and emphysematous cholecystitis are surgical emergencies. Preferred methods for diagnosis of these conditions are US and CT, respectively.

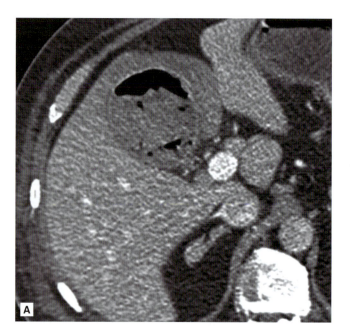

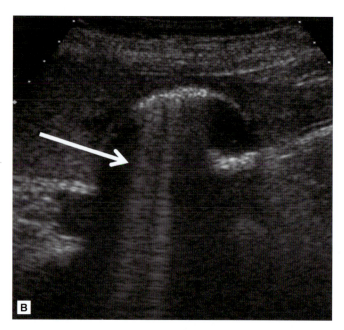

1. A. Contrast-enhanced CT image shows gas and debris in the lumen of the gallbladder. **B.** Transverse US image demonstrates a highly echogenic crescentic focus in the nondependent aspect of the gallbladder, casting a broad "dirty" shadow (arrow). These findings are characteristic of emphysematous cholecystitis.

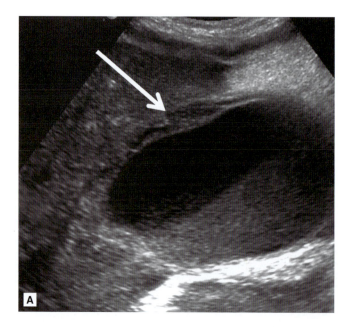

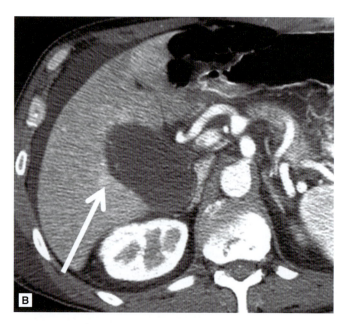

2. A. On this longitudinal US image the wall of the gallbladder has a multilayered, striated appearance (arrow), with mucosal sloughing. **B.** The CT image obtained with intravenous contrast shows no enhancement of the gallbladder wall, with hyperemia of the adjacent liver parenchyma (arrow). These findings are typical of gangrenous cholecystitis.

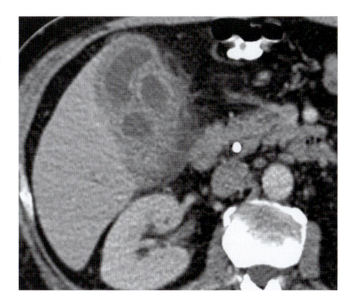

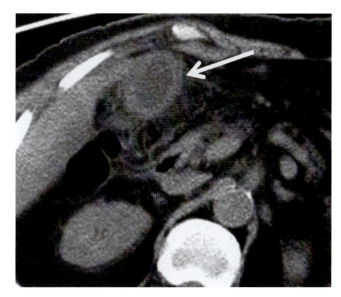

3. The contrast-enhanced CT image demonstrates multiple intramural and pericholecystic fluid collections, consistent with abscesses. The gallbladder itself is poorly defined. Advanced cholecystitis with perforation and walled-off abscesses were found at laparotomy.

4. Noncontrast CT image shows diffuse thickening and hyperdensity (arrow) within the gallbladder wall. This finding is indicative of intramural hemorrhage, associated with advanced acute cholecystitis.

PRESENTATION

- Acute: fever and right upper quadrant abdominal pain (cholangitis)
- Chronic: constitutional symptoms, weight loss, fatigue, jaundice

FINDINGS

US, CT, and MR show biliary ductal dilatation with intrahepatic calculi and pneumobilia. Other findings include lobar or segmental atrophy (most commonly the lateral segments of the left lobe), patchy or segmental fatty infiltration, and enhancement of bile duct wall.

DIFFERENTIAL DIAGNOSIS

- Ascending cholangitis
- Acute cholecystitis
- Choledocholithiasis
- Pyogenic liver abscess
- Biliary ascariasis and other parasitic infections

COMMENTS

Recurrent pyogenic cholangitis or cholangiohepatitis (RPC) occurs most commonly in inhabitants of or immigrants from Southeast Asia, where predisposing helminthic infections and malnutrition are endemic. Malnutrition leads to a deficiency of enzymes in bile that favors the accumulation of unconjugated bile and the formation of calcium bilirubinate complexes. These concretions of bilirubinate and/or biliary parasites, such as *Ascaris lumbricoides* or *Clonorchis sinensis* act as the nidus for formation of pigmented stones. The disease affects men and women equally and is characterized by recurrent episodes of ascending cholangitis secondary to intrahepatic biliary obstruction caused by these intrahepatic pigment stones. Over time, recurrent bile duct inflammation leads to fibrotic changes, stricture formation, multiple hepatic abscesses, progressive hepatic parenchymal destruction, cirrhosis, and portal hypertension. Cholangiocarcinoma is another potential long-term complication of RPC.

US, CT, and MR provide accurate noninvasive anatomic evaluation of the location, stage, and severity of the biliary ductal findings associated with RPC. Appropriate medical and/or surgical treatment can also be planned. All modalities typically show biliary ductal dilatation, often with disproportionate dilatation of the extrahepatic and central intrahepatic ducts relative to the more peripheral biliary ducts. On US, periportal hyperechogenicity is a frequent finding. Intrahepatic calculi and pneumobilia are both frequent findings as well, but may be difficult to differentiate from each other as both are associated with acoustic shadowing. On CT, intrahepatic bile duct stones are more easily identified on noncontrast CT because 90% of the stones are hyperattenuating relative to the normal unenhanced liver parenchyma. Pneumobilia is a frequent finding and is usually secondary to prior history of endoscopic intervention or surgery. If there is no such history, passage of calculi through the ampulla with reflux of enteric gas or cholangitis caused by gas-forming organisms are other possibilities. Other CT findings include lobar or segmental atrophy (most commonly the lateral segments of the left lobe) and patchy or segmental fatty infiltration. Enhancement of bile duct walls may also be identified on contrast-enhanced CT and is generally indicative of acute cholangitis.

MR and magnetic resonance cholangiopancreatography (MRCP) provide excellent quality images that display the characteristic findings of RPC. Rapid sequences and technical developments such as parallel imaging allow image acquisition in short breath-hold periods. The main advantage over endoscopic retrograde cholangiopancreatography (ERCP) is the ability to depict ducts proximal to stenotic segments without the risk of causing or aggravating biliary sepsis. MRCP has been reported to show 100% of confirmed dilated duct segments, 96% of focal strictures, and 98% of calculi. Duct strictures in RPC are usually short and usually less than 1 cm in length. Noncalcified calculi are more clearly visualized with MR than CT, but differentiating between biliary stones and gas may be difficult. Although gas is usually nondependent, there are multiple exceptions to this "rule." The current role of ERCP is all but limited to providing a means for therapeutic interventions, dictated by findings on other imaging tests (especially MRCP).

Noninvasive tests are also used to monitor the progression of the disease and to detect developing complications, such as abscess formation, intrahepatic bilomas, portal vein thrombosis, and cholangiocarcinoma. Cholangiocarcinoma occurs in approximately 5% of patients with the disease and occurs more commonly in atrophied segments or segments with a heavy stone burden. The typical appearance of hilar or extrahepatic cholangiocarcinoma is a focal area of wall thickening and enhancement with narrowing of the affected duct. RPC also increases the risk of hepatocellular carcinoma, likely related to the development of cirrhosis in severe cases.

REFERENCES

1. Park MS, Yu JS, Kim KW, et al. Recurrent pyogenic cholangitis: comparison between MR cholangiography and direct cholangiography. *Radiology.* 2001;220:677-682.
2. Heffernan EJ, Geoghegan T, Munk PL, Ho SG, Harris AC. *AJR.* 2009;192:W28-W35.

PEARLS

- Occurs most commonly in inhabitants of or immigrants from Southeast Asia, where predisposing helminthic infections and malnutrition are endemic.

- Characterized by recurrent episodes of ascending cholangitis secondary to intrahepatic biliary obstruction caused by these intrahepatic pigment stones.

- US, CT, and MR typically show biliary ductal dilatation, often with disproportionate dilatation of the extrahepatic and central intrahepatic ducts relative to the more peripheral biliary ducts, intrahepatic calculi, and pneumobilia.

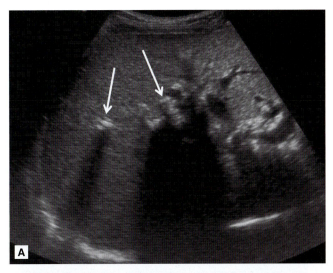

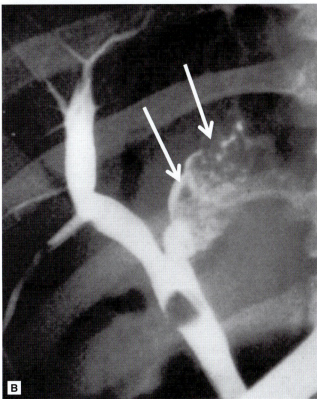

1. A. Transverse US image demonstrates multiple echogenic stones (arrows) with acoustic shadowing in the left hepatic lobe. **B.** ERCP image of the same patient shows the dilated left intrahepatic ducts with multiple intraluminal filling defects (arrows), representing stones and sludge.

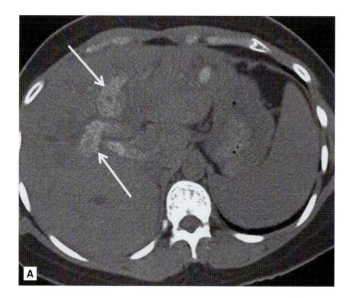

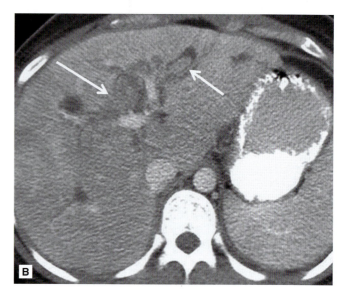

2. Unenhanced (**A**) and contrast-enhanced (**B**) CT images show multiple, large, partially calcified casts of stones and sludge (**A** and **B**, arrows) filling multiple intrahepatic bile ducts. The stones are more easily appreciated on the noncontrast-enhanced image (**A**).

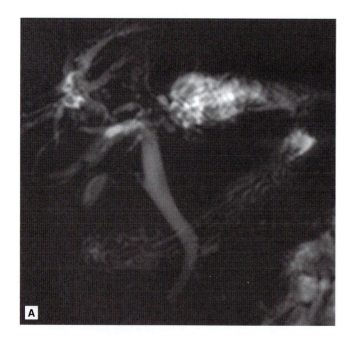

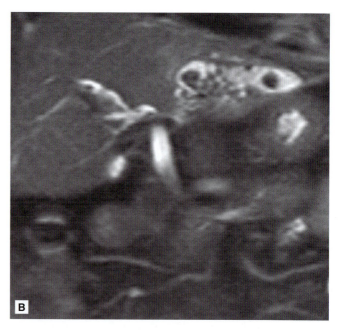

3. Oblique coronal MRCP (**A**, thick slab and **B**, thin section) images show characteristic findings of RPC. The intrahepatic ducts are massively dilated and contain multiple large hypointense filling defects.

PRESENTATION

- Usually asymptomatic, incidental imaging finding
- Occasionally: palpable mass in right upper quadrant

FINDINGS

The hallmark of porcelain gallbladder is multifocal or diffuse calcification of the gallbladder wall. On US, differentiation from large gallstones can be difficult. On MR, the calcified wall is seen as a diffusely hypointense gallbladder wall, especially on T2-weighted images.

DIFFERENTIAL DIAGNOSIS

CALCIFICATIONS IN RIGHT UPPER QUADRANT

- Cholelithiasis
- Right kidney stone
- Calcified renal cyst
- Calcified right adrenal gland
- Hepatic calcification: echinococcal cyst, schistosomiasis, old infarct
- Emphysematous cholecystitis (ultrasonography)
- Gallbladder carcinoma

COMMENTS

The term *porcelain gallbladder* is most often used to describe nonspecific calcifications of the gallbladder wall, which can occur as single or multiple deposits of calcium, or can be diffuse and concentric. Other names given to a calcified gallbladder include calcifying cholecystitis and cholecystopathia chronica calcarea. Over 90% of porcelain gallbladders are associated with gallstones. Most pathologists consider the gallbladder wall calcifications to occur as a response to a low-grade chronic inflammation. On histology, the chronically inflamed muscular layer of the gallbladder wall undergoes fibrosis and subsequently develops deposits of dystrophic calcification. There is a known and well-documented association between porcelain gallbladder and gallbladder carcinoma, cited at approximately 20%.

Some studies suggest that the pattern of calcification determines the risk of associated carcinoma: Selective (focal) calcification is more likely to harbor cancerous cells than diffuse intramural calcifications. Most carcinomas associated with porcelain gallbladder are diffusely infiltrating adenocarcinomas, although squamous cell carcinoma has been described as well.

Patients with porcelain gallbladder are usually asymptomatic, and the finding is often incidental on an imaging study: CT, abdominal radiograph, or ultrasonography. Although the vast majority of patients are asymptomatic, it is usually agreed upon that carcinoma occurs in association with porcelain gallbladder with sufficient frequency to warrant prophylactic cholecystectomy. Therefore, cholecystectomy is usually recommended for individuals with a porcelain gallbladder, even if completely asymptomatic.

The diagnosis of a porcelain gallbladder on CT is usually straightforward. However, on US, a porcelain gallbladder must be distinguished from large solitary gallstones. Gallstones are mobile, but this determination can be difficult in patients with contracted gallbladders filled with stones. Although from the therapeutic point of view this differentiation may not be important, since symptomatic patients with gallstones and patients with porcelain gallbladders usually require cholecystectomy, CT may help in the differential diagnosis in specific cases. On MR, the calcified wall is seen as a diffusely hypointense gallbladder wall, especially on T2-weighted images.

PEARLS

- The term *porcelain gallbladder* describes nonspecific calcifications of the gallbladder wall, which can occur as single or multiple deposits of calcium, or can be diffuse and concentric.

- Porcelain gallbladder is associated with cholelithiasis and gallbladder carcinoma.

- On US, porcelain gallbladder should be distinguished from a single large gallstone and emphysematous cholecystitis. CT is the best modality to detect gallbladder wall calcifications.

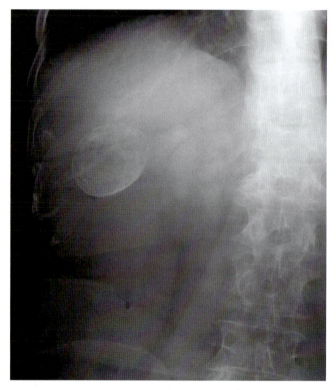

1. Abdominal radiograph demonstrates a peripherally calcified, oval shape, structure in the right upper quadrant. Appearance and location are characteristic of a porcelain gallbladder.

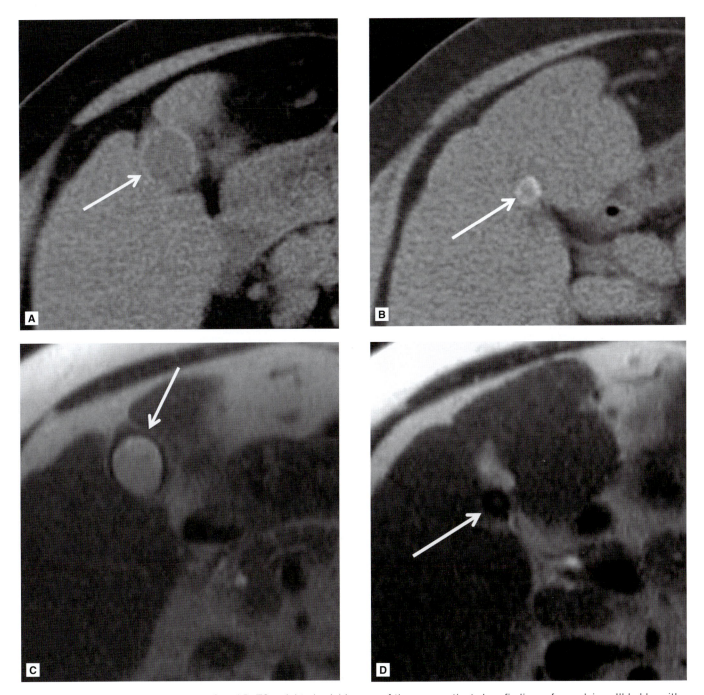

2. A and **B**. Noncontrast CT images and **C** and **D**. T2-weighted axial images of the same patient show findings of porcelain gallbladder with associated cholelithiasis. The gallbladder wall contains a thin rim of calcification (**A**, arrow), seen as homogeneously hypointense on **2D** (arrow). The partially calcified gallstone (**B**, arrow) is also hypointense on MR (**C**, arrow).

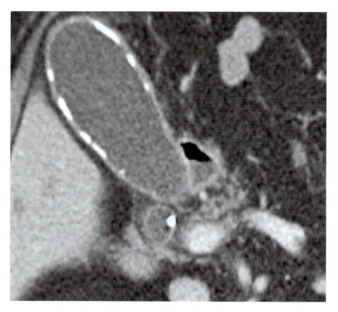

3. Dense, but discontinuous, calcifications in the wall of the gallbladder seen on a contrast-enhanced CT image. This finding is typical of porcelain gallbladder.

PRESENTATION

- Fatigue, fevers, weight loss

- Intermittent jaundice, hepatomegaly, abnormal liver function test results

- Cholestasis with pruritus and fat malabsorption

- Cirrhosis and complications of portal hypertension

FINDINGS

US may show intra- and extrahepatic ductal dilatation, increased bile duct wall echogenicity and heterogeneous liver parenchyma. On cholangiography (MRCP or ERCP), generalized beading and multifocal stenoses of the intrahepatic and extrahepatic are characteristic findings. CT and MR demonstrate abnormal wall thickening and enhancement of the biliary ductal wall.

DIFFERENTIAL DIAGNOSIS

- Chronic viral or autoimmune hepatitis

- Choledocholithiasis

- Cholangiocarcinoma

- Traumatic or iatrogenic biliary tract strictures

- Congenital anomalies of the biliary tract

COMMENTS

Primary sclerosing cholangitis (PSC) is a chronic cholestatic liver disease that affects primarily individuals in their third and fourth decade of life, with a slight male predominance. However, the disease is being increasingly recognized in children. It is frequently seen in association with inflammatory bowel disease (IBD), especially ulcerative colitis (UC), which is present in 70% to 80% of patients who have PSC. Conversely, 2.5% to 7.5% of patients with IBD eventually develop PSC. It may precede the onset of UC or may develop following proctocolectomy.

The mechanisms responsible for the development of PSC are unknown, but bacterial and viral infections, toxins, and immunologic and genetic factors have been suggested as etiologic agents. The relationship of PSC with IBD helps understand the potential etiology of the disease. It is believed that a transient bacterial or viral infection, or the absorption of bacterial byproducts in patients with colonic disease who are genetically predisposed may elicit an immune-mediated destruction of the hepatobiliary tract.

Other autoimmune disorders occur in approximately 25% of patients with PSC. Also, there is an increased expression of the HLA-B8, a gene that has been linked to other autoimmune disorders, in patients with PSC. This supports the theory of an immune-mediated pathogenesis.

The diagnosis of PSC is made on the basis of a combination of clinical features, characteristic biochemical profile abnormalities indicative of cholestasis and typical findings on cholangiography, but always requires confirmation with liver biopsy and histology. US may show intra- and extrahepatic ductal dilatation, increased bile duct wall echogenicity and heterogeneous liver parenchyma. On cholangiography (MRCP or ERCP), a generalized beading and multifocal stenoses of the intrahepatic and extrahepatic biliary is the characteristic finding of PSC. CT and MR may demonstrate abnormal wall thickening and enhancement of the biliary ductal wall. T2-weighted MR images can also show peripheral wedge-shaped areas of high–signal intensity which may be related to underlying perfusion changes caused by the bile duct inflammation. The diagnostic accuracy of magnetic resonance cholangiography (MRC) in patients with PSC is 90%, compared to 97% for ERCP. ERCP is potentially risky in patients with multifocal intrahepatic strictures, as adequate depiction of the abnormalities often requires overfilling and forceful injection of contrast material with the potential for development of bacterial cholangitis and sepsis. MRC is particularly advantageous in this circumstance.

PSC is usually progressive, leading to cirrhosis, portal hypertension, and liver failure. Effective medical treatment modalities for childhood PSC are undetermined. Liver transplantation remains the only effective therapeutic option for patients with end-stage liver disease from PSC.

PEARLS

- Approximately 70% of patients with PSC have ulcerative colitis and 10% of patients with ulcerative colitis have PSC.

- Usually progressive, leading to cirrhosis, portal hypertension, and liver failure. Cholangiocarcinoma complicates long-standing PSC.

- The diagnosis is made on the basis of clinical features, characteristic biochemical profile abnormalities indicative of cholestasis and typical findings on cholangiography, but liver biopsy is required for confirmation.

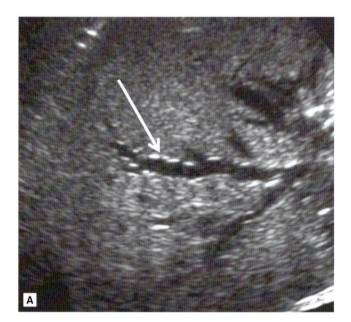

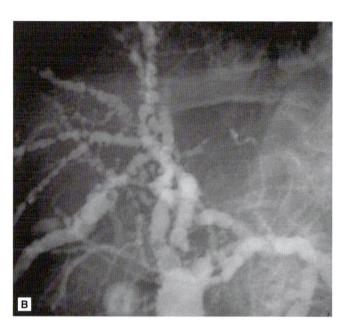

1. A. Transverse US image demonstrates beading and wall thickening of intrahepatic bile ducts in the right hepatic lobe (arrow). **B.** ERCP image confirms beading of multiple intrahepatic ducts. These findings are characteristic of PSC.

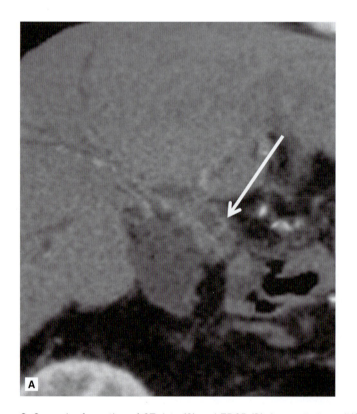

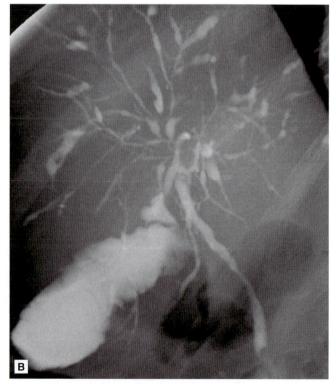

2. Coronal reformation of CT data (**A**) and ERCP (**B**) demonstrate multifocal strictures in the intrahepatic ducts, typical of PSC. Note also bile duct wall thickening and enhancement in **A** (arrow).

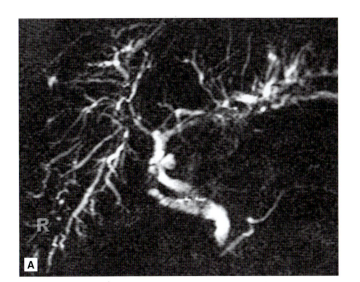

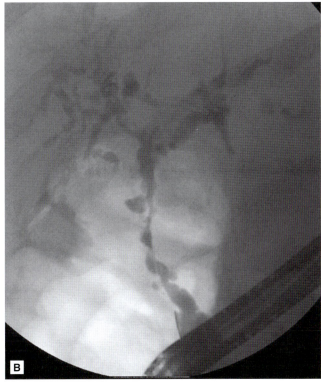

3. A. MRCP image (thick-slab sequence), and **B.** ERCP show wall irregularity with beading and multifocal strictures of the intrahepatic and extrahepatic bile ducts. These findings are typical of PSC.

PRESENTATION

- Usually asymptomatic
- Incidental finding on imaging studies
- Often coexists with cholelithiasis
- Occasionally, nonspecific abdominal pain

FINDINGS

The main finding is cyst-like spaces (diverticula) in a thickened gallbladder wall. US shows echogenic intramural foci located within these diverticula (Rokitansky-Aschoff sinuses), from which V-shaped "comet tail" reverberation artifacts emanate.

DIFFERENTIAL DIAGNOSIS

- Gallbladder cancer
- Metastatic melanoma
- Acalculous cholecystitis
- Polyposis, papillomatosis, adenoma, and cystadenoma

COMMENTS

Adenomyomatosis is a common benign condition characterized by hyperplastic changes of unknown etiology involving the gallbladder wall and causing overgrowth of the mucosa, thickening of the muscular wall, and formation of intramural diverticula or sinus tracts termed Rokitansky-Aschoff sinuses. Morphologically, adenomyomatosis is tumor-like, but has no malignant potential and may involve the gallbladder in focal, segmental, or diffuse forms. Some form of adenomyomatosis is found in 1% to 8.7% of cholecystectomy specimens.

Adenomyomatosis is most often an incidental imaging finding and usually does not require any specific treatment. Although adenomyomatosis frequently coexists with cholelithiasis, no direct causative relationship has been proved. Adenomyomatosis occasionally is found in patients with nonspecific or biliary-type abdominal pain, and in some cases cholecystectomy may be considered for relief of symptoms.

On imaging, adenomyomatosis is typically seen as focal or diffuse thickening of the gallbladder wall. US is the primary modality used for biliary tract imaging, and adenomyomatosis is frequently identified as nonspecific finding of gallbladder wall thickening, often with sludge and calculi. The finding of cyst-like spaces (diverticula) in a thickened gallbladder wall is usually an indication of adenomyomatosis. Echogenic intramural foci, usually located within these diverticula, from which a V-shaped "comet tail" reverberation artifacts emanate are highly specific for adenomyomatosis. These echogenic foci represent cholesterol crystals within the lumina of Rokitansky-Aschoff sinuses, characteristic of adenomyomatosis. If large enough, Rokitansky-Aschoff sinuses can be identified on CT and MR. A "rosary sign" has been described, formed by enhancing epithelium within intramural diverticula surrounded by the relatively unenhanced hypertrophied gallbladder muscularis. MR images demonstrate wall thickening and intramural T2 hyperintense, T1 hypointense, nonenhancing foci, which correspond to the Rokitansky-Aschoff sinuses. Oral cholecystography (now performed very rarely) and MRCP occasionally show the "pearl necklace sign," which describes the characteristically curvilinear arrangement of multiple rounded bright intraluminal cavities.

PEARLS

- Characterized by gallbladder wall thickening and intramural diverticula (Rokitansky-Aschoff sinuses).
- Common benign may be associated with cholelithiasis.
- US shows echogenic intramural foci producing V-shaped "comet tail" artifacts.

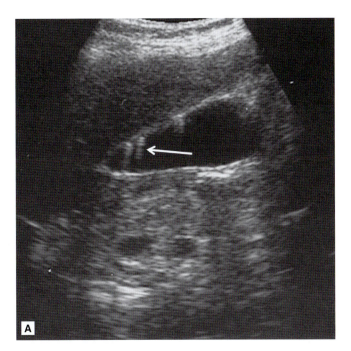

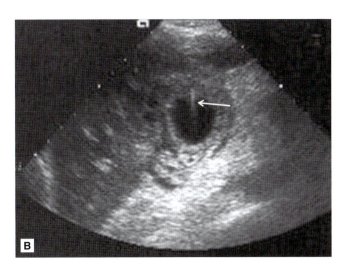

1. US images of the gallbladder of two different patients demonstrate echogenic foci with reverberation ("comet tail") artifact (arrows), characteristic of adenomayomatosis. Wall thickening is more pronounced on **B** than **A**.

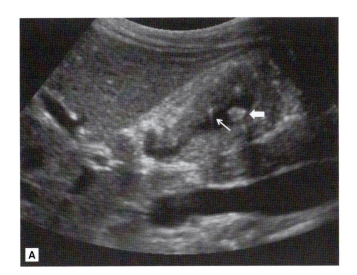

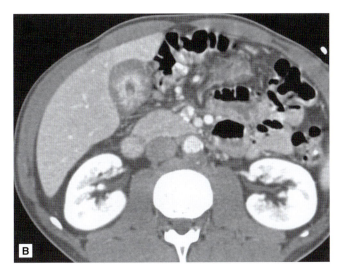

2. US (**A**) and CT (**B**) images of a patient with adenomyomatosis of the gallbladder. There is severe wall thickening, echogenic foci with "comet tail" artifact (narrow white arrow) and an associated gallstone (broad white arrow), a common concomitant finding in this condition.

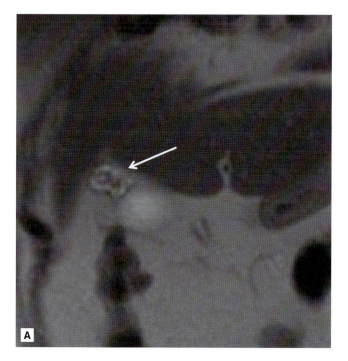

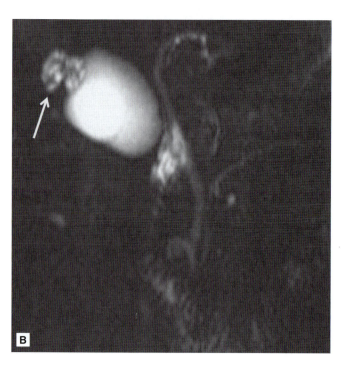

3. MR images (**A**, coronal T2-weighted image and **B**, MRCP image) demonstrate findings of focal adenomyomatosis in the gallbladder fundus. There is focal wall thickening and intramural hyperintense foci (**A** and **B**, arrows), representing the Rokitansky-Aschoff sinuses.

PRESENTATION

- Episodic colicky abdominal pain after cholecystectomy
- Dyspepsia
- Abnormal liver function tests

FINDINGS

US and CT usually demonstrate nonspecific dilatation of the common bile duct. MRCP shows a focal blunted or tapered stricture at the ampulla and the pancreatic duct may also be dilated. ERCP may show delayed emptying of injected contrast from the common bile duct.

DIFFERENTIAL DIAGNOSIS

- Choledocholithiasis
- Ampullary carcinoma
- Chronic pancreatitis
- Gastritis, peptic ulcer

COMMENTS

Ampullary stenosis (or "sphincter of Oddi dysfunction") is usually a diagnostic consideration in patients with recurrent colicky-type pain in the right upper quadrant of the abdomen after cholecystectomy. Many of these patients have abnormal results of their laboratory studies (ie, elevated liver enzymes) or imaging studies (dilated biliary ductal system) and are found to have a small fibrotic or dysfunctional sphincter of Oddi on ERCP. These patients are usually treated with biliary sphincterotomy, often with relief of symptoms.

Unfortunately, many patients present with less specific symptoms and only minimal laboratory imaging abnormalities (or none at all). These patients are a real diagnostic dilemma and their pain and complaints often are treated as secondary to a broader problem of visceral motility or hypersensitivity, or even psychiatric in nature. The need for ERCP in this subgroup of patients with little objective evidence of a biliary tract disease is uncertain, and the therapeutic value of a sphincterotomy is also very questionable.

Imaging studies are of critical importance in determining which patients with postcholecystectomy pain do have a biliary cause for their symptoms, such that appropriate therapy can be instituted. After other potential causes of the patient's symptoms are excluded, such as musculoskeletal, functional digestive or pancreatic diseases are excluded, it is legitimate to consider ampullary stenosis, especially if there is elevation of the liver enzymes and/or amylase and lipase levels within 24 hours of any acute pain attack. Ultrasonography and CT usually demonstrate nonspecific dilatation of the common bile duct, perhaps with mildly dilated intrahepatic ducts as well. MRCP is an excellent test for evaluating the biliary ductal system in this setting. In addition to the dilated ducts, MRCP excludes a bile duct stone with a high degree of certainty and may show a focal blunted or tapered stricture at the ampulla, suggesting the diagnosis of ampullary stenosis. The pancreatic duct may also be dilated. However, endoscopy with direct visualization should always be recommended, especially if the patient is jaundiced, as the MRCP appearance may be very similar to an ampullary carcinoma. Pharmacologic-enhanced MRCP with secretin or cholecystokinin may provide additional evidence of ampullary obstruction, but this is not usually necessary.

ERCP may show delayed emptying of injected contrast from the common bile duct, but this is a subjective sign. Sphincter manometry is widely regarded as the gold standard for the diagnosis of ampullary stenosis or sphincter of Oddi dysfunction, but the evidence supporting its use and potential complications is not very strong.

PEARLS

- Typical presentation is biliary-type colicky pain in patients postcholecystectomy.

- MRCP and ERCP demonstrate dilated bile ducts, with distal tapering at the ampulla, but no mass.

- Sphincterotomy may be curative in appropriately selected patients.

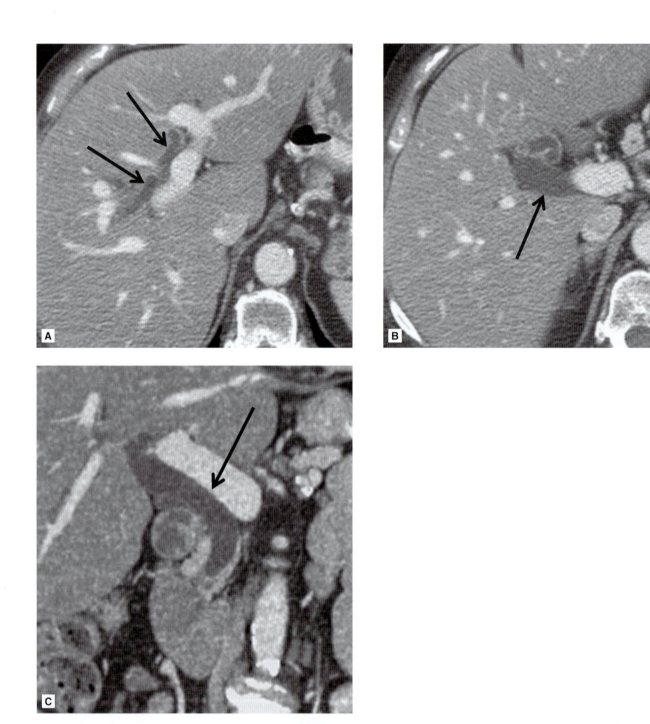

1. A and **B.** Two axial CT images demonstrate dilated intrahepatic ducts (**A**, arrows) as well as a dilated common bile duct (**B** and **C**, arrow), which measures 11 mm in diameter. **C.** Thin section minimum intensity projection (MinIP) reformation of the same CT data shows the dilated common bile duct with distal tapering. These findings are characteristic of ampullary stenosis.

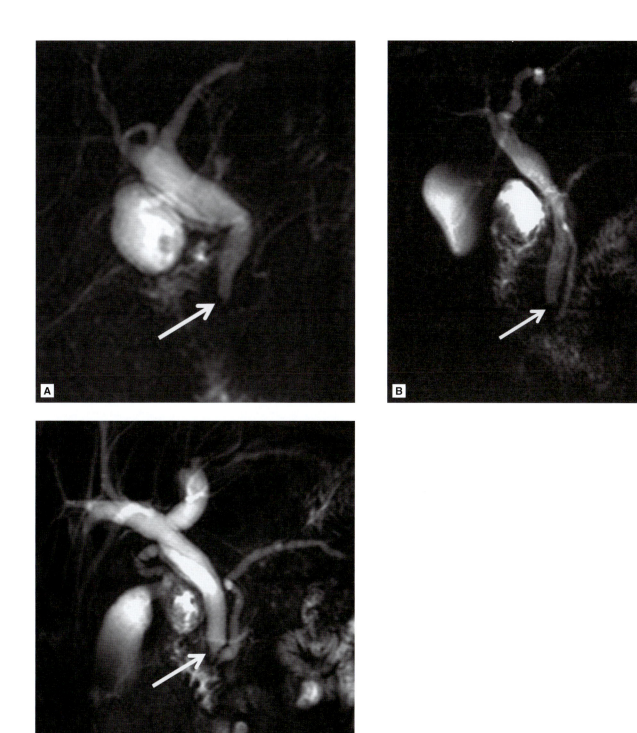

2. **A**, **B**, and **C**. Thick-section MRCP images of three different patients with ampullary stenosis. The bile duct is dilated in the patients and the pancreatic duct is dilated in **A** and **B**. **C**. The distal ducts have a tapered appearance (arrows) and there is no mass effect to suggest a malignant lesion. There is no evidence to suggest presence of an impacted stone.

PRESENTATION

- Recurrent colicky right upper quadrant pain.
- Nausea, vomiting is unusual.
- Mild right upper quadrant tenderness.

FINDINGS

Hepatobiliary scintigraphy with hydroxy iminodiacetic acid (HIDA) shows a gallbladder ejection fraction of less than 35%. Administration of cholecystokinin may recreate the patient's pain.

DIFFERENTIAL DIAGNOSIS

- Cholelithiasis, choledocholithiasis
- Acute cholecystitis
- Hepatitis
- Gastritis
- Peptic ulcer disease
- Pancreatitis

COMMENTS

The main characteristic of biliary dyskinesia (also frequently called acalculous cholecystopathy) is recurrent right upper quadrant pain in the absence of gallstones. The painful episodes characteristically occur in the right upper quadrant 30 to 60 minutes after meals and usually last 1 to 4 hours. An abnormal gallbladder function, with incomplete emptying with contractions, is the most accepted theory. These patients frequently undergo extensive, often invasive and expensive, testing prior to receiving definitive therapy. The exact pathophysiology is unknown but likely is due to an abnormal gallbladder motility that possibly causes a relative obstruction of the cystic duct. Biliary dyskinesia does not progress to more serious conditions, such as acute cholecystitis. Although the treatment of choice is laparoscopic cholecystectomy, the rates of symptomatic improvement are not as favorable as in patients with biliary colic and gallstones.

The true incidence of acalculous cholecystopathy is unknown. With the advent of laparoscopic cholecystectomy, there are data to suggest an increased rate of cholecystectomy in the population. In general, 10% to 15% of patients undergoing laparoscopic cholecystectomy have biliary dyskinesia. As with calculous biliary disease, biliary dyskinesia occurs with higher frequency in women than in men, especially between the ages of 40 and 60 years. The increased incidence of biliary dyskinesia in women suggests an association with female sex hormones.

No laboratory studies specific for biliary dyskinesia exist. Instead, the studies (liver function tests, amylase levels, upper gastrointestinal [GI] endoscopy) help rule out other conditions that are part of the differential diagnosis. US is most useful to rule out conditions in the differential diagnosis such as gallstones, cholecystitis, and biliary ductal obstruction. Hepatobiliary scintigraphy with hydroxy iminodiacetic acid (HIDA) is used to assess gallbladder function and to select patients who may benefit from cholecystectomy. After the gallbladder fills with the radioisotope, cholecystokinin (or an analog) is administered to induce emptying of the gallbladder, allowing an ejection fraction to be calculated. In general, a gallbladder ejection fraction of less than 35% is considered abnormal as indicative of biliary dyskinesia. Administration of cholecystokinin may also recreate the patient's pain, and provide further evidence that cholecystectomy may be indicated.

PEARLS

- **Presents with recurrent episodes of colicky (biliary type) right upper quadrant pain.**
- **US, CT, and MRCP usually demonstrate normal gallbladder and bile ducts.**
- **HIDA scan with administration of cholecystokinin is best test for diagnosis, demonstrating a decreased ejection fraction of the gallbladder (< 35%).**

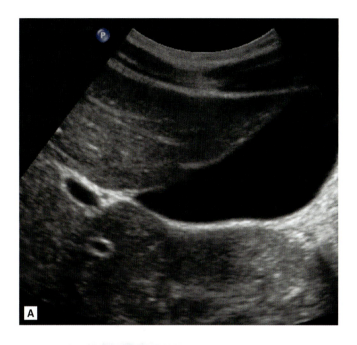

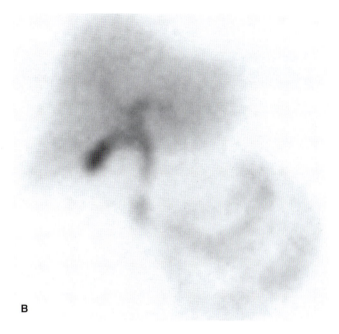

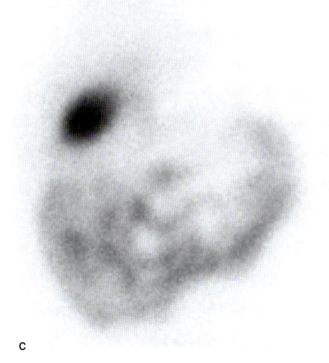

1. A. US image in a patient with colicky right upper quadrant demonstrates a normal-appearing gallbladder. **B** and **C.** HIDA scan planar images obtained 10 minutes after injection of the radiotracer (**B**) and 60 minutes after administration of intravenous cholecystokinin. The calculated ejection fraction was 15%.

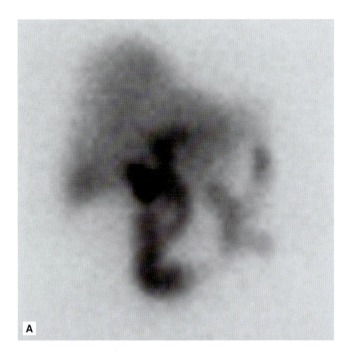

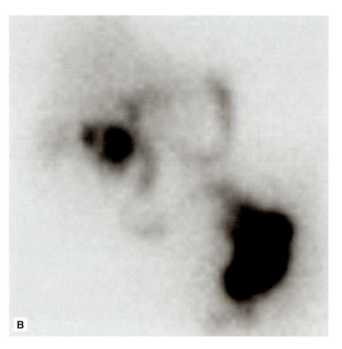

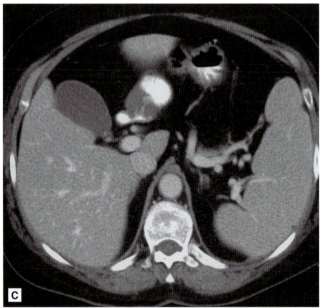

2. A. Contrast-enhanced CT image demonstrates a normal gallbladder. **B** and **C.** HIDA scan planar images obtained 10 minutes after injection of the radiotracer (**B**) and 60 minutes after administration of intravenous cholecystokinin. There is persistent radiotracer in the gallbladder; calculated ejection fraction was 7%. These findings are characteristic of biliary dyskinesia. The patient's symptoms resolved after cholecystectomy.

STONE DISEASE

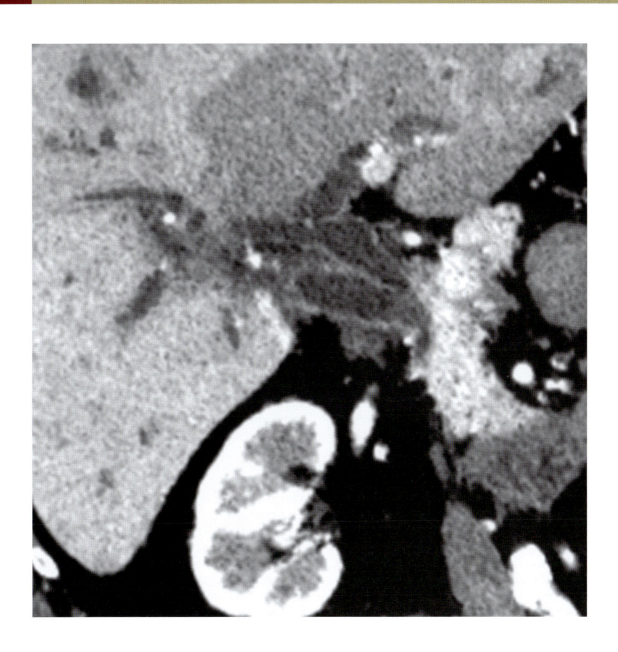

PRESENTATION

- Colicky right upper quadrant pain, with nausea and vomiting

- Jaundice, which can be episodic

- Fever (usually an indication of superimposed ascending cholangitis) and sepsis

- Acute pancreatitis

FINDINGS

US demonstrates a focus of hyperechogenicity within the bile duct, with associated acoustic shadowing. On CT, stones may appear hypo-, iso- or hyperattenuating relative to surrounding bile. On heavily T2-weighted MR images, all stones are depicted as low–signal intensity intraductal foci.

DIFFERENTIAL DIAGNOSIS

- Acute cholecystitis

- Hepatic abscess

- Acute hepatitis

- Malignant biliary obstruction

COMMENTS

Symptomatic cholelithiasis is a very common medical problem affecting patients of all ages, gender (although the disease is more common in women) and nationalities. Choledocholithiasis complicates 10% to 15% of these cases, but the frequency may be even higher in patients older than 60 years. The clinical suspicion of choledocholithiasis complicates the workup and management of simple cholelithiasis, leading to additional diagnostic and therapeutic procedures, and contributes to increased morbidity and mortality associated with gallstone disease. The vast majority of cases of choledocholithiasis are secondary, and usually occur as a result of the passage of stones from the gallbladder through the cystic duct into the common bile duct (CBD) (secondary choledocholithiasis). Primary formation of stones within the CBD is much less common.

Multiple factors, such as bile stasis with sludge formation, chemical and pH imbalances, and increased bilirubin excretion have been linked to the formation of these stones. Gallstones vary in their chemical composition. Cholesterol stones are composed mainly of cholesterol, black pigment stones are mainly pigment, and brown pigment stones are made up of a mix of pigment and bile lipids.

Patients with choledocholithiasis may be completely asymptomatic; in approximately 7% of cases, the stones are found incidentally during cholecystectomy. Approximately 25% to 50% of CBD stones eventually cause symptoms and require treatment. Patients become symptomatic after biliary obstruction ensues and the clinical presentation will depend on the degree of obstruction and on the presence or absence of biliary infection. Laboratory tests, such as elevated bilirubin, alkaline phosphatase, and gamma-glutamyl transpeptidase levels can suggest biliary obstruction but the results are not specific. The white blood cell count is elevated in patients with associated ascending cholangitis

Although US is highly accurate for detecting biliary ductal dilatation, direct depiction of bile duct stones as intraductal echogenic foci with acoustic shadowing is often suboptimal. The reported sensitivity of US for the detection of CBD stones is variable (15%-70%). Duodenal gas frequently limits the ability to visualize the distal CBD. CT is equally useful for detecting ductal dilatation, and is more precise than US for identifying the site and the cause of the obstructing lesion. The sensitivity of CT for detection of choledocholithiasis varies between 60% and approximately 90%. Multidetector CT technology with thin slices and high spatial resolution improves the ability to detect small stones. The appearance of biliary stones on CT depends upon stone composition: Pigment is associated with higher content of calcium and a hyperattenuating appearance, while cholesterol stones are low in attenuation. As mentioned previously, most stones contain both pigment and cholesterol and, therefore, their appearance on CT is variable. CT acquisition parameters, especially the kilovoltage, also determine the appearance of biliary stones. Although oral and intravenous contrast may obscure small intraductal stones, the clinical indication of CT usually mandates the administration of one or both contrast materials. MR cholangiography is the ultimate noninvasive test for detecting bile duct stones. It is a noninvasive tool with very high sensitivity and specificity (~ 95%-98%, comparable to endoscopic retrograde cholangiopancreatography [ERCP]). On heavily T2-weighted images, all stones, regardless of their composition, are depicted as low–signal intensity intraductal foci, completely or partially surrounded by high–signal intensity bile. State of the art MR scanners and pulse sequences allow the acquisition of fast sequences for magnetic resonance cholangiography (MRC), during short breath-hold periods. Although rare, radiologists must be aware of potential causes of false-negative and false-positive MR cholangiographic images and interpretations.

Currently, ERCP is usually reserved for patients with confirmed bile duct stones demonstrated on other imaging tests. In this scenario, ERCP serves to confirm the diagnosis and, especially, as the preferred means for therapy of retained bile duct stones. More recently, other tests such as endoscopic ultrasonography and choledochoscopy have been introduced into clinical practice. The role that these tests may play in the preinterventional diagnosis of choledocholithiasis has not been firmly established.

PEARLS

- Choledocholithiasis occurs in 10% to 15% or patients with cholelithiasis.

- Affected patients present with abdominal pain and signs of biliary obstruction.

- US and CT can demonstrate findings of choledocholithiasis, but MRCP is the most accurate noninvasive test for diagnosis and ERCP is reserved for therapy.

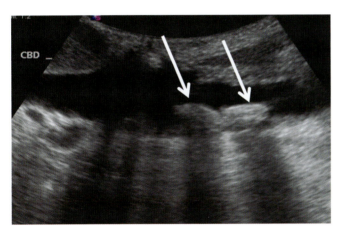

1. US image, obtained along the long axis of the CBD, demonstrates a dilated bile duct with two intraluminal echogenic stones (arrows) with acoustic shadowing.

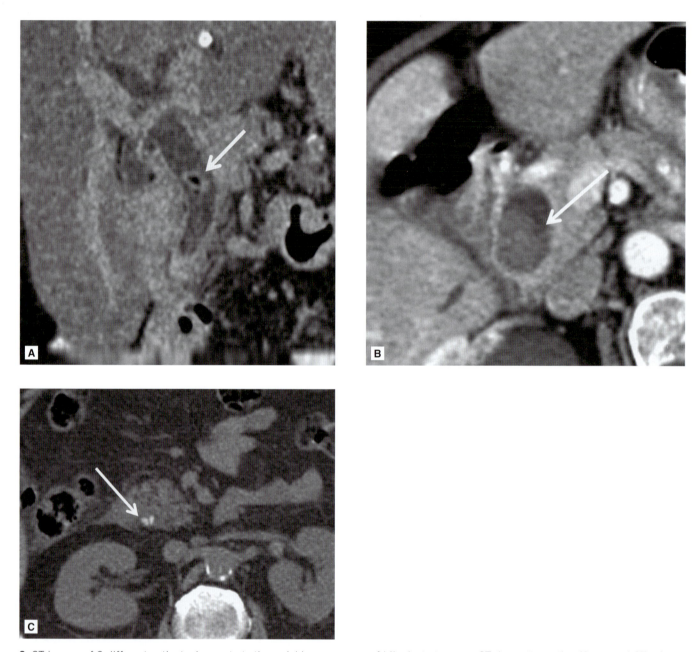

2. CT images of 3 different patients demonstrate the variable appearance of bile duct stones on CT: hypoattenuating (**A**, coronal CT reformation), homogeneous soft tissue attenuation (**B**), and hyperattenuating (**C**). The arrows point to the stones on the 3 images.

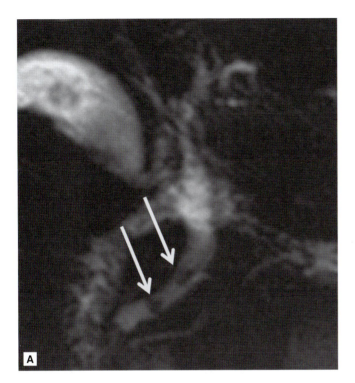

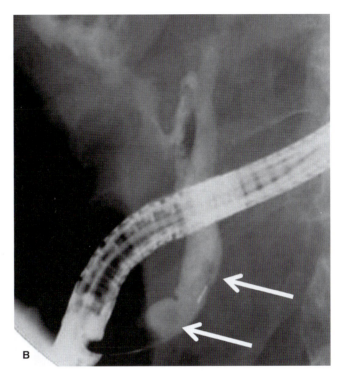

3. A. MR cholangiography (single-shot thick slab) image demonstrates multiple hypointense stones (arrows) in the distal CBD. **B.** ERCP performed as a therapeutic intervention confirms presence of multiple stones (arrows).

PRESENTATION

- Right upper quadrant pain
- Fever
- Jaundice
- Elevated alkaline phosphatase and bilirubin levels

FINDINGS

Imaging studies demonstrate an impacted stone in the gallbladder neck, with dilated intrahepatic ducts, dilatation of the common hepatic duct, and a normal caliber distal common bile duct. The gallbladder may be distended.

DIFFERENTIAL DIAGNOSIS

- Recurrent cholangitis
- Acute pancreatitis
- Acute cholecystitis

COMMENTS

Mirizzi syndrome occurs when a large gallstone (or multiple small gallstones) becomes impacted in the cystic duct or Hartmann pouch. This is a result of chronic and/or acute cholecystitis that leads to contraction of the gallbladder. The inflammatory process extends beyond the gallbladder to involve the hepatoduodenal ligament, which then causes secondary stenosis of the common hepatic duct. Anatomic variants such as a long cystic duct coursing parallel with the common hepatic duct or a low insertion of the cystic duct into the common bile duct increase the risk of developing Mirizzi syndrome in patients with cholelithiasis. A fistulous communication between the two involved ducts may develop as well.

Accurate presurgical diagnosis of Mirizzi syndrome determines the patient's prognosis. Chronic inflammation with extensive fibrosis and scarring can lead to serious surgical complications if not detected before the intervention. Adhesions may make visualization of the biliary anatomy at laparotomy extremely difficult, especially within the hepatoduodenal ligament. The common bile duct may be mistaken for the cystic duct, and ligation or permanent injury may occur during surgery.

Imaging studies are critical for a precise preoperative diagnosis of Mirizzi syndrome. US demonstrates the impacted stone with dilated intrahepatic ducts, dilatation of the common hepatic duct, and a normal caliber distal common bile duct. Similar findings may be seen on CT,

although direct visualization of the impacted stone is less predictable. MRCP is the most accurate noninvasive test for diagnosing Mirizzi syndrome. Findings include the impacted stone in the gallbladder neck or junction of the cystic duct with the common hepatic duct and a dilated biliary system above the level of impaction. The gallbladder may be distended. On direct cholangiography (ERCP or percutaneous transhepatic cholangiography [PTC]), a filling defect representing the calculus in the expected position of the cystic duct and/or a smooth extrinsic compression of the common hepatic duct are seen.

PEARLS

- Mirizzi syndrome occurs when a large gallstone (or multiple small gallstones) becomes impacted in the cystic duct or Hartmann pouch.

- Clinical presentation includes pain, jaundice, and fever.

- Findings on CT, US, MRCP, or ERCP include a smooth extrinsic compression of the common hepatic duct caused by the impacted stone in the gallbladder neck or distal cystic duct and a dilated biliary system above the level of impaction.

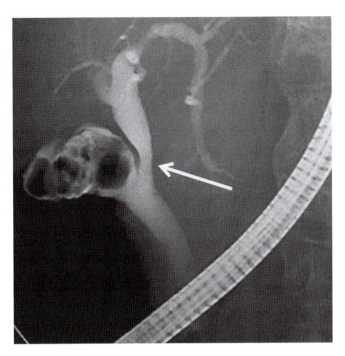

1. ERCP demonstrates multiple large filling defects within a contracted gallbladder. One of the stones is impacted in Hartmann pouch. There is a smooth narrowing of the common hepatic duct (arrow) proximal to the insertion of the cystic duct, caused by the extrinsic compression by the impacted stone. The intrahepatic ducts are dilated. The combination of findings is characteristic of Mirizzi syndrome.

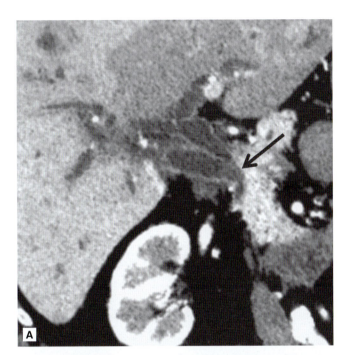

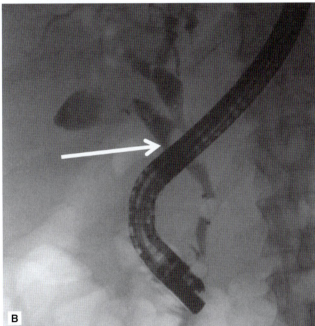

2. A. Coronal reformation of contrast-enhanced CT examination demonstrates a soft tissue attenuation stone (arrow) impacted at the junction of the cystic duct and common hepatic duct, with marked intrahepatic bile duct dilatation. Regional differences in hepatic parenchymal enhancement are caused by complicating ascending cholangitis and hyperemia of the right lobe. **B.** ERCP confirms the CT findings and the diagnosis of Mirizzi syndrome. Note the stone (arrow) impacted at the junction of the common hepatic and cystic ducts.

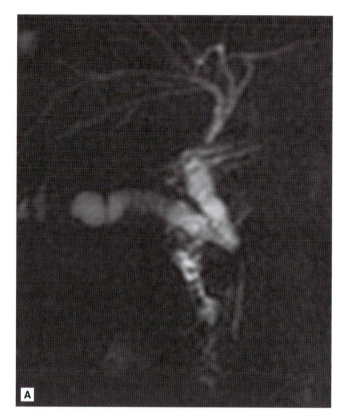

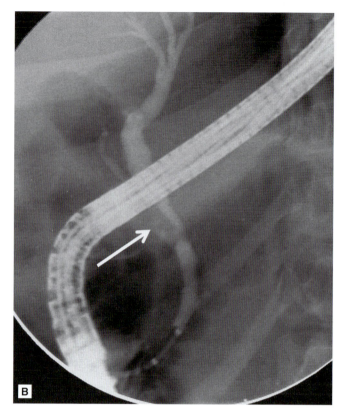

3. A. Thick-slab MRCP demonstrates the dilated common hepatic duct and cystic duct, with a normal-caliber common bile duct. **B.** ERCP demonstrates the filling defect (stone, arrow), at the junction of the common hepatic and cystic ducts. The findings represent Mirizzi syndrome.

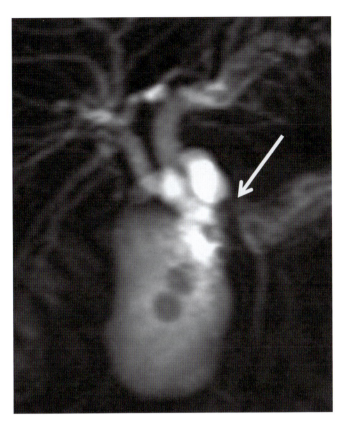

4. Thick-slab MRCP shows dilated intrahepatic ducts, common hepatic duct and cystic duct, with a signal intensity gap at the junction of these two ducts (arrow). This gap represents an impacted stone. The caliber of the common bile duct is normal. Note also stones in the dilated gallbladder.

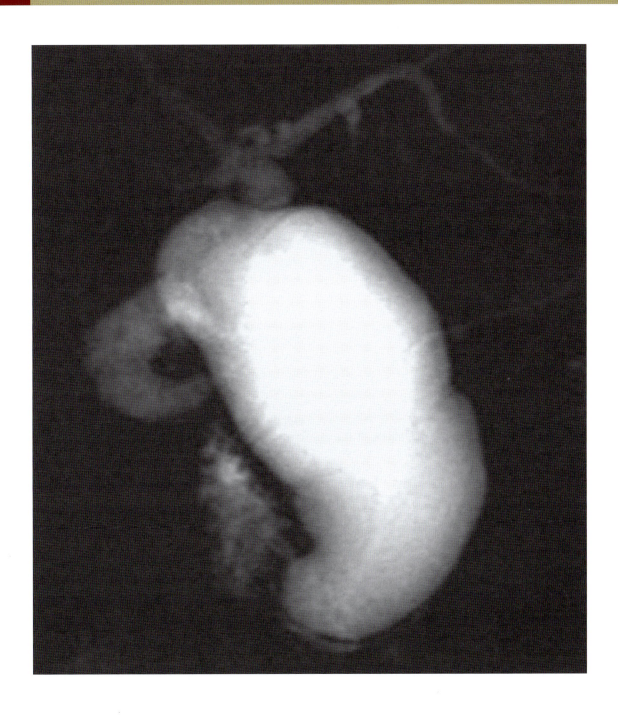

PRESENTATION

- Intermittent abdominal pain
- Jaundice
- Fever, hepatic abscesses
- Palpable abdominal mass (infants and children)

FINDINGS

The main findings on imaging include biliary ductal dilatation and a cystic mass in the vicinity of the porta hepatis and/or the head of the pancreas. Communication of the cyst with the biliary tree can be confirmed with CT cholangiography, biliary scintigraphy, hepatobiliary contrast-enhanced MR cholangiography, or ERCP.

DIFFERENTIAL DIAGNOSIS

- Hepatic cyst
- Hepatic abscess
- Pancreatic pseudocyst
- Enteric duplication cyst
- Gallbladder duplication
- Mesenteric cyst

COMMENTS

Choledochal cysts are congenital cystic dilatations of the extrahepatic biliary tree, intrahepatic biliary ducts, or both. They are slightly more common in women and in individuals of Asian descent, especially Japanese. Most patients with choledochal cysts have some clinical manifestation of the disease in childhood (before 10 years of age). However, some choledochal cysts do not become clinically apparent until early adulthood. The pathogenesis of choledochal cysts is most likely multifactorial. The majority (~ 90%) of patients with choledochal cysts have an anomalous pancreaticobiliary junction (APBJ) of the common bile duct with the pancreatic duct. An APBJ is characterized by the entry of the pancreatic duct into the common bile duct 1 cm or more proximal to where the common bile duct reaches the ampulla of Vater. The APBJ allows pancreatic secretions and enzymes to reflux into the common bile duct, resulting in inflammation and weakening of the bile duct wall, eventually leading to the formation of a choledochal cyst.

The preferred classification of choledochal cysts is the one refined by Todani and colleagues, which divides them into five major types. Type I choledochal cysts are the most common, representing 80% to 90%. Type I cysts are fusiform (more commonly) or saccular dilatations of the entire common hepatic and common bile ducts or of segments of each. Type II choledochal cysts are isolated protrusions or diverticula that project from the common bile duct wall, usually connected to the common bile duct by a narrow stalk. Type III choledochal cysts are found in the intraduodenal portion of the common bile duct. Type IVA cysts are characterized by multiple dilatations of the intrahepatic and extrahepatic biliary tree. Type IVB choledochal cysts consist of multifocal dilatations of the extrahepatic bile duct. Type V choledochal cysts are defined by isolated dilatation of the intrahepatic biliary radicles typically affecting both hepatic lobes, but occasionally involving predominantly one lobe, more commonly the left lobe.

The clinical presentation of choledochal cysts varies with the age of the patient. In early infancy, a workup to exclude biliary atresia may be initiated. Infants can have a palpable mass in the right upper abdominal quadrant. Children in whom the diagnosis is made after infancy present with intermittent bouts of biliary obstructive symptoms, a palpable mass in the right upper quadrant and recurrent episodes of acute pancreatitis. Often, however, the only clinical symptom may be intermittent colicky abdominal pain. An analysis of biochemical laboratory values reveals elevations in amylase and lipase levels which lead to the proper diagnostic imaging workup. Some patients do not present with the disease until adulthood, in which case the presenting symptoms are vague epigastric or right upper quadrant abdominal pain and jaundice. Adults with choledochal cysts can also present with hepatic abscesses, cirrhosis, recurrent pancreatitis, cholelithiasis, and portal hypertension. Complications of untreated choledochal cysts include stone formation, severe pancreatitis, cholangitis and hepatic abscesses, cirrhosis, and portal hypertension. However, the most dreaded complication is cholangiocarcinoma, which is reported rate to occur in 9% to 28% of patients.

US is the initial examination of choice in patients with choledochal cysts. Findings include a cystic mass seen in the vicinity of the porta hepatis and/or the head of the pancreas. In some cases, the specific type of choledochal cyst may be suggested or diagnosed with certainty. Furthermore, advances in US technology have enabled to make the diagnosis in the antenatal period. Although US scan findings are diagnostic in many patients, detailed depiction of the anatomy (such as the location of an APBJ) during the preoperative evaluation often requires complementary studies, such as CT, MRI, MRCP, or ERCP. CT scans demonstrate a low-attenuation (similar to bile) cystic mass that is clearly separate from the gallbladder. The wall of the cyst can appear thickened if episodes of inflammation and cholangitis have occurred. MR cholangiography is the preferred confirmatory imaging study because it does not require breath-holding, is noninvasive, and is not associated with ionizing radiation. Cysts appear as large fusiform or saccular masses that may be extrahepatic, intrahepatic, or both, depending on the type. Associated anomalies of the pancreatic duct, its junction with the common bile duct, and the long common channel formed by the two are usually well demonstrated on MRI or MRCP images. If necessary, communication of the cyst with the biliary tree can be confirmed with CT cholangiography, biliary scintigraphy, hepatobiliary contrast-enhanced MR cholangiography or ERCP. CT and MR help to confirm the diagnosis and provide information about the relationships of the cyst to surrounding structures such as the portal vein, pancreas, duodenum, and liver. Cross-sectional imaging studies are also helpful for detecting associated conditions and complications of choledochal cysts, such as choledocholithiasis, intrahepatic biliary dilatation, portal vein thrombosis, gallbladder or biliary neoplasms, pancreatitis, and hepatic abscesses.

PEARLS

- A choledochal cyst is a congenital cystic dilatation of the extrahepatic and/or intrahepatic biliary tree.

- Affected patients usually become symptomatic in childhood: abdominal pain, jaundice, palpable mass.

- Diagnosis is made with US, CT, MRCP, or ERCP.

- Five different types, classified with the Todani classification.

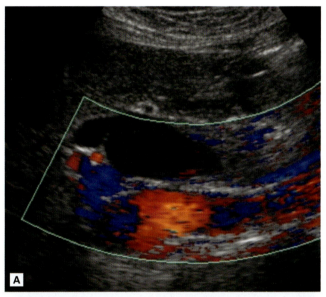

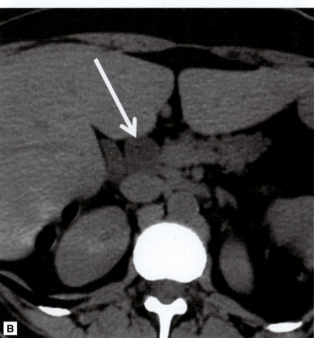

1. A. Color Doppler US image demonstrates marked fusiform dilatation of the extrahepatic bile duct. **B.** Unenhanced axial CT image of the same patient shows a dilated common bile duct (arrow), with normal-caliber intrahepatic ducts. These findings are characteristic of a Todani type I choledochal cyst.

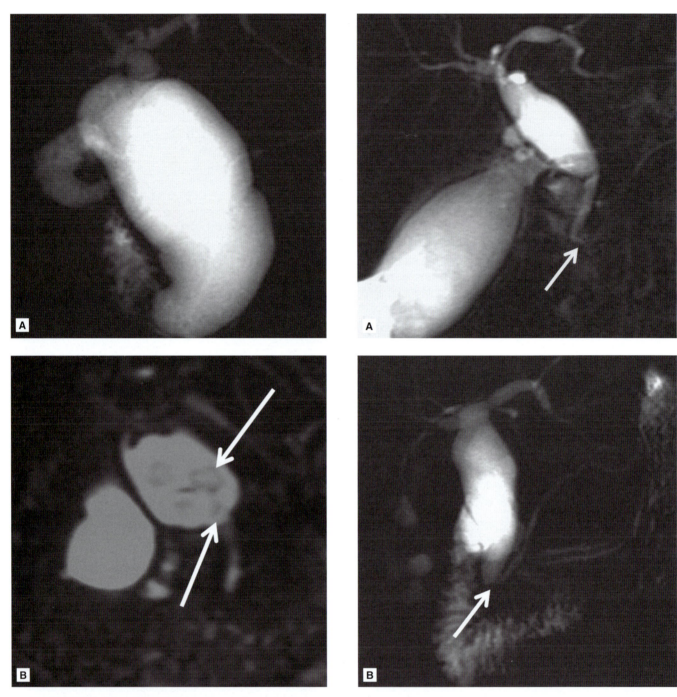

2. A and **B** demonstrate MRCP findings of two different patients with type I choledochal cysts. The intrahepatic bile ducts are not dilated in both cases, despite the massive fusiform dilatation of the common bile duct. Note also filling defects within the choledochal cyst in **B** (arrows). These represent stones or sludge.

3. A and **B** show MRCP findings in two different patients with choledochal cysts and abnormal pancreaticobiliary junction (arrows).

PRESENTATION

- Hyperbilirubinemia
- Abdominal pain
- Fever
- Nausea and vomiting
- Hepatomegaly

FINDINGS

Imaging tests show cystic lesions which communicate with the bile ducts, often with complicating stones. Direct cholangiography reveals saccular dilatation of segmental intrahepatic biliary radicles in which the contrast medium collects, without obstruction.

DIFFERENTIAL DIAGNOSIS

- Biliary atresia
- Choledochal cyst
- Hepatic fibrosis
- Primary sclerosing cholangitis
- Recurrent pyogenic cholangitis

COMMENTS

Caroli disease, also known as communicating cavernous ectasia of the intrahepatic biliary tree, is characterized by nonobstructive cystic dilatation of the intrahepatic bile ducts. It is believed to have an autosomal recessive inheritance pattern and may be associated with autosomal recessive polycystic kidney disease and hepatic fibrosis. Morphologically, the affected intrahepatic bile ducts are saccular and dilated, usually in a segmental distribution. Caroli disease is usually diagnosed in young adulthood, although presentations in childhood are not uncommon and even prenatal diagnosis has been reported.

Morbidity is common and is related to complications of the disease. These include recurrent ascending cholangitis with hepatic abscess, sepsis, choledocholithiasis, portal hypertension, and cholangiocarcinoma, which occurs in 5% to 8% of the patients. After cholangitis occurs, a large proportion of patients die within 10 years. Therapy includes treatment of complications, biliary drainage and, ultimately, liver transplantation. If the process is segmental or lobar, partial liver resections may be therapeutic as well. Patients with Caroli disease often have abnormalities in the results of their liver function tests, especially the alkaline phosphatase levels. Elevated white blood cell counts and positive blood cultures suggest superimposed cholangitis.

Imaging studies play a major role in the diagnosis of Caroli disease. Ultrasonography and/or CT are usually the initial test/s obtained. Intrahepatic cystic lesions which communicate with the bile ducts are the hallmark imaging finding. Nuclear scintigraphy, if performed, confirms absence of significant obstruction, which may be suggested by cross-sectional examinations. MRCP exquisitely demonstrates the cystic, dilated, intrahepatic ducts as well as the complicating stones. CT and MR are also useful for detecting developing cholangiocarciomas. Direct cholangiography via PTC or ERCP is ultimately necessary to confirm the diagnosis and to provide a means for biliary drainage and stone removal. Direct cholangiography reveals dilated segmental intrahepatic biliary radicles with outpouchings in which the contrast medium collects, without obstruction. The extrahepatic bile duct is usually normal or only minimally dilated. Stones may be noted as well.

PEARLS

- **Characterized by nonobstructive cystic dilatation of the intrahepatic bile ducts.**

- **Morbidity related to complications: recurrent ascending cholangitis with hepatic abscess, sepsis, stones, portal hypertension, and cholangiocarcinoma.**

- **Intrahepatic cystic lesions which communicate with the bile ducts is the hallmark imaging finding.**

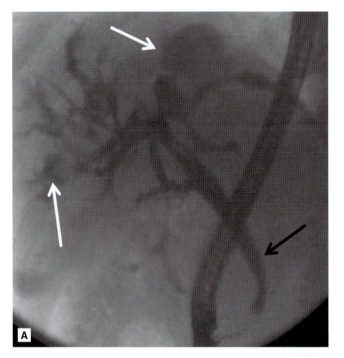

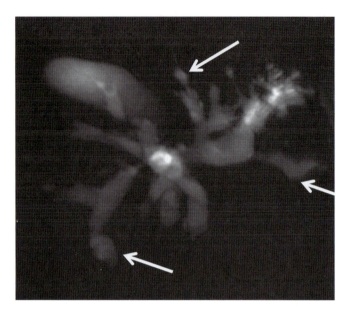

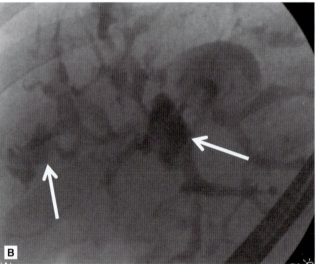

1 and **2.** Endoscopic retrograde cholangiography (**1A** and **1B**) and MR cholangiography (Fig. **2**) images of two different patients demonstrate typical findings of Caroli disease, with cystic dilatation of the communicating intrahepatic ducts (white arrows). The extrahepatic duct is clearly normal (black arrow) in **1A**.

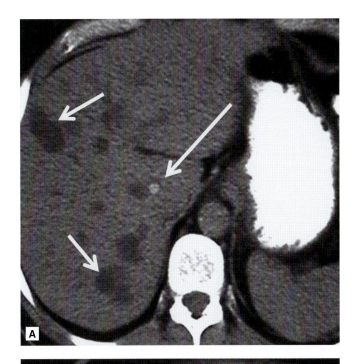

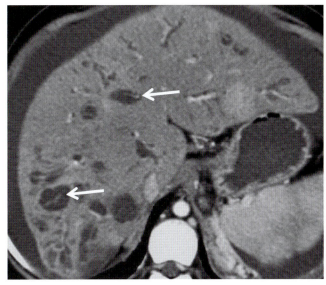

4. CT image obtained with intravenous contrast demonstrates multiple cystic structures, representing dilated bile ducts, centered around the portal venous branches "central dot sign" (arrows). Note also the cirrhotic appearance of the liver and findings of portal hypertension (ascites and splenomegaly).

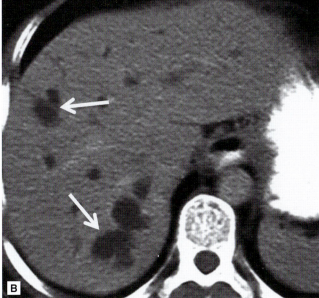

3. CT images obtained without (**A**) and with (**B**) intravenous contrast demonstrates multiple dilated intrahepatic biliary ducts with a saccular configuration (short arrows) and a calcified stone (**A**, long arrow) inside one of the dilated ducts.

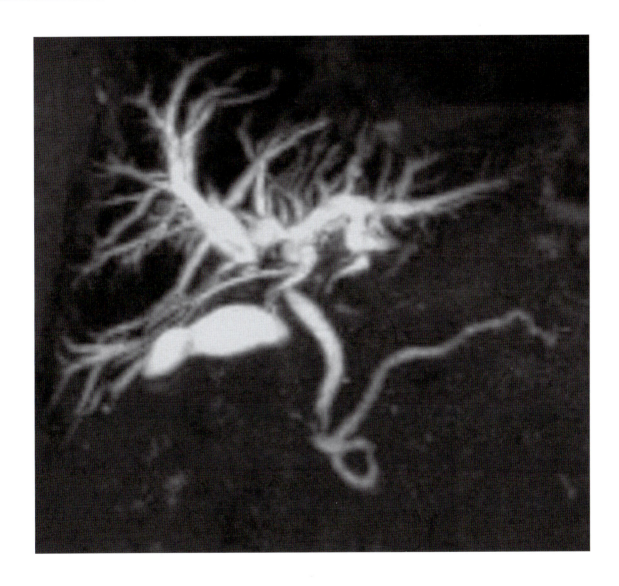

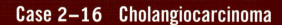

PRESENTATION

- Jaundice
- Clay-colored stools, dark urine
- Pruritus
- Weight loss
- Abdominal pain

FINDINGS

Imaging tests show biliary ductal dilatation with an obstructing tumor lesion. The fibrous nature of these tumors is responsible for a highly characteristic feature: Contrast retention on delayed CT or MR images acquired 10 to 15 minutes after injection.

DIFFERENTIAL DIAGNOSIS

- Pancreatic cancer
- Metastatic lymphadenopathy with biliary obstruction
- Gallbladder cancer
- Advanced hepatocellular carcinoma
- Chronic benign biliary obstruction

COMMENTS

Cholangiocarcinomas are primary malignancies of the biliary duct system that may originate in the liver or, more commonly in the perihilar (also called Klatskin tumors) or extrahepatic bile ducts. More than 90% of these tumors are ductal adenocarcinomas. The etiology of most bile duct cancers is uncertain, but chronic inflammation, such as occurs with primary sclerosing cholangitis (PSC) or chronic parasitic infection (eg, *Clonorchis sinensis*, a hepatobiliary fluke) predispose to the development of this tumor. The lifetime risk of developing this cancer in the setting of PSC is 10% to 20%. Most patients present with advanced disease and are not eligible for curative resection. Prognosis is dismal, with a median survival of 8 to 10 months.

On histology, classic cholangiocarcinomas are well to moderately differentiated adenocarcinomas. A dense fibrous stroma is characteristic and may be the predominant feature. Cholangiocarcinomas tend to grow slowly, infiltrating the walls of the ducts and dissecting along tissue planes. Local extension occurs into the liver, vascular structures at the porta hepatis, and regional lymph nodes

of the celiac and pancreaticoduodenal chains. Peritoneal seeding is also common.

Laboratory tests typically demonstrate evidence of extrahepatic cholestasis, with elevated bilirubin, alkaline phosphatase, and gamma-glutamyltransferase levels. With prolonged biliary obstruction, the prothrombin time can become elevated because of vitamin K malabsorption. An elevated serum CA 19-9 level greater than 100 U/mL is an indirect marker of cholangiocarcinoma in patients with PSC.

Multiple imaging tests are available for the diagnosis and stating of cholangiocarcinoma. On US, the biliary ductal system is dilated and, if performed with careful attention, the obstructing lesion can be depicted as well. In some practices, contrast-enhanced US is used routinely for staging hilar cholangiocarcinomas. Multidetector CT demonstrates ductal dilatation and large mass lesions and has the capability to evaluate for intra-abdominal lymphadenopathy and peritoneal seeding. MR cholangiography enables imaging of bile ducts and permits accurate staging of the extent of bile duct involvement (ie, Bismuth classification). CT or MR angiography using current techniques are used for detecting vascular invasion and preoperative evaluation. The characteristic fibrous nature of these tumors is responsible for a highly characteristic feature: contrast retention on delayed CT or MR images, acquired 10 to 15 minutes after injection.

Preliminary evaluation with positron emission tomography (PET) has shown promise in diagnosing cholangiocarcinoma in patients with underlying PSC. Endoscopic ultrasonography enables both bile duct visualization and nodal evaluation. This technique, although not widely available, also has the capability to aspirate for cytologic studies. Percutaneous transhepatic cholangiography and ERCP are usually reserved for patients with a confirmed diagnosis who require palliative drainage or stent placement for relief of cholestatic symptoms.

PEARLS

- **Most common type is perihilar (Klatskin tumor).**
- **Growth is slow and infiltration along bile duct walls and vessels is common.**
- **Extent of bile duct involvement determined with Todani classification; MRCP and ERCP are the imaging tests used for this staging.**

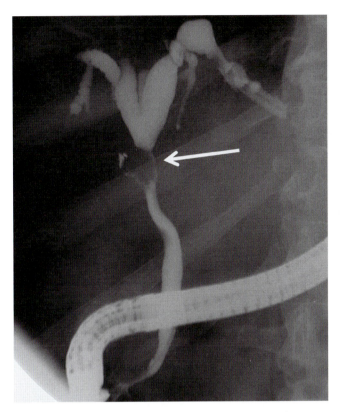

1. ERCP demonstrates typical findings of a hilar cholangiocarcinoma (Klatskin tumor). There is a short segment malignant stricture (arrow) involving the proximal common hepatic duct. However, the primary biliary ductal confluence is preserved (Bismuth I).

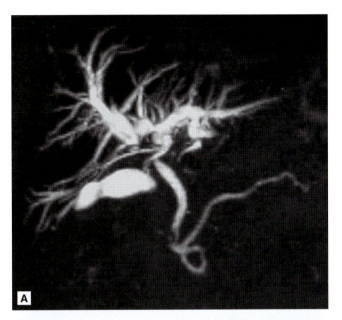

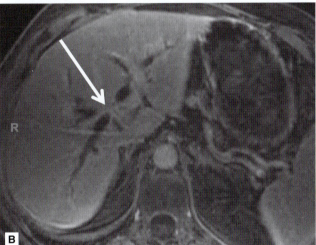

2. A. MRCP image demonstrates characteristic findings of Klatskin tumor, with markedly dilated intrahepatic ducts and normal-appearing common bile duct and pancreatic duct. Since the primary biliary confluence and both secondary confluences (right and left) appear to be involved, this tumor would be classified as a Bismuth IV. The portal venous phase image of the contrast-enhanced MR sequence (**B**) demonstrates dilated intrahepatic bile ducts converging toward the hilum, where there is an abrupt cutoff (arrow) of these ducts. This cutoff represents the location of the Klatskin tumor.

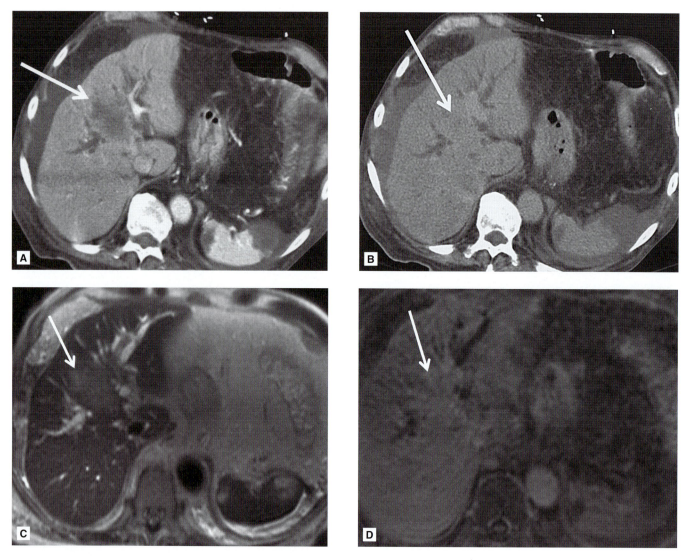

3. Contrast-enhanced CT images (**A.** portal venous phase and **B.** 15-minute delayed phase) demonstrate characteristic findings of cholangiocarcinoma. On **A**, the infiltrating tumor (arrow) has irregular borders and is predominantly hypoattenuating. The obstructed intrahepatic ducts are dilated. The delayed-phase image (**B**) shows retention of contrast material throughout the majority of the tumor (arrow). On the fast spin-echo (FSE) T2-weighted MR image (**C**) the tumor (arrow) is slightly hyperintense relative to liver parenchyma. On **D**, a delayed-phase of contrast-enhanced image, the tumor (arrow) also shows central retention of contrast. ERCP (**E**), performed prior to palliative treatment of obstructive jaundice confirms the malignant narrowing of the confluence of the bile ducts at the hilum. The cholangiographic appearance is consistent with a Bismuth IV tumor.

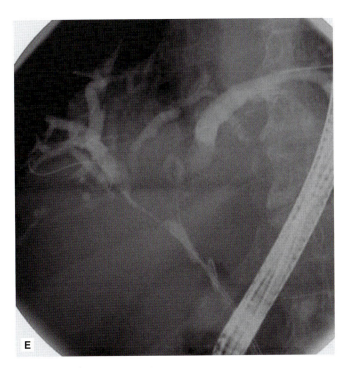

E

3. (*continued*)

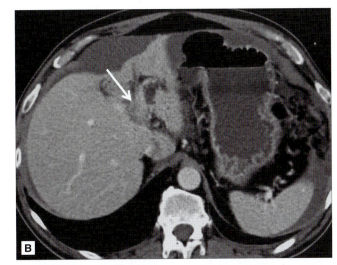

B

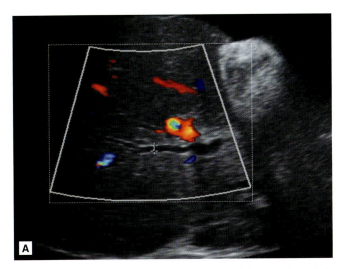

A

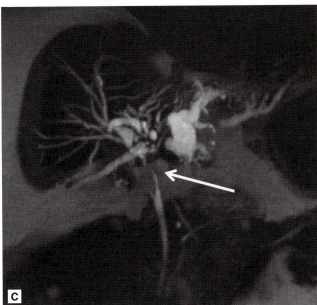

C

4. Color Doppler US image (**A**) demonstrates mild-to-moderate intrahepatic biliary ductal dilatation. Contrast-enhanced CT image obtained in the portal venous phase (**B**) demonstrates an irregular, poorly enhancing, mass in the perihilar region (arrow) causing obstruction of the left hepatic lobe biliary ducts. Note also the volume loss in the left hepatic lobe, with capsular retraction. This is an indication of chronic biliary obstruction. **C.** MRCP image demonstrates the typical appearance of a stricture from hilar cholangiocarcinoma (Klatskin tumor, arrow) causing biliary obstruction. **B** and **C** also demonstrate a large amount of ascites and omental disease, secondary to extrahepatic extension of the tumor.

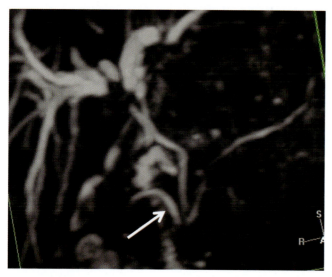

5. The MRCP image shows typical cholangiographic findings of a Bismuth stage IV hilar cholangiocarcinoma. However, there are also findings of an annular pancreas, with the ventral pancreas component (arrow) located to the right of the duodenum and joining the common bile duct at the major papilla. This case illustrates the great value of MRCP for proper planning of palliative therapy in hilar cholangiocarcinoma.

PRESENTATION

- Abdominal pain
- Jaundice
- Weight loss, anorexia
- Palpable mass

FINDINGS

Appearances on US, CT, or MR include an extensive mass that partially or totally replaces the gallbladder lumen, a focal polypoid mass arising from the wall of the gallbladder and focal or diffuse irregular thickening of the gallbladder wall.

DIFFERENTIAL DIAGNOSIS

- Cholelithiasis
- Cholecystitis
- Hepatitis
- Cirrhosis
- Cholangiocarcinoma
- Porta hepatis lymphadenopathy

COMMENTS

Gallbladder cancer is the most common type of cancer of the biliary tract. Adenocarcinoma is the most common histologic type followed by squamous cell carcinoma. Gallbladder cancer incidence increases with age and is more common in women. Also, incidence varies substantially with racial and ethnic groups. Rates are highest among American Indians and Hispanics. The tumor usually arises in the setting of chronic inflammation of the gallbladder, which in the vast majority of patients is secondary to gallstone disease. Other factors that have been implicated in the development of gallbladder cancer include certain hereditary syndromes, obesity, chemical and occupational exposures, and ingestion of certain medications. The tumor is usually located in the fundus of the gallbladder. Unfortunately, the tumor is often advanced at the time of diagnosis. Common sites of spread beyond the gallbladder include regional lymphadenopathy, the liver parenchyma directly, the hepatoduodenal ligament, transperitoneal spread, stomach, colon, and the extrahepatic bile duct. The prognosis in gallbladder disease is poor, with 5-year survival rates of 15% to 20%. Definitive therapy for localized gallbladder carcinoma is surgical (cholecystectomy).

Early-stage carcinoma is typically diagnosed incidentally on specimens from cholecystectomy performed for cholelithiasis or cholecystitis. One percent of patients undergoing cholecystectomy for cholelithiasis have an incidental gallbladder carcinoma.

Results of laboratory tests are not specific. CA 19-9 may be elevated in patients with gallbladder cancer. Patients with advanced disease often have elevated alkaline phosphatase and bilirubin levels. However, the specific diagnosis of gallbladder cancer is usually suggested by results of imaging tests. On gross pathology, gallbladder carcinoma presents as diffusely infiltrating lesions or as polypoid masses with intraluminal growth. Imaging tests reflect these pathological presentations. The most common appearance on US, CT, or MR is an extensive mass that partially or totally replaces the gallbladder lumen. A polypoid mass arising from the wall of the gallbladder accounts for approximately one-third of cases. The remaining patients have focal or diffuse irregular thickening of the gallbladder wall. Almost all patients will have stones as well. The main differential diagnostic considerations in these patients with focal or diffuse gallbladder wall thickening are adenomyomatosis, cholecystitis, hepatitis, and edematous states with secondary thickening. Signs of more advanced disease that can be seen on US, CT, MR, or MRCP include a mass that replaces the gallbladder lumen, with biliary obstruction at the level of the porta hepatis and secondary ductal dilation, lymphadenopathy, and direct hepatic invasion. Cholangiography, via the percutaneous of retrograde routes, confirms the location of the biliary obstruction and may establish the definitive diagnosis through bile cytology.

PEARLS

- **Predilection for elderly, women, American Indians and Hispanics, and the majority of patients have associated gallstones.**

- **The different morphologic types of gallbladder carcinoma include an extensive mass that partially or totally replaces the lumen, a polypoid mass arising from the wall of the gallbladder and focal or diffuse irregular thickening of the gallbladder wall.**

- **The tumor is often advanced at the time of diagnosis and common sites of spread include regional lymphadenopathy, the liver parenchyma directly, the hepatoduodenal ligament, transperitoneal spread, stomach, colon, and the extrahepatic bile duct.**

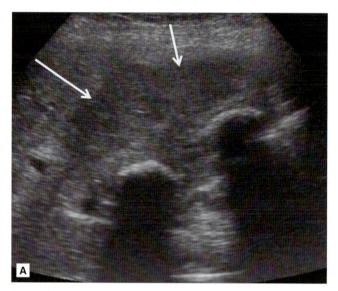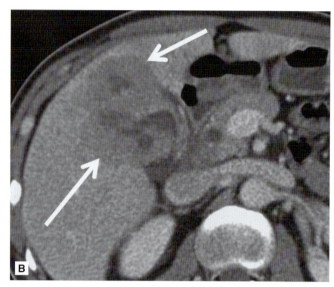

1. A. US image demonstrates a large heterogeneous mass replacing the lumen of the gallbladder and surrounding two large stones. The mass has invaded the liver parenchyma anteriorly (arrows). **B.** Contrast-enhanced CT image of the same patient shows the mass arising from the gallbladder wall and invading the livery parenchyma (arrows).

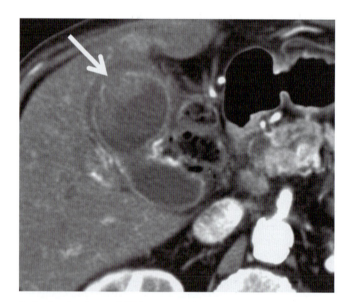

2. Contrast-enhanced CT image demonstrates a polypoid mass originating from the gallbladder fundus (arrow) and invading the adjacent liver parenchyma.

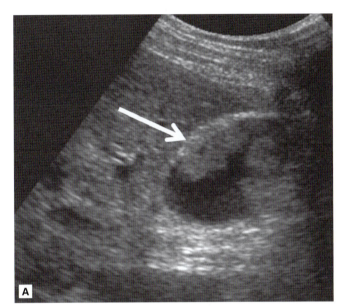

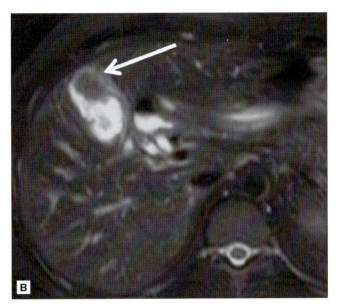

3. US image (**A**) and T2-weighted MR image (**B**) show a polypoid lesion (arrows) arising from the gallbladder wall. No evidence of spread beyond the gallbladder was seen on preoperative imaging. Gallbladder cancer was found at cholecystectomy.

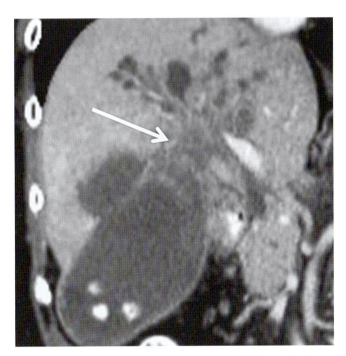

4. A coronal reformation of a contrast-enhanced CT examination shows an ill-defined mass in the neck of the gallbladder. The mass has invaded the porta hepatis (arrow) and is causing biliary ductal obstruction. Note also dependent calcified gallstones.

PRESENTATION

- Nausea, vomiting
- Jaundice
- Pruritus
- Weight loss
- Abdominal pain
- Diarrhea

FINDINGS

Imaging shows dilatation of the biliary and pancreatic ducts and an irregular mass in the region of the ampulla. Positron emission tomography (PET) imaging can detect a hypermetabolic lesion.

DIFFERENTIAL DIAGNOSIS

- Pancreatic cancer
- Malignant perihilar adenopathy with biliary obstruction
- Impacted stone with obstruction

COMMENTS

Adenocarcinomas arising from or around the ampulla of Vater are uncommon, accounting for approximately 0.5% of gastrointestinal tract malignancies. The periampullary region is anatomically complex, representing the junction of 3 epithelial-lined structures: pancreatic duct, bile duct, and duodenum. The pancreatic and common bile ducts merge and exit through the ampulla into the duodenum. Although distinguishing between true ampullary cancers and periampullary tumors is important in order to understand the biology of these tumors (with prognostic implications), this differentiation is not generally possible on the basis of imaging features alone.

Patients usually present with symptoms, signs, and laboratory test results suggesting malignant biliary obstruction. Symptoms are not specific, but painless jaundice is a common presentation. Physical examination may disclose a Courvoisier gallbladder (ie, a distended, palpable gallbladder in a patient with obstructive jaundice). Routine laboratory studies typically disclose a rising bilirubin level. Serum alkaline phosphatase and other liver function tests are usually elevated as well. Serum levels of cancer antigen 19-9 (CA 19-9) and carcinoembryonic antigen (CEA), two nonspecific tumor markers, may be elevated.

An abdominal ultrasound is usually the initial study to evaluate the common bile duct and/or pancreatic duct for evidence of obstruction. The finding of dilatation of these ducts is essentially diagnostic for extrahepatic obstruction. Since the periampullary region is particularly difficult to explore with US, most patients subsequently undergo a contrast-enhanced CT examination (MR is also an option). In addition to the dilated bile and pancreatic ducts, CT scan often demonstrates a low-attenuation mass but is not helpful in differentiating ampullary carcinoma from tumors of the head of the pancreas. If the tumor is less than 2 cm in diameter, ductal dilatation may be the only abnormality noted on CT. CT and MR evaluate the local region of interest for possible spread of the tumor (lymph nodes, vasculature) and also evaluate the liver for possible metastases. PET imaging (usually with CT) can detect metabolically active, tumor-invaded, lymph nodes that are still within normal CT size criteria. The current role of ERCP is mostly limited to providing a means for palliative treatment of jaundice. Surgery, with pancreaticoduodenectomy, remains as the best treatment option to achieve definitive cure. Prognosis of ampullary carcinoma is better than that of pancreatic ductal adenocarcinoma, and depends on the stage of the tumor and the histology (as mentioned above).

PEARLS

- **Commonly presents as painless jaundice and other signs of malignant biliary obstruction.**

- **Prognosis is better than pancreatic ductal adenocarcinoma, but differentiating between the two tumors can be problematic.**

- **Images typically show marked biliary ductal dilatation (and often pancreatic ductal as well), with abrupt obstruction at the ampulla.**

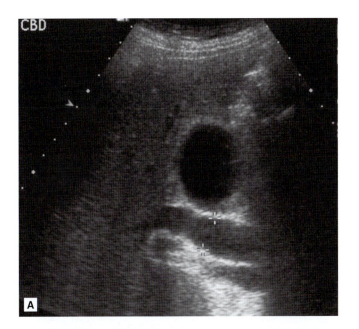

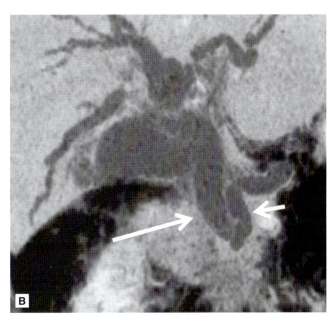

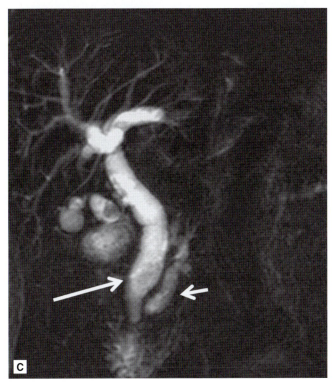

1. US image obtained in the plane of the extrahepatic bile duct (**A**) demonstrates a dilated proximal common bile duct (calipers), but the distal segment is obscured by the dark shadow created by the echogenic bowel anteriorly. **B.** CT image (minimal intensity projection [minIP] reformation of the contrast-enhanced CT data) **C.** MR cholangiopancreatography image, demonstrate markedly dilated bile ducts (**B** and **C**, long arrows) and pancreatic duct (**B** and **C**, short arrows), with abrupt obstruction at the ampulla.

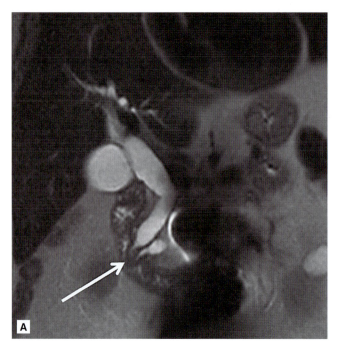

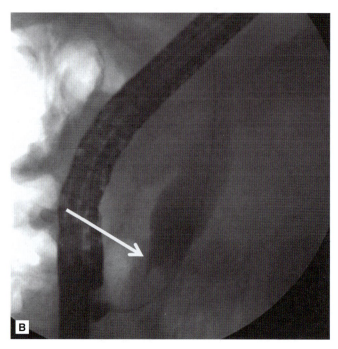

2. A. MR cholangiopancreatography image demonstrates typical findings of ampullary carcinoma, with markedly dilated common bile duct and pancreatic duct and a short stricture (arrow) affecting both ducts at the ampulla. There is a suggestion of a small low–signal intensity mass surrounding both ducts, in the medial wall of the duodenum. **B.** Endoscopic retrograde cholangiography was performed for further evaluation and temporary decompression of the bile ducts with a stent. Note the short area of narrowing with a malignant appearance affecting the distal duct (arrow).

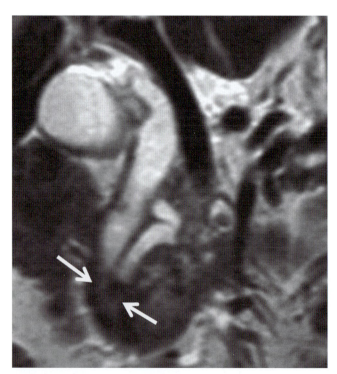

3. MR cholangiopancreatography image in a different patient demonstrates typical findings of ampullary carcinoma, with dilated common bile duct and pancreatic duct and short distal strictures (arrows).

PRESENTATION

- Usually asymptomatic
- Nonspecific abdominal or right upper quadrant pain

FINDINGS

Imaging findings include focal polypoid lesions adhered to the wall, without acoustic shadow on US. Multiple cholesterol polyps may produce a "strawberry" gallbladder appearance. Larger polyps may enhance with contrast on CT or MR.

DIFFERENTIAL DIAGNOSIS

- Gallbladder carcinoma
- Adenomyomatosis
- Metastatic disease
- Cholelithiasis

COMMENTS

Gallbladder polyps are much less common than gallstones. The lifetime prevalence of gallbladder polyps ranges between 1% and 4%, approximately. Polyps are usually discovered as an incidental finding when an US of the abdomen is performed for an unrelated reason.

Five different types of polyps can be found in the gallbladder. Three of the types are not neoplastic and, collectively, account for more than 95% of all gallbladder polyps: cholesterol polyps, adenomyomas (adenomyomatosis), and inflammatory polyps. Cholesterol polyps account for 60% of all gallbladder polyps. They can be single, but are usually multiple and range in size from 2 to 10 mm. When these cholesterol polyps are generalized, the process is called cholesterolosis of the gallbladder. Cholesterol polyps are not neoplastic and are usually asymptomatic. In cholesterolosis, triglycerides and cholesterol esters are deposited in the lamina propria of the gallbladder wall. Grossly, the gallbladder wall has a strawberry-like appearance—hence, the term "strawberry" gallbladder. Occasionally, cholesterol polyps can slough off and cause biliary colic from cystic duct obstruction. Adenomyomatosis represents the second most common type of gallbladder polyps. This condition is covered in a separate, dedicated, chapter in this book. Inflammatory polyps are the third most common type. These polyps consist of granulation tissue and fibrous tissue mixed with chronic inflammatory cells. They are generally solitary, and range in size from 5 to 10 mm.

Adenomas represent 4% of gallbladder polyps, while other rare miscellaneous neoplastic lesions (neurofibromas, carcinoids, leiomyomas, etc) account for the remainder. Adenomas of the gallbladder range in size from 5 to 20 mm and are usually pedunculated. These lesions are potentially premalignant, but the evolution of adenoma to carcinoma is less predictable than for colonic adenomas progressing to colon carcinoma. Almost all adenomas that contain foci of cancer are larger than 12 mm in size. Adenomas greater than 18 mm have a higher likelihood of containing invasive gallbladder cancer. However, the majority of gallbladder carcinomas probably do not appear to arise from previously benign gallbladder adenomas.

Since most gallbladder polyps are asymptomatic, management is usually guided by the characteristic appearance on US, CT, and MR. On US, polyps are echogenic, adhered to the wall and do not cast an acoustic shadow. Cholesterol polyps tend to be highly echogenic and, if multiple, the gallbladder may have the typical "strawberry" appearance, characteristic of cholesterolosis. Larger polyps, especially adenomas, may enhance with contrast on CT or MR or may demonstrate internal vascularity with Doppler US. The best treatment for gallbladder polyps is to perform cholecystectomy when polyp size is larger than 10 mm, since most cholesterol and inflammatory polyps do not reach this size. Polyps 4 mm or smaller can be ignored and polyps measuring between 5 and 9 mm should be followed periodically with US.

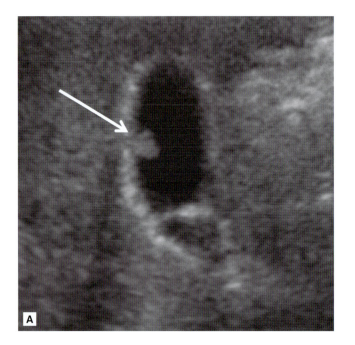
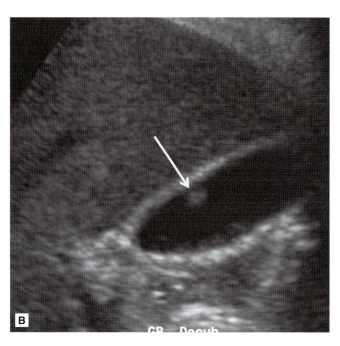

1. Transverse (**A**) and longitudinal (**B**) US images of the gallbladder demonstrate a single, small, echogenic lesion (arrows) without associated acoustic shadowing. The lesion did not move with changes in the patient's position. Thus, the findings are characteristic of a gallbladder polyp.

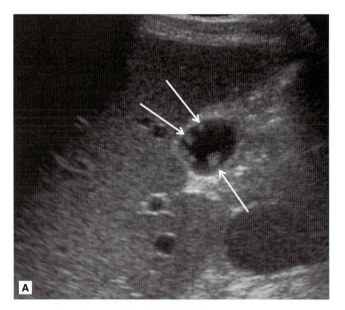
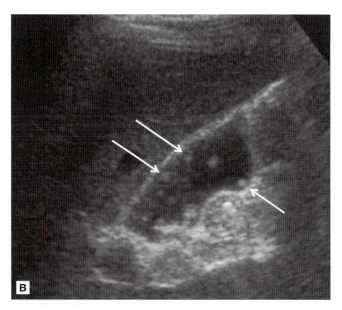

2. Transverse (**A**) and longitudinal (**B**) US images of the gallbladder show multiple, small, echogenic lesions (arrows) arising from the wall, without associated acoustic shadowing. The lesions are fairly uniform in size. This appearance is characteristic of cholesterolosis.

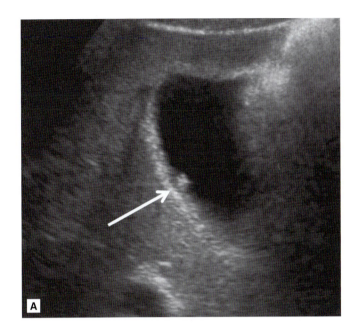

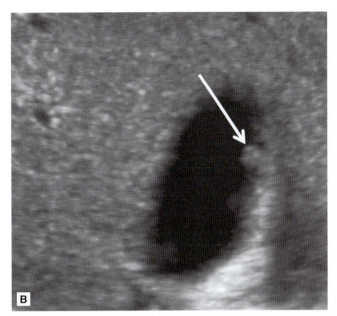

3. Transverse (**A**) and longitudinal (**B**) US images demonstrate an echogenic lesion (arrows) without associated acoustic shadowing arising from the wall of the gallbladder. This lesion was found to be a small adenomatous polyp after cholecystectomy.

CHAPTER 3

PANCREAS

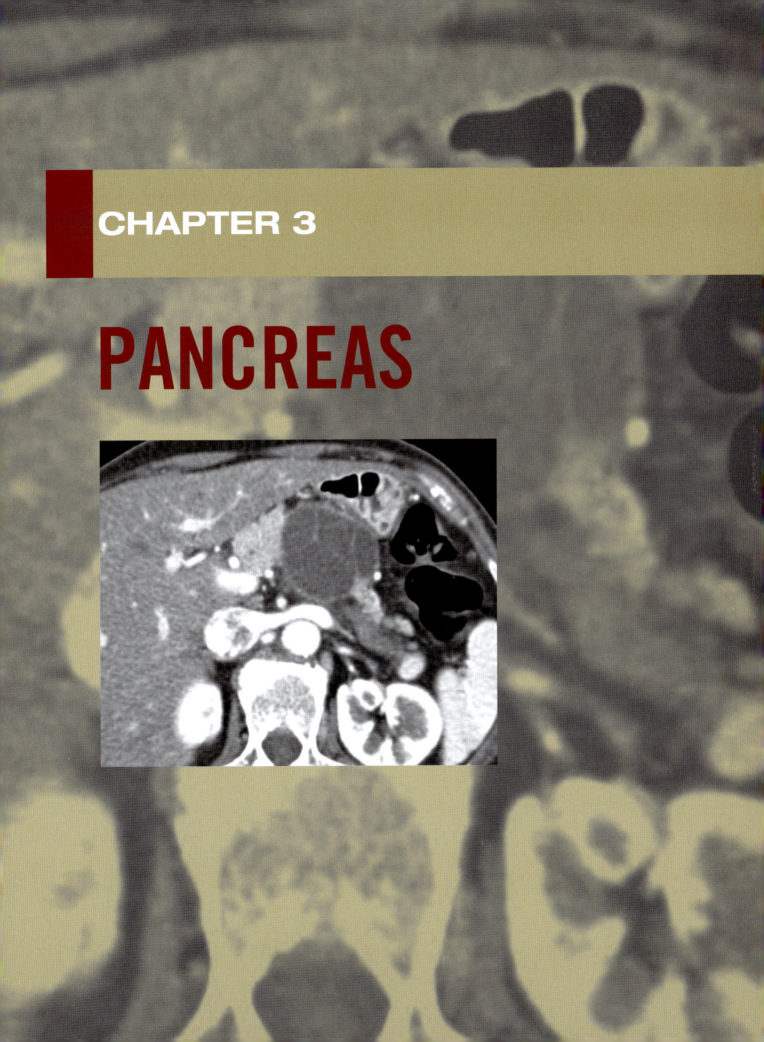

PANCREATIC NEOPLASMS

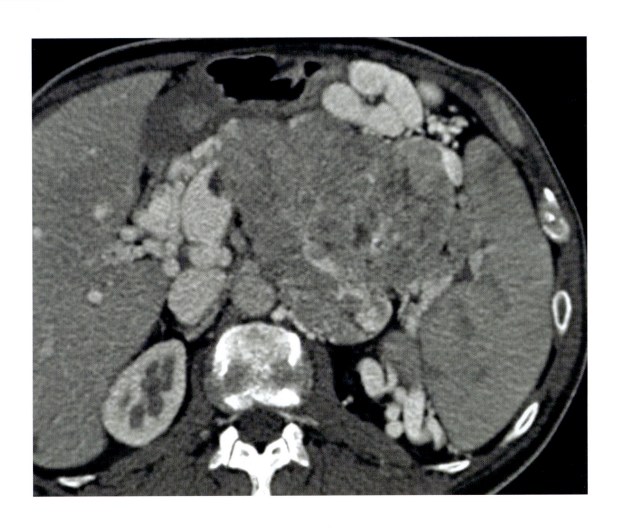

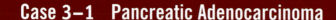

PRESENTATION

Patients may present with painless jaundice, abdominal pain radiating to the back, weight loss, or nausea and vomiting.

FINDINGS

Pancreatic adenocarcinomas are typically identified on computed tomography (CT) as ill-defined, hypoattenuating mass lesions resulting in biliary and/or pancreatic ductal dilatation.

DIFFERENTIAL DIAGNOSIS

- Focal pancreatitis
- Pancreatic metastases
- Neuroendocrine tumor
- Pancreatic lymphoma

COMMENTS

Pancreatic adenocarcinoma is the fourth leading cause of malignancy-related death in the United States with risk factors for its development including cigarette smoking, alcohol use, chronic pancreatitis, as well as diabetes, among others. The overall 5-year survival rate of pancreatic adenocarcinoma approximates 5%, related to the aggressive nature of this malignancy as well as the typical late stage clinical presentations. In fact, approximately 50% of patients present with distant metastases and only 20% are amenable to radical surgery aimed at curative resection.

The role of imaging in pancreatic adenocarcinoma is to stage the tumor and determine whether it is amenable to operative resection based on the extent of the local disease, in the absence of distant metastases. While ultrasound (US) may be employed as the initial imaging modality in patients presenting with signs and symptoms suspicious for a pancreatic malignancy and may identify ductal dilatation (biliary and/or pancreatic) as well, in some cases, the primary tumor itself, CT is the imaging modality of choice for definite staging and characterization of pancreatic adenocarcinoma.

On CT, following the administration of intravenous contrast material with widely employed biphasic acquisitions (typically 45 seconds and 65-70 seconds following contrast administration), pancreatic adenocarcinomas are typically hypoattenuating with respect to the normal gland,

especially on the earlier, parenchymal (45 seconds) phase of enhancement. In some cases, however, the tumor may remain isoattenuating to the pancreatic parenchyma on all phases of contrast enhancement. In these cases, identifying secondary signs such as pancreatic or biliary ductal obstruction is critical in diagnosing the underlying tumor. Upstream pancreatic parenchymal atrophy is also another potential useful imaging finding related to an underlying pancreatic adenocarcinoma.

Following the identification and characterization of the primary tumor, CT is useful in assessing for evidence of distant metastases which preclude curative surgery. Thus, the presence of metastases (especially hepatic) and intraperitoneal tumor spread, as evidenced by omental caking, peritoneal nodularity, and ascites should be sought. When assessing local disease, evaluating for evidence of vascular invasion is of paramount importance. Unequivocal CT findings of vascular involvement include encasement, contiguity with the tumor along greater than 50% of the circumference of a vascular structure, and wall irregularity or deformation of the vessel; direct involvement of the celiac axis, superior mesenteric and gastroduodenal arteries as well as the superior mesenteric and portal veins typically precludes an attempt at curative resection. In addition to the evaluation of vascular structures in the vicinity of the tumor, regional lymph nodes, while not a contraindication to curative resection, should be scrutinized and abnormalities described for guidance of operative resection, if applicable. Finally, gross local invasion of adjacent local structures, such as the stomach and bowel should be evaluated as these findings may have important implications for attempted curative resection.

PEARLS

- In the minority of cases, pancreatic adenocarcinomas remain isoattenuating to the adjacent pancreatic parenchyma on all phases; in these cases, secondary signs such as biliary and pancreatic ductal dilatation may be useful in diagnosing the underlying tumor.

- The assessment of local vascular involvement is critical in assessing patients for potential curative resection.

- Diagnosing subtle intraperitoneal metastases or small hepatic metastases is important as these findings preclude attempts at curative resection.

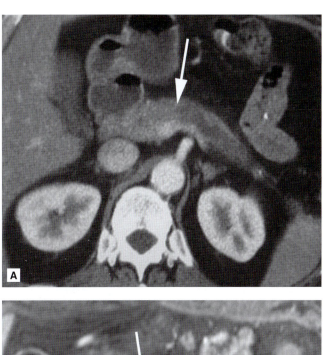

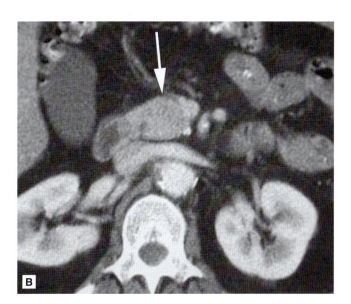

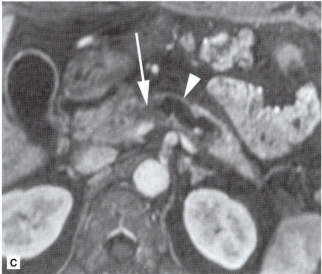

1. A. Axial, contrast-enhanced CT image demonstrates an ill-defined, hypoattenuating pancreatic mass lesion (arrow) in the pancreatic body with abrupt termination of the dilated pancreatic duct at the level of the tumor. **B.** Axial, contrast-enhanced CT image demonstrates normal attenuation of the pancreatic head (arrow), in contrast to the tumor located within the pancreatic body. **C.** Axial, contrast-enhanced magnetic resonance imaging (MRI) image demonstrates the hypoenhancing tumor (arrow) with abrupt termination of the dilated pancreatic duct (arrowhead) at the level of the tumor.

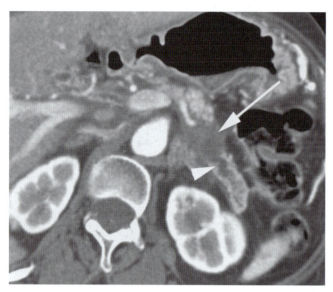

2. Axial, contrast-enhanced CT image demonstrates an ill-defined, hypoattenuating pancreatic mass lesion (arrow) in the pancreatic tail causing moderate upstream ductal dilatation (arrowhead), classic features of a pancreatic adenocarcinoma.

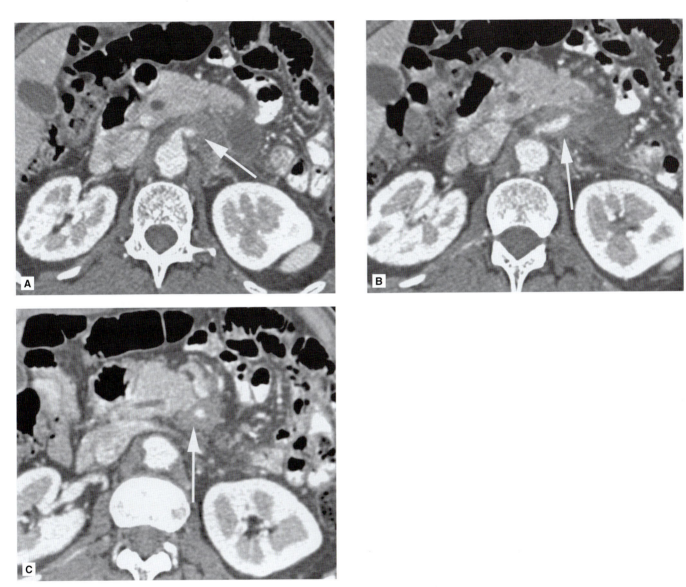

3. A. Axial, contrast-enhanced CT image demonstrates tumoral encasement (arrow) of the origin of the superior mesenteric artery. **B.** Axial, contrast-enhanced CT image demonstrates soft tissue (arrow) surrounding the proximal spinal muscular atrophy (SMA), consistent with tumoral encasement. **C.** Axial, contrast-enhanced CT image demonstrates tumor (arrow) surrounding the SMA, a finding which precludes attempts at curative operative resection.

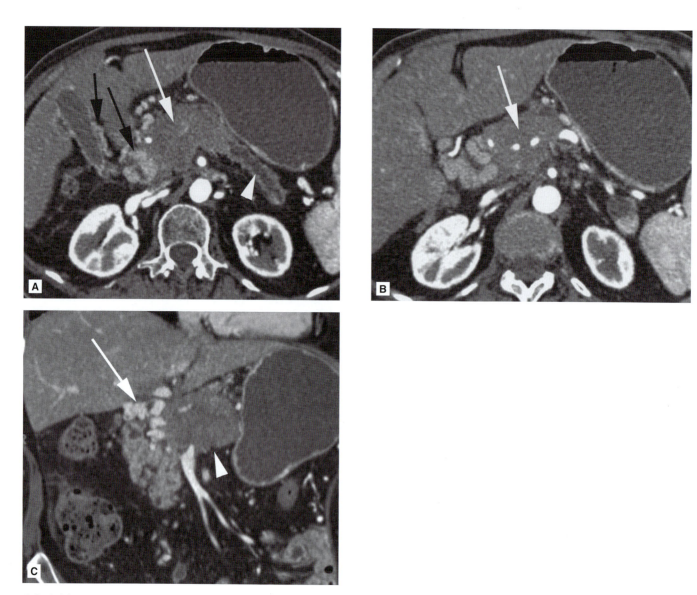

4. A. Axial, contrast-enhanced CT image demonstrates a large pancreatic mass in the head and body of the pancreas (white arrow) causing moderate pancreatic ductal dilatation (arrowhead). In addition, the portal vein is thrombosed as evidenced by cavernous transformation with several small varices noted (black arrows). **B.** Axial, contrast-enhanced CT image demonstrates the large pancreatic mass surrounding the major branches of the celiac axis (arrow). **C.** Coronal, contrast-enhanced CT image demonstrates the large pancreatic mass lesion (arrowhead) which obstructs the superior mesenteric vein and which has thrombosed the portal vein with multiple varices identified (arrow).

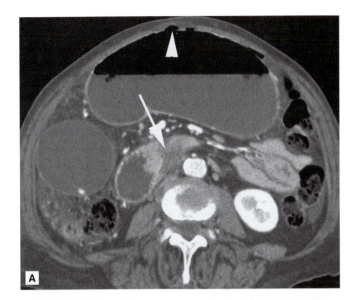

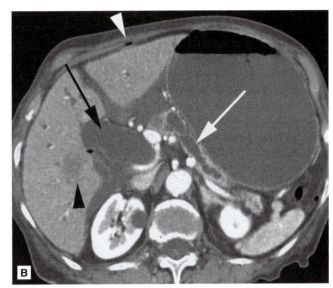

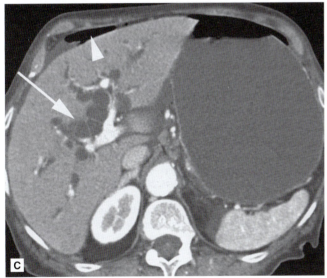

5. A. Axial, contrast-enhanced CT image demonstrates an ill-defined pancreatic mass lesion in the uncinate process (arrow) which is invading the duodenum, resulting in obstruction of the proximal gastrointestinal (GI) tract. As a result of this obstruction, the stomach has perforated, as evidenced by several foci of free intraperitoneal along its anterior extent (arrowhead). **B.** Axial, contrast-enhanced CT image demonstrates marked dilatation of the common bile (black arrow) and pancreatic (white arrow) ducts secondary to the pancreatic mass lesion. Free intraperitoneal air noted secondary to the stomach perforation (white arrowhead) as well as hepatic metastases (black arrowhead). **C.** Axial, contrast-enhanced CT image demonstrates marked dilatation of the intrahepatic bile ducts (arrow) secondary to the obstructing tumor. Free intraperitoneal air (arrowhead) is again noted, related to the perforation of the obstructed stomach.

PRESENTATION

Often incidentally detected; may present with vague abdominal pain or symptoms related to mass effect.

FINDINGS

Mucinous cystic neoplasms generally manifest as a unilocular cystic lesion or may be composed of several larger (> 2 cm) cysts separated by septations.

DIFFERENTIAL DIAGNOSIS

- Serous cystic neoplasm
- Pancreatic pseudocyst
- Solid and papillary epithelial neoplasm
- Pancreatic adenocarcinoma

COMMENTS

Mucinous cystic neoplasm, also referred to macrocystic cystadenomas or cystadenocarcinomas, is a rare tumor, more commonly seen in women with the average age at presentation reported to be 55 years. Mucinous cystic neoplasms account for approximately half of all cystic pancreatic neoplasms.

Histologically, mucinous cystic neoplasms can be divided into non-neoplastic cysts, cystadenomas, and cystadenocarcinomas. These lesions are differentiated from intraductal papillary mucinous neoplasms (IPMN) by the lack of communication with the pancreatic ductal system. Non-neoplastic cysts are considered to have no malignant potential and lack the characteristic ovarian stroma surrounding the epithelial lining which does demonstrate mucinous differentiation in this entity. Mucinous cystadenomas are lined by mucin-producing columnar epithelium with surrounding ovarian-type stroma. Cystadenomas do have a malignant potential depending on whether foci of dysplasia or carcinoma in situ are present in the epithelial lining of the cyst. When invasive elements are seen at histology, these lesions are termed mucinous cystadenocarcinomas.

On imaging, mucinous cystic neoplasms generally manifest as a unilocular cystic lesion or may be composed of several larger (> 2 cm) cysts separated by septations. Non-neoplastic mucinous cysts and cystadenomas are similar in their imaging appearance though the wall of cystadenomas is typically thick and demonstrates enhancement after intravenous contrast administration during a delayed phase of image acquisition on CT and MRI. When present, septations may also demonstrate enhancement. Typically, mucinous cystic neoplasms demonstrate imaging features of simple cysts on US, CT, and MRI. T1 hyperintensity within the cysts has been described. When soft tissue nodules are identified within the cysts, this imaging finding is indicative of carcinoma. As expected, these soft tissue nodules demonstrate enhancement after intravenous contrast administration on CT and MRI.

PEARLS

- **Mucinous cystic neoplasms account for approximately half of all cystic pancreatic neoplasms.**

- **Mucinous cystic neoplasms can be divided into non-neoplastic cysts, cystadenomas, and cystadenocarcinomas.**

- **Typically, mucinous cystic neoplasms demonstrate imaging features of simple cysts on US, CT, and MRI.**

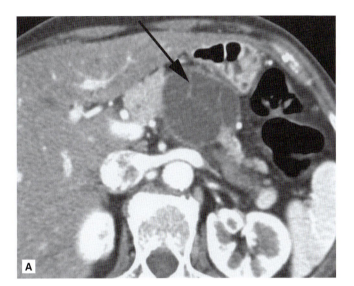

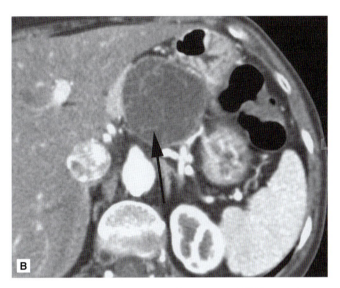

1. A. Axial, enhanced CT image demonstrates a large cystic lesion with several thin septations (arrow). **B.** Axial, enhanced CT image demonstrates a large cystic lesion with several thin septations (arrow).

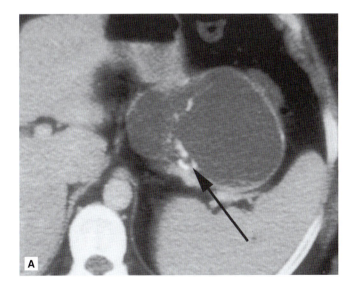

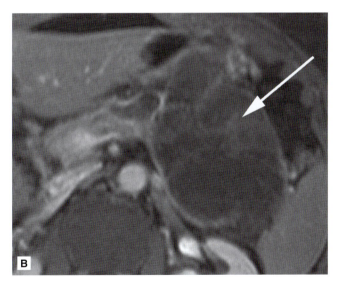

2. A. Axial, enhanced CT image demonstrates a large cystic lesions with several thin septations, some of which are partially calcified (arrow). **B.** Axial, enhanced CT image demonstrates a large cystic lesion with multiple thin septations (arrow).

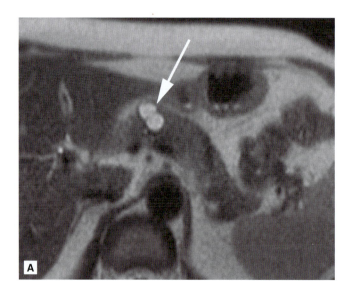

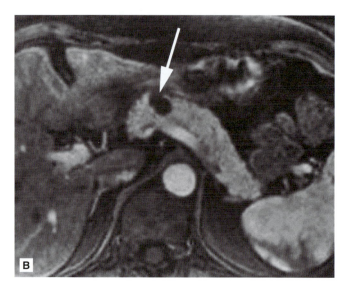

3. A. Axial T2-weighted MRI image reveals a small multilocular cystic lesion in the pancreatic head (arrow). **B.** Axial, enhanced T1-weighted MRI image reveals a small multilocular cystic lesion in the pancreatic head (arrow).

PRESENTATION

Typically nonspecific abdominal or possibly back pain, nausea, and vomiting

FINDINGS

The most common morphology of serous cystadenomas is the polycystic type in which numerous small (< 2 cm) cysts separated by fine septations are identified. These septations may coalesce, resulting in a central scar which may calcify.

DIFFERENTIAL DIAGNOSIS

- Mucinous cystic neoplasm
- Pancreatic pseudocyst
- Solid and papillary epithelial neoplasm
- Pancreatic adenocarcinoma

COMMENTS

Pancreatic serous cystadenoma, previously referred to as glycogen-rich cystadenoma and microcystic cystadenoma, is a rare tumor, more commonly seen in women with the average age at presentation reported to be 62 years. Serous cystic neoplasms of the pancreas are most commonly benign; however, serous cystadenocarcinoma does occur and accounts for approximately 3% of serous cystic neoplasms in the pancreas. Though seen more frequently with increased utilization of imaging, serous cystadenomas remain a rare lesion of the pancreas. Serous cystadenomas occur with increased frequency in patients with von Hippel-Lindau (VHL) disease.

Serous cystadenomas are typically large at presentation, with size in the range of 5 to 8 cm but these lesions may become quite large with reports up to 20 cm in size. Typically, serous cystadenomas are solitary but rarely, multiple synchronous lesions are seen. On gross tissue specimen evaluation, serous cystadenomas are composed of numerous smaller cysts, giving the morphologic patterns seen at imaging detailed below. The cystic spaces are lined by cuboidal epithelium, the cytoplasm of which is rich in glycogen but, importantly, does not contain mucin.

On imaging, serous cystadenomas have three different morphologic patterns: polycystic, honeycomb, and oligocystic. The most common morphology is the polycystic type in which numerous small (< 2 cm) cysts separated by fine septations are identified. These septations may coalesce, resulting in a central scar which may calcify. In the honeycomb pattern, innumerable subcentimeter cysts are present but not individually delineated on imaging resulting in a soft tissue or heterogenous attenuation appearance on CT. The oligocysts morphologic pattern is the least frequent, seen in less than 10% of cases. In oligocystic cystadenomas, larger (> 2 cm) cysts are identified and there is considerable overlap with mucinous cystic tumors. The lobulated contour of a serous cystadenoma may be useful in differentiating this entity from mucinous cystic neoplasms which often have a smoothly marginated contour. Solid variants of serous cystadenomas are exceedingly rare but have been reported. On ultrasound multilocular cysts may be seen but an echogenic, solid appearance is also often encountered secondary to the numerous tissue interfaces related to the small, discrete cysts. Mixed cystic and echogenic, solid-appearing pattern is also described. On CT, discrete cysts are identified in the polycystic and oligocystic types but, as noted, soft tissue attenuation with the honeycomb pattern may be seen. The central scar calcification, seen in up to 20% of cases, is readily seen at CT. Similar imaging features are identified on MRI with the honeycomb pattern having been reported to be characterized as a cystic lesion when a solid appearance is identified on ultrasound or CT.

PEARLS

- Serous cystic neoplasms of the pancreas are most commonly benign; however, serous cystadenocarcinoma does occur and accounts for approximately 3% of serous cystic neoplasms in the pancreas.

- Serous cystadenomas are typically large at presentation, with size in the range of 5 to 8 cm.

- On imaging, serous cystadenomas have three different morphologic patterns: polycystic, honeycomb, and oligocystic.

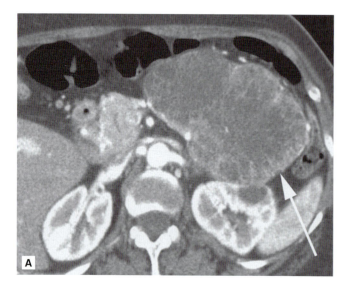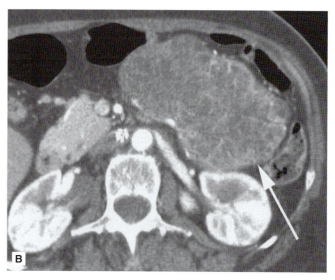

1. A. Axial, enhanced CT image demonstrates a large cystic pancreatic lesion with multiple fine septations consistent with a polycystic morphology of a serous cystadenoma (arrow). **B.** Axial, enhanced CT image demonstrates a large cystic pancreatic lesion with multiple fine septations consistent with a polycystic morphology of a serous cystadenoma (arrow).

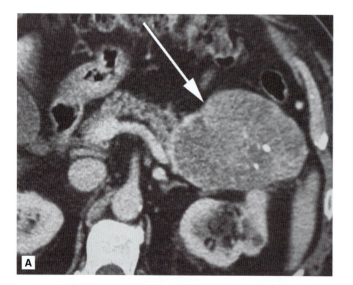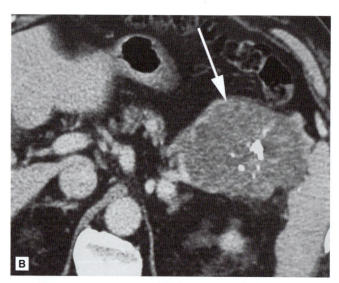

2. A. Axial, enhanced CT image demonstrates a cystic lesion with fine septations some of which are calcified (arrow). **B.** Axial-enhanced CT image demonstrates a cystic lesion with fine septations some of which are calcified centrally, a typical finding of serous cystadenomas (arrow).

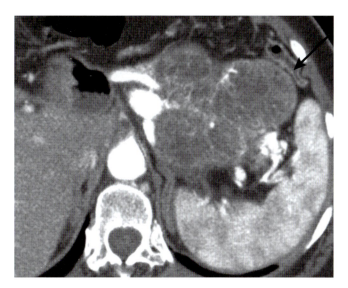

3. Axial, enhanced CT image demonstrates multiloculated serous cystadenoma of the pancreas (arrow).

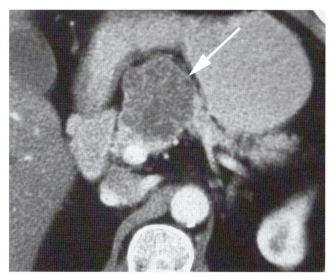

4. Axial, enhanced CT image demonstrates serous cystadenoma of the pancreas with numerous fine septations (arrow).

PRESENTATION

Typically nonspecific abdominal fullness possibly with pain, nausea, and vomiting

FINDINGS

Solid and papillary epithelial neoplasms (SPENs) are usually quite large at presentation with a mean diameter of 9 cm and have a range of appearances from predominately cystic to solid and are typically surrounded by a well-defined rim.

DIFFERENTIAL DIAGNOSIS

- Mucinous cystic neoplasm
- Pancreatic pseudocyst
- Serous cystic neoplasm
- Pancreatic adenocarcinoma

COMMENTS

SPENs of the pancreas are also known as solid and pseudopapillary epithelial neoplasms as well as papillary and cystic tumors and solid-cystic tumors. SPEN arises from totipotential pancreatic cells that have the potential to differentiate into exocrine or endocrine elements of the pancreas. Though the majority of SPEN are diagnosed in the pancreas, these lesions have been reported to occur in ectopic locations of pancreatic tissue including the retroperitoneum, liver, and mesocolon.

SPEN is a rare clinical entity, having been reported to account for up to 2.7% of pancreatic neoplasms. The mean age of patients diagnosed with SPEN is 27 years and the majority of the lesions are diagnosed within the first three decades of life. SPEN are most commonly identified in adolescent girls and young women of non-Caucasian ethnicity. These tumors have a favorable prognosis with a low malignant potential with 5-year survival rates reported to be 97%. Malignant SPEN are typically identified in older patients, the majority of which are men.

SPENs are usually quite large at presentation with a mean diameter of 9 cm. On imaging, SPENs have a range of appearances from predominately cystic to solid and are typically surrounded by a well-defined rim. Variable degrees of hemorrhage, calcification, and necrosis within the tumor may result in various degrees of heterogeneity. On US, variable echotexture is reported with increased through transmission in cases in which cystic components are identified. On CT, after intravenous contrast administration, the solid, enhancing components, when present, have been described to be predominately in the periphery of the lesions. Calcifications are reported in nearly one-third of patients with SPEN on CT. on MRI, SPEN demonstrates variable imaging characteristics depending on the mixture of solid, cystic, or hemorrhagic components. Areas of T1 hyperintensity are often identified related to areas of hemorrhage. On all modalities, fluid-debris levels may be identified usually corresponding to cystic cavities at histology.

PEARLS

- SPENs have a favorable prognosis with a low malignant potential with 5-year survival rates reported to be 97%.

- The mean age of patients diagnosed with SPEN is 27 years and are most commonly identified in adolescent girls and young women of non-Caucasian ethnicity.

- Variable degrees of hemorrhage, calcification, and necrosis within a SPEN may result in various degrees of heterogeneity on imaging.

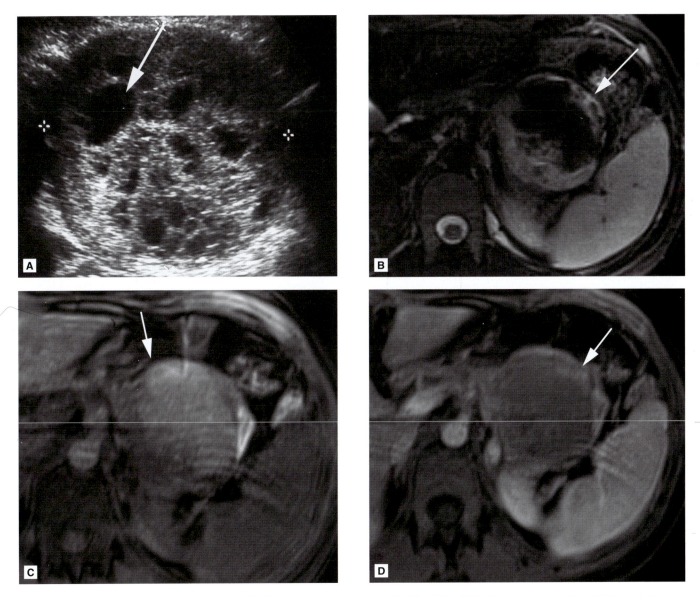

1. A. US image reveals a large solid and cystic SPEN of the pancreas (arrow). **B.** Axial T2-weighted image reveals a large T2 hyperintense SPEN (arrow). **C.** Axial, unenhanced T1-weighted image reveals T1 hyperintensity suggestive of hemorrhage within the SPEN (arrow). **D.** Axial, enhanced T1-weighted image reveals enhancing components within the periphery of the SPEN (arrow).

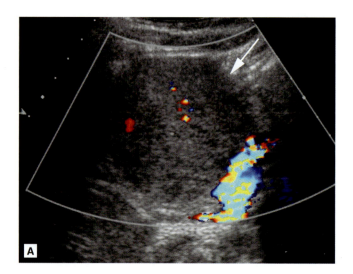
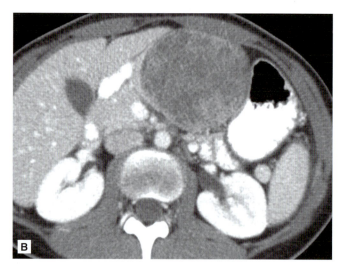

2. A. US image reveals a large solid and cystic SPEN of the pancreas with minimal vascularity (arrow). **B.** Axial, enhanced CT image reveals a SPEN involving the pancreatic head.

PRESENTATION

Typically asymptomatic

FINDINGS

An imaging feature useful in distinguishing an intraductal papillary mucinous neoplasm (IPMN) from other cystic pancreatic lesions is the visualization of direct communication between the cystic lesion and the main pancreatic duct. With multidetector computed tomography (MDCT) and MRI, this finding has been reported to be visible in the majority of IPMNs.

DIFFERENTIAL DIAGNOSIS

- Mucinous cystic neoplasms
- Serous cystic neoplasms
- Pancreatic pseudocysts

COMMENTS

IPMNs of the pancreas were relatively recently described and have been recognized with increasing frequency. In some populations such as liver transplant recipients, the incidental finding of pancreatic cystic lesions, the majority of which are likely IPMNs, exceeds 50%. A slight female predominance has been reported in this tumor which is most commonly seen in an older population (60-80 years).

Pathologically, IPMNs range from benign adenomas to frank malignancy. In malignant IPMNs, approximately half are conventional tubular adenocarcinomas while the rest others are colloid carcinomas which have a slightly more favorable prognosis. Overall, malignant IPMNs have been reported to have a better 5-year survival than pancreatic endocrine tumors, mucinous tumors, or adenocarcinomas. IPMNs originate from the main pancreatic duct, a side branch of the main duct, or a combination of the two. Unlike mucinous cystic neoplasms, IPMNs lack ovarian-type stroma. IPMNs typically produce a large degree of extracellular mucin which is often retained in and results in distention of the pancreatic ducts.

Based on the site of origin, IPMNs are divided into main duct, side branch, or combined types. Numerous imaging features have been reported to increase the likelihood of malignant IPMN. These include an IPMN of the main duct or combined type, diffuse dilatation of the main duct, significant dilatation of the main duct (approximating or exceeding 1 cm), mural nodules or solid components, and obstruction of the common bile duct. A useful imaging feature in distinguishing an IPMN from the remaining cystic tumors in the differential is the visualization of direct communication between the cystic lesion and the main pancreatic duct. With MDCT and MRI, this finding has been reported to be visible in the majority of IPMNs. The finding of communication with the main duct is highly specific; though pancreatic pseudocysts may communicate with the main duct, the degree of communication is typically not large enough to visualize on noninvasive imaging. Another common imaging finding in IPMNs is seen when the main duct distended with mucin is bulging of the papilla of Vater. In patients with incidentally noted side branch IPMNs which are the most common type, the risk of developing pancreatic ductal adenocarcinoma distinct from the IPMN has been reported to be not insignificant with reports of this occurring in 4% to 8% of patients. Thus in patients with IPMNs being observed with serial imaging follow-up, the remainder of the pancreatic parenchyma should be carefully scrutinized as well. Currently, the long-term follow-up data continues to be accrued to eventually develop evidence-based imaging follow-up recommendations for this prevalent incidental finding.

PEARLS

- Pathologically, IPMNs range from benign adenomas to frank malignancy.

- Based on the site of origin, IMPNs are divided into main duct, side branch, or combined types.

- Imaging findings which are suggestive of a possible malignant IPMN include the presence of an IPMN of the main duct or combined type, diffuse dilatation of the main duct, significant dilatation of the main duct (approximating or exceeding 1 cm), mural nodules or solid components, and obstruction of the common bile duct.

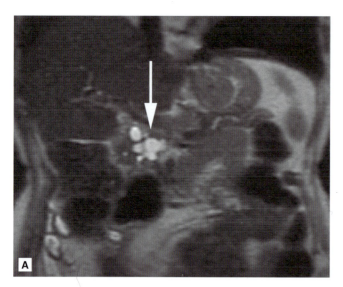 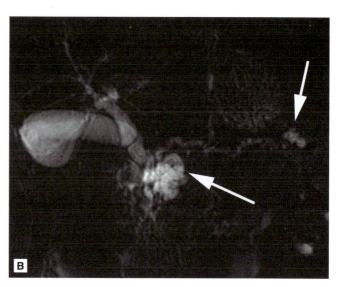

1. A. Coronal T2-weighted MRI image demonstrates multiple cystic lesions within the pancreatic head (arrow). **B.** Coronal magnetic resonance cholangiopancreatography (MRCP) image again reveals multiple cystic lesions within the pancreatic head as well as additional lesions in the region of the tail (arrows).

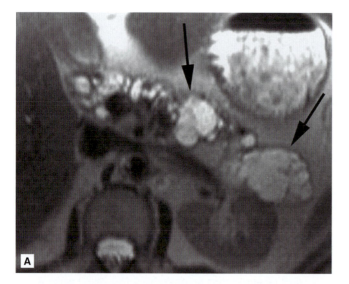 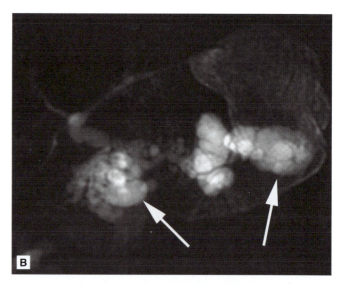

2. A. Axial T2-weighted MRI image demonstrates numerous cystic lesions throughout the pancreas (arrows). **B.** Coronal MRCP image again reveals numerous cystic lesions throughout the pancreas (arrows).

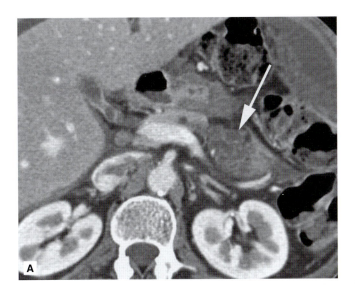

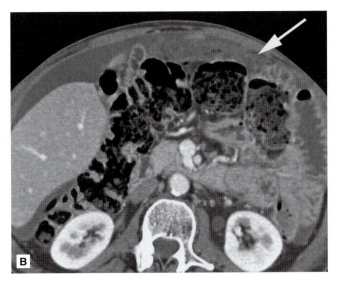

3. A. Axial contrast-enhanced CT demonstrates a cystic lesion within the pancreas which demonstrates multiple thick, enhancing septations, suggestive of possible malignancy (arrow). **B.** Axial contrast-enhanced CT reveals intraperitoneal spread of malignancy in this case of a malignant IPMN as evidence by ascites and omental caking (arrow).

Case 3–6 Pancreatic Endocrine Tumor

PRESENTATION

It varies depending on whether the tumor is functional as well as the specific endocrine tumor cell type. Range of symptoms includes hypoglycemia (insulinoma), epigastric pain (gastrinoma), migratory rashes (glucagonoma) as well as asymptomatic, incidentally discovered tumors, among others.

FINDINGS

Syndromic endocrine tumors are typically smaller and hyperenhancing and more readily identified on the arterial phase of image acquisition. Necrosis, cystic degeneration, as well as calcification have been described and are more frequently encountered in larger tumors.

DIFFERENTIAL DIAGNOSIS

• Pancreatic adenocarcinoma

• Cystic pancreatic neoplasms

• Pancreatic metastases

COMMENTS

Pancreatic endocrine tumors may be classified into syndromic (functioning) and nonsyndromic (nonhyperfunctioning) and nonfunctional types. Pancreatic endocrine tumors are often referred to as islet cell tumors though this may be a misnomer as many of the tumors are not directly derived from islet cells. Though pancreatic endocrine tumors usually occur sporadically, these tumors are associated with genetic syndromes including von Hippel-Lindau disease, multiple endocrine neoplasia type 1 (MEN 1), neurofibromatosis type 1 (NF 1), and tuberous sclerosis.

The syndromic endocrine tumors are usually diagnosed at a smaller size than their nonsyndromic counterparts given the symptomotology related to the hormone production. The most common syndromic tumor is the insulinoma which may present with the classic Whipple triad of symptoms of hypoglycemia, relief of symptoms with glucose administration and fasting glucose levels less than 50 mg/dL. Gastrinomas are the second most common syndromic endocrine tumor of the pancreas and patients often present with elevated gastrin levels and Zollinger-Ellison syndrome. Glucagonoma is an uncommon endocrine tumor and patients may present with a typical migratory rash termed necrolytic migratory erythema. Vipomas secrete, among others, vasoactive intestinal peptide (VIP) hormone which may lead to a characteristic watery diarrhea. The secretion of VIP may lead to Verner-Morrison syndrome or watery diarrhea, hypokalemia, and achlorhydria

(WDHA) syndrome. Finally, somatostatinoma represents a rare variety of endocrine tumor which secretes somatostatin, often leading to hyperglycemia, gallstones, and steatorrhea. The majority of insulinomas (90%) and gastrinomas (70%) are benign while the majority of the less commonly encountered endocrine tumors are malignant. Nonsyndromic islet cell tumors represent approximately 50% of all pancreatic endocrine tumors and, while hormonally active, do no present with clinical sequela of hormone production and, thus, may present later than syndromic tumors.

CT is considered the imaging modality of choice for diagnosis and staging as well as follow-up imaging in patients with pancreatic endocrine tumors though these tumors are also readily identified on MRI. Dual-phase imaging with both arterial and portal venous phases of image acquisition is important in optimizing sensitivity as a fraction of pancreatic endocrine tumors may only be clearly identified on one of these phases. Syndromic endocrine tumors are typically smaller and hyperenhancing and more readily identified on the arterial phase of image acquisition. Necrosis, cystic degeneration, as well as calcification have been described and are more frequently encountered in larger tumors. When imaging pancreatic endocrine tumors, it should be kept in mind that gastrinomas are often multiple and extrapancreatic in location, typically occurring within the gastrinoma triangle which is defined as the confluence of the neck and body of the pancreas medially, the cystic and common bile ducts superiorly, and the second and third portions of the duodenum inferiorly. The majority of insulinomas, glucagonomas, vipomas, and somatostatinomas are pancreatic in location though extrapancreatic location of these tumors is well described. Given that the majority of glucagonomas, vipomas, and somatostatinomas are malignant, a large fraction of patients with these tumors present with metastases at the time of diagnosis.

PEARLS

• **Pancreatic endocrine tumors may be classified into syndromic (functioning) and nonsyndromic (nonhyperfunctioning) and nonfunctional types.**

• **The syndromic endocrine tumors are usually diagnosed at a smaller size than their nonsyndromic counterparts given the symptomotology related to the hormone production.**

• **CT is considered the imaging modality of choice for diagnosis and staging as well as follow-up imaging in patients with pancreatic endocrine tumors though these tumors are also readily identified on MRI.**

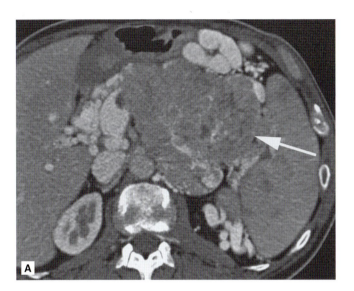

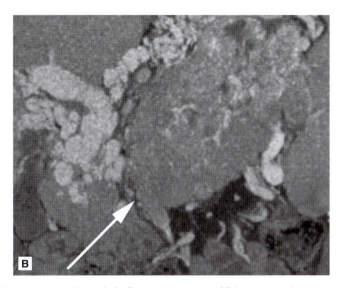

1. A. Axial, enhanced CT image reveals a large neuroendocrine tumor of the pancreas (arrow). **B.** Coronal, enhanced CT image reveals a large neuroendocrine tumor of the pancreas (arrow).

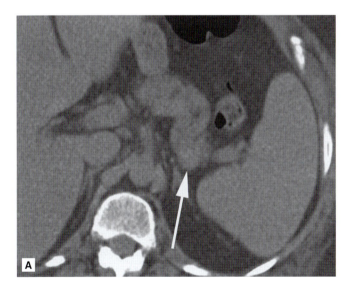

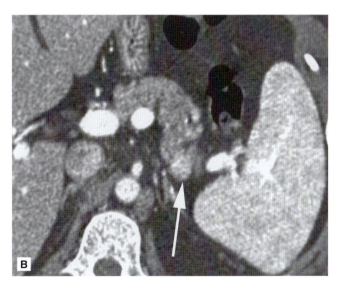

2. A. Axial, unenhanced CT image reveals a small, relatively hyperattenuating insulinoma of the pancreas (arrow). **B.** Axial, arterial phase CT image reveals a small, hypervascular insulinoma of the pancreas (arrow).

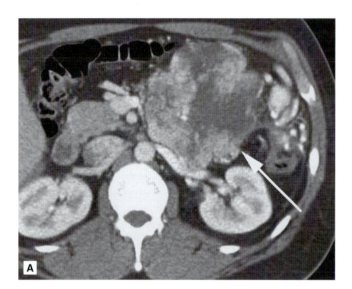

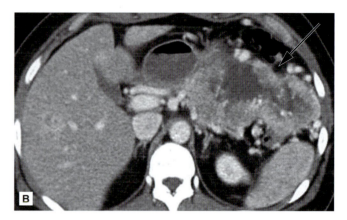

3. A. Axial, enhanced CT image reveals a large neuroendocrine tumor of the pancreatic tail (arrow). **B.** Axial, enhanced CT image reveals a large neuroendocrine tumor of the pancreatic tail (white arrow in **A**, and hypervascular hepatic metastasis black arrow in **B**).

PRESENTATION

Back pain, abdominal pain, weight loss, jaundice, nausea, gastrointestinal obstruction

FINDINGS

Metastases may be solitary or multifocal in nature and diffuse enlargement of the parenchyma has also been described. Larger tumors (> 1.5 cm) have typically been reported to demonstrate a peripheral rim of enhancement and hypervascular metastases may demonstrate brisk enhancement on the early phases of image acquisition. On MRI, metastases to the pancreas typically appear relatively T1 hypointense, T2 hyperintense, and demonstrate peripheral enhancement when larger.

DIFFERENTIAL DIAGNOSIS

- Pancreatic adenocarcinoma
- Cystic pancreatic tumors
- Pancreatic endocrine tumors
- Focal pancreatitis

COMMENTS

Metastases to the pancreas are uncommon but when they do occur, the common primary tumors include lung cancer, renal cell carcinoma, breast cancer, prostate cancer, gastrointestinal (GI) tract malignancy, and melanoma. In autopsy series, metastases of the pancreas have been reported to account for between 3% and 12% of pancreatic malignancies. Significantly higher frequency has been reported in clinical series in subgroups in which patients had been previously treated for an extrapancreatic malignancy.

Though metastases to the pancreas are often asymptomatic, when signs and symptoms are present, they are similar to those in patients with primary pancreatic malignancies and include abdominal pain, back pain, jaundice, and weight loss, among others. In addition, though uncommon, elevated amylase levels have been reported.

On imaging, metastases may be solitary or multifocal in nature and diffuse enlargement of the parenchyma has also been described. Typically, the lesions appear slightly hypoattenuation or relatively isoattenuation to the pancreatic parenchyma on unenhanced CT images. Following the administration of intravenous contrast, larger tumors (> 1.5 cm) have typically been reported to demonstrate a peripheral rim of enhancement. Hypervascular metastases such as those related to primary renal cell carcinoma may demonstrate brisk enhancement on the early phases of image acquisition.

On MRI, metastases to the pancreas typically appear relatively T1 hypointense, T2 hyperintense, and demonstrate peripheral enhancement when larger, similar to CT. In addition, similar to primary pancreatic malignancy, secondary imaging features which may be seen include obstruction of the pancreatic or biliary ducts as well as atrophy of the more distal aspects of the pancreatic parenchyma. In cases of solitary metastases to the pancreas, no specific imaging features have been described which definitively differentiate metastases from a primary malignancy. In cases of multifocal involvement, on the other hand, metastases to the pancreas should be strongly considered as an underlying etiology.

PEARLS

- Metastases to the pancreas are uncommon but when they do occur, the common primary tumors include lung cancer, renal cell carcinoma, breast cancer, prostate cancer, GI tract malignancy, and melanoma.

- Similar to primary pancreatic malignancy, secondary imaging features which may be seen in pancreatic metastases include obstruction of the pancreatic or biliary ducts as well as atrophy of the more distal aspects of the pancreatic parenchyma.

- Though solitary metastases may appear similar to primary pancreatic malignancy, in cases of multifocal involvement, on the other hand, metastases to the pancreas should be strongly considered as an underlying etiology.

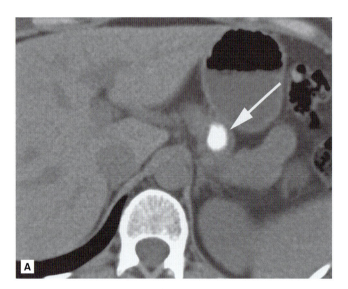
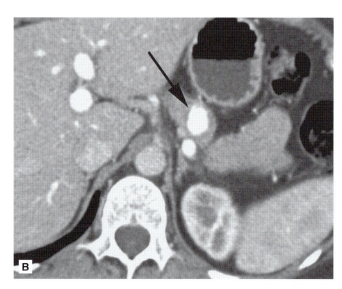

1. A. Axial, unenhanced CT image reveals a focal calcification within the pancreatic parenchyma, in this case related to an osteosarcoma metastasis (arrow). **B.** Axial, enhanced CT image demonstrates the presence of a solitary, calcified osteosarcoma metastasis in the pancreas (arrow).

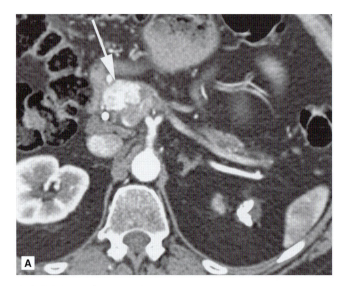
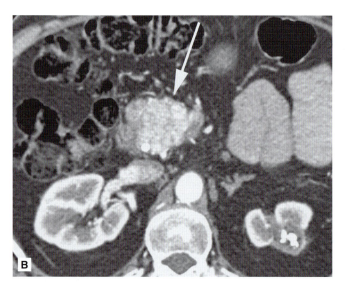

2. A. Axial, arterial phase CT image demonstrates a hypervascular metastasis in the region of the pancreatic head in this case of renal cell carcinoma metastasis to the pancreas (arrow). **B.** Axial, arterial phase CT image demonstrates a large hypervascular metastasis in the pancreas in this case of renal cell carcinoma metastasis to the pancreas (arrow).

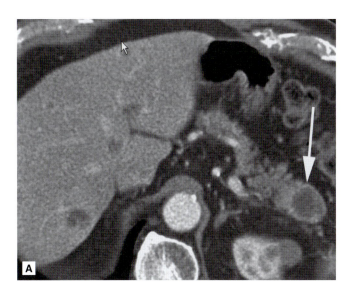

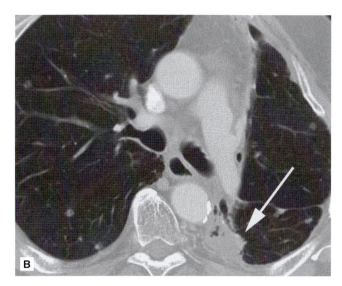

3. A. Axial, enhanced CT image reveals a solitary metastasis in the pancreatic tail (arrow). Incidental note is made of metastasis to the liver. **B.** Axial CT image reveals primary pulmonary malignancy (arrow), in this case an adenocarcinoma responsible for the pancreatic metastasis.

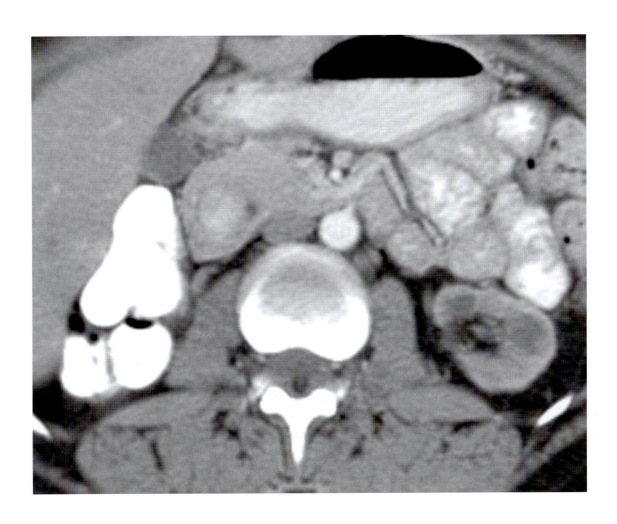

Case 3-8 Pancreas Divisum

PRESENTATION

Typically asymptomatic, incidental finding on imaging. However, in some patients, pancreas divisum may contribute to chronic abdominal pain and acute, recurrent pancreatitis.

FINDINGS

The caliber of the dorsal pancreatic duct is seen to be larger than that of the ventral duct. In addition, the dorsal and ventral ducts do not appear to communicate with each other.

DIFFERENTIAL DIAGNOSIS

- Annular pancreas
- Dominant duct of Santorini

COMMENTS

Pancreas divisum is due to a failure of fusion between the ventral and dorsal ducts of the pancreas, a finding which has been reported to occur between 4% and 10% of the general population. In cases of pancreas divisum, the duct of Wirsung, or ventral duct, serves only to drain the ventral aspect of the pancreas (a portion of the pancreatic head and the uncinate process) which represents the minority of the pancreatic parenchyma. The duct of Wirsung, or dorsal duct, serves to drain the majority of the pancreatic parenchyma through the minor papilla. While typically an asymptomatic, incidental imaging finding, there is a higher incidence of pancreas divisum in patients with chronic abdominal pain and recurrent bouts of acute pancreatitis.

It has been hypothesized that the relative obstruction to the flow of pancreatic secretions through the minor papilla may lead to chronic pain and pancreatitis.

Multidetector-row CT may identify cases of pancreas divisum as evidenced by a dominant dorsal duct without direct evidence of communication between the ventral and dorsal ducts. The use of multiplanar reformations has been suggested to improve the diagnostic capability of CT with regard to pancreas divisum. MR pancreatography has been reported to be highly sensitive to the detection of pancreas divisum, as evidenced by a dominant dorsal duct and lack of communication between dorsal and ventral ductal systems. In addition, the use of secretin-enhanced MR pancreatography has been reported to be useful in more clearly delineating pancreatic ductal anatomy as well as related findings in patients with pancreas divisum. For instance, focal dilatation of the terminal dorsal duct secondary to a degree of mechanical obstruction, termed a santorinicele, has been reported to be readily diagnosed with secretin-enhanced MR pancreatography.

PEARLS

- **Pancreas divisum is the most common congenital anomaly of the pancreatic ductal system, reportedly affecting between 5% and 10% of the general population.**

- **CT and MR pancreatography may readily identify cases of pancreas divisum in which a dominant dorsal duct is found to lack communication with the ventral duct.**

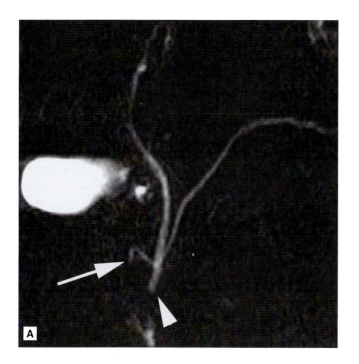

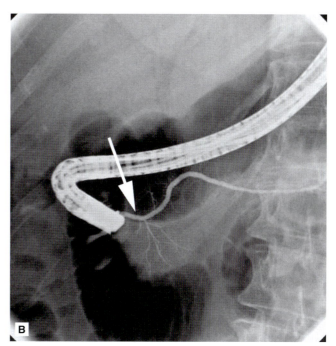

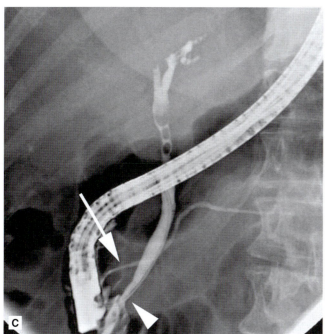

1. A. MRCP image demonstrates abnormal course of the main pancreatic duct which is draining via the minor papilla in this case of pancreas divisum (arrow in **A**, **B**, **C**). **B.** Opacification of the dorsal pancreatic duct via the minor papilla is seen in this case of pancreas divisum. Note the abnormally large size of the dominant dorsal duct in this case. **C.** The abnormal relationship between the drainage of the main pancreatic and common bile duct (arrowhead in **A**, **C**) is well seen in this endoscopic retrograde cholangiopancreatography (ERCP) image in a patient with pancreas divisum.

PRESENTATION

Majority are asymptomatic adults but patients may present with nonspecific abdominal pain, vomiting, and pancreatitis.

FINDINGS

Annular pancreas is diagnosed based on findings of a ring of pancreatic tissue and an annular duct surrounding the second portion of the duodenum.

DIFFERENTIAL DIAGNOSIS

- Pancreatic adenocarcinoma

COMMENTS

Annular pancreas is a rare congenital abnormality which results from the absence of rotation of the ventral anlage of the pancreas resulting in a portion of the pancreas encircling the second portion of the duodenum. Normally, the pancreas develops from dorsal and ventral anlage. Initially, the ventral anlage is bifid with subsequent atrophy of one of the anlages followed by fusion with the dorsal anlage. Theories as to the development of annular pancreas include failure of atrophy of the bifid ventral anlage (Baldwin's theory) resulting in pancreatic tissue encircling the duodenum or abnormal adherence of the ventral anlage to the duodenum (Lecco's theory) with resultant incomplete rotation resulting in an annular configuration. Four types of annular pancreas are described based on the pattern of drainage of the annular duct. In type I, the annular duct drains into the duct of Wirsung; type II annular duct drains into the common bile duct; type III annular duct drains into the major papilla with absence of the duct of Wirsung; type IV annular duct drains into the duct of Santorini.

Annular pancreas occurs with prevalence reported in autopsy studies of 5 to 15 patients per 100,000 while ERCP studies have reported the prevalence to be 400 cases per 100,000, likely under- and overestimations of the true prevalence, respectively. Of the symptomatic cases, approximately 50% present with biliary or gastrointestinal obstruction in neonates, possibly with associated pancreatitis. In adults, annular pancreas may present with duodenal obstruction or pancreatitis. In addition, adult patients may present with gastrointestinal hemorrhage related to peptic ulceration. Rarely, biliary obstruction has been reported in adult patients.

Annular pancreas may be diagnosed on CT- or MRI-based findings of a ring of pancreatic tissue and an annular duct surrounding the second portion of the duodenum. It has been shown that direct visualization of the entirety of the encircling ring on CT and MRI is not requisite for the diagnosis of annular pancreas. In the proper clinical scenario, such as unexplained chronic pancreatitis, pancreatic parenchyma extending along the anterior and posterolateral aspect of the second portion of the duodenum should be viewed with suspicion, even if complete surrounding tissue is not seen. In these cases, the pancreatic ring may be too thin to visualize on imaging at some points throughout its course as it may extend in the duodenal wall. In some cases, depending on the quality of the CT images, the fullness of the pancreatic head may be mistaken as an underlying mass lesion and MRCP may offer further characterization of the congenital ductal anomaly. A high association with pancreas divisum approaching 40% of patients with annular pancreas has been reported and may be seen on CT or MRI. There is also association with chronic pancreatitis and calcifications may thus be identified in the pancreas.

PEARLS

- Annular pancreas is a rare congenital abnormality which results from the absence of rotation of the ventral anlage of the pancreas resulting in a portion of the pancreas encircling the second portion of the duodenum.

- In adults, annular pancreas may present with duodenal obstruction or pancreatitis.

- There is a high association with pancreas divisum and annular pancreas; up to 40% of patients with annular pancreas are found to have pancreas divisum.

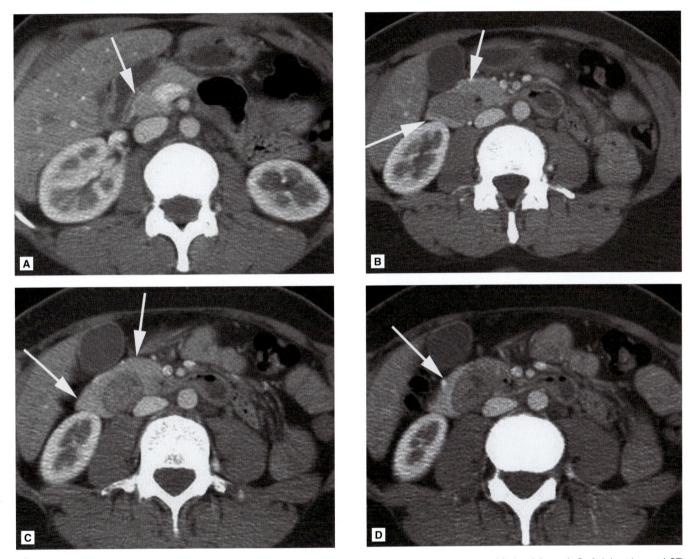

1. **A.** Axial, enhanced CT image demonstrates a normal appearance and position of the pancreas at this level (arrow). **B.** Axial, enhanced CT image more inferiorly demonstrates a portion of the pancreatic parenchyma posterolateral to the duodenum (arrows). **C.** Axial, enhanced CT image more inferiorly now demonstrates the pancreas to nearly completely encircle the second portion of the duodenum (arrows). **D.** Axial, enhanced CT image more inferiorly reveals a portion of the pancreas lateral to the duodenum (arrow). **E.** Coronal, enhanced CT image illustrates the pancreas, a portion of which is seen inferolateral to the second portion of the duodenum (arrows).

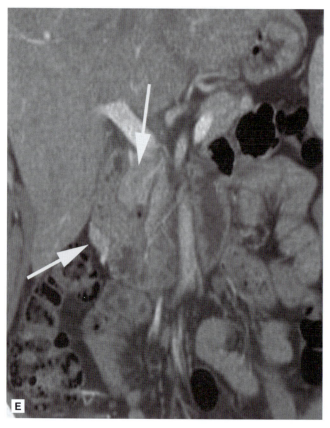

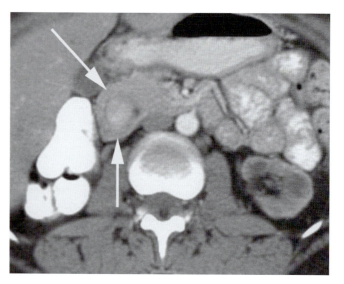

2. Axial, enhanced CT image demonstrates the pancreas completely encircling the second portion of the duodenum (arrows).

1. (*continued*)

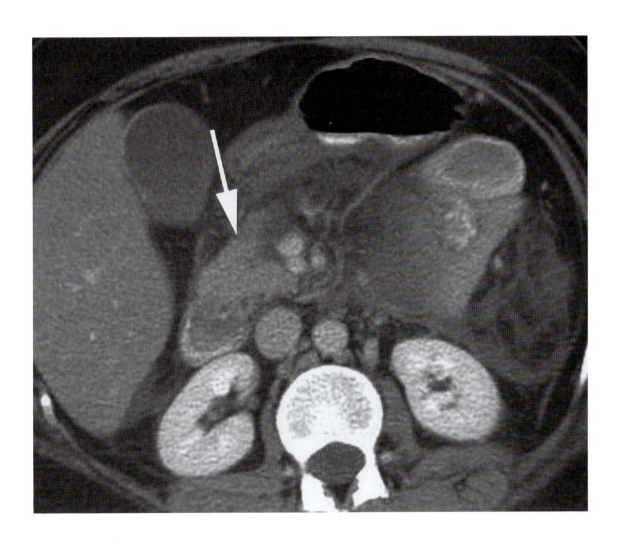

Case 3–10   Acute Pancreatitis

PRESENTATION

Patients typically present with nausea, vomiting, and mild-to-severe epigastric pain which is often described as radiating to the back.

FINDINGS

Depending on the severity of the acute pancreatitis, the imaging findings may range for pancreatic enlargement to pancreatic and peripancreatic inflammation, pseudocyst formation, and necrosis.

DIFFERENTIAL DIAGNOSIS

- Groove pancreatitis
- Autoimmune pancreatitis
- Pancreatic adenocarcinoma

COMMENTS

Acute pancreatitis is defined as acute inflammation of the pancreas, the severity of which ranges from mild inflammation of the gland to frank pancreatic necrosis. The most common causes of acute pancreatitis include alcohol abuse as well as gallstone-related pancreatitis in which biliary stones serve to obstruct the distal common bile duct and pancreatic duct, resulting in pancreatitis. Other less common etiologies of acute pancreatitis include iatrogenic causes, such as ERCP, inherited forms of pancreatitis, certain drugs including antimicrobials, hypertriglyceridemia and hypercalcemia, congenital anomalies such as pancreas divisum, and autoimmune pancreatitis, among myriad others.

The pathophysiology of acute pancreatitis involves an initial injury of the pancreatic acinar cells, resulting in the release of pancreatic enzymes into the interstitial and endothelial spaces of the gland. The resulting enzymatic degradation of the gland yields a vascular injury which ultimately produces tissue edema and oxidative stress. The vascular injury also leads to increased permeability which may yield thrombosis, hemorrhage, and glandular necrosis.

Patients with acute pancreatitis typically present with nausea, vomiting, and epigastric pain. In severe cases with pancreatic hemorrhage, Turner sign which is defined as flank bruising or Cullen sign, defined as bruising about the umbilicus, may be identified. In addition to the more mild presentations with epigastric pain, patients with severe acute pancreatitis may present with hypotension, metabolic acidosis, respiratory and renal failure related to a systemic inflammatory response syndrome. In addition, elevation of serum amylase and lipase is also typically observed in patients with acute pancreatitis.

In patients with clinically suspected complicated acute pancreatitis, CT is the imaging modality of choice for the assessment of the gland and the evaluation of any potential complications. Nevertheless, initial plain radiographs may demonstrate secondary findings such as the presence of a localized functional ileus, termed a "sentinel loop," as evidenced by small or large bowel dilatation in the vicinity of the pancreatic inflammation as well as the so called "colon cutoff" sign in which spasm of the colon in the region of the splenic flexure yields an abrupt termination of the upstream, air-filled colon. In addition, pancreatic calcifications may be seen on plain radiographs suggesting a history of chronic pancreatitis.

CT with intravenous contrast is typically employed to characterize the gland and assess for any complications in cases of moderate and severe acute pancreatitis. With intravenous contrast, it is critical to assess for pancreatic necrosis, defined as focal or diffuse zones of nonenhanced pancreatic parenchyma, the extent of which is typically further characterized. On CT, parenchymal enlargement as well as peripancreatic inflammation and fluid are typically identified in cases of acute pancreatitis. Also, the presence of pseudocysts is readily identified on CT. While typically located about the pancreatic parenchyma in the retroperitoneum, pancreatic pseudocysts may invaginate into atypical locations such as the gastric wall as well as the splenic hilum or splenic parenchyma. Other complications related to acute pancreatitis which should be sought on CT imaging include venous thromboses which typically affect the splenic vein but may extend into the portal venous system or involve the superior mesenteric vein. In addition to venous complications, arterial pseudoaneurysms may form secondary to acute pancreatitis; while splenic arterial pseudoaneurysms are typical, pseudoaneurysms may involve other branches of the celiac axis or superior mesenteric artery. Given their inherent instability, arterial pseudoaneurysms may lead to significant hemorrhage within the abdomen.

PEARLS

- In patients with clinically suspected complicated acute pancreatitis, CT is the imaging modality of choice for assessing the gland and evaluating for any potential complications.

- The identification of pancreatic necrosis and the assessment of its degree of parenchymal involvement are critical in determining appropriate management in cases of severe acute pancreatitis.

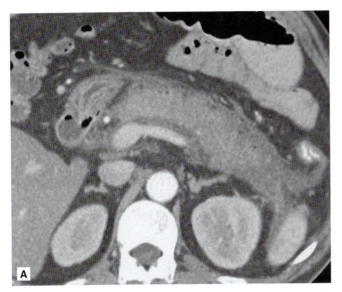

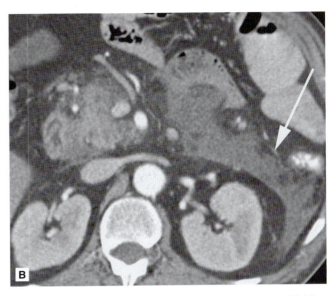

1. **A.** Axial, contrast-enhanced CT image demonstrates enlargement of the pancreas with moderate peripancreatic inflammation and fluid. **B.** Axial, contrast-enhanced CT image demonstrates inferior extension of the peripancreatic inflammation and fluid along the retroperitoneum (arrow).

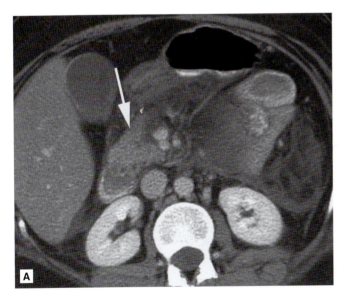

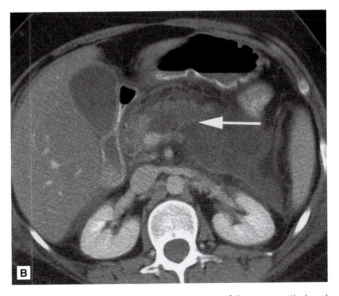

2. **A.** Axial, contrast-enhanced CT image demonstrates peripancreatic inflammation and fluid with normal enhancement of the pancreatic head (arrow). **B.** Axial, contrast-enhanced CT image demonstrates peripancreatic inflammation and fluid with abnormally decreased enhancement of the pancreatic body (arrow) consistent with pancreatic necrosis.

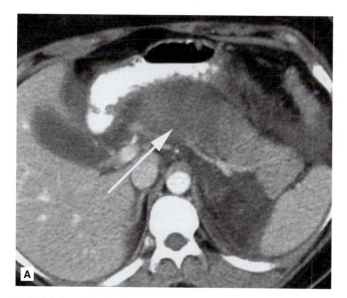

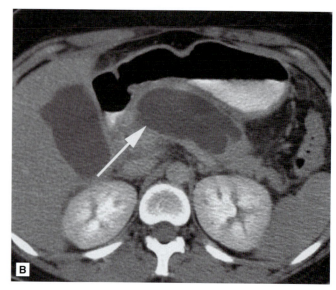

3. A. Axial, contrast-enhanced CT image demonstrates pancreatic enlargement, peripancreatic inflammation and fluid, and abnormally decreased enhancement of the pancreatic body (arrow) consistent with pancreatic necrosis. **B.** Axial, contrast-enhanced CT image from examination performed at a later date demonstrates resolution of the peripancreatic inflammation and interval development of a pancreatic walled off necrosis (arrow).

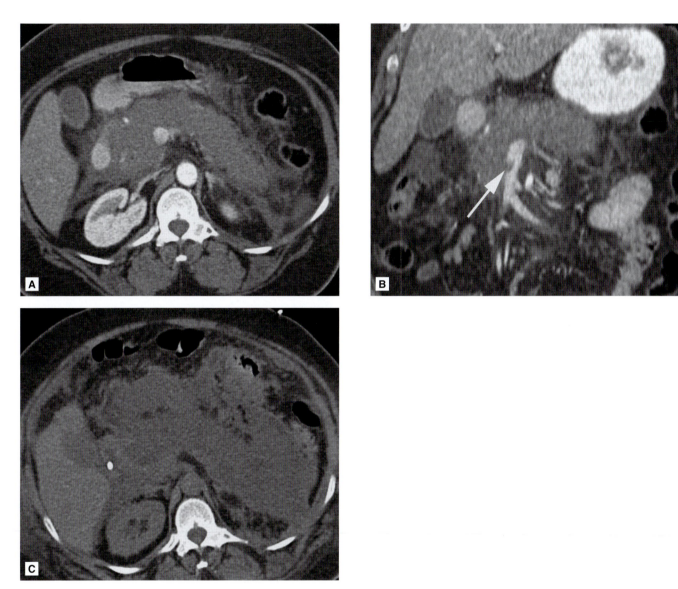

4. A. Axial, contrast-enhanced CT image demonstrates pancreatic enlargement and peripancreatic inflammation and fluid consistent with acute pancreatitis. **B.** Coronal, contrast-enhanced CT image demonstrates partially occlusive superior mesenteric vein (SMV) thrombus (arrow) related to the acute pancreatitis. **C.** Axial, unenhanced CT image from examination performed at a later date demonstrates marked enlargement and hypoattenuation of the pancreas suggesting diffuse glandular and extra-pancreatic necrosis.

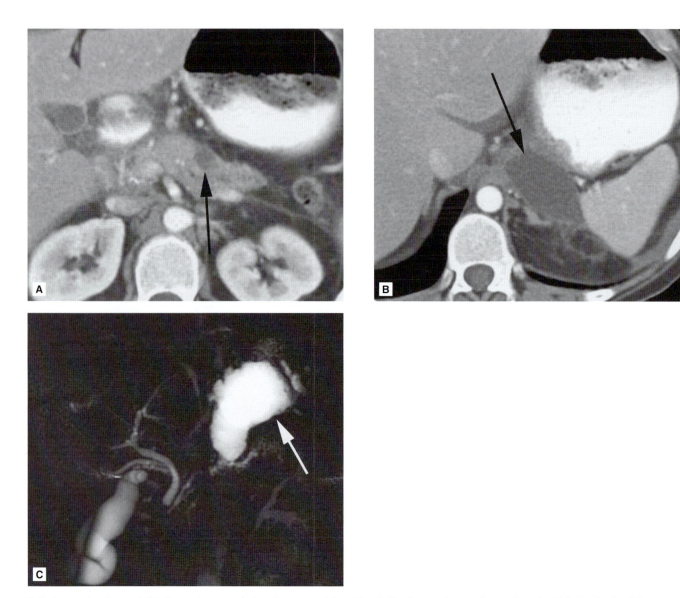

5. A. Contrast-enhanced CT shows changes of chronic pancreatitis with calcification and a small pseudocyst within the body of the pancreas (arrow). **B.** Shows a large pseudocyst replacing the body of the pancreas (arrow). **C.** Thick slab MRCP shows a large T2 bright pseudocyst communicating with the pancreatic duct (arrow).

PRESENTATION

Recurrent abdominal pain, epigastric tenderness, fever, sepsis, shock

FINDINGS

The term necrotizing pancreatitis commonly refers to pancreatic necrosis with infection with gas-forming organisms, thus, the presence of gas within an inflamed pancreas is pathognomonic in the proper clinical setting.

DIFFERENTIAL DIAGNOSIS

- Acute pancreatitis though the presence of gas is pathognomonic in the proper clinical setting of acute pancreatitis.

COMMENTS

Emphysematous pancreatitis is a rare, severe complication of acute pancreatitis which is characterized by the presence of gas within the pancreatic parenchyma. When compared to acute pancreatitis, the mortality and morbidity are markedly elevated with mortality rates reported to approach 50%. There have been reported associations between necrotizing pancreatitis and diabetes as well as other etiologies of immune compromise such as human immunodeficiency virus (HIV) and chronic renal failure.

Though gas within the pancreas may be associated with penetrating duodenal ulcers, prior instrumentation, patulous ampulla of Vater, as well as enteropancreatic fistulae, the term necrotizing pancreatitis commonly refers to pancreatic necrosis with infection with gas-forming organisms.

Typically, the infection results from gram-negative organisms such as *Escherichia coli* though often the source of infection is polymicrobial.

CT is the modality of choice for the diagnosis and characterization of the location and extent of gas within and around the pancreatic parenchyma. The gas may be confined to the pancreatic parenchyma but often tracks throughout the anterior pararenal space and other regions of the retroperitoneum and may extend into the lesser sac and peritoneal cavity. Though intravenous contrast is not necessary to diagnose and evaluate the extent of gas in the pancreas, its administration may be useful to evaluate the degrees of pancreatic necrosis. Imaging findings associated with acute pancreatitis are typically present including peripancreatic stranding and fluid with possible pseudocyst formation, among others.

PEARLS

- Emphysematous pancreatitis is a rare, severe complication of acute pancreatitis which is characterized by the presence of gas within the pancreatic parenchyma with mortality rates reported to approach 50%.

- Typically, necrotizing pancreatitis results from gram-negative organisms such as *E coli* though often the source of infection is polymicrobial.

- CT is the modality of choice for the diagnosis and characterization of the location and extent of gas within and around the pancreatic parenchyma.

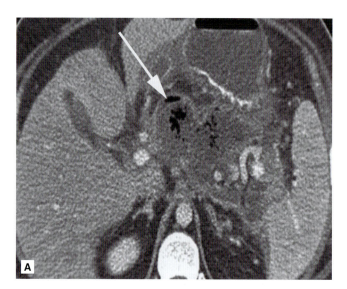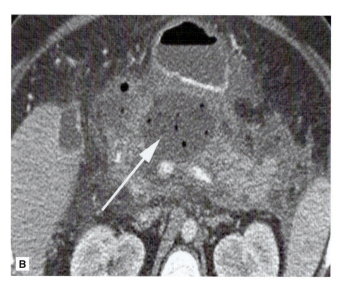

1. A. Axial, enhanced CT image demonstrates hypoattenuating area of pancreatic necrosis containing gas (arrow) consistent with pancreatic necrosis. **B.** Axial, enhanced CT image demonstrates a region of pancreatic necrosis containing gas (arrow) consistent with pancreatic necrosis.

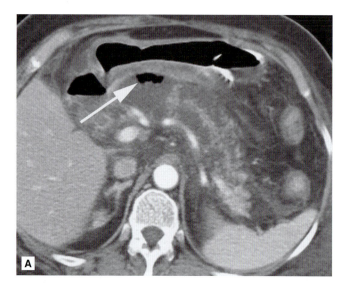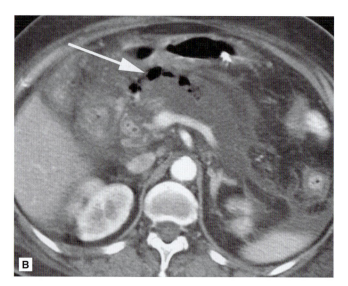

2. A. Axial, enhanced CT image reveals large areas of pancreatic necrosis, portions of which contain gas (arrow). **B.** Axial, enhanced CT image reveals a large area of pancreatic necrosis containing gas (arrow).

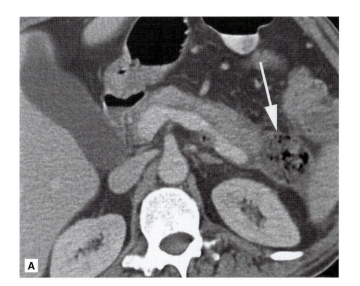

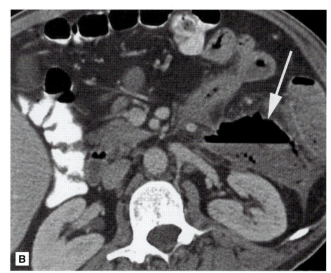

3. A. Axial, enhanced CT image reveals a focal area of pancreatic necrosis containing gas (arrow) within the region of the pancreatic tail.
B. Axial, enhanced CT image reveals a focal area of pancreatic necrosis containing gas (arrow) in the region of the pancreatic tail.

PRESENTATION

Chronic, intermittent abdominal pain, diarrhea, and weight loss

FINDINGS

Imaging findings of chronic pancreatitis typically include pancreatic atrophy, the presence of calcification, and the main pancreatic duct may be noted to be irregularly strictured with intermittent areas of dilatation.

DIFFERENTIAL DIAGNOSIS

- Pancreatic atrophy unrelated to chronic pancreatitis (eg, malignancy with obstruction of pancreatic duct)

COMMENTS

The most common etiology of chronic pancreatitis is excessive alcohol consumption, accounting for greater than 50% of cases. In up to 30% of patients with chronic pancreatitis, the etiology is unknown and these cases are considered idiopathic though it is postulated that a certain portion of these cases may be due to atypical genetic mutations. Both congenital and acquired mechanical obstruction to the outflow of pancreatic exocrine secretions may result in chronic pancreatitis. Thus, pancreas divisum and annular pancreas are considered congenital etiologies while acquired etiologies include traumatic pancreatic duct stricture or stricture related to long-standing inflammation in adjacent organs such as the duodenum. Other, less common etiologies of chronic pancreatitis include hyperlipidemia and hypercalcemia, cystic fibrosis, nutritional (ie, tropical) pancreatitis, hereditary pancreatitis, autoimmune pancreatitis, as well as medication use. The mean age of patients affected with chronic pancreatitis is approximately 45 years with a bimodal age distribution seen in patients with idiopathic pancreatitis.

In contradistinction to acute pancreatitis, chronic pancreatitis represent chronic, irreversible inflammation which leads to fibrosis and calcification. As such, patients often complain of chronic pain and exhibit normal or only minimally elevated pancreatic enzymes. In long-standing cases of chronic pancreatitis, signs and symptoms related to exocrine and endocrine insufficiency may be seen such as steatorrhea and diabetes mellitus, respectively. The pathophysiology of chronic pancreatitis is related to intraductal obstruction, the direct toxin effecting fibrosis and inflammation, the presence of necrosis and fibrosis, as well as ischemia related to fibrosis and obstruction.

Using CT, the findings in patients with chronic pancreatitis typically include pancreatic atrophy and the presence of calcification. When clearly seen, the main pancreatic duct may be noted to be irregularly strictured with intermittent areas of dilatation. In addition, the fibrosis may result in narrowing and relative obstruction of the distal, intrapancreatic common bile duct. On MRI, the findings of chronic pancreatitis include low signal on T1-weighted images related to the decreased protein content of the parenchyma, decreased and delayed enhancement after intravenous contrast administration, as well as the presence of dilated side branches of the pancreatic duct. In addition, pancreatic atrophy and calcification as well as stricturing with intermittent dilatation of the main pancreatic duct, which may contain stones, are readily identified when present. On both CT and MRI, areas of acute chronic pancreatitis or focal areas of mass-like fibrosis may pose a diagnostic dilemma given a similar imaging appearance to pancreatic adenocarcinoma.

PEARLS

- Chronic pancreatitis represents chronic, irreversible inflammation which leads to fibrosis and calcification of the parenchyma.

- Findings of chronic pancreatitis include low signal on T1-weighted MRI images, decreased and delayed enhancement after intravenous contrast administration, as well as the presence of dilated side branches of the pancreatic duct.

- Areas of acute chronic pancreatitis or focal areas of mass-like fibrosis may pose a diagnostic dilemma given a similar imaging appearance to pancreatic adenocarcinoma.

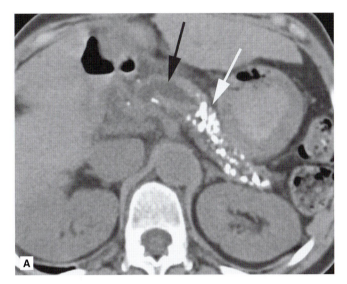
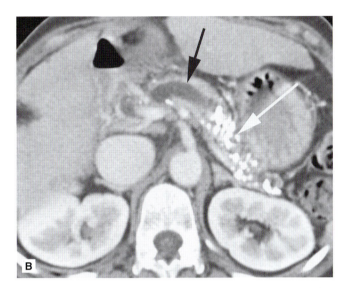

1. A. Axial, unenhanced CT image demonstrates pancreatic parenchymal calcifications (white arrow) as well as dilatation of the pancreatic duct (black arrow) related to fibrosis and structuring of the main duct. **B.** Axial, enhanced CT image demonstrates pancreatic parenchymal calcifications (white arrow) as well as dilatation of the pancreatic duct (black arrow) related to fibrosis and structuring of the main duct. Also note the atrophy of the residual pancreatic parenchyma.

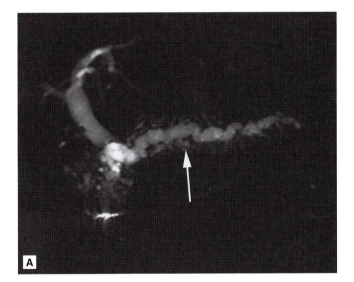
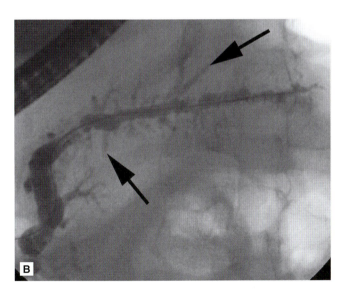

2. A. MRCP image reveals dilatation of both the main pancreatic duct as well as the common bile duct related to chronic pancreatitis and pancreatic fibrosis. Also, numerous dilated side branches are seen (arrow). **B.** ERCP image reveals irregular dilatation of the main pancreatic duct and numerous dilated side branches are seen (arrows).

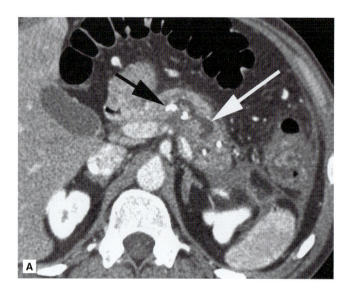
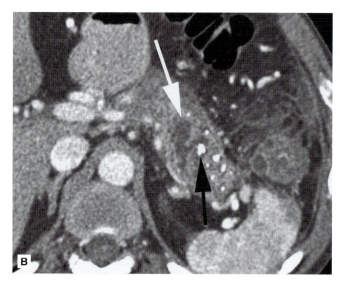

3. A. Axial, enhanced CT image demonstrates pancreatic parenchymal calcifications (black arrow) as well as dilatation of the pancreatic duct (white arrow). Incidental note is made of active inflammation consistent with acute on chronic pancreatitis as evidenced by peripancreatic inflammation which also involves the adjacent colon. **B.** Axial, enhanced CT image again demonstrates pancreatic parenchymal calcifications (black arrow) as well as dilatation of the pancreatic duct (white arrow).

PRESENTATION

Chronic abdominal pain and jaundice. Severe abdominal pain associated with acute pancreatitis is rare.

FINDINGS

The typical features associated with autoimmune pancreatitis include diffuse enlargement of the pancreatic parenchyma with loss of the typical lobular contour as well as a surrounding, peripancreatic "halo" of hypoattenuation on CT. Extrapancreatic manifestations include lung and renal lesions as well as the presence of biliary ductal strictures.

DIFFERENTIAL DIAGNOSIS

- Chronic pancreatitis related to other etiologies such as alcohol

- Pancreatic adenocarcinoma in cases of focal pancreatitis

COMMENTS

Autoimmune pancreatitis is a rare cause of chronic pancreatitis, reportedly responsible for 5% to 10% of all cases of chronic pancreatitis. Though patients' age on diagnosis of autoimmune pancreatitis varies widely, patients are typically greater than 50 years of age; men are more commonly affected than women. Similar to other autoimmune diseases, autoimmune pancreatitis is often associated with other immune diseases including inflammatory bowel disease, sarcoidosis, and rheumatoid arthritis, among others. Autoimmune pancreatitis has been associated with hypergammaglobulinemia and elevated levels of immunoglobulin G4 (IgG4) though the latter may be a secondary response to the inflammation associated with this disease.

Patients with autoimmune pancreatitis typically present with chronic, mild abdominal pain, jaundice, and weight loss.

The symptoms of autoimmune pancreatitis may be intermittent with periods or remission; severe abdominal pain typically seen with acute pancreatitis is rare. Patients with autoimmune pancreatitis are often responsive to corticosteroid therapy and this fact has been used as a diagnostic criterion for this disease.

On imaging, the typical features associated with autoimmune pancreatitis include diffuse enlargement of the pancreatic parenchyma with loss of the typical lobular contour as well as a surrounding, peripancreatic "halo" of hypoattenuation on CT. Additionally, atrophy of the distal pancreas may be seen along with enlargement of regional lymph nodes. Though typically diffuse, autoimmune pancreatitis may be focal and the distinction between autoimmune pancreatitis and pancreatic adenocarcinoma may be challenging though diffuse, irregular ductal narrowing as well as extrapancreatic manifestations (see later) may be helpful in diagnosing autoimmune pancreatitis. In addition to the aforementioned pancreatic findings, autoimmune pancreatitis may present with biliary ductal narrowing which may result in upstream biliary dilatation. Also, masslike pulmonary and renal lesions as well as periaortic soft tissue infiltration have been associated with autoimmune pancreatitis.

PEARLS

- Autoimmune pancreatitis is typically responsive to corticosteroid therapy.

- Hypergammaglobulinemia and elevated IgG4 levels are associated with autoimmune pancreatitis.

- In cases of autoimmune pancreatitis, a diffusely enlarged, "sausage-shaped" pancreas with surrounding "halo" of low attenuation is often seen on CT.

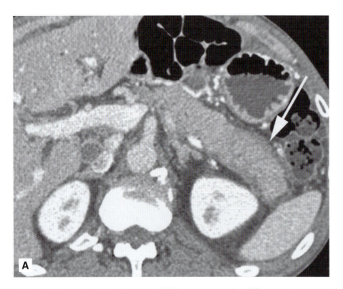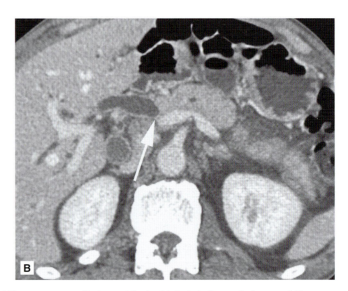

1. **A.** Axial, contrast-enhanced CT image reveals diffuse enlargement of the pancreas with loss of typical lobulated morphology and the presence of a low-attenuation "halo" (arrow). **B.** Axial, contrast-enhanced CT image reveals diffuse enlargement of the pancreas with dilatation of the suprapancreatic common bile duct (arrow).

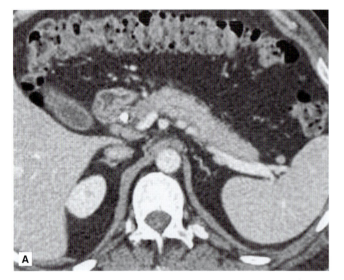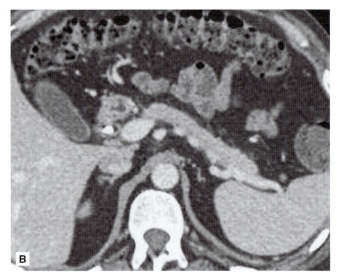

2. **A.** Axial, contrast-enhanced CT image reveals mild, diffuse enlargement of the pancreas and the presence of a low-attenuation "halo". **B.** Axial, contrast-enhanced CT image demonstrates the near-complete resolution of the findings of autoimmune pancreatitis after approximately 8 weeks of corticosteroid therapy.

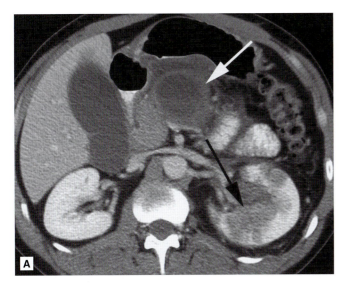

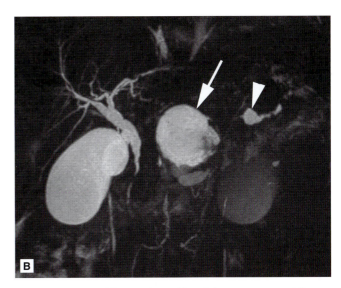

3. A. Axial, contrast-enhanced CT image demonstrates a pancreatic pseudocyst (white arrow) in a patient with autoimmune pancreatitis, an uncommon finding. Also, note the ill-defined renal mass lesions (black arrow), a well-described association with autoimmune pancreatitis. **B.** Coronal MRCP image demonstrates a pancreatic pseudocyst (arrow) as well as irregular dilatation of the distal pancreatic duct (white arrowhead). Also, biliary dilatation related to the pancreatic inflammation is well seen.

PRESENTATION

Recurrent abdominal pain, vomiting, and patients rarely present with jaundice

FINDINGS

The classic imaging finding in cases of groove pancreatitis is the presence of soft tissue attenuation within the pancreaticoduodenal groove. In addition, small cystic lesions may be identified within the duodenal wall and groove region.

DIFFERENTIAL DIAGNOSIS

- Focal pancreatitis
- Pancreatic adenocarcinoma
- Groove carcinoma
- Groove neuroendocrine tumors
- Ampullary or periampullary tumors

COMMENTS

Groove pancreatitis represents a rare form of focal, chronic pancreatitis in which the pancreaticoduodenal groove is involved. The pancreaticoduodenal groove represents the potential space bordered by head of the pancreas, the common bile duct, and the duodenum. Two forms of this disease process have been described, the pure form in which the chronic inflammation affects the pancreaticoduodenal groove while sparing the pancreatic head and the segmental form which involves the pancreatic head in addition to involvement of the pancreaticoduodenal groove. The underlying etiology of groove pancreatitis remains controversial though several factors including biliary disease, gastric resections, peptic ulcer disease, and pancreatic heterotopia in the duodenum, among others have been related to this disease process.

The hallmark of groove pancreatitis is the formation of fibrous scar tissue in the pancreaticoduodenal groove and pancreatic head in cases of the segmental form of the disease. Given the location of this disease, the duodenum is also affected by chronic inflammation resulting in scar and the development of stenosis which may become severe and symptomatic. In addition, there is the formation of cystic lesions within the duodenal wall and pancreaticoduodenal groove which are theorized to be secondary to cystic dystrophy of heterotopic pancreatic tissue within the duodenal wall. Finally, Brunner gland hyperplasia in the duodenum is typical in groove pancreatitis.

On imaging, the classic finding on CT is the presence of soft tissue attenuation within the pancreaticoduodenal groove which may display relative delayed enhancement after intravenous contrast administration. In addition, small cystic lesions may be identified within the duodenal wall and groove region. On MRI, multiple imaging features have been described and may be useful in differentiating groove pancreatitis from pancreatic adenocarcinoma which shares many similar imaging features and may pose a diagnostic dilemma. As on CT, groove pancreatitis demonstrates soft tissue within the groove, typically hypointense on T1 and variable on T2-weighted images. Similar to CT, delayed enhancement of this fibrotic mass may be seen. Cystic lesions within the duodenal wall and pancreatic groove are readily appreciated on MRI. Pancreatic edema, thickening and stenosis of the duodenum, as well as tapering of the distal common bile duct and main pancreatic duct have been described in groove pancreatitis and may be well seen on MRI. The smoothly tapering distal common bile duct and lack of vascular invasion have been described as usual differentiating features of groove pancreatitis from pancreatic adenocarcinoma.

PEARLS

- Groove pancreatitis represents a rare form of focal, chronic pancreatitis in which the pancreaticoduodenal groove is involved.

- The hallmark of groove pancreatitis is the formation of fibrous scar tissue in the pancreaticoduodenal groove and pancreatic head.

- On imaging, the classic findings include the presence of soft tissue attenuation within the pancreaticoduodenal groove which may display relative delayed enhancement after intravenous contrast administration as well as small cystic lesions within the duodenal wall and groove region.

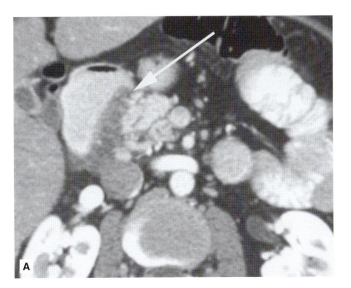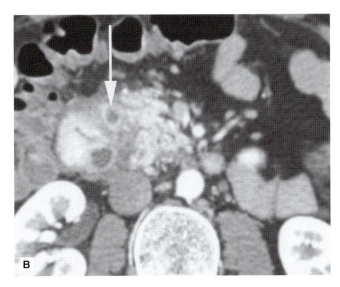

1. A. Axial, enhanced CT image demonstrates focal, relatively hypoattenuating region of soft tissue in the pancreaticoduodenal groove (arrow).
B. Axial, enhanced CT image demonstrates focal, relatively hypoattenuating region of soft tissue in the pancreaticoduodenal groove containing several cystic areas (arrow).

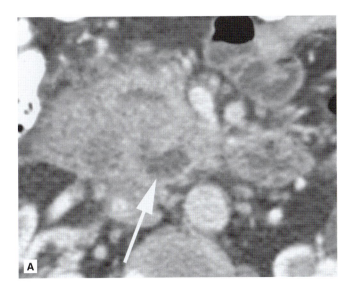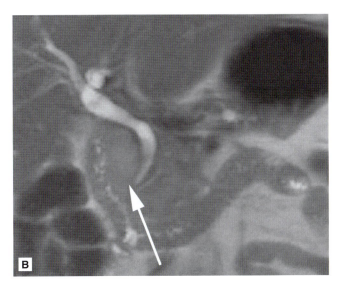

2. A. Axial, enhanced CT image demonstrates focal, relatively hypoattenuating region of soft tissue in the pancreaticoduodenal groove containing a cystic area (arrow). **B.** Coronal T2-weighted MRI image reveals a focal, relatively hyperintense area of soft tissue in the pancreaticoduodenal groove (arrow).

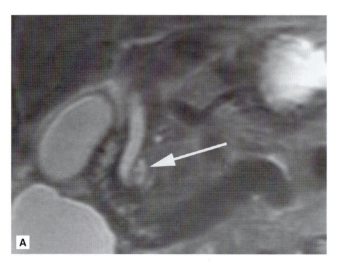

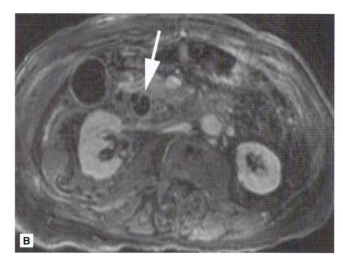

3. A. Coronal T2-weighted MRI image reveals several small cystic areas in the region of the pancreaticoduodenal groove (arrow). **B.** Axial, enhanced T1-weighted image demonstrates several cysts in the pancreaticoduodenal groove (arrow).

CHAPTER 4

SPLEEN

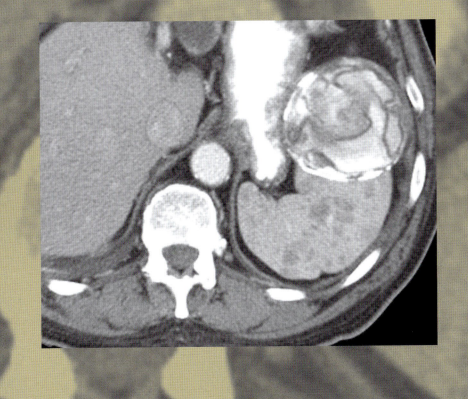

BENIGN SPLENIC LESIONS

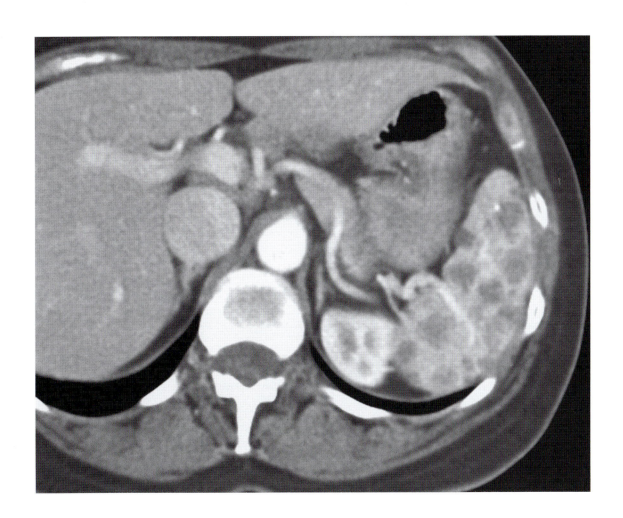

PRESENTATION

- Incidental finding

FINDINGS

Imaging findings are typically that of a simple cyst; internal septations are frequently identified.

DIFFERENTIAL DIAGNOSIS

- Splenic lymphangioma
- Splenic hamartoma
- Splenic hemangioma

COMMENTS

True (primary) splenic cysts are epithelial-lined lesions, in contradistinction to splenic pseudocysts. The epithelial lining of true splenic cysts suggests a developmental origin and several hypotheses as to their pathogenesis have been posited, including infolding of the peritoneal mesothelium after rupture of the splenic capsule, origin from normal lymph spaces of the splenic parenchyma, as well as peritoneal mesothelium cells sequestered in a splenic sulcus, among others. True splenic cysts may be categorized, depending on the lining, as epidermoid, dermoid, or mesothelial.

Though often asymptomatic and incidentally discovered, true splenic cysts may become quite large and patients may present with symptoms referable to the left upper quadrant including pain and abdominal fullness. True cysts, given their developmental origin are often encountered in a younger patient population, with the average age of the patient approaching 20 years, though the age ranges from infants to older adults. Complications of splenic cysts include infection, hemorrhage, as well as rupture.

Imaging characteristics are consistent with those of a cyst. On ultrasound (US), splenic cysts typically demonstrate the classic features of a simple cyst, lacking internal architecture. Though less common in splenic pseudocysts, calcification may be associated with primary splenic cysts. Also, thin internal septations as well as internal echoes and layering debris may be seen on US, possibly related to prior episodes of hemorrhage. On computed tomography (CT), similar findings of a cyst are seen, that is, an avascular, well-circumscribed, relatively hypoattenuating lesion. Internal septations are often frequently identified at CT as well. As on US, areas of calcification may be identified in cases of true splenic cysts, though less commonly than in splenic pseudocysts. The water content on splenic cysts results in hypointense T1 and hyperintense T2 signal on magnetic resonance imaging (MRI) with respect to normal splenic parenchyma with no enhancement after contrast administration. The presence of hemorrhage, however, may increase the expected signal of the cyst on T1-weighted MRI.

PEARLS

- **True splenic cysts are epithelial-lined lesions; the epithelial lining of true splenic cysts suggests a developmental origin.**

- **May become quite large and cause symptoms related to mass effects in addition to complications such as infection, hemorrhage, as well as rupture.**

- **Imaging findings are typically that of a simple splenic cyst.**

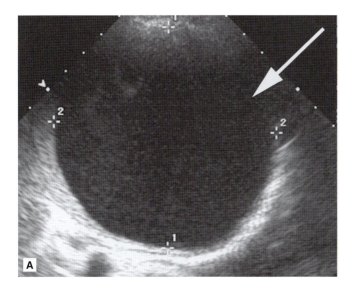
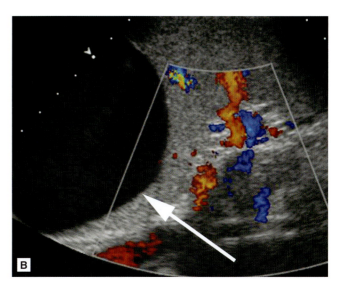

1. A. US image demonstrates the presence of a large, simple epithelial cyst within the spleen (arrow). **B.** Doppler US image demonstrates the presence of a large epithelial cyst with expected avascularity within the spleen (arrow).

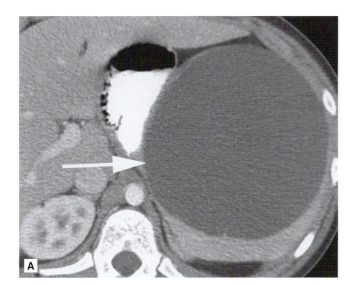
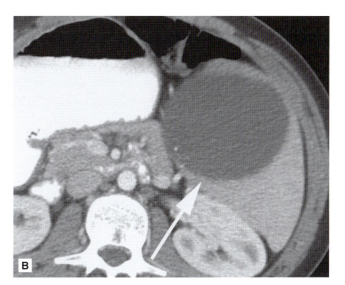

2. A. Axial, portal venous phase CT image demonstrates the presence of a large, simple epithelial splenic cyst (arrow). **B.** Axial, portal venous phase CT image more inferiorly demonstrates the presence of a large, simple epithelial splenic cyst (arrow).

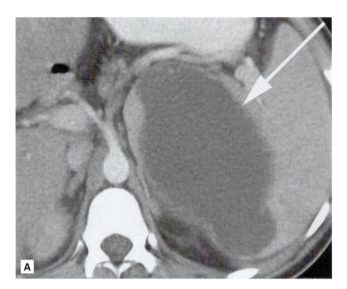

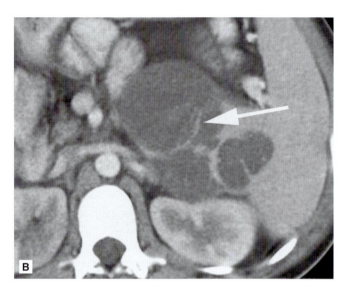

3. A. Axial, portal venous phase CT image demonstrates the presence of a large, simple epithelial splenic cyst with several thin septations (arrow). **B.** Axial, portal venous phase CT image more inferiorly demonstrates the presence of multiple lobulations and septations within an epithelial splenic cyst (arrow).

PRESENTATION

Typically, incidental finding but may present with left upper quadrant fullness and pain.

FINDINGS

The variability of pathological features in splenic hemangiomas leads to varied appearances with several patterns of enhancement as well as the possibility of calcification and cystic areas.

DIFFERENTIAL DIAGNOSIS

- Splenic lymphangioma
- Splenic metastases
- Splenic angiosarcoma
- Splenic hamartoma

COMMENTS

Splenic hemangioma, though representing the most common benign primary splenic neoplasm is, nevertheless, rare. Splenic hemangiomas are thought to be of congenital origin and represent a proliferation of vascular channels, heterogeneous in their size from capillary to cavernous, lined by a single layer of endothelium. Typically, these vascular channels may be separated by splenic pulp tissue or fibrous septae. Splenic hemangiomas may be intrasplenic or exophytic and, though size is variable, are typically less than 2 cm in size. Though lesions may be cystic or solid, smaller lesions tend to be solid. Larger, cavernous hemangiomas may develop areas of thrombosis and infarction.

The incidence of splenic hemangiomas reportedly ranges from less than 1% to nearly 15% in autopsy studies and is similar in men and women, though possibly with a slight male predominance. Typically, splenic hemangiomas are single, small, asymptomatic, incidentally discovered lesions. Splenic hemangiomas may be seen in the setting of diffuse hemangiomatosis such as Klippel-Trénaunay syndrome. However, with progressive enlargement, patients may present with signs and symptoms referable to the left upper quadrant such as a palpable mass and abdominal pain. Though splenomegaly may be seen with splenic hemangiomas, it is an uncommon finding. Complications from splenic hemangiomas, though rare, include rupture, hypersplenism and malignant degeneration.

Malignant degeneration is reportedly more frequent in cases of large splenic hemangiomas or multiple hemangiomas. Kassabach-Merritt, a consumptive coagulopathy occurring in vascular tumors, has been reported in large splenic hemangiomas.

Given the variability in their pathologic features, splenic hemangiomas may have a somewhat variable imaging appearance, though the majority presents as predominately solid lesions with cystic areas. On US, splenic hemangiomas are commonly seen as echogenic lesions, often with cystic areas. When present, calcification of the lesion is identified as echogenic, shadowing areas. At unenhanced CT, splenic hemangiomas are typically hypo- or isoattenuating with respect to normal splenic parenchyma and demonstrate a mottled pattern of enhancement after contrast administration, likely due to the cystic, nonenhancing portions of the tumor. Centripetal enhancement patterns similar to hepatic hemangiomas have also been described. Areas of calcification ranging from thin, curvilinear areas to coarser calcification related to necrosis may also be clearly seen on CT. On MRI, splenic hemangiomas are typically isointense on T1 and hyperintense on T2 with respect to normal splenic parenchyma. Several enhancement patterns on MRI have been described, including early homogeneous enhancement which persist, early, peripheral enhancement with delayed homogeneous enhancement, as well as progressive centripetal enhancement with persistent lack of enhancement of a central scar. As with CT, larger lesions demonstrate more variable enhancement patterns, likely related to the variability on pathological features including areas of thrombosis and infarction. This variability and the subsequent lack of specificity of the imaging findings of larger splenic hemangiomas may preclude a definitive imaging diagnosis.

PEARLS

- **Though representing the most common primary benign splenic neoplasm, hemangiomas are rare.**
- **Typically represent single, small, incidentally discovered splenic lesions.**
- **Varied imaging appearance given variability of pathological features.**

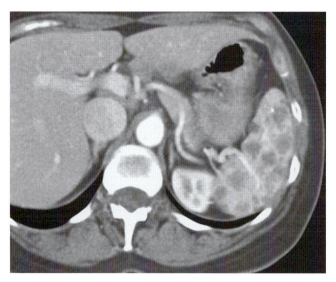

1. Axial, contrast-enhanced CT image in a patient with hemangiomatosis demonstrates numerous relatively hypoattenuating splenic lesions.

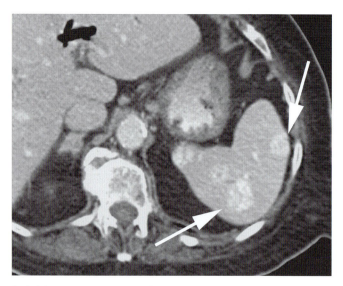

2. Axial, contrast-enhanced CT image demonstrates several splenic hemangiomas which are seen to avidly enhance relatively homogeneously (arrows).

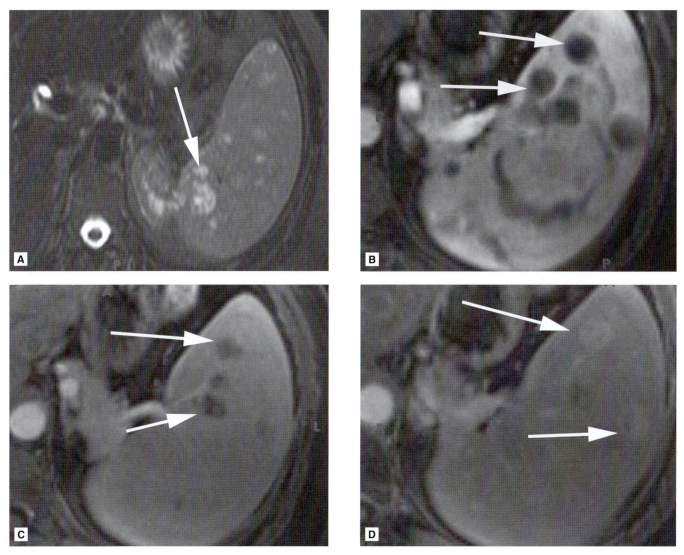

3. A. Axial, T2-weighted MRI image demonstrates several T2-hyperintense splenic hemangiomas (arrow). **B.** Axial, T1-weighted contrast-enhanced, arterial phase image demonstrates hypointense splenic hemangiomas (arrows). **C.** Axial, T1-weighted contrast-enhanced, portal venous phase image demonstrates hypointense splenic hemangiomas with patchy areas of enhancement noted (arrows). **D.** Axial, T1-weighted contrast-enhanced, delayed phase image demonstrates hyperintense splenic hemangiomas (arrows).

PRESENTATION

• Incidental finding

FINDINGS

Lymphangiomas are typically identified as cystic, avascular lesions in which internal septations or calcifications may be seen.

DIFFERENTIAL DIAGNOSIS

• Splenic angiosarcoma

• Splenic metastases

• Splenic hamartoma

• Splenic hemangioma

• Splenic cyst

COMMENTS

Lymphangiomas represent a relatively rare, benign splenic lesion consisting of endothelium-lined spaces containing proteinaceous material, in contradistinction to splenic hemangiomas which contain blood. Both splenic lymphangiomas and hemangiomas are vasoformative with hemangiomas being more common. Lymphangiomas of the spleen may present as discrete, single nodules, multiple discrete nodules or diffuse lymphangiomatosis. Lymphangiomas are typically solid or microcystic and a central scar may be present. Based on the location and size of the endothelial-lined channels, lymphangiomas are categorized into capillary, cavernous, and cystic types. Though single lymphangiomas may be intraparenchymal, a subcapsular location is more common owing to the concentration of the splenic lymphatics. When multifocal, lymphangiomas are typically separated by distinct areas of normal-appearing splenic parenchyma. Finally, lymphangiomas may present as large cystic lesions or as more diffuse involvement of the spleen in which little splenic parenchyma is spared, termed lymphangiomatosis.

Lymphangiomas of the spleen are more commonly identified in children. Typically, these are incidentally discovered, asymptomatic lesions; however, increasing size may lead to symptoms related to compression of adjacent structures. Additionally, larger lesions have been associated with hypersplenism, portal hypertension, and consumptive coagulopathy. Though lymphangiomas may be single or multiple discrete lesions, lymphangiomatosis represents a systemic disorder, more commonly seen in children, whereby the neck, axilla, lungs, mediastinum, pericardium, liver, and osseous structures are reportedly involved. A rare, reported complication of splenic lymphangiomas is degeneration into lymphangiosarcomas.

Imaging findings reflect the cystic, avascular nature of splenic lymphangiomas. On US, lymphangiomas are typically identified as single or multiple cystic lesions, which may contain internal septations or echogenic debris. Punctate calcifications associated with lymphangiomas have also been described on US. On CT, well-defined, low-attenuation lesions, typically subcapsular in location, are identified. Given their cystic nature, these lesions lack enhancement after contrast administration. The presence of mural calcification suggests the cystic type of splenic lymphangioma. On MRI, lymphangiomas may have variable appearances on T1-weighted images from hypointense to hyperintense depending on the degree of intracystic protein content or hemorrhage. Lymphangiomas are typically hyperintense on T2 with respect to adjacent splenic parenchyma with internal septations readily visualized. Though exceedingly rare, solid components seen at imaging, should raise the suspicion for malignant degeneration.

PEARLS

• Rare, benign spleen lesions with endothelial lining and proteinaceous content.

• More commonly seen in children in whom lymphangiomatosis may be seen as systemic disease with lymphangiomas throughout the body, including the neck, axilla, lungs, mediastinum, pericardium, liver, and osseous structures.

• Cystic imaging appearance in which septations or calcification may be identified.

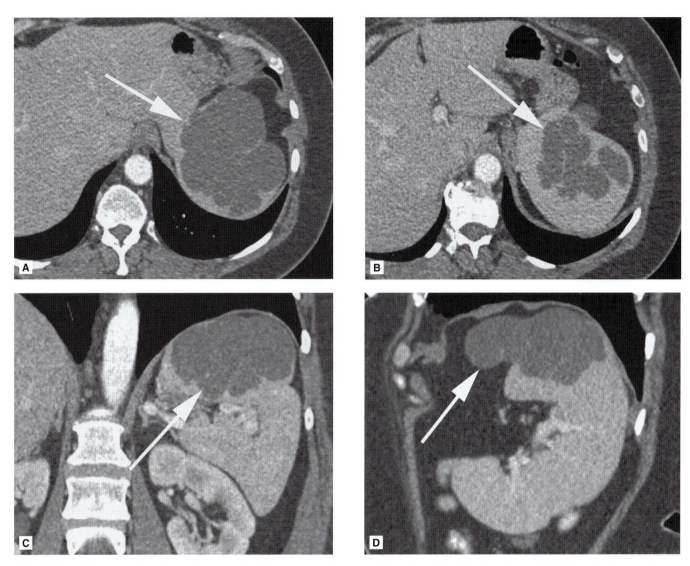

1. A. Axial, portal venous phase image demonstrates the presence of a large, minimally septated lymphangioma within the splenic parenchyma (arrow). **B.** Axial, portal venous phase image more inferiorly demonstrates the presence of a large, minimally septated, lobulated lymphangioma within the splenic parenchyma (arrow). **C.** Coronal, portal venous phase image demonstrates the presence of a large, minimally septated lymphangioma within the splenic parenchyma (arrow). **D.** Sagittal, portal venous phase image demonstrates the presence of a large, minimally septated lymphangioma within the splenic parenchyma (arrow).

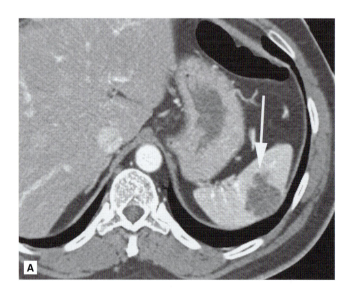

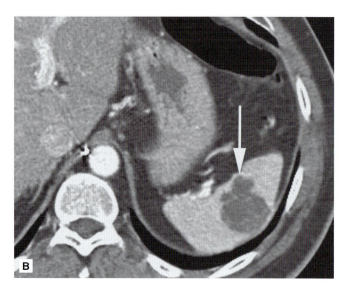

2. A. Axial, portal venous phase image demonstrates the presence of lymphangioma within the spleen with several septations clearly identified (arrow). **B.** Axial, portal venous phase image more inferiorly demonstrates the presence of lymphangioma within the spleen with several septations clearly identified (arrow).

PRESENTATION

- Incidental finding

FINDINGS

Hamartomas of the spleen may be subtle and identified secondary to contour abnormality and heterogeneous enhancement after contrast administration.

DIFFERENTIAL DIAGNOSIS

- Splenic lymphangioma
- Splenic metastases
- Splenic angiosarcoma
- Splenic hemangioma

COMMENTS

Hamartomas are rare, benign splenic lesions which are thought to be congenital in origin, related to a focal area of abnormal development of splenic parenchyma. An alternative theory of the origin of splenic hamartomas is that they are related to an acquired, focal, proliferative process. Nevertheless, splenic hamartomas represent an admixture of normal splenic red pulp. Typically, hamartomas are solitary, though multiple lesions may be identified.

Commonly splenic hamartomas are asymptomatic, incidentally discovered lesions which occur without age or sex predilection. Splenic hamartomas have been associated with the presence of hamartomas elsewhere in the body such as in patients with tuberous sclerosis and Wiskott-Aldrich–like syndrome. Also, strong associations with neoplastic disease or hematologic abnormalities have been described and, thus, the theory of their acquired etiology. Rare complications of splenic rupture associated with hamartomas have been described, the risk of which may be exacerbated by underlying liver disease and portal hypertension.

On US, splenic hamartomas have been described as relatively hyperechoic, hypervascular masses. Infrequently, cystic areas and calcification are seen. On CT, hamartomas may be subtle and nearly isoattenuating to surrounding splenic parenchyma both prior to and after intravenous contrast administration. Heterogenous enhancement and focal contour abnormalities, may, however permit the localization of splenic hamartomas on CT. On MRI, splenic hamartomas are commonly, with respect to normal splenic parenchyma, isointense on T1 and heterogeneously hyperintense on T2. After contrast administration, early, diffuse, heterogeneous enhancement is described with increasing uniformity on delayed images.

PEARLS

- **Hamartomas are rare, benign splenic lesions felt to be of congenital origin.**

- **Splenic hamartomas have been associated with tuberous sclerosis, Wiskott-Aldrich–like syndrome, as well as neoplastic disease and hematologic abnormalities.**

- **Hamartomas of the spleen may be subtle on imaging but heterogeneous enhancement and deformation of the splenic contour may be useful imaging findings.**

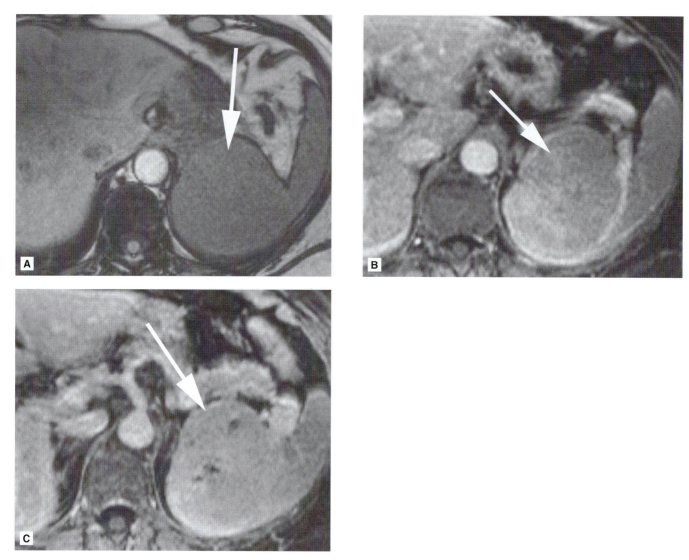

1. A. Axial T1-weighted image demonstrates a large, relatively isointense splenic mass lesion (arrow). **B.** Axial, contrast-enhanced, late-arterial phase T1-weighted MRI image demonstrates an enhancing mass lesion which is relatively isointense to the splenic parenchyma with minimal heterogeneity (arrow). **C.** Axial, contrast-enhanced, portal venous phase T1-weighted MRI image demonstrates a slightly heterogeneously enhancing mass lesion (arrow).

MALIGNANT SPLENIC LESIONS

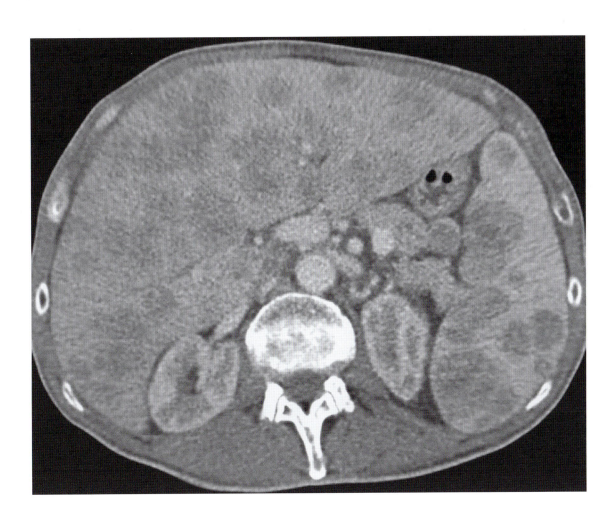

PRESENTATION

Abdominal pain and constitutional symptoms (fever and weight loss) as well as splenomegaly and possible left upper quadrant mass on palpation

FINDINGS

Imaging findings are that of a nonspecific, aggressive-appearing mass lesion which demonstrates cystic areas, necrosis, hemorrhage, and heterogeneous enhancement.

DIFFERENTIAL DIAGNOSIS

- Splenic lymphangioma
- Splenic metastases
- Splenic hamartoma
- Splenic hemangioma
- Splenic cyst
- Splenic abscess

COMMENTS

Angiosarcomas are rare, vascular tumors representing the most common tumor of the spleen which is not of hematologic or lymphoid origin. The histologic features of angiosarcoma of the spleen are similar to those in other organs: a mass of disorganized vascular channels lined by atypical cells. The degree of cellular differentiation may be somewhat heterogeneous throughout the tumor with more well-differentiated areas approximating splenic sinus tissue and more poorly differentiated areas demonstrating sarcomatous features. Typically, the spleen is markedly enlarged often with diffuse involvement of significant portions of the splenic parenchyma though more well-defined solitary mass lesions are also described.

Patients with splenic angiosarcomas tend to be older as this tumor is rarely seen in patients less than 40 years of age. Patients are typically symptomatic with abdominal pain and constitutional symptoms and may present with hematologic disorders including thrombocytopenia and anemia. Associations with a history of chemotherapy for lymphoma as well as radiation for breast cancer have been described but, unlike hepatic angiosarcoma, exposure to carcinogens such as thorium dioxide, arsenic, and vinyl chloride have not been reported. Complications of splenic angiosarcoma include rupture and patients may initially present with a spontaneous hemoperitoneum related to splenic angiosarcoma. Prognosis in patients diagnosed with splenic angiosarcoma is poor and metastatic disease is commonly seen to involve the liver, lungs, osseous structures, and lymphatic system.

The imaging features of a splenic angiosarcoma are that of a nonspecific aggressive-appearing mass lesion. On US, a heterogeneous, ill-defined mass lesion is typically seen, often with cystic areas related to areas of focal hemorrhage and necrosis. Doppler analyses often reveal relative hypervascularity of the solid aspects of the mass lesion. On CT, an ill-defined, aggressive-appearing mass lesion demonstrating heterogeneous early enhancement is typically identified. Given areas of necrosis and hemorrhage, calcification may be seen; massive radial calcification has been reported. Complications of spontaneous hemoperitoneum related to splenic rupture as well as hypervascular metastases may clearly be identified on CT. The imaging appearance of a splenic angiosarcoma on MRI reflects areas of hemorrhage and, thus, the mass is often hypointense on T1 and T2 relative to splenic parenchyma. Similar enhancement patterns to CT are seen, that is, heterogeneous early enhancement.

PEARLS

- Splenic angiosarcomas are rare but represent the most common primary tumor of the spleen not of lymphoid or hematologic origin.

- Metastatic disease is commonly seen with this aggressive tumor and complications include splenic rupture.

- Imaging findings typically reveal a large, aggressive-appearing mass lesion with necrosis and hemorrhage.

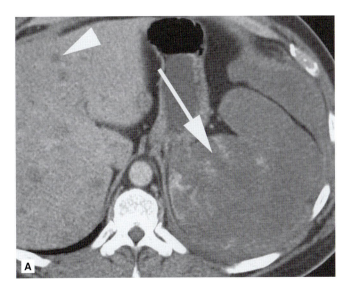

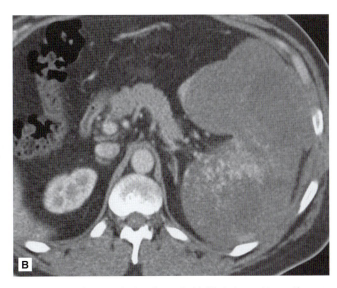

1. A. Axial, enhanced CT image demonstrates a large, heterogeneously enhancing splenic mass lesion (arrow). Multiple hypoattenuating liver metastases are also noted (arrowhead). **B.** Axial, enhanced CT image demonstrates a large, heterogeneously enhancing splenic mass lesion with marked enlargement of the spleen.

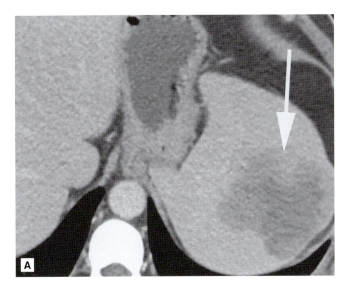

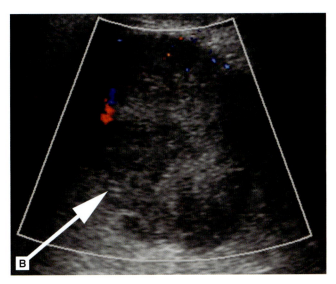

2. A. Axial, enhanced CT image demonstrates a large, relatively hypoattenuating enhancing splenic mass lesion (arrow). **B.** US image reveals a large relatively hypoechoic mass lesion (arrow) corresponding to the hypoattenuating mass seen on CT.

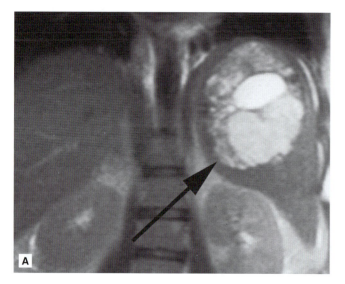

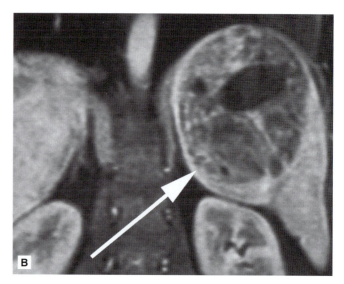

3. A. Coronal, T2-weighted MRI image demonstrates a cystic, multiseptated, hyperintense mass lesion within the spleen (arrow A, B).
B. Coronal, contrast-enhanced, T1-weighted MRI image demonstrates a relatively hypointense splenic mass lesion.

PRESENTATION

Clinical presentation is variable, ranging from asymptomatic to left upper quadrant pain, splenomegaly, or palpable left upper quadrant mass.

FINDINGS

On CT, splenic metastases are typically well-defined, hypoattenuating, solid-appearing lesions.

DIFFERENTIAL DIAGNOSIS

- Splenic lymphoma
- Primary splenic neoplasms; benign and malignant
- Splenic infection
- Splenic granulomatous disease

COMMENTS

Splenic metastases are rare and are usually seen in patients with widespread disseminated tumor involvement. Metastases typically arise from hematogenous spread of primary malignancies, the most common of which include melanoma, lung, and breast cancers. Splenic lymphoma is the most common splenic malignancy and typically presents as multiple discrete lesions or diffuse splenic involvement. Hodgkin or non-Hodgkin lymphoma may involve the spleen as the primary site or as a site of metastatic involvement. Other primary malignancies which may result in splenic metastases include ovarian, gastric, and prostate carcinoma. Splenic metastases can also arise from retrograde involvement via the splenic vein or lymphatics or by direct tumor extension. Metastases to the spleen typically present as multiple discrete lesions; however, they may present as single lesions, confluent, or diffuse lesions.

Both benign splenic neoplasms, such as hemangiomas or hamartomas, and malignant neoplasms such as primary angiosarcoma can mimic splenic metastasis. Fungal or pyogenic infections and granulomatous diseases may have imaging appearances similar to splenic metastases.

The imaging appearance of splenic metastases depends on whether the lesions are multiple, single, or infiltrative and is also dependent on the underlying primary malignancy. On US, while the appearance may be variable, the most common US manifestation of a metastatic splenic lesion is the appearance of a discrete hypoechoic lesion with a surrounding hyperechoic "halo." On CT, splenic metastases are typically well-defined, hypoattenuating, solid-appearing lesions, though rarely, the lesions may appear cystic. After the administration of contrast, central or peripheral enhancement can be identified. On MRI, metastatic lesions are T1 hypo- to isointense and T2 hyperintense relative to normal splenic parenchyma. The appearance on T2 images may be useful in differentiating metastases related to splenic lymphoma from other primary malignancies as lymphoma within the spleen may be T2 hypointense, a rare feature of metastases related to other primary malignancies.

PEARLS

- Metastases typically arise from hematogenous spread of primary malignancies, the most common of which include melanoma, lung, and breast cancers.

- Splenic lymphoma is the most common splenic malignancy which may involve the spleen as the primary site or as a site of metastatic involvement.

- On MRI, metastatic lesions are T1 hypo- to isointense and T2 hyperintense relative to normal splenic parenchyma.

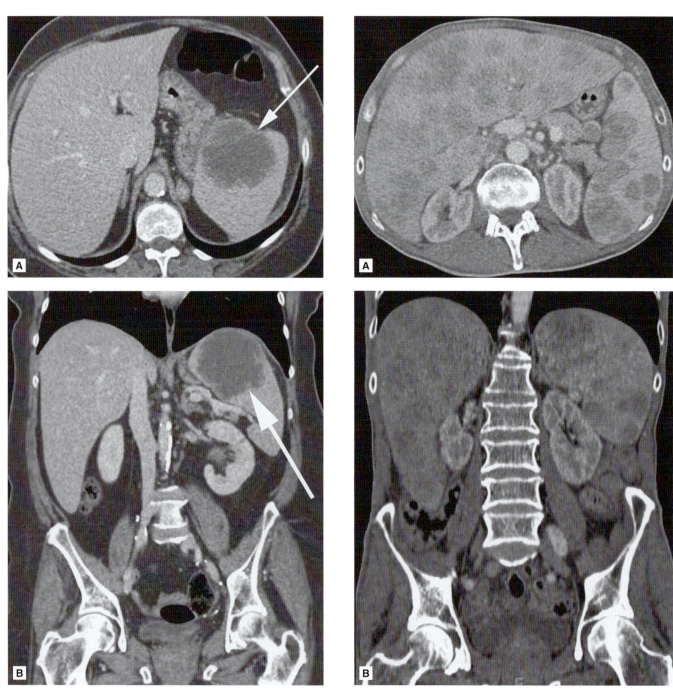

1. A. Axial, contrast-enhanced CT image demonstrates a large, relatively hypoattenuating lesion in the spleen (arrow), secondary to endometrial cancer metastasis. **B.** Coronal, contrast-enhanced CT image demonstrates a single, large endometrial cancer metastasis in the spleen (arrow).

2. A. Axial, contrast-enhanced CT image demonstrates innumerable hypoattenuating lesions in the spleen as well as the liver, secondary to melanoma metastases. **B.** Coronal, contrast-enhanced CT image demonstrates innumerable melanoma metastases throughout the liver and spleen.

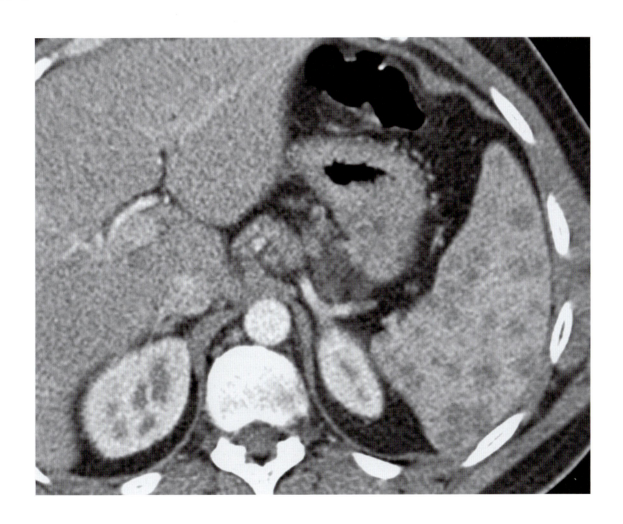

Case 4–7 Splenic Granulomatous Disease

PRESENTATION

Varies depending on etiology, often indolent, low-grade fevers, and weight loss

FINDINGS

Typically, numerous small lesions are identified throughout the splenic parenchyma (often also the liver), the spleen may be enlarged, and calcification may occur over time depending on the etiology.

DIFFERENTIAL DIAGNOSIS

- Splenic infection (fungal)
- Splenic metastases

COMMENTS

Granulomatous diseases of the spleen are characterized by inflammation and the formation of splenic granulomas. There are myriad etiologies of granulomatous diseases of the spleen, most commonly, sarcoidosis, tuberculosis, and histoplasmosis.

Sarcoidosis is a systemic disease which results in non-caseating granulomas which can affect any portion of the body. While the most commonly involved organ is the lungs, up to 15% of patients may develop abdominal involvement. Tuberculous infection of the spleen is rare and often involves concurrent infection of the liver with primary infection of the lung or gastrointestinal tract. Histoplasmosis is the most common granulomatous disease in North America as this organism thrives in soil containing excrement from birds and bats. Histoplasmosis involvement of the spleen preferentially affects immunocompromised patients though infection in patients with competent immune systems is also found.

Granulomatous diseases of various etiologies result in an immune inflammatory response which leads to granuloma formation and the typical imaging appearance of numerous small splenic lesions which may calcify over time. The most common finding in patients with splenic involvement in sarcoidosis is splenomegaly, often with concurrent hepatomegaly and lymphadenopathy. Less commonly, innumerable small hypoattenuating nodules of varying size may be identified in the spleen on CT, often with similar findings in the liver. The splenic nodules in sarcoidosis may coalesce, resulting in confluent, hypoattenuating regions. In patients with tuberculosis or histoplasmosis involving the spleen, hepatosplenomegaly may also be identified, possibly along with multiple well-circumscribed nodules. On MRI in granulomatous diseases, numerous small, T1- and T2-hypointense lesions may be seen on T1- and T2-weighted images. As chronic granulomas may calcify, characteristic areas of hypointense signal demonstrating blooming on gradient-echo images may be identified. Often, the hepatosplenic findings in granulomatous diseases are associated with intra-abdominal lymphadenopathy.

PEARLS

- Granulomatous diseases are characterized by inflammation and the formation of granulomas in the splenic parenchyma.

- Common etiologies of splenic granulomatous disease include sarcoidosis, tuberculosis, and histoplasmosis.

- Commonly, innumerable small lesions are seen throughout the splenic parenchyma in cases of granulomatous disease; often the liver is also involved.

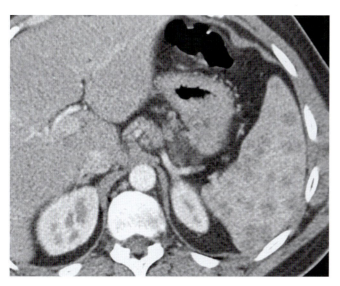

1. Axial, enhanced arterial phase CT image demonstrates numerous focal, hypoattenuating areas in the splenic parenchyma in a patient with splenic sarcoidosis.

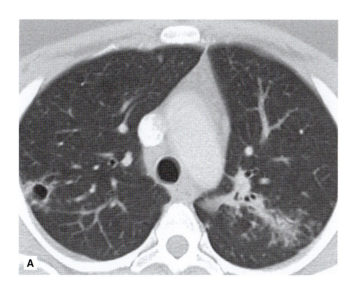

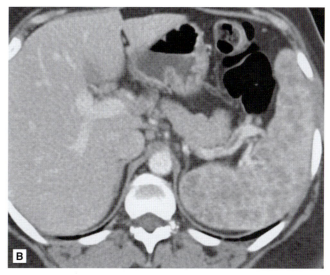

2. A. Axial CT of the chest demonstrates areas of consolidation and cavitation in a patient with sarcoidosis. **B.** Axial, enhanced portal venous phase CT image demonstrates numerous focal, hypoattenuating areas in the splenic parenchyma in a patient with splenic sarcoidosis.

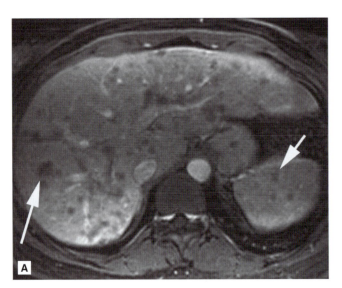

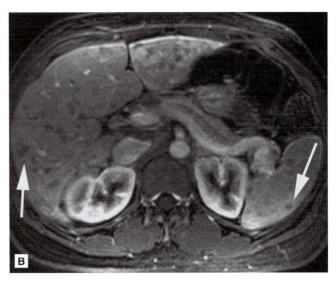

3. A. Axial, T1-weighted contrast-enhanced MRI image reveals multiple hypoattenuating areas in the liver and splenic parenchyma in a patient with histoplasmosis (arrows). **B.** Axial, T1-weighted contrast-enhanced MRI image reveals multiple hypoattenuating areas in the liver and splenic parenchyma in a patient with histoplasmosis (arrows).

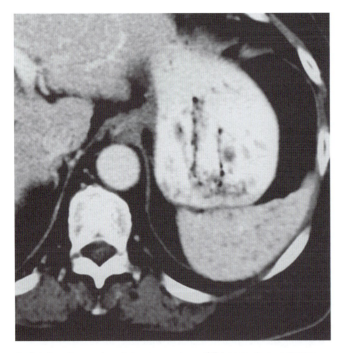

4. Axial, enhanced portal venous phase CT image demonstrates numerous focal, hypoattenuating areas in the splenic parenchyma in a patient with splenic tuberculosis.

PRESENTATION

Fever, left upper quadrant pain, and splenomegaly

FINDINGS

Relatively hypoattenuating collection with respect to the splenic parenchyma on CT. Peripheral enhancement and internal septations may be seen and, though more specific for infection, the presence of air is rare.

DIFFERENTIAL DIAGNOSIS

- Splenic lymphangioma
- Splenic metastases
- Splenic angiosarcoma
- Splenic hemangioma
- Splenic cyst

COMMENTS

Splenic abscesses are typically a result of aerobic pathogens, but in up to 50% of cases the infections are polymicrobial. Most commonly, splenic abscesses are a result of hematogenous seeding from an infection elsewhere, including endocarditis, pneumonia, urinary tract infections, osteomyelitis, among myriad others. Contiguous spread of infection also may result in a splenic abscess from subphrenic abscesses, diverticulitis, as well as pancreatic infections. Finally, splenic trauma as well as infarction may result in splenic abscesses.

Splenic abscesses, though rare, carry a high mortality rate, reportedly approaching 50%. Patients with splenic abscesses are often immunocompromised, such as patients with diabetes, human immunodeficiency virus (HIV), those undergoing chemotherapy, as well as alcoholics. The classic presentation of left upper quadrant pain, fever, and splenomegaly is only seen in approximately one-third of patients with splenic abscesses. The majority of patients will be febrile and present with abdominal pain, however, the presentation is often nonspecific. The so-called Kehr sign results from irritation of the diaphragmatic pleura, causing associated referred shoulder pain.

Splenic abscesses are typically heterogeneously hypoechoic on US with hypervascularity reflecting the underlying inflammation. The early, phlegmonous stages of a splenic abscess may be relatively isoechoic to the adjacent splenic parenchyma, becoming increasingly hypoechoic as the infection evolves into a discrete abscess. On CT, splenic abscesses are relatively hypoattenuating, especially centrally where they are fluid containing and necrotic. If a capsule has developed in response to a splenic abscess, mild peripheral enhancement of the surrounding splenic parenchyma may be visualized. Internal septations may be visualized and, though pathognomonic for a splenic abscess, the presence of air is rarely identified. On MR, imaging characteristics of splenic abscesses should include increased T2 signal as well as possible peripheral enhancement after intravenous contrast administration.

PEARLS

- **Typically results from anaerobic pathogens, but in up to 50% of cases infections are polymicrobial.**
- **The mortality of splenic abscesses is high with common presentation including abdominal pain and fever.**
- **US, CT, and MRI offer utility in diagnosing splenic abscesses.**

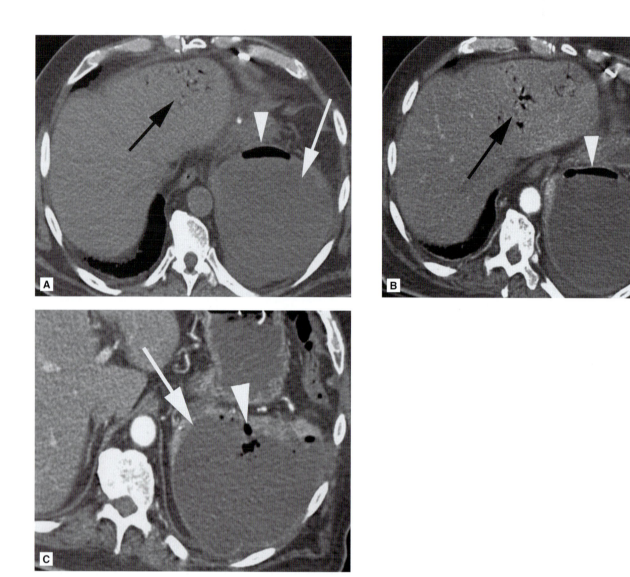

1. A. Axial, unenhanced CT image demonstrates a large, relatively hypoattenuating splenic abscess (white arrow) which contains gas, a rare imaging finding (arrowhead). In addition, portal venous air is identified within the liver (black arrow). **B.** Axial, enhanced CT image demonstrates a large, relatively hypoenhancing splenic abscess (white arrow) which contains gas (arrowhead). In addition, portal venous air is identified within the liver (black arrow). **C.** Axial, enhanced CT image demonstrates a large, relatively hypoenhancing splenic abscess (arrow) containing multiple foci of gas (arrowhead).

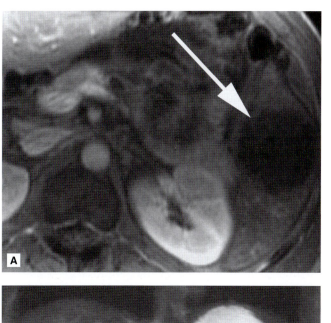

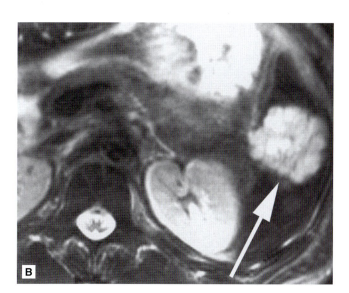

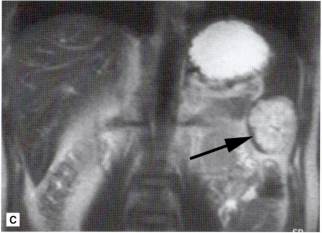

2. A. Axial, T1-weighted, gadolinium-enhanced image demonstrates a relatively hypointense splenic abscess (arrow). **B.** Axial, T2-weighted image demonstrates a relatively hyperintense splenic abscess (arrow). **C.** Coronal, T2-weighted image demonstrates a relatively hyperintense splenic abscess (arrow).

PRESENTATION

- Incidental finding

FINDINGS

Typically, cystic lesions with internal septations and possible calcification. The presence of daughter cysts is less common in splenic hydatid cysts.

DIFFERENTIAL DIAGNOSIS

- Splenic lymphangioma
- Splenic metastases
- Splenic hemangioma
- Splenic cyst

COMMENTS

Echinococcal infection is a result of infection by the larval form of the cestode *Echinococcus* with *Echinococcus granulosus* accounting for the majority (95%) of these cases. Echinococcal disease is highly endemic in portions of South America, Africa, Europe, and Asia though there is a worldwide distribution. Echinococcal disease most commonly affects the liver, followed by the lungs. Splenic hydatid disease is uncommon and isolated splenic infection is exceedingly rare. The wall of the hydatid cyst is composed of an inner germinal layer and an outer laminated membrane, both of which are surrounded by a layer of compressed, fibrotic splenic parenchyma termed as pericyst.

Typically, hydatid disease of the spleen is asymptomatic, however, mild symptoms related to compression of adjacent structures may become manifest. Hydatid cysts are slow growing, increasing in size by approximately 2 to 3 cm per year. Patients with hydatid disease of the spleen will be found to have eosinophilia up to 30% of the time but currently available enzyme-linked immunosorbent and immunoelectrophoresis assays offer markedly increased sensitivities greater than 95%. Complications related to echinococcal disease of the spleen include superinfection as well as cyst rupture. Subcapsular cysts are at increased risk for rupture, a complication which may result in anaphylactic shock. Both superinfection and cyst rupture also typically result in significant pain. The chronic pericyst inflammation related to hydatid disease may result in adhesion and fistulization with adjacent structures including the left kidney or colon, liver and bile ducts, pancreas, thoracic cavity, and airways.

The imaging features of splenic hydatid disease reflect its cystic nature and, therefore, on US, well-defined anechoic lesions are typically seen. In splenic hydatid disease, the lesions are usually solitary and the finding of daughter cysts is atypical. Associated calcification may also be seen on US and, when present, collapsed membranes within a cystic lesion, termed the water lily sign, increase specificity and are virtually pathognomonic for the diagnosis of hydatid disease. Internal debris, so-called hydatid sand, reflects scolices and portions of the germinal layer. The attenuation on CT is somewhat variable reflecting the internal contents of the cyst. Though typically hypoattenuating, the expecting attenuation may be increased by the presence of internal debris, hydatid sand, detached membranes, as well as the presence of daughter cysts. Also, calcification of the periphery of the hydatid cysts may be well seen on CT. MRI features are that expected from a cystic lesion such that the lesions are T1 hypointense and T2 hyperintense with respect to splenic parenchyma, though the T1 signal is somewhat variable depending on the internal contents of the cyst. The cyst contents, including the presence of daughter cysts or hydatid sand are also well delineated on MRI, especially T2-weighted images.

PEARLS

- *E granulosus* accounts for the majority of infections and is endemic in portions of South America, Africa, Europe, and Asia.

- Typically asymptomatic, though may have symptoms of mass effect from larger lesions and other complications such as superinfection, cyst rupture, and fistulization with adjacent structures.

- Cystic lesions identified on imaging with collapse of membranes is a pathognomonic imaging finding in splenic hydatid disease.

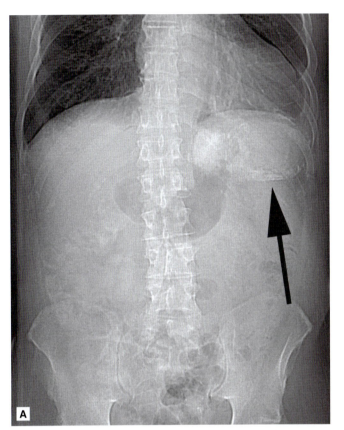

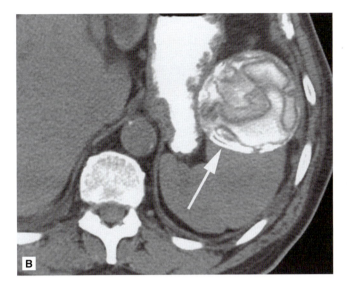

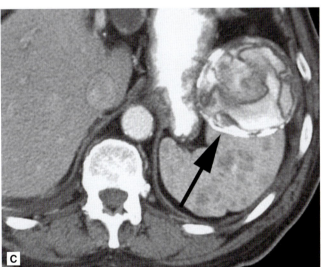

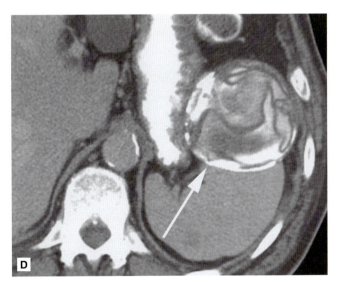

1. A. Abdominal plain radiograph demonstrates a large, rounded area of calcification overlying the expected location of the spleen in the left upper quadrant (arrow), in this case representing a calcified hydatid cyst. **B.** Axial, unenhanced CT image demonstrates a heavily calcified echinococcal cyst (arrow) with collapsed membranes seen within this lesion, an imaging finding which is virtually pathognomonic of this diagnosis. **C.** Axial, portal venous phase–enhanced CT image demonstrates a heavily calcified echinococcal cyst (arrow) with collapsed membranes seen within this lesion, an imaging finding which is virtually pathognomonic of this diagnosis. Additional, smaller, hypoattenuating lesions within the spleen are also noted. **D.** Axial, delayed phase–enhanced CT image demonstrates a heavily calcified echinococcal cyst (arrow). *(Case courtesy of Alvaro Huete, MD)*

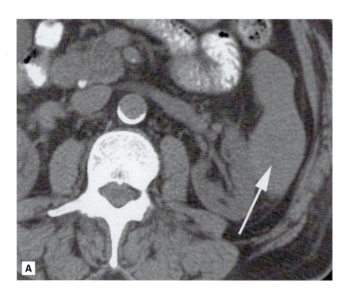

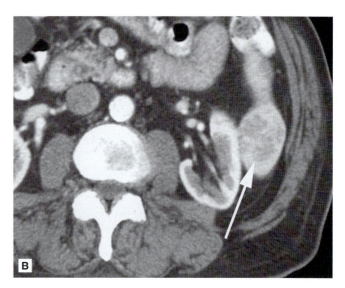

2. A. Axial, unenhanced CT image reveals a subtle area of hypoattenuation within the posterior aspect of the inferior portion of the spleen (arrow). **B.** Axial, enhanced CT image reveals a focal cystic area within the posterior aspect of the inferior portion of the spleen, in this case a hydatid cyst (arrow). *(Case courtesy of Alvaro Huete, MD)*

PRESENTATION

Fever and abdominal pain in neutropenic patients

FINDINGS

Hepatosplenomegaly may be the only imaging finding but when resolves, microabscesses are seen as innumerable small lesions throughout the spleen and often the liver.

DIFFERENTIAL DIAGNOSIS

- Splenic granulomatous disease

- Splenic metastases

COMMENTS

Fungal infections involving the spleen occur in cases of disseminated fungal disease which occur in patients with hematologic malignancy or immune compromise. In immunocompromised patients, candidiasis is the most common infection of the liver and spleen. However, other fungal infections including histoplasmosis [see Splenic Granulomatous Disease (case 4-7)], *Aspergillus*, *Cryoptococcus*, mucormycosis, among others may occur.

In certain patient populations, invasive fugal infections are increasing in incidence with up to 50% of patients developing a fungal infection after bone marrow transplantation. Additionally, an increasing number of diseases are being treated with immunosuppression, likely to result in increased incidence of fungal infection. In the appropriate patient population, abdominal pain, nausea, vomiting, elevated alkaline phosphatase levels raise the suspicion of hepatosplenic fungal infection. Fungal abscesses have been reported to account for 20% to 40% of splenic abscesses.

Even in cases of widely disseminated fungal infection, the microabscesses may be below the resolution of imaging and, thus, hepatosplenomegaly may be the only imaging finding, if any. It has been well reported that fungal lesions in the spleen may not be visible until the patient recovers from the neutropenic stage of their disease as the host inflammatory response influences the imaging appearance. When identified, splenic microabscesses are well-circumscribed, round, lesions typically with concurrent similar liver findings. Four US patterns of hepatosplenic candidiasis have been described: (1) central hypoechoic necrosis surrounded by an echogenic zone of inflammation, termed the wheel-within-a-wheel appearance; (2) central echogenic focus surrounded by peripheral hypoechoic rim; (3) homogeneously hypoechoic lesion, the most common US manifestation; (4) echogenic lesion demonstrating a component of acoustic shadowing. On CT, fungal microabscesses are seen as multiple low-attenuation nodules, the size of which is typically in the range of 5 to 10 mm. In some cases, a central hyperechoic focus may be identified (wheel-within-a-wheel appearance). After intravenous contrast administration, nodules have bee reported to enhance centrally with peripheral enhancement also having been described. On MRI, fungal microabscesses typically demonstrate hypo- to isointense T1 signal, hyperintense T2 signal with enhancement after gadolinium contrast administration. There are several published reports in which MRI is shown to be superior to CT and US in detecting fungal microabscesses.

PEARLS

- **Typically results from disseminated fungal infections in immunocompromised patients or those with hematologic malignancies.**

- ***Candida* is the most common fungal infection of the spleen and liver.**

- **Microabscesses, when identified at imaging, are seen as innumerable small lesions throughout the spleen and often the liver, concurrently.**

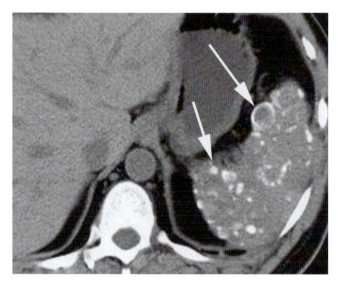

1. Axial, unenhanced CT image reveals multiple areas of calcification within the spleen in a patient with a history of histoplasmosis, a common sequela of prior granulomatous infection (arrows).

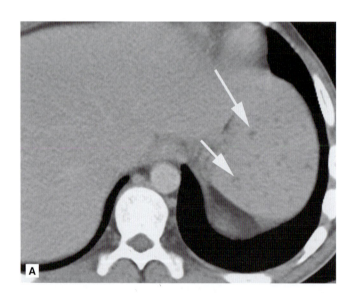

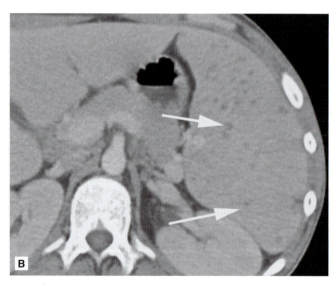

2. A. Axial, enhanced CT image demonstrates multiple small hypoattenuating areas within the splenic parenchyma in a patient with splenic candidiasis (arrows). **B.** Axial, enhanced CT image more inferiorly demonstrates multiple small hypoattenuating areas within the splenic parenchyma in a patient with splenic candidiasis (arrows).

MISCELLANEOUS

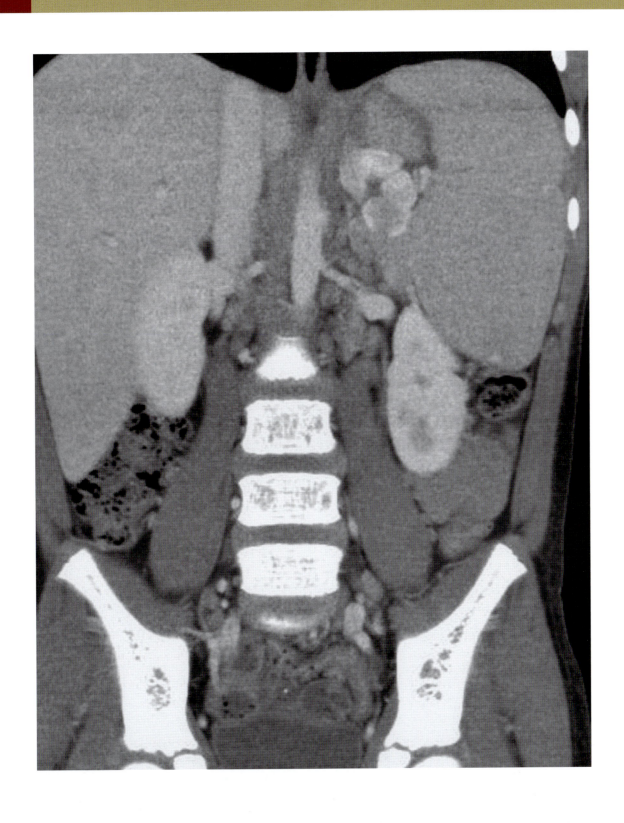

PRESENTATION

Left upper quadrant pain, splenomegaly, fever, possibly hypovolemic shock in acute cases

FINDINGS

Splenomegaly and mottled areas of heterogeneity are often seen in cases of splenic sequestration.

DIFFERENTIAL DIAGNOSIS

• Splenic infarct

COMMENTS

Acute splenic sequestration is a complication of sickle cell disease and results in rapid trapping of a large amount of blood within the splenic parenchyma leading to rapid decrease in hematocrit and possibly hypovolemia. The pathophysiology of acute sequestration is unknown but the triggering event is hypothesized to be acute obstruction to venous outflow resulting in acute sequestration of red cells and platelets in the splenic parenchyma.

As a certain distensibility of the splenic parenchyma is requisite to acute sequestration, acute splenic sequestration crises (ASSC) typically occur in infants and young children with homozygous sickle cell disease. However, in adults with heterozygous sickle cell disease, splenic distensibility is preserved and, thus, ASSC is a complication, albeit rare, in this patient population as well. Patients with hemoglobin S-C have been reported to suffer ASSC into the eighth decade of life.

On US, the imaging findings of splenic sequestration include splenomegaly as well as multiple, peripherally located, relatively hypoechoic areas corresponding to infarction and hemorrhage. Similarly, on CT, areas of peripheral hypoattenuation may be seen. On CT, the areas of hypoattenuation may appear mottled with areas of relative hyperattenuation corresponding to hemorrhage. On MRI, hyperintense areas corresponding to the hypoechoic or hypoattenuating areas on US and CT, respectively, are seen on T1- and T2-weighted images. The hyperintense signal reflects the underlying hemorrhage associated with ASSC. Peripheral low intensity may be seen in areas of splenic sequestration on MRI related to the presence of hemosiderin.

PEARLS

• **In patients with homozygous sickle cell disease, ASSC typically occurs in infants and young children while in those patients with heterozygous sickle cell disease, this may occur in adults.**

• **The spleen is typically enlarged with mottled heterogeneity related to infarction and hemorrhage.**

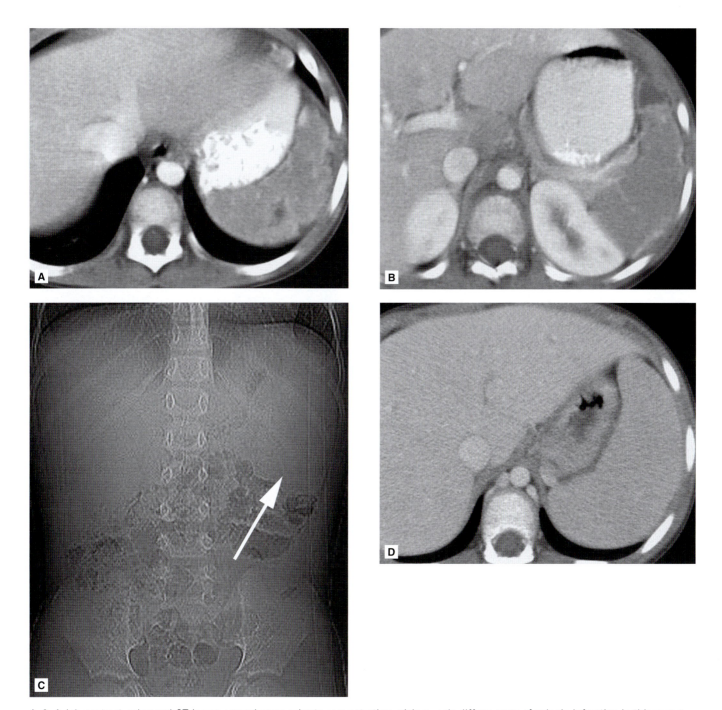

1. A. Axial, contrast-enhanced CT image several years prior to sequestration crisis reveals diffuse areas of splenic infarction in this young child with sickle cell disease. **B.** Axial, contrast-enhanced CT image more inferiorly several years prior to sequestration crisis reveals diffuse areas of splenic infarction in this young child with sickle cell disease. **C.** Scout topogram demonstrates markedly enlarged spleen in this young child with ASSC (arrow). **D.** Axial, contrast-enhanced CT image demonstrates a markedly enlarged spleen in this young child with ASSC. **E.** Axial, contrast-enhanced CT image more inferiorly demonstrates a markedly enlarged spleen in this young child with ASSC. **F.** Coronal, contrast-enhanced CT image demonstrates a markedly enlarged spleen in this young child with ASSC.

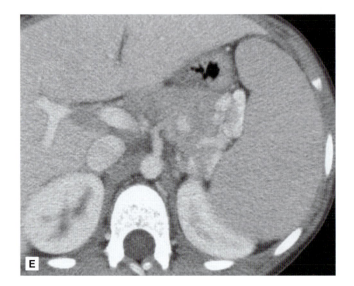

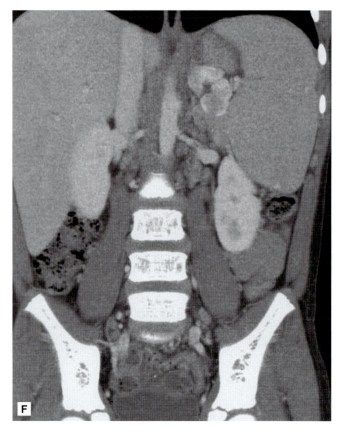

1. (*continued*)

PRESENTATION

Clinical presentation ranges from asymptomatic to symptoms such as left upper quadrant pain, fevers, chills, nausea, vomiting, and left shoulder pain (Kehr sign) to shock related to hemorrhage and splenic rupture.

FINDINGS

Peripheral, wedge-shaped areas of infarction are seen as hypo- or anechoic areas on US and demonstrate relative hypoenhancement on CT and MRI.

DIFFERENTIAL DIAGNOSIS

- Splenic hematoma or contusion
- Infiltrating malignancy (lymphoma, etc)
- Splenic abscess

COMMENTS

Splenic infarction is caused by a compromise of vascular supply of the spleen leading to subsequent ischemia and necrosis. The insult to the vascular supply of the spleen may be secondary to either arterial or venous occlusion. The splenic parenchyma is supplied by both the splenic artery as well as the short gastric arteries, which are branches of the gastroepiploic artery. The short gastric arteries typically supply the upper portions of the spleen. Even with occlusion of the main splenic artery, the short gastric arterial blood supply often preserves a large majority of the splenic parenchyma. The intrasplenic arterial vasculature is segmental, leading to classic imaging features detailed below.

Common etiologies of splenic infarcts are hematologic disorders, including benign hypercoagulable states, sickle cell disease, as well as malignant hematologic disorders such a leukemia, lymphoma, and myelofibrosis, among others. Splenic infarcts may be caused by thromboemboli from various sources such as endocarditis and atrial fibrillation, among others. Trauma, including iatrogenic injury, may result in splenic infarction. Myriad other etiologies of splenic infarction are known and include pancreatitis, pancreatic malignancy, depositional diseases, collagen vascular diseases, among numerous others. Complications of splenic infarction include splenic abscess formation as a result of infection of areas of parenchymal necrosis or as a result of septic thromboemboli causing the initial insult. Though rare, splenic infarction may lead to parenchymal and subcapsular hemorrhage and can lead to spontaneous splenic rupture.

The imaging appearance of splenic infarcts is related to the splenic arterial anatomy which results in peripheral, wedge-shaped areas of ischemia and necrosis. On US, splenic infarcts appear as peripheral, wedge-shaped, round, or irregular hypoechoic or anechoic areas. On CT, the classic imaging appearance is that of peripheral, wedge-shaped areas of hypoattenuation, though often the areas of infarction are less regular and more round. These imaging findings are best appreciated after intravenous contrast enhancement and may be subtle on unenhanced images. After contrast administration, splenic infarcts may appear heterogenous and mottled with mixed areas of residual perfusion. In cases in which there is a component of hemorrhage, heterogenous hyperattenuation may be appreciated on unenhanced images. The expected temporal progression of a splenic infarct results in progressive diminution of size, possibly with calcification caused by fibrosis in the area of infarct. On MRI, imaging appearances are similar and infarcts appear as peripheral, wedge-shaped defects which exhibit decreased T1 and T2 signal and lack enhancement after gadolinium contrast administration.

PEARLS

- Splenic infarcts may be caused by hypercoagulable states, thromboemboli, or trauma, among other etiologies.

- Imaging findings of peripheral, wedge-shaped areas of relative hypoenhancement are well seen after contrast administration using CT and MRI.

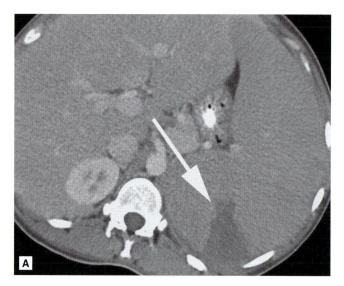
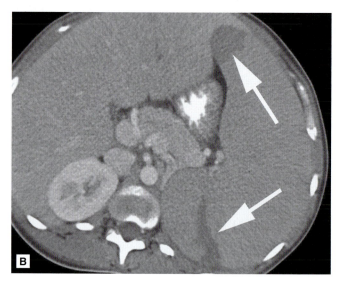

1. A. Axial, enhanced CT image demonstrates peripheral areas of infraction (arrow) in a patient with marked splenomegaly related to chronic myeloblastic leukemia (CML). **B.** Axial, enhanced CT image demonstrates peripheral areas of infraction (arrows) in a patient with marked splenomegaly related to CML.

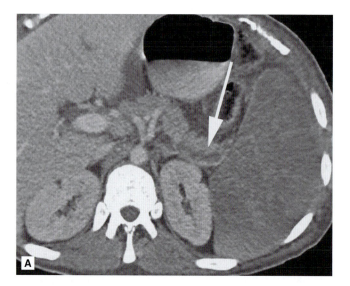
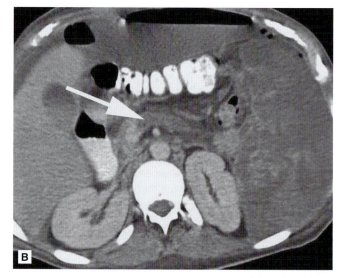

2. A. Axial, enhanced CT image demonstrates mottled enhancement of a massively infarcted spleen related to thrombosis of the splenic vein (arrow) in a patient with hypercoagulability related to Crohn disease. **B.** Axial, enhanced CT image demonstrates mottled enhancement of a massively infarcted spleen related to thrombosis of the splenic vein (arrow) in a patient with hypercoagulability related to Crohn disease.

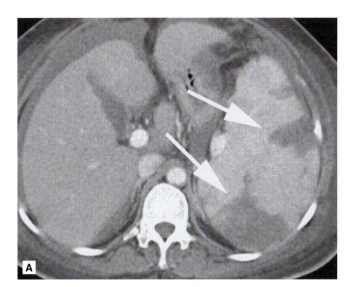

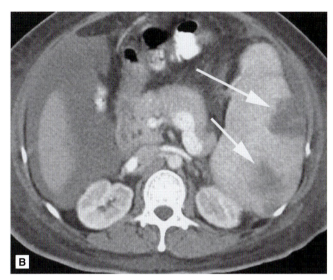

3. A. Axial, enhanced CT image reveals multiple, peripheral wedge-shaped infarcts (arrows) related to thromboembolic disease. **B.** More inferior, axial, enhanced CT image reveals multiple, peripheral wedge-shaped infarcts (arrows) related to thromboembolic disease.

PRESENTATION

Acute and/or recurrent abdominal pain

FINDINGS

Hypoechoic, hypovascular appearance of the spleen on US with enlargement and decreased or absent enhancement on CT.

DIFFERENTIAL DIAGNOSIS

- Splenic infarct, not otherwise specified (NOS)
- Wandering spleen

COMMENTS

Splenic torsion is a rare cause of abdominal pain which is related to the suspensory ligaments of the spleen which, when absent, underdeveloped, or hypermobile, predispose to splenic torsion. The suspensory ligaments of the spleen include the splenorenal, also known as the lienorenal, ligament which attaches the spleen to the posterior abdominal wall overlying the left kidney and the gastrolienal ligament which attaches the spleen to the greater curvature of the stomach. The phrenicocolic ligament extends from the splenic flexure of the colon to the diaphragm and aids in supporting the spleen inferiorly. Abnormal development or laxity of these ligaments may result in an ectopic, "wandering" spleen which may undergo torsion with subsequent ischemia and infarction. Other causes of hypermobility which may predispose to splenic torsion include laxity of suspensory ligaments related to pregnancy, splenomegaly, as well as a history of abdominal surgery or trauma.

Splenic torsion is rare, having been reported in 0.3% of patients undergoing splenectomy in one large series. The symptoms of splenic torsion are related to the degree to which the spleen is torsed. Thus, in mild cases, patients may report chronic abdominal pain while in moderate cases in which the spleen torses to a greater degree, patients may report more severe pain which may be intermittent in nature reflecting lesser or greater degrees of rotation as the spleen torses and detorses. In severe cases in which the spleen is infarcted, patients may present with an acute abdomen. Alternatively, patients may present with an abdominal or pelvic mass secondary to torsion of the spleen with parenchymal congestion. The splenomegaly related to torsion may result in pancytopenia, though typically this diagnosis is not associated with laboratory abnormalities.

The imaging manifestations of splenic torsion depend both on the underlying etiology and the degree of torsion. As splenic torsion is often related to wandering spleen, the spleen may be seen in an ectopic location. On US, the echotexture may be heterogeneous related to congestion and possible areas of infarction. The spleen may be quite enlarged secondary to vascular congestion. Decreased vascular perfusion may be seen with Color Doppler US. Similarly, on CT, the spleen, which is often enlarged, may be identified as a mass in an ectopic location with decreased or possibly absent enhancement after the administration of intravenous contrast depending on the degree of torsion. In cases of wandering spleen with torsion, the elongated vascular pedicle is clearly seen on CT. Twisting of the vascular pedicle, possibly with involvement of the pancreatic tail, has been described as having a whorled appearance on CT.

PEARLS

- **Splenic torsion is due to abnormality of the suspensory ligaments of the spleen.**

- **Symptomatology and imaging findings relate to the degree of splenic torsion.**

- **As the suspensory ligaments of the spleen are abnormal, a torsed spleen may be located in an ectopic location.**

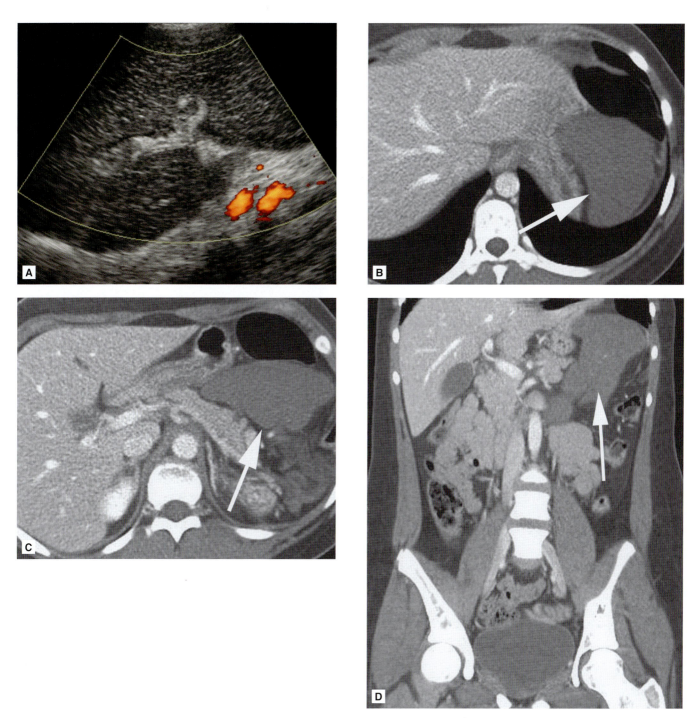

1. A. Color Doppler US image demonstrates an enlarged, hypoechoic spleen with no demonstrable vascularity consistent with infarction. **B.** Axial, enhanced CT image reveals no discernable enhancement of the spleen (arrow), consistent with infarction, in this case related to splenic torsion. **C.** Axial, enhanced CT image reveals no discernable enhancement of the spleen (arrow), consistent with infarction, in this case related to splenic torsion. **D.** Coronal, enhanced CT image reveals diffuse hypoattenuation of the splenic parenchyma with no discernable enhancement of the spleen (arrow), consistent with infarction.

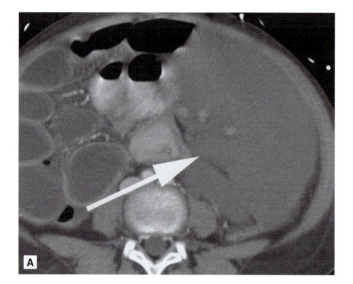

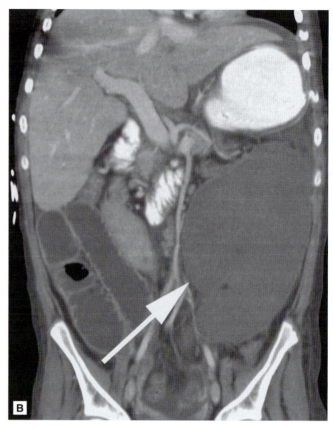

2. A. Axial, enhanced CT image reveals no discernable enhancement of the spleen (arrow) which is noted to be in an ectopic location. This finding is consistent with infarction, in this case related to splenic torsion. **B.** Coronal, enhanced CT image reveals no discernable enhancement of the spleen (arrow), consistent with infarction, in this case related to splenic torsion. Abnormal, ectopic location of the spleen is also appreciated in this image.

PRESENTATION

Typically incidentally detected though may cause pain related to infarction of splenules, bowel obstruction, and enlarging abdominal mass lesions have been described.

FINDINGS

Scattered deposits of soft tissue, typically within the peritoneal cavity; nuclear medicine techniques such as technetium-99m-labeled heat-damaged red blood cells or Indium-111-labeled platelets offer additional specificity.

DIFFERENTIAL DIAGNOSIS

- Lymphoma
- Metastatic disease related to several primary malignancies

COMMENTS

Splenosis is defined as autotransplanation of splenic tissue to various compartments of the body, typically related splenic rupture due to trauma or iatrogenic etiologies. Often, many discrete nodules of splenic tissue are present which commonly may number approximately 100 discrete nodules though a case in which greater than 400 nodules of splenic tissue were present has been reported. The histology of splenosis-related splenic tissue varies but typically, absent or deficient white pulp is reported as well as absence of trabecular structures.

Two mechanisms for the formation of splenosis are hypothesized: seeding of splenic pulp related to rupture as well as hematogenous spread of splenic pulp. In seeding related to traumatic or iatrogenic rupture, the degree of splenosis is postulated to be related to the severity of rupture and amount of pulp deposited throughout the peritoneal cavity or, in cases of severe trauma, in other compartments of the body. Cases of splenosis related to hematogenous dissemination of splenic pulp afford an explanation of intraparenchymal splenosis (liver, etc) as well as distant sites of splenosis (intracranial, etc).

The average delay between the inciting traumatic event and discovery of abdominopelvic splenosis is 10 years

with approximately 20 years for intrathoracic splenosis. As splenosis is commonly asymptomatic, cases are typically discovered incidentally on imaging evaluations for other clinical indications. Cases of rare complications related to splenosis which have been reported include infarction of splenosis with pain, hydronephrosis related to mass effect, and an enlarging abdominal mass lesion.

Cross-sectional imaging may identify splenosis as irregular tissue, often with distorted morphology lacking a hilum. The blood supply in splenic tissue related to splenosis originates from nearby vasculature and often does not originate from the splenic artery. Most commonly, splenosis is identified along the peritoneum, mesentery, or omentum. However, the splenic tissue in splenosis has been described throughout much of the body, including the thorax and even in subcutaneous tissue and brain. Though splenosis is typically a benign process, it can pose a diagnostic dilemma when identified incidentally on imaging. As such, it may be mistaken for malignancy such as lymphoma, among others, depending on its location. On CT and conventional MRI, splenosis demonstrates relatively nonspecific imaging features. Currently, the imaging modalities of choice are nuclear medicine. Technetium-99mm sulfur colloid is often employed in evaluating suspected splenosis though technetium-99m-labeled heat-damaged red blood cells or Indium-111-labeled platelets afford greater sensitivity and specificity.

PEARLS

- Autotransplantation of splenic tissue from a number of etiologies including splenic rupture and hematogenous spread.

- Delay between inciting event and the detection of splenosis is typically 10 to 20 years.

- Nonspecific soft tissue deposits are seen at imaging though nuclear medicine imaging may afford greater specificity.

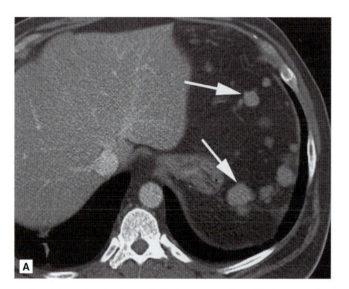

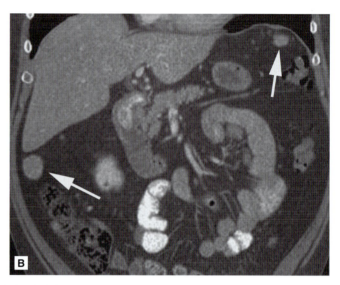

1. A. Axial, contrast-enhanced CT image reveals multiple areas of splenosis in the left upper quadrant (arrows). **B.** Coronal, contrast-enhanced CT image reveals multiple areas of splenosis in the upper abdomen (arrows).

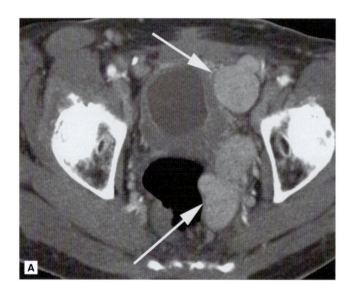

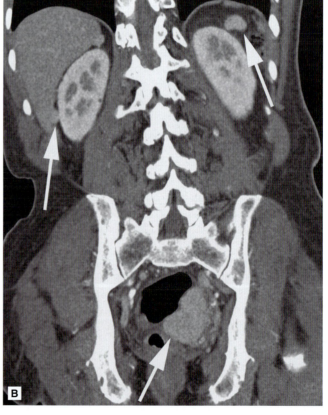

2. A. Axial, contrast-enhanced CT image reveals multiple areas of splenosis in the pelvis (arrows). **B.** Coronal, contrast-enhanced CT image reveals multiple areas of splenosis in the upper abdomen and pelvis (arrows).

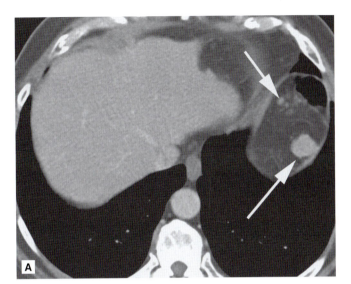

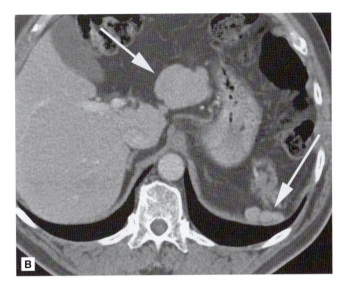

3. A. Axial, contrast-enhanced CT image reveals multiple areas of splenosis in the left upper quadrant (arrows). **B.** Axial, contrast-enhanced CT image more inferiorly reveals multiple areas of splenosis in the left upper quadrant and mid-abdomen (arrows).

CHAPTER 5

ESOPHAGUS

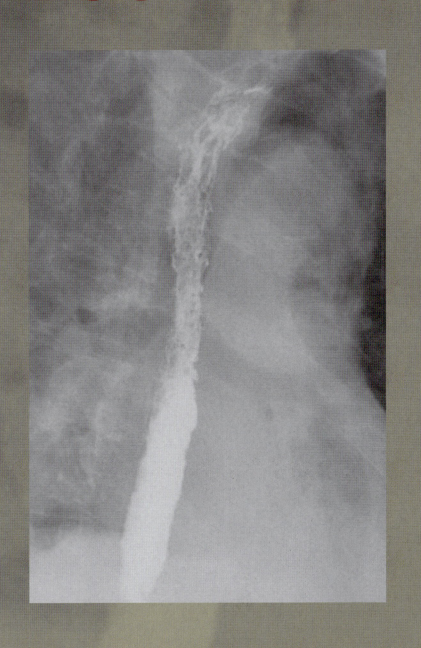

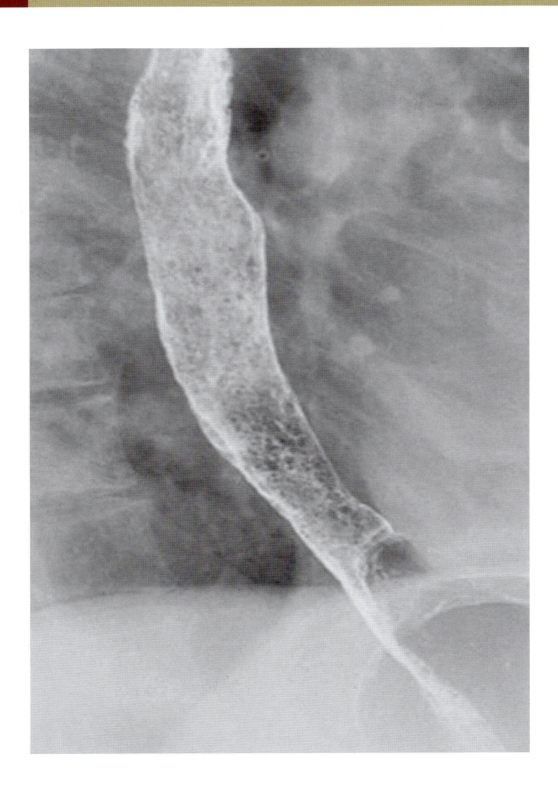

PRESENTATION

Dysphagia, retrosternal pain or odynophagia within several hours to days after taking the medication

FINDINGS

Imaging findings on double-contrast esophagram typically include several discrete ovoid or linear superficial ulcers in proximal or mid-esophagus with surrounding edema.

DIFFERENTIAL DIAGNOSIS

- Infectious esophagitis caused by herpes simplex virus I (HSV1), cytomegalovirus (CMV), human immunodeficiency virus (HIV)
- Reflux esophagitis
- Early esophageal carcinoma

COMMENTS

A number of drugs have been described to be associated with drug-induced esophagitis (DIE) since its original description in 1970. The most common drugs that cause DIE include tetracycline, doxycycline, potassium chloride, quinidine, aspirin and other nonsteroidal anti-inflammatory drugs (NSAIDs), ferrous sulphate, ascorbic acid, and alendronate. Typically patients have a history of taking offending drugs. DIE is a focal contact esophagitis with ulceration of adjacent mucosa by the ingested dissolving tablet. The mid-esophagus is the most common site of involvement, the reason being that it is the transition zone between skeletal and smooth muscle and also due to the external compression by the adjacent aortic arch or left mainstem bronchus, thus leading to abnormal peristaltic activity which permits lengthened mucosal contact with ingested medications.

The radiological finding in DIE depends on the degree of involvement of the esophagus which is again related to the nature of the offending drug. Double-contrast esophagram is the choice of the study. Tetracycline and doxycycline cause superficial ulcerations without permanent damage whereas quinidine, NSAIDs, potassium chloride, and alendronate are associated with more aggressive esophagitis leading to formation of deep ulcers and strictures. The affected segments of the esophagus show single or multiple shallow ulcerations over an edematous background mucosa. These ulcers may be punctate, linear, ovoid, stellate, or serpiginous shape involving either one wall or the entire circumference. A repeat esophagram 7 to 10 days after withdrawal of the offending drug shows dramatic healing of the ulcerations.

Mid-esophagus at the level of aortic arch or left main bronchus is the most common site of involvement as it is being the transition zone between skeletal and smooth muscle and thus leads to discoordinate peristaltic activity which permits lengthened mucosal contact with ingested medication. Less frequently pre-existing conditions of the esophagus like motility disorders, strictures, or compression by enlarged heart on esophagus can also lead to increased transit time and thus subject to prolonged retention of the medication within the esophagus.

PEARLS

- **DIE is a focal contact esophagitis with ulceration of the adjacent mucosa in patients taking the offending drug.**
- **Double-contrast esophagram shows single or multiple ovoid or linear superficial ulcers in the mid-esophagus with surrounding edema, which returns to a normal mucosal pattern once the offending drug is withdrawn.**
- **Viral esophagitis often mimics DIE. However, clinical history and temporal relation of drug ingestion and onset of symptoms help to differentiate the two.**

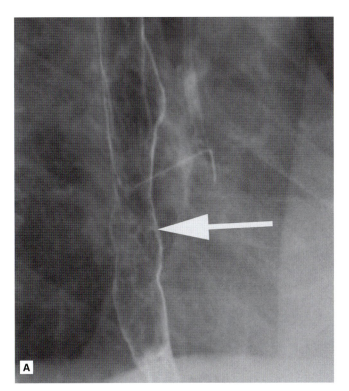

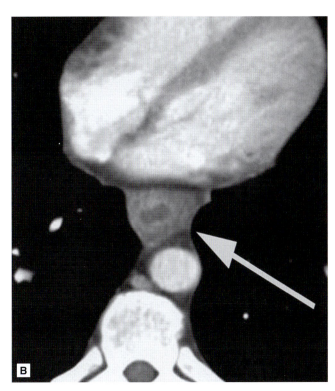

1. A. Fluoroscopic image from barium-swallow examination reveals multiple, small, ovoid ulcerations (arrow) in a patient with cisplatin-induced esophagitis. **B.** Axial, contrast-enhanced CT image demonstrates significant esophageal edema (arrow) related to cisplatin-induced esophagitis.

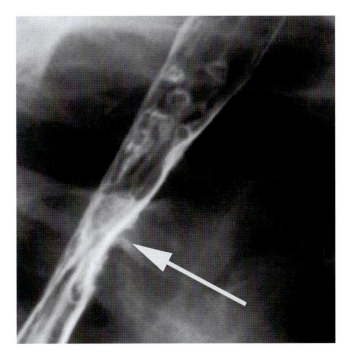

2. Fluoroscopic image from barium-swallow examination reveals multiple, small, ovoid, and linear ulcerations (arrow) in a patient with NSAID-induced esophagitis.

PRESENTATION

Dysphagia, after several months following radiation treatment

FINDINGS

Esophagram shows a long smooth tapered stricture in the mid-esophagus.

DIFFERENTIAL DIAGNOSIS

- Infectious esophagitis
- Esophageal involvement by mediastinal tumors

COMMENTS

Mediastinal radiation therapy for malignant tumors of the lungs, mediastinum, or thoracic spine can lead to radiation-induced esophageal damage. Radiation doses in the range of 20 to 45 Gy lead to a self-limited esophagitis, whereas high doses greater than 50 Gy frequently cause severe esophagitis with irreversible stricture formation. Patients who receive high-dose radiation encompassing the esophagus usually develop an acute, self-limited esophagitis within 1 to 4 weeks which subsequently leads to chronic radiation esophagitis characterized by progressive submucosal scarring and fibrosis. Chronic radiation esophagitis usually manifests 4 to 8 months following radiation therapy as a long, smooth, tapered stricture.

Acute radiation esophagitis is characterized by mucosal edema and inflammation, sometimes with small discrete ulcers within the known radiation portal. Double-contrast esophagram shows mucosal granularity and decreased distensibility of the involved segment of the esophagus. After 4 to 8 weeks following radiation therapy, the esophagus typically demonstrates abnormal motility with poor peristalsis. Subsequent submucosal scarring and fibrosis leads to a long, relatively smooth and tapered stricture of the esophagus several months after completion of therapy. In patients with severe disease, a fistulous communication may develop between the airway and the esophagus, due to radiation-induced necrosis and/or from erosion by the primary tumor.

PEARLS

- Dysphagia in a patient with past history of radiation therapy to the chest should always raise the suspicion of radiation-induced esophageal injury.

- Acute radiation esophagitis causes mucosal edema and inflammation with small discrete ulcers, submucosal scarring and fibrosis, and in the later period causes luminal narrowing.

- Esophagogram demonstrates a long segment with a relatively smooth, tapered, stricture.

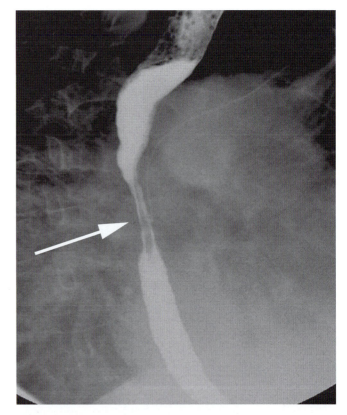

1. Barium swallow demonstrates a long stricture in mid-esophagus (arrow) with smoothly tapered margins secondary to radiation.

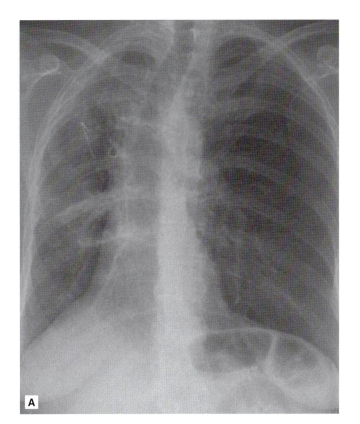

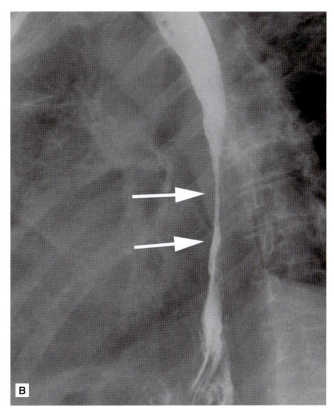

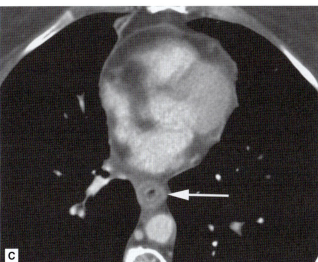

2. A. Frontal chest radiograph reveals linear paramediastinal fibrosis and right-sided volume loss related to radiation. **B.** Barium swallow shows a long, smoothly tapered stricture in mid-esophagus (arrows) secondary to radiation. **C.** Axial, contrast-enhanced CT image reveals circumferential thickening of the esophagus (arrow) related to radiation esophagitis.

PRESENTATION

Heartburn, retrosternal burning, and pain that tends to radiate into the neck and is worse after eating.

FINDINGS

Findings on barium esophagram vary with severity but typically include thickened and nodular mucosal folds with superficial ulcerations in the distal esophagus.

DIFFERENTIAL DIAGNOSIS

- Herpes esophagitis
- *Candida* esophagitis
- Feline esophagus
- Glycogen acanthosis

COMMENTS

Failure of the lower oesophageal sphincter to act as an effective barrier to prevent gastric contents from entering the distal esophagus leads to reflux esophagitis. The severity of reflux esophagitis depends on multiple factors like the frequency and duration of reflux episodes, the content of the refluxed material, and the status of the esophageal mucosa. Several predisposing factors have been described as causing reflux esophagitis, including primary gastroesophageal reflux disease, repeated prolonged vomiting secondary to peptic ulcer disease, biliary colic, intestinal obstruction, acute alcoholic gastritis, repeated vomiting, hormonal effect during third trimester of pregnancy, scleroderma, and medications such as anticholinergics, nitrites, and beta-adrenergic agents.

Reflux esophagitis is best evaluated with a biphasic fluoroscopic examination consisting of upright double-contrast esophagography for the assessment of the esophageal mucosa and prone single-contrast esophagography for demonstrating areas of decreased distensibility of the distal esophagus. However, endoscopy is the most definitive test for reflux esophagitis. A fine nodular or granular appearance due to mucosal edema and inflammation in the distal third or half of the esophagus is the earliest sign of reflux esophagitis on double-contrast esophagram. As the disease progresses, shallow ulcers and erosions are seen with surrounding edematous mucosa, radiating folds, and puckering and sacculation of the esophageal wall on double-contrast images. With the single-contrast technique, the esophagus may show decreased distensibility with a thickened wall and grossly irregular contours with serrated or speculated margins resulting from extensive ulcerations, edema, and spasm. Some patients may develop scarring from reflux esophagitis, which leads to focal outpouchings or sacculations and fixed transverse folds in the distal esophagus.

In more chronic cases, circumferential scarring of the distal esophagus leads to formation of a peptic stricture which appears as smooth, tapered area of concentric narrowing in the distal esophagram, characteristically located above a sliding hiatal hernia.

PEARLS

- Failure of the lower sphincter to act as a barrier to stomach contents entering the distal esophagus leads to reflux esophagitis.

- A biphasic examination with upright double-contrast esophagography and prone single-contrast esophagography is the best test for complete assessment.

- On double-contrast imaging, findings include shallow ulcers and erosions in the distal esophagus with surrounding edematous mucosa and radiating folds.

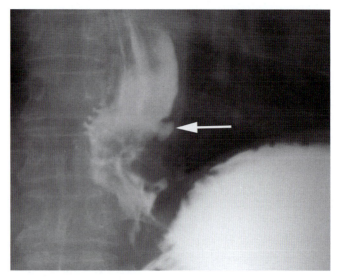

1. Esophagram demonstrates thickened longitudinal folds and multiple deep ulcers (arrow) in distal esophagus secondary to reflux esophagitis.

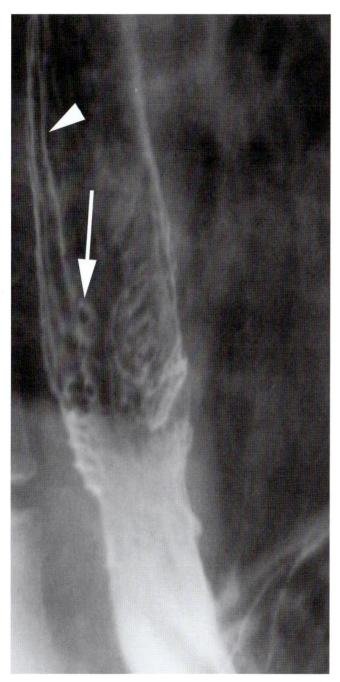

2. Double-contrast image from a barium swallow demonstrates thickened folds (arrowhead) and multiple shallow ulcers (arrow) in the distal esophagus secondary to reflux esophagitis.

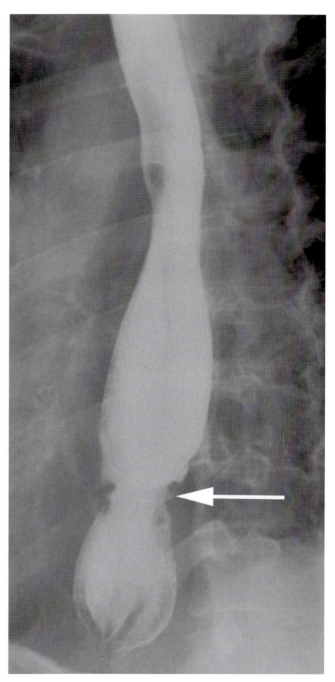

3. Double-contrast image from a barium swallow reveals asymmetric narrowing and ulcerations (arrow) in distal esophagus related to reflux esophagitis.

PRESENTATION

Odynophagia is the most common presenting symptom while, occasionally, patients may present with chest pain, gastrointestinal bleeding, and dysphagia.

FINDINGS

The appearance of viral esophagitis varies based on the underlying etiology and ranges from multiple small, discrete ulcers in herpes simplex virus (HSV) esophagitis to giant ulcers greater than 1 cm in size in cytomegalo virus (CMV) esophagitis.

DIFFERENTIAL DIAGNOSIS

- *Candida* esophagitis
- Reflux esophagitis
- Drug-induced esophagitis

COMMENTS

Viral esophagitis is the second most common type of infectious esophagitis, trailing only *Candida* esophagitis. The three most common causes of viral esophagitis are HSV, CMV, and human immunodeficiency virus (HIV). Patients at risk for developing viral esophagitis often have underlying conditions that predispose the esophageal mucosa to infection such as an immunocompromised state or prior radiation therapy. Typically, the infection is the result of reactivation of a latent virus rather than exogenous infection.

The diagnosis of esophagitis is typically made via a double-contrast esophagram. HSV is the most common viral esophagitis and is usually found in immunocompromised patients, although on occasion, normal hosts can also be infected. HSV is characterized by multiple small, discrete ulcers with a punctate, linear, or stellate shape. There is often a surrounding halo of edema and a background of normal mucosa. Advanced cases may have plaques and the appearance of a shaggy mucosa, similar to *Candida* esophagitis. If imaging findings are equivocal or response to treatment is inadequate, tissue sampling can be done for definitive diagnosis. Pathologically, early disease is characterized by esophageal blisters or vesicular rupture, while later disease will appear as fibrinous exudates forming pseudomembranes over the ulcers.

Unlike HSV, CMV esophagitis almost never occurs in immunocompetent hosts. CMV esophagitis is characterized by giant ulcers, usually greater than 1 cm in size, that are relatively flat. Occasionally there are small satellite lesions as well. HIV esophagitis also has flat giant ulcers that can be indistinguishable from CMV, and tissue diagnosis may be needed to establish a definitive etiology. Other less common viral causes of esophagitis include Epstein-Barr virus (EBV) (deep linear ulcers) and human papillomavirus (HPV) (multiple papillary excrescences).

PEARLS

- HSV esophagitis, the most common etiology of viral esophagitis, is characterized by multiple small, discrete ulcers with a punctate, linear, or stellate shape.

- CMV esophagitis is characterized by giant ulcers, usually greater than 1 cm in size, that are relatively flat and is almost never seen in immunocompetent hosts.

- HIV esophagitis has flat giant ulcers that can be indistinguishable from CMV infection.

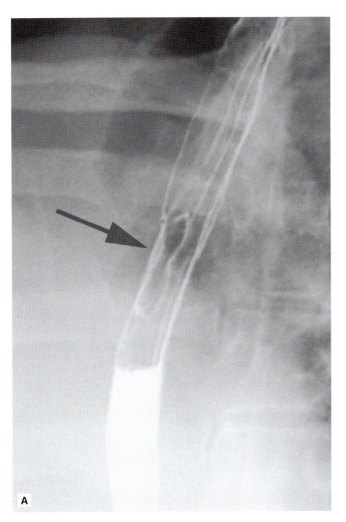

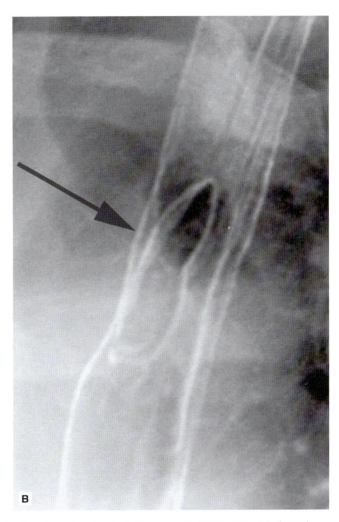

1. A. Fluoroscopic image from a barium swallow examination demonstrates the characteristic giant ulcer seen in CMV esophagitis (arrow).
B. The characteristic giant ulcer seen in CMV esophagitis (arrow) is well seen in this fluoroscopic image from a barium swallow examination.

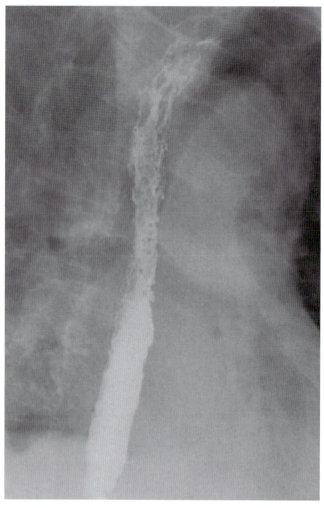

2. Fluoroscopic image from a barium swallow examination demonstrates numerous small discrete punctuate and linear ulcers characteristic of HSV esophagitis.

PRESENTATION

Acute or insidious onset of dysphagia and retrosternal pain in patients who are immunocompromised

FINDINGS

Double-contrast esophagram demonstrates esophageal dysmotility, fold thickening, ulcerations with discrete plaque-like lesions, and mucosal nodularity and/or granularity.

DIFFERENTIAL DIAGNOSIS

- Reflux esophagitis
- Herpes esophagitis
- Glycogen acanthosis
- Superficial spreading carcinoma

COMMENTS

Candida esophagitis is the most common infectious esophagitis and is caused by *Candida albicans*, a commensal inhabitant of the pharynx. *Candida* esophagitis occurs predominantly in patients who are immunocompromised because of an underlying malignancy, such as leukemia or lymphoma, and in patients receiving radiation therapy, chemotherapy, corticosteroids or any other immunosuppressant drug. Chronic debilitating diseases like diabetes, multiple myeloma, lupus erythematosus, primary hypothyroidism, and renal failure are additional factors that predispose to candidal infection. Esophageal candidiasis is also found in patients with local esophageal stasis secondary to functional or mechanical disturbances.

Typically, patients present with acute onset of dysphagia or odynophagia. Oropharyngeal involvement is seen in up to 75% of the patients with *Candida* esophagitis. Double-contrast esophagram is the preferred imaging method to demonstrate the mucosal involvement. Dysmotility may be the only finding on early stages. However, as the disease progresses, small marginal filling defects are produced with fine serrations along the outer border. With further involvement of mucosa, discrete plaque-like lesions consisting of longitudinally oriented area of mucosal ulcerations covered with necrotic epithelial debris and moulds of fungi will develop, with normal intervening mucosa. Nodularity, granularity, and fold thickening may occur due to mucosal inflammation and edema. In severe *Candida* esophagitis, the esophagus becomes grossly irregular with a shaggy marginal contour because of coalescent plaques, deep ulcerations, and sloughing of mucosa. In some patients, barium may penetrate under the plaques or pseudomembranes producing a radiographic appearance of double-barrelled esophagus or intramural tracking.

Candida esophagitis secondary to local esophageal stasis (particularly in patients with achalasia or scleroderma) appears as tiny nodular defects, polypoid folds, or a distinctive lacy pattern on double-contrast esophagram. A "foamy" esophagus refers to innumerable tiny rounded bubbles on the top of the barium column from extrinsic production of CO_2 by the yeast form of the fungus.

PEARLS

- *Candida* esophagitis is the most common cause of esophagitis caused by *C albicans* in immunocompromised patients.

- Typical findings on double-contrast esophagram include multiple discrete plaque-like filling defects with shaggy, irregular luminal contours. Early stages present with multiple discrete small ulcers.

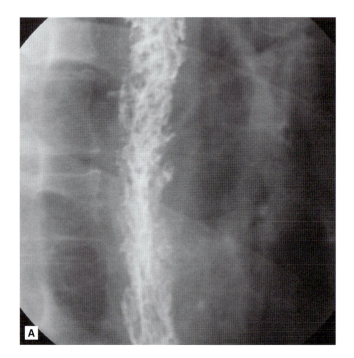

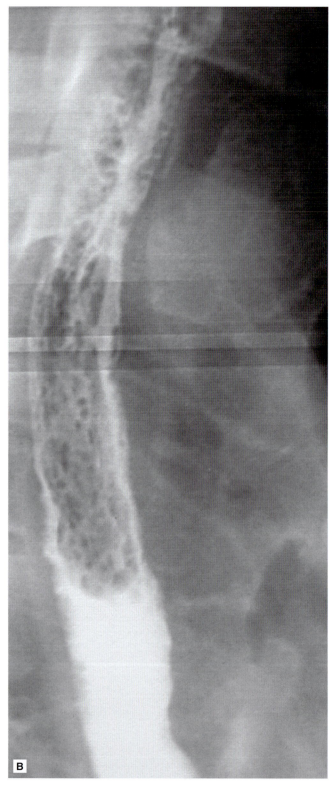

1. A. Barium study in a patient with AIDS shows shaggy irregular contour from coalescent plaque-like mucosal ulceration. **B.** Double-contrast image reveals multiple discrete and confluent plaque-like ulcers of various shapes in a patient with *Candida* esophagitis.

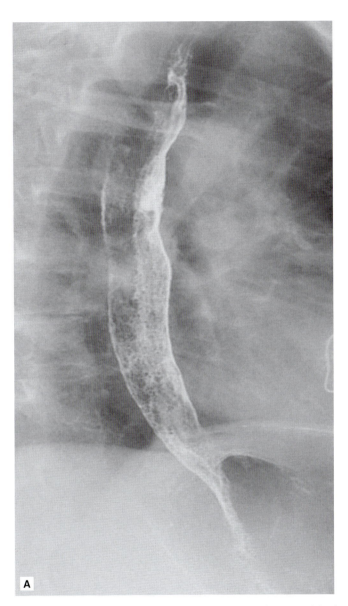

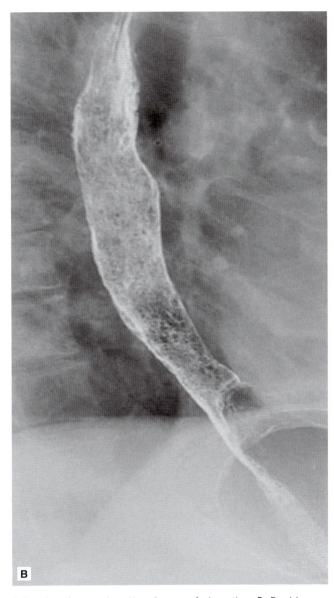

2. A. Double-contrast view of esophagus illustrates innumerable tiny nodular elevations and scattered areas of ulceration. **B.** Double-contrast view of the esophagus reveals numerous small filling defects, an early finding in patients with *Candida* esophagitis.

ESOPHAGEAL DIVERTICULA

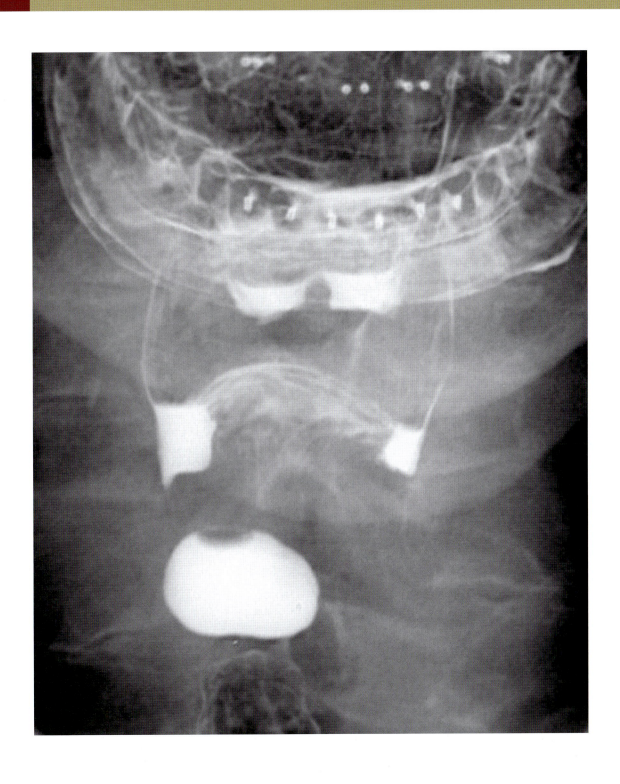

PRESENTATION

Usually presents with suprasternal dysphagia, reflux or regurgitation, cough, aspiration pneumonia.

FINDINGS

Zenker diverticula are identified as round or oval, smoothly marginated outpouchings of the posterior portion of the pharyngoesophageal segment.

DIFFERENTIAL DIAGNOSIS

- Killian-Jamieson diverticulum
- Pseudo-Zenker diverticulum

COMMENTS

A Zenker diverticulum is mucosal hernia of the cervical esophagus through an anatomically weak muscular gap in the posterior portion of the cricopharyngeus muscle. This area is located between the horizontal and oblique fibers of the pharyngoesophageal segment above the cricopharyngeus muscle called the Killian dehiscence or Killian triangle. Zenker diverticula are pulsion diverticula resulting from increased esophageal pressure related to failure of the cricopharyngeus muscle to relax during swallowing. Prominence of the cricopharyngeal muscle is invariably seen. Hypertrophy of the cricopharyngeus muscle may occur with gastroesophageal reflux which contributes to the formation of Zenker diverticula. Esophageal spasm or dysmotility and other associated abnormalities such as hiatal hernia may predispose to diverticular formation.

Zenker diverticula are more common than Killian-Jamieson diverticula and are more commonly symptomatic. Suprasternal dysphagia and retention of undigested food within the diverticulum can cause halitosis and choking with possible aspiration. These diverticula typically occur in older patients and can be seen in patients with esophageal dysmotility disorders or abnormal swallowing.

During swallowing on a fluoroscopic barium examination, Zenker diverticula appear as round or oval, smoothly marginated outpouchings of the posterior portion of the pharyngoesophageal segment with the neck originating above the cricopharyngeus muscle. A thickened cricopharyngeus muscle is seen inferior to the diverticulum and is best visualized on the lateral projection. Emptying of the barium-filled diverticulum or regurgitation is seen after swallowing during the barium examination. Pseudo-Zenker diverticula are a potential imaging pitfall and result from a pharyngeal peristaltic wave and a prominent cricopharyngeus muscle which can appear as a transient small bulge emanating from the posterior pharyngeal wall caudal to the cricopharyngeus muscle, however, after the peristaltic wave passes, the trapped barium is cleared.

PEARLS

- A Zenker diverticulum is mucosal hernia of the cervical esophagus through an anatomically weak muscular gap in the posterior portion of the cricopharyngeus muscle.

- Zenker diverticula appear as round or oval, smoothly marginated outpouchings of the posterior portion of the pharyngoesophageal segment, at the level of the cricopharyngeus muscle.

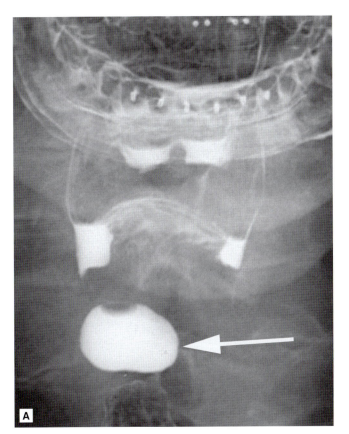

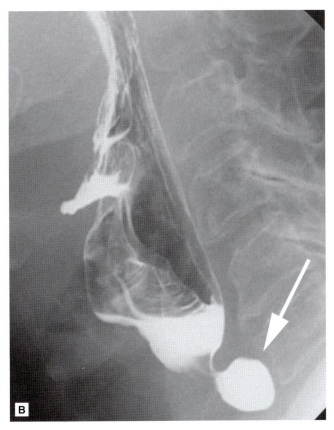

1. A. Frontal fluoroscopic image from a barium-swallow examination demonstrates a barium-filled outpouching from the pharyngoesopha-geal segment (arrow). **B.** Lateral fluoroscopic image from a barium-swallow examination confirms the presence of a Zenker diverticulum as evidenced by its posterior location (arrow), at the level of the cricopharyngeus muscle.

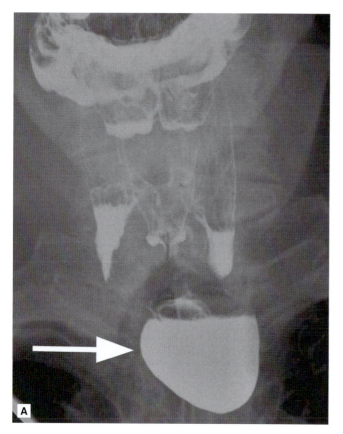

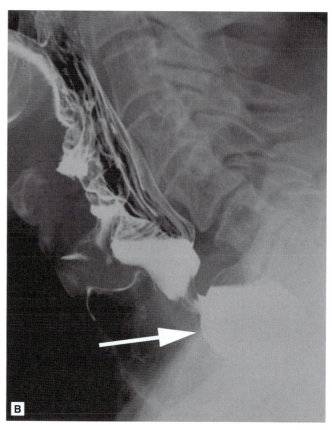

2. A. Frontal fluoroscopic image from a barium-swallow examination demonstrates the presence of a large air and barium-filled outpouching from the pharyngoesophageal segment (arrow). **B.** Lateral fluoroscopic image from a barium-swallow examination confirms the presence of a large Zenker diverticulum as evidenced by its posterior location (arrow).

PRESENTATION

While usually asymptomatic, patients may occasionally present with regurgitation or dysphagia.

FINDINGS

On fluoroscopic esophagram, traction diverticula are typically located in the mid-esophagus with a tented or triangular shape and a wide mouth.

DIFFERENTIAL DIAGNOSIS

- Zenker diverticulum
- Pulsion diverticulum
- Esophageal ulcer
- Esophageal perforation

COMMENTS

Esophageal traction diverticula represent a relatively rare type of esophageal outpouching caused by acutely inflamed and enlarged subcarinal lymph nodes. These inflamed lymph nodes adhere to the walls of the esophagus during the initial inflammatory process, and subsequently, as the inflammation subsides, retract the esophageal wall. This process produces an outpouching of all three layers of the esophagus, usually along the right anterior wall at the level of the carina. Tuberculosis is the most common cause, but other granulomatous infections such as sarcoidosis and histoplasmosis may have a similar consequence. Typically, small diverticula are asymptomatic but larger diverticula may lead to symptoms such as regurgitation and dysphagia. While uncommon, potential complications of traction diverticula include their progression to esophageal perforation as well as the formation of fistula to adjacent structures including airways and vasculature.

The presence of a traction diverticulum may be suggested on plain radiography by calcification of perihilar nodes and thickening of the posterior tracheal stripe. Confirmation of a suspected traction diverticulum requires a fluoroscopic esophagram study which typically demonstrates a mid-esophageal diverticulum with a tented or triangular shape and a wide mouth. Traction diverticula tend to empty when the esophagus is collapsed given the presence of muscular layers in these true diverticula. Traction diverticula may range from a few millimeters to several centimeters in size.

PEARLS

- **Traction diverticula are typically caused by acutely inflamed and enlarged subcarinal lymph nodes.**

- **On fluoroscopic esophagography, pulsion diverticula are typically identified as mid-esophageal diverticulum with a tented or triangular shape and a wide mouth.**

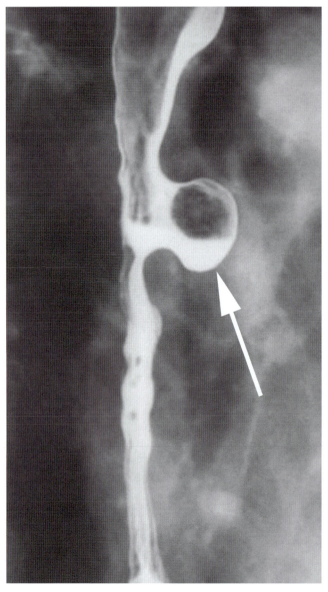

1. Fluoroscopic image during a barium-swallow examination demonstrates a small mid-esophageal, air- and contrast-containing diverticulum, the imaging features of which are consistent with a traction diverticulum (arrow).

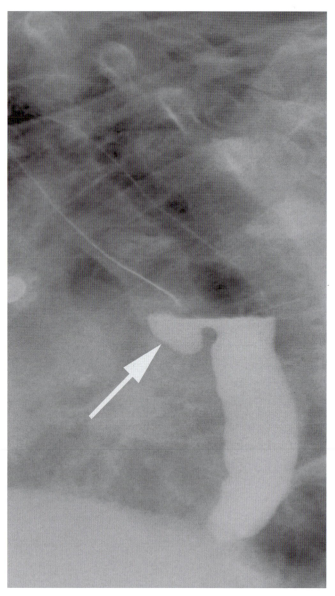

2. Fluoroscopic image acquired during a barium-swallow examination demonstrates a mid-esophageal traction diverticulum (arrow).

PRESENTATION

While typically asymptomatic, patients may present with regurgitation, halitosis, chest pain, or aspiration.

FINDINGS

Pulsion diverticula are often found in an epiphrenic location and are associated with abnormal esophageal motility or peristalsis (ie, diffuse spasm, presbyesophagus, achalasia).

DIFFERENTIAL DIAGNOSIS

- Traction diverticulum
- Esophageal web
- Esophageal ring
- Hiatal hernia
- Killian-Jamieson diverticulum

COMMENTS

Pulsion diverticula are often large and saccular esophageal outpouchings (false diverticula) of mucosa and submucosa through the oblique and transverse layers of the cricopharyngeal muscles. Pulsion diverticula are caused by high intraluminal pressures resulting in an outpouching through an area of relative mural weakness. Pulsion diverticula may be located anywhere along the esophagus, but are often found in an epiphrenic location and are associated with abnormal esophageal motility or peristalsis (ie, diffuse spasm, presbyesophagus, achalasia). In an epiphrenic location, pulsion diverticula are commonly found on the lateral wall of the esophagus and are more frequently seen on the right side of the esophagus. In contradistinction to traction diverticulum, pulsion diverticula contain no muscle within their walls, and therefore tend to retain undigested food contents, leading to complaints of regurgitation of undigested food, halitosis, globus sensation and increased rates of dysphagia, gastroesophageal reflux, and aspiration pneumonia. Potential complications of pulsion diverticula, while uncommon, include gastrointestinal hemorrhage as well as the development of malignancy within a diverticulum.

As pulsion diverticula are false diverticula and lack muscular layers, they are readily identified on fluoroscopic studies given an inability to contract and expel retained contrast material. Fluoroscopic studies may also reveal an etiology of increased intraluminal pressure leading to the pulsion diverticulum such as achalasia. On CT, pulsion diverticula are typically thin-walled and well circumscribed and may contain variable amounts of oral contrast, debris, and air.

PEARLS

- **Pulsion diverticula are caused by high intraluminal pressures, typically related to abnormal esophageal motility or peristalsis, resulting in an outpouching through an area of relative mural weakness.**

- **Pulsion diverticula may be located anywhere along the esophagus, but are often found in an epiphrenic location.**

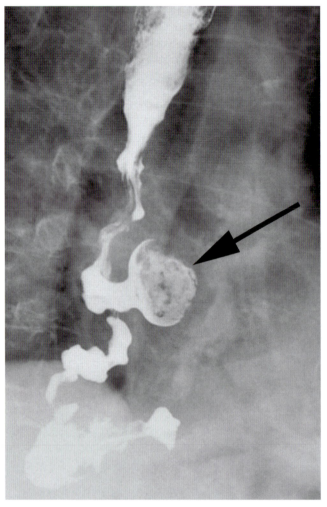

1. Fluoroscopic image from a barium-swallow examination demonstrates a pulsion diverticulum (arrow) in the distal esophagus in a patient with severe esophageal dysmotility.

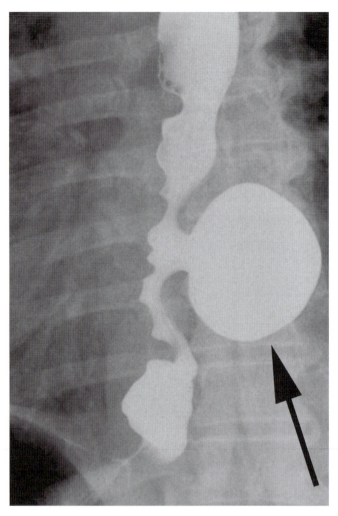

2. Fluoroscopic image from a barium-swallow examination demonstrates a pulsion diverticulum (arrow) in the typical epiphrenic location in the distal esophagus. Note the severe esophageal dysmotility, a common underlying etiology.

PRESENTATION

While pseudodiverticula are typically incidental and asymptomatic, patients may present with dysphagia or epigastric pain due to associated esophageal strictures or esophagitis.

FINDINGS

Tiny, innumerable, barium-filled outpouchings in longitudinal rows parallel to esophageal wall are typically appreciated on barium studies.

DIFFERENTIAL DIAGNOSIS

• Drug-induced esophagitis

• Reflux esophagitis

• Infectious esophagitis

COMMENTS

Esophageal intramural pseudodiverticulosis is a benign condition characterized by multiple flask-shaped outpouchings in the esophageal wall. Pseudodiverticulosis is thought to result from dilation of excretory ducts of deep mucous glands. Some believe that this ductal dilatation results from plugging and obstruction of ducts by thick, viscous mucous, inflammatory material, and/or desquamated epithelium. Others believe that the ducts may be externally compressed by periductal inflammation and fibrosis that results from chronic esophagitis. Pseudodiverticulosis itself rarely causes problems but the patients usually have associated chronic esophagitis, gastroesophageal reflux, and candida colonization, or motility disorders. In fact, up to 80% to 90% of patients with esophageal pseudodiverticulosis are found to have endoscopic and/or histologic evidence of esophagitis. Strictures coexist in 90% of the reported cases, most frequently in the upper third of the esophagus. Endoscopy and biopsy are required to rule out malignancy when a stricture is present. Pseudodiverticulosis usually occurs in the elderly, with a slight male predominance and most patients present with intermittent or slowly progressive dysphagia and/or heartburn due to associated strictures and/or esophagitis. Complications related to pseudodiverticula are rare and include pseudodiverticulosis, abscess formation, perforation, and mediastinitis.

The pseudodiverticula form in the wall of the esophagus with diffuse involvement in half of the patients and segmental involvement in the other half. The outpouchings are typically tiny, ranging in size from 1 to 4 mm. Single-contrast barium esophagograms readily demonstrate tiny, innumerable, barium-filled outpouchings in longitudinal rows parallel to esophageal wall. Thin barium better demonstrates the pseudodiverticula compared to thick barium given its ability to penetrate the necks of these tiny outpouchings. Inflammatory debris may fill the necks of the pseudodiverticula, preventing the entry of barium, resulting in failure to visualize them on imaging. Intramural bridging between the adjacent pseudodiverticula appears as intramural tracks which may be mistaken for large flat ulcers or extramural barium collections. On CT, tiny foci of intramural gas, esophageal wall thickening and mucosal irregularity may be seen.

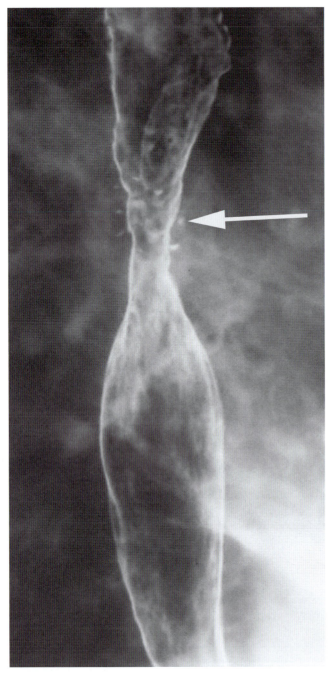

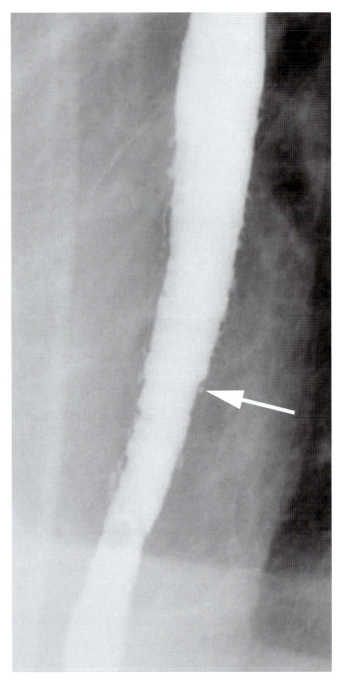

1. Fluoroscopic image from a barium-swallow examination demonstrates numerous small outpouchings of the esophagus immediately proximal to an esophageal stricture, consistent with pseudodiverticula (arrow).

2. Fluoroscopic image from a barium-swallow examination demonstrates innumerable small outpouchings throughout the esophagus consistent with pseudodiverticula (arrow).

PRESENTATION

Usually asymptomatic, however, can present with dysphagia or regurgitation.

FINDINGS

A Killian-Jamieson diverticulum is identified on a barium examination as a round or oval, smoothly marginated, barium-filled diverticulum from the anterolateral wall of the cervical esophagus.

DIFFERENTIAL DIAGNOSIS

• Zenker diverticulum

COMMENTS

A Killian-Jamieson diverticulum is a saccular protrusion of the anterolateral esophagus through an area of muscular weakness known as the Killian-Jamieson space. The Killian-Jamieson space is located inferior to the cricopharyngeus muscle attachment on the cricoid cartilage and lateral to the suspensory ligaments of the esophagus. Killian-Jamieson diverticula project anteriorly and laterally, off midline, in the proximal cervical esophagus and are located below the cricopharyngeus muscle.

Typically Killian-Jamieson diverticula are asymptomatic and are incidentally found; however, they may occasionally present with dysphagia and regurgitation. They typically occur in older patients and in patients with esophageal dysmotility disorders or abnormal swallowing. The diverticula are usually bilateral but can be unilateral and Killian-Jamieson diverticula may coexist with Zenker diverticula. The Killian-Jamieson diverticula tend to be smaller in size and are less likely to be symptomatic compared to Zenker diverticula.

The esophageal protrusion of the Killian-Jamieson diverticulum is identified on a barium examination as a round or oval, smoothly marginated, barium-filled diverticulum of variable size protruding from the anterolateral wall of the cervical esophagus, in contradistinction to a Zenker diverticulum which is located in the midline and protrudes posteriorly. On CT, air, oral contrast, and fluid can be seen in a Killian-Jamieson diverticulum.

PEARL

• A Killian-Jamieson diverticulum is identified on a barium examination as a round or oval, smoothly marginated, barium-filled outpouching of variable size protruding from the anterolateral wall of the cervical esophagus.

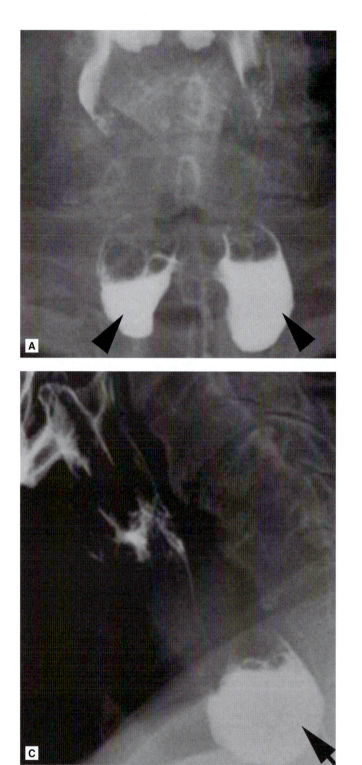

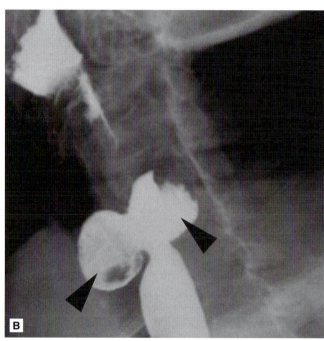

1. A. Frontal fluoroscopic image from a barium-swallow examination demonstrates bilateral Killian-Jamieson diverticula extending laterally from the cervical esophagus (arrowheads). **B.** Oblique fluoroscopic image from a barium-swallow examination demonstrates bilateral Killian-Jamieson diverticula extending laterally from the cervical esophagus (arrowheads). **C.** Lateral fluoroscopic image from a barium-swallow examination demonstrates bilateral Killian-Jamieson diverticula extending laterally from the cervical esophagus (arrow).

ESOPHAGEAL NEOPLASMS

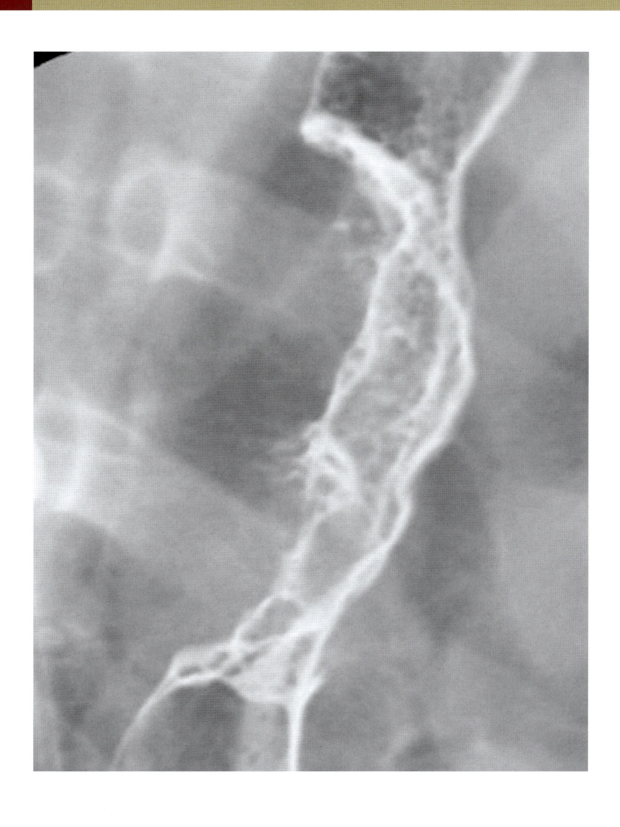

PRESENTATION

Most patients, especially the elderly, present with long-standing dysphagia. Fewer patients present with regurgitation of the mass into the pharynx or mouth.

FINDINGS

Fibrovascular polyp is diagnosed based on finding a fat density lesion within the expanded lumen of the esophagus, with a thin rim of contrast surrounding the polyp. Barium esophagram reveals a large, smooth, intraluminal mass with a stalk.

DIFFERENTIAL DIAGNOSIS

- Fibrovascular polyp
- Adenomatous polyp
- Spindle cell carcinoma
- Intraluminal gastrointestinal stromal tumor
- Primary malignant melanomas of the esophagus

COMMENTS

Fibrovascular polyps are pedunculated intraluminal mass lesions with a potential to grow to a large size. Histologically, these polyps are covered by normal squamous epithelium with a central core of fibrovascular tissue, adipose cells and stroma that develop in loose mucosa or submucosa of the cervical esophagus. Esophageal peristalsis drags them toward the stomach as they grow over a period of time. Patients are usually elderly, men, and asymptomatic initially. As the polyps grow, they become large and obstruct, ulcerate or bleed. Occasionally, they may prolapse into the mouth or even into larynx, causing asphyxia.

On barium esophagram, a bulky, smooth, sausage-shaped intraluminal mass that arises in the cervical esophagus and extends into the upper or middle third of the thoracic esophagus is seen. It is often difficult to demonstrate the cervical attachment of the fibrovascular polyp on barium studies. CT and MRI demonstrate the fat-containing lesion within the esophageal lumen, with a thin rim of contrast surrounding the polyp.

PEARLS

- Fibrovascular polyps are solitary, pedunculated, intraluminal lesions arising from the upper cervical esophagus.

- These tumors are covered by squamous epithelium and have a vascular core of fibrous and adipose tissue.

- Barium studies show a mobile intraluminal mass and CT and MRI demonstrate a fat-containing lesion within the esophageal lumen.

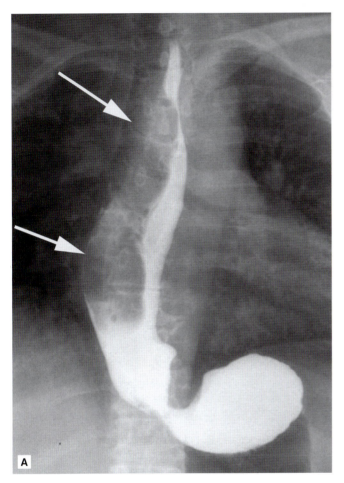

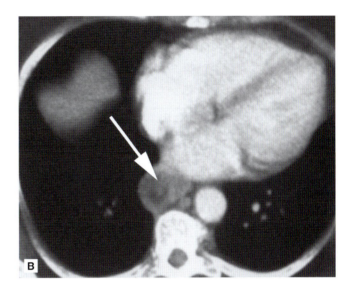

1. A. Esophagram image reveals a large, smooth, filling defect within the esophagus (arrows). **B.** Axial, contrast-enhanced CT image reveals a filling defect within the esophageal lumen (arrow) with soft tissue and fat attenuation representing a fibrovascular polyp.

PRESENTATION

Esophageal leiomyomas are usually asymptomatic. Symptomatic patients present with intermittent, slowly worsening dysphagia.

FINDINGS

En face barium esophagram demonstrates a smooth, rounded intramural defect. Profile images demonstrate with margins that make right or slightly obtuse angles with the adjacent normal esophageal wall.

DIFFERENTIAL DIAGNOSIS

Intramural tumors (lipoma, granular cell tumor, hemangioma, fibroma, neurofibroma), congenital duplication and acquired retention cysts, Kaposi sarcoma, lymphomatous or leukemic infiltration, and any extramural lesions.

COMMENTS

Leiomyoma is a well-encapsulated smooth muscle submucosal tumor. It is the most common benign tumor of the esophagus and is most often found in the lower two-thirds, as this portion has abundant smooth muscle. They usually attain a size of 2 to 8 cm and giant tumors may grow up to 20 cm. Leiomyomas are often seen as solitary lesions, but multiple tumors are present in 3% to 4% of cases. Occasionally, leiomyomas show amorphous or punctuate calcification. Esophageal leiomyomas have been described in association with vulval leiomyomas and with hypertrophic osteoarthropathy.

Leiomyomas of the esophagus are often asymptomatic. When these patients are symptomatic, they present with intermittent, slowly worsening dysphagia or, less commonly, with substernal discomfort, vomiting, or weight loss. Esophageal leiomyomas rarely ulcerate or bleed and a very small fraction undergoes malignant degeneration over a period. Asymptomatic patients may never require any aggressive treatment.

Exophytic esophageal leiomyomas may appear as mediastinal masses on chest radiographs. Barium esophagram demonstrates a discrete smooth, round or ovoid filling defect. When viewed in profile, the lesion has a smooth, rounded surface and their superior and inferior margins form right or obtuse angles with the adjacent esophagus, suggesting an intramural origin. Typically, leiomyomas appear as homogenous ovoid masses of soft tissue density eccentric to the lumen on CT but differentiation from other esophageal tumors is often difficult.

PEARLS

- **Leiomyoma is a well-encapsulated smooth muscle submucosal tumor and is most often found in the lower two-thirds of the esophagus.**

- **Often asymptomatic, but when symptomatic, they present with intermittent, slowly worsening dysphagia.**

- **The typical appearance on barium esophagram is of an intramural lesion with margins that make an obtuse angle with the normal adjacent esophageal wall.**

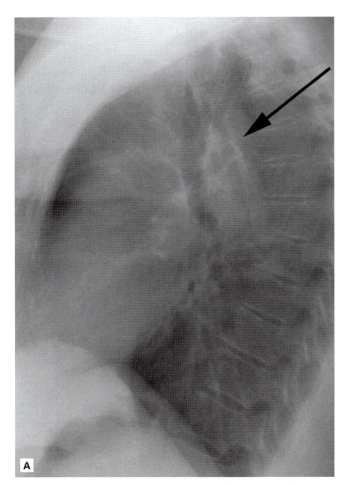

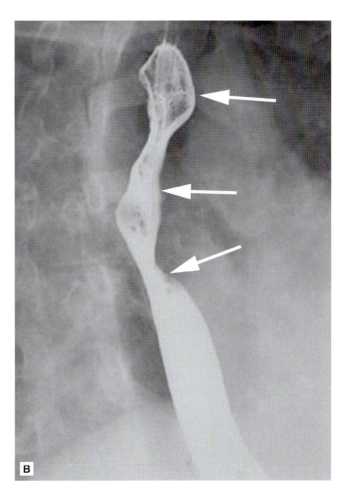

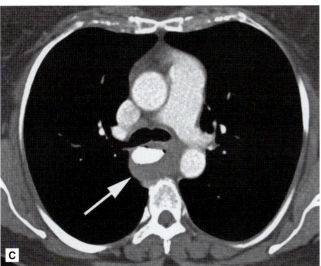

1. **A.** Lateral chest radiograph reveals an opacity overlying the expected course of the esophagus (arrow). **B.** Esophagram image reveals a well-defined, smooth distortion of the barium column (arrows) with obtuse angles with respect to the esophageal lumen. **C.** Axial, contrast-enhanced CT image reveals an intramural mass lesion (arrow) within the esophagus representing an esophageal leiomyoma.

Case 5–13   Esophageal Carcinoma

PRESENTATION

Dysphagia, odynophagia, and weight loss

FINDINGS

Barium studies demonstrate a large centrally ulcerated or polypoid mass with irregular luminal contour and abruptly shouldering edges in the esophagus.

DIFFERENTIAL DIAGNOSIS

- Spindle cell carcinoma
- Lymphoma
- Esophageal leiomyoma
- Metastasis

COMMENTS

Primary esophageal carcinoma accounts for approximately 7% of all gastrointestinal (GI) malignancies and constitutes only 1% of all cancers. Two major histologic types include squamous cell carcinoma and adenocarcinoma. Squamous cell carcinoma is most often affects mid-esophagus and is associated with alcohol and tobacco consumption. Conditions like achalasia, lye stricture, head and neck tumors, celiac disease, Plummer-Vinson syndrome, radiation, and tylosis are thought to predispose patients to develop squamous cell carcinoma. Adenocarcinoma most often occurs in the distal esophagus and is increasing in frequency due to its association with Barrett esophagus and subsequent dysplasia. A variety of morphologic appearances that include ulcerative, polypoid, nodular, and irregular structuring are known to be associated with both histologic types. Other less common types include varicoid and superficial spreading. Most of the esophageal carcinomas are detected in a stage of advanced narrowing or stricture. Barium studies demonstrate a malignant stricture with nodular and irregular margins due to tumor infiltration. As the disease advances, the esophageal lumen may become obliterated and total dysphagia develops. It is also common for the tumor to spread through the muscular layers and then infiltrate adjacent structures in the mediastinum, such as the aorta. Further growth and deep extension leads to fistulization with the trachea and bronchial tree. Early mediastinal extension has been attributed to the lack of a serosal layer in the esophagus.

CT typically demonstrates asymmetric thickening of the esophageal wall or polypoid growth filling the lumen along with a dilated esophagus proximal to the lesion. CT is a better tool for assessment of mediastinal extension and staging such as metastatic involvement of lungs, liver, and lymph nodes.

PEARLS

- Alcohol and tobacco consumption increases the risk of developing squamous cell cancer, whereas Barrett metaplasia in the distal esophagus predisposes patients to develop adenocarcinoma.

- Squamous cell carcinoma occurs in mid-esophagus and does not cross the gastroesophageal junction, whereas adenocarcinoma arising in pre-existing Barrett esophagus frequently extends to the stomach.

- Barium swallow demonstrates infiltrative ulcer or polypoid growth with nodular and irregular margins leading to stricture formation. CT helps in assessment of tumor extent and distant metastasis.

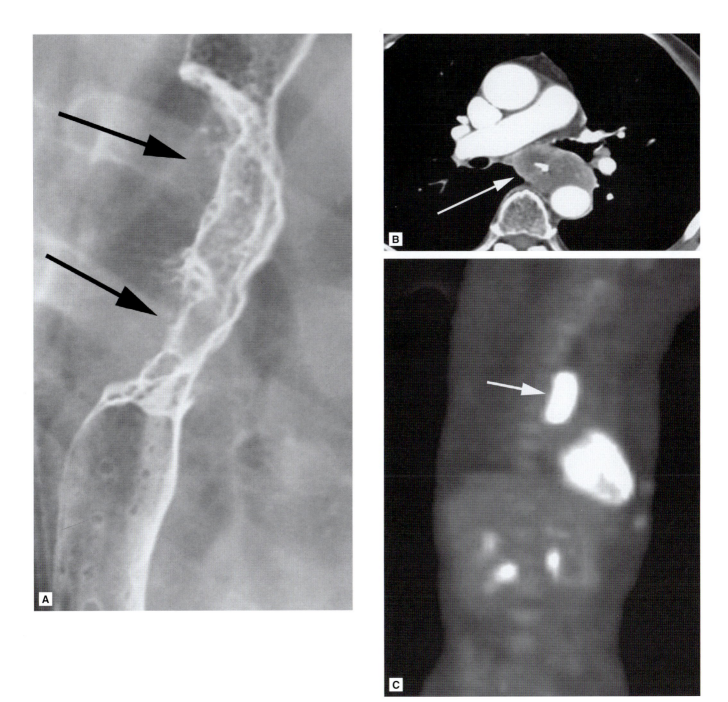

1. **A.** Double-contrast barium study demonstrates infiltrative lesion in mid-esophagus with an irregular luminal contour and shelf-like proximal and inferior borders (arrows). **B.** Axial, contrast-enhanced CT image reveals circumferential thickening of the esophagus (arrow) related to an esophageal carcinoma. **C.** Fluorodeoxyglucose positron emission tomography (FDG-PET) image reveals marked FDG avidity related to the esophageal carcinoma (arrow).

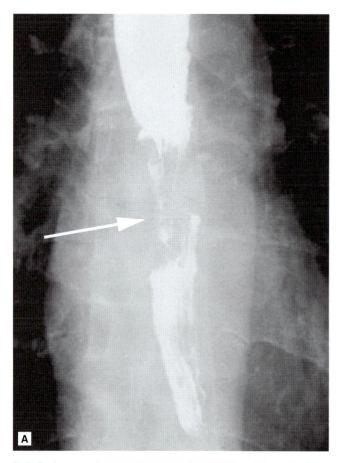

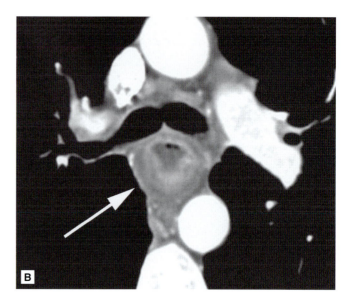

2. A. Barium esophagram shows a polypoid filling defect with irregular borders and abruptly shouldering edges in mid-esophagus (arrow).
B. Axial, contrast-enhanced CT image reveals circumferential thickening of the mid-esophagus (arrow) related to an esophageal carcinoma.
C and **D.** Fused PET/CT images reveals marked FDG avidity related to the esophageal carcinoma (arrow).

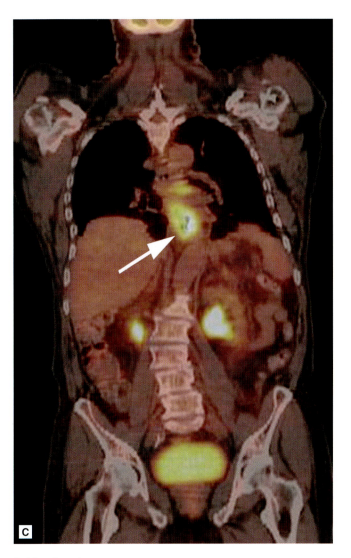

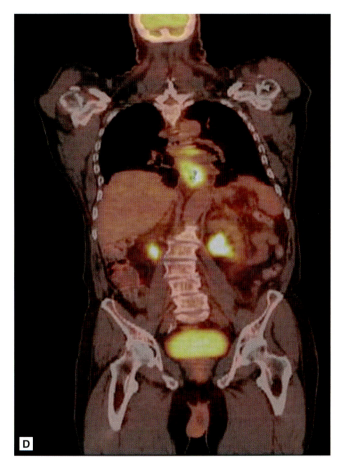

2. (*Continued*)

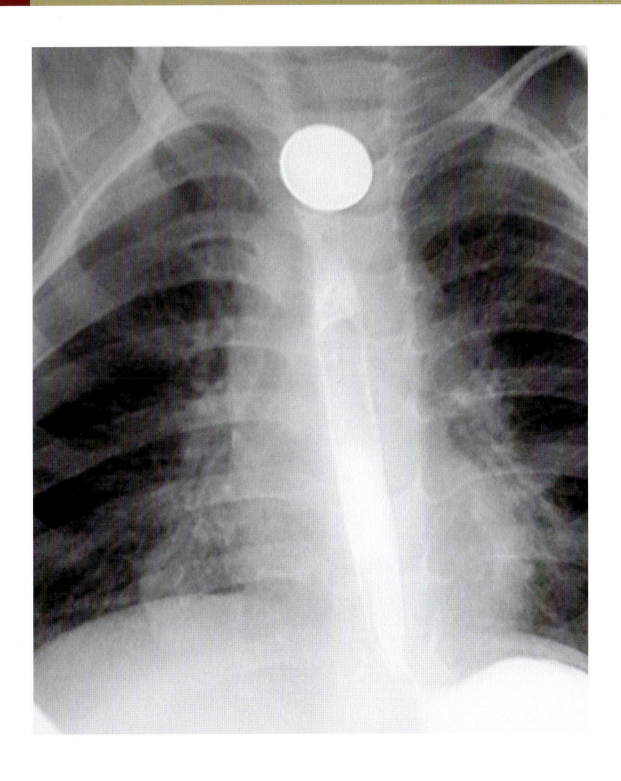

PRESENTATION

Classically presents with a combination of vomiting, chest pain, and subcutaneous emphysema, also known as Mackler triad.

FINDINGS

CT scan demonstrates periesophageal air collection, para-aortic air tracking, pneumomediastinum, pneumothorax, and free leakage of oral contrast from the esophagus.

DIFFERENTIAL DIAGNOSIS

- Mallory-Weiss syndrome
- Epiphrenic pulsion diverticulum
- Traumatic or iatrogenic injury from prior instrumentation

COMMENTS

Boerhaave syndrome refers to a spontaneous full thickness rupture of the esophagus due to barogenic trauma induced by uncoordinated vomiting with pyloric closure and diaphragmatic contraction against a closed cricopharyngeus. It was first described in 1724 by Herman Boerhaave, a famous Dutch professor of medicine. Boerhaave found remnants of the meal in the left pleural cavity following rupture of the distal esophagus in a 50-year-old naval officer, who died after a period of self-induced vomiting after eating a rich meal. This condition still is named after Boerhaave to distinguish a spontaneous esophageal rupture from traumatic ruptures.

The esophagus differs from the rest of the alimentary tract by the lack of a serosal layer which predisposes it to rupture at lower pressures than other segments of the digestive tube. The distal left posterolateral region is the most commonly perforated site, seen in up to 85% of cases. This may be attributed to a number of anatomic reasons, such as the lack of adjacent supporting structures, thinning of the musculature in the lower esophagus, weakening of the esophageal wall by the entrance of vessels and nerves, and the anterior angulation of the esophagus at the left diaphragmatic crus. Other less common sites of perforation include the right lateral region in up to 20% of cases, followed by anterior and posterior perforations accounting for less than 10%. Esophageal rupture leads to mediastinal emphysema and formation of fluid collection as the gastric contents of air and fluid pass through the tear. Subsequently, a large left hydropneumothorax develops.

The chest radiograph remains the initial imaging test in most patients with Boerhaave syndrome. The most common findings are mediastinal widening and mediastinal emphysema followed by left-sided pleural effusion and atelectasis. Esophagography using water-soluble contrast is the study of choice for suspected esophageal perforation. The examination usually shows leakage of contrast from the distal esophagus into the mediastinum and details of the site of involvement and extent of perforation. Water-soluble contrast agents are generally safe on the extraluminal tissues. When adequate esophagograms cannot be obtained, a noncontrast CT scan offers advantage with higher sensitivity for detection of mediastinal air and fluid, and can also be used to monitor response if the perforation was treated nonoperatively. A major drawback to noncontrast CT is that the exact site of perforation cannot always be localized definitively. CT esophagogram with dilute water-soluble contrast can be used to overcome this issue to some extent.

PEARLS

- Boerhaave syndrome is a spontaneous perforation of the distal esophagus following barogenic trauma, like vomiting or other violent straining.

- The left posterolateral aspect of the distal esophagus is the most common site of rupture with periesophageal, pleural, pericardial air and fluid collections.

- Fluoroscopic or CT esophagram with a water-soluble contrast agent shows leakage from the distal esophagus into the mediastinum, along with other signs of perforation.

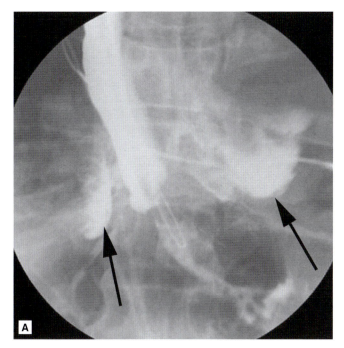

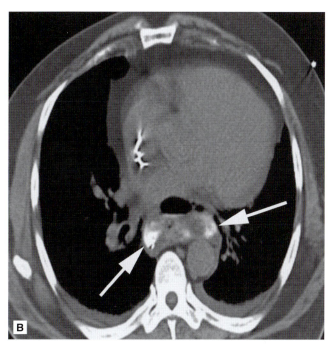

1. **A.** Frontal image obtained during barium swallow demonstrates leakage of oral contrast from the distal esophagus in a patient with Boerhaave syndrome (arrows). **B.** Axial CT image demonstrates extraluminal air and contrast within the mediastinum surrounding the distal esophagus (arrows).

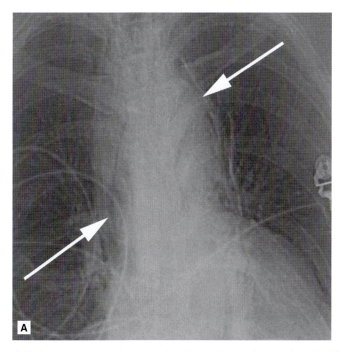

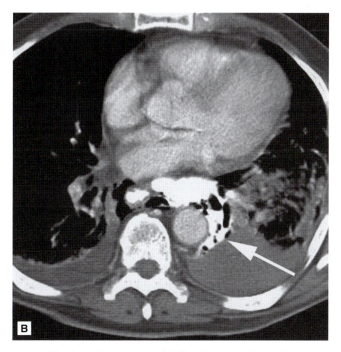

2. **A.** Scout topogram demonstrates streaky lucencies consistent with pneumomediastinum in a patient with Boerhaave syndrome (arrows). **B.** Axial CT image reveals a large degree of leakage of oral contrast from the distal esophagus (arrow). Note the large left-sided pleural effusion, a common finding in patients with Boerhaave syndrome.

Case 5–15 Esophageal Foreign Body (Food Impaction)

PRESENTATION

Patients usually present with sudden onset of substernal chest pain, odynophagia, or dysphagia after food ingestion.

FINDINGS

Esophagogram demonstrates an impacted food (typically meat) bolus in the distal esophagus as a polypoid filling defect.

DIFFERENTIAL DIAGNOSIS

- Esophageal tumor

COMMENTS

The majority of pharyngeal or esophageal foreign body impactions occur in the pediatric population. The most common foreign bodies are coins or parts of toys ingested accidentally or intentionally. In the adult population, animal or fish bones and unchewed boluses of meat are commonly encountered foreign bodies in the esophagus. Sharp objects, such as bones, tend to lodge in the pharynx at the level of the cricopharyngeus and the meat bolus usually impacts in the distal esophagus. Foreign body impactions tend to occur more commonly in patients with pre-existing esophageal strictures or rings, psychiatric disorders, mental retardation, or impairment caused by alcohol, and those seeking some secondary gain from access to a medical facility. In many instances, the impaction resolves spontaneously. The onset of symptoms may be delayed for hours or days after the ingestion.

Persistent impaction of foreign body causes transmural esophageal inflammation and subsequent pressure necrosis leading to perforation. Extravasation of luminal contents can initiate mediastinitis which may lead to sudden, rapid clinical deterioration with sepsis and shock. Uncommonly, a foreign body can erode through the wall of the esophagus causing an aortoesophageal, esophagobronchial, or esophagopericardial fistula. Sharp, pointed, or elongated foreign bodies are associated with increased risk of perforation, vascular injuries, and fistula formation.

Plain radiographs of the neck and chest can be used to identify true radiopaque foreign objects and free mediastinal air. The lateral projection of the neck confirms the location of foreign bodies in the upper esophagus. However, less radiodense objects like fish or chicken bones, wood, plastic, most glass and thin metallic objects are not readily seen and difficult to differentiate from overlying calcified thyroid or cricoid cartilage. A swallow with barium-soaked cotton ball or marshmallow may get entangled in the foreign body and helps to identify nonopaque, small foreign bodies.

The next best study to perform is a barium swallow to determine whether a foreign body is present and is causing obstruction. Animal or fish bones in the pharynx or cervical esophagus appear as a linear filling defect in the vallecula, piriform sinus, or cricopharyngeal region. However, they can be easily obscured by barium. Foreign body impaction in the thoracic esophagus is seen as a polypoid filling defect, with an irregular meniscus resulting from barium outlining the superior border of the impacted bolus. The incompletely distended esophagus below the impaction or tiny leakage of barium around the impacted foreign body may erroneously suggest a stricture. When esophageal perforation is suspected, appropriate choice of contrast medium is very important because patients with food impaction are also at high risk for aspiration. Therefore, to avoid the risk of pulmonary edema from aspiration, it is safe to use low-osmolar water-soluble contrast agents. A noninvasive method to relieve symptoms of distal esophageal impaction is to administer 1 mg of glucagon to relax the lower esophageal sphincter. This method may not be helpful for the upper- and mid-esophagus as glucagon does not affect the motor activity in the proximal esophagus. Gas-forming agents can distend the esophagus above the obstruction and facilitate the distal passage of the foreign body. However, due to the risk of perforation, these agents should not be used if the impaction has been present for more than 24 hours duration. Invasive therapeutic interventions include extraction using endoscopy or via the use of a wire basket or a Foley catheter under fluoroscopic guidance. Persistent symptoms related to the esophagus in cases of suspected foreign body ingestion should be pursued with endoscopy even after an apparently unrevealing radiographic evaluation.

PEARLS

- Pharyngeal or esophageal foreign body impaction is seen most commonly in the pediatric population following an accidental ingestion, In adults, animal or fish bones and unchewed boluses of meat are commonly impacted foreign bodies.

- Foreign bodies may be radiopaque or radiolucent and appear as a linear filling defect or as a polypoid filling defect with irregular meniscus on imaging.

- Endoscopic removal is the treatment of choice if the impacted bolus fails to pass spontaneously or by noninvasive methods due to the risk of potential life-threatening complications from perforation.

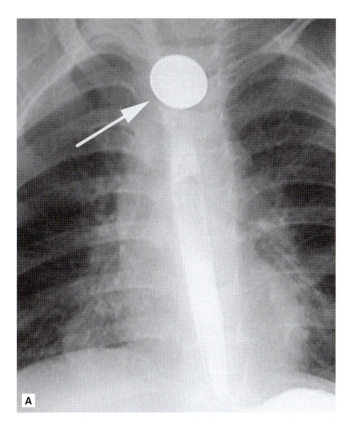

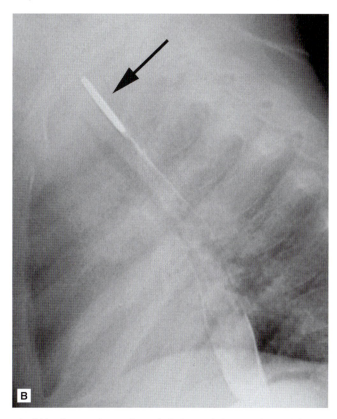

1 A. Frontal chest radiograph in a pediatric patient reveals a coin impacted within the esophagus (arrow). **B.** Lateral chest radiograph in a pediatric patient reveals the orthogonal view of the coin lodged within the esophagus (arrow).

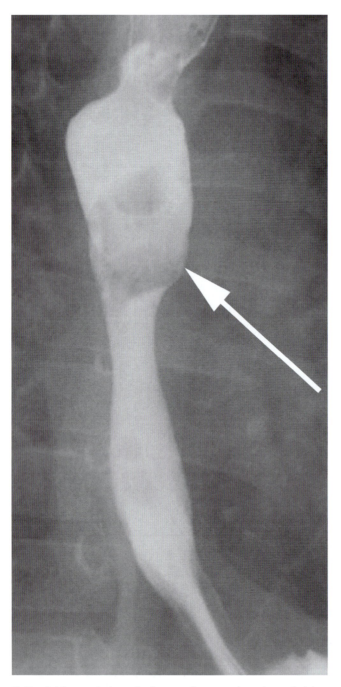

2. Frontal image during a barium swallow reveals an impacted foreign body within the esophagus (arrow); in this case, the foreign body turned out to be a meatball.

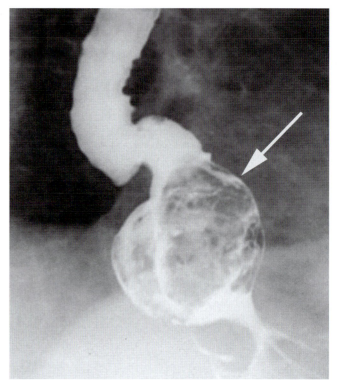

3. Frontal image during a barium swallow reveals a large impacted portion of steak within the distal esophagus (arrow).

PRESENTATION

Typical clinical presentation is slowly progressive dysphagia for both solids and liquids with symptoms of regurgitation like cough, choking, aspiration, and pneumonia.

FINDINGS

Dynamic, contrast esophagogram demonstrates absence of primary peristalsis with gross dilatation of esophagus and smooth, tapered, beak-like appearance at the level of the esophagogastric junction.

DIFFERENTIAL DIAGNOSIS

- Esophagitis with stricture (peptic stricture)
- Complicated scleroderma
- Esophageal carcinoma
- Chagas disease
- Postvagotomy effect

COMMENTS

Achalasia is a motility disorder of the esophagus characterized by aperistaltic esophageal dilatation with lower esophageal sphincter dysfunction. The actual cause is unknown, but histologic examination usually demonstrates degenerative changes in the dorsal vagal nucleus, vagal trunk, and myenteric plexus in the region of the gastroesophageal junction. Achalasia usually affects both genders equally, and generally between the ages of 20 and 40 years. The earliest changes are characterized by a defective or absent distal peristalsis, associated with a normal or slightly narrowed gastroesophageal junction. Occasionally, the early stages may demonstrate high amplitude, simultaneous, repetitive nonpropulsive contractions; this condition is often referred to as *vigorous achalasia*.

At initial presentation patients with achalasia may complain of a combination of three classical symptoms: dysphagia, noncardiac chest pain and/or reflux-like symptoms (possibly due to fermentation of the food material retained in the esophagus and production of lactic acid). The precise pattern of these symptoms varies from patient to patient. Some cases of achalasia are relatively asymptomatic and are found incidentally as a megaesophagus with a large air-fluid level on routine chest radiographs.

Regardless of initial presentation, the diagnosis of achalasia requires careful investigation using a variety of techniques. Full investigation should include esophageal manometry, imaging examinations such as barium swallow, endoscopic US, and endoscopy. Esophageal manometry is the most sensitive diagnostic modality to detect the early motility changes of the achalasic esophagus, which occur before anatomical changes develop. Dynamic barium swallow under fluoroscopy demonstrates lack of peristalsis, proximal esophageal dilatation and a typical "bird's beak" appearance of the distal esophagus, indicating impaired lower esophageal sphincter relaxation. Timed barium swallow can aid in evaluation and quantification of esophageal emptying for the purposes of comparing findings before and after treatment, as well as to assess the relative severity. Delayed emptying is diagnosed by calculating either the volume or the surface area of retained barium, which correlates well with both basal tone and relaxation pressure of the lower esophageal sphincter. Radionuclide transit studies may also help in quantifying esophageal retention. Administration of an isotope-labelled meal, either solid or liquid, followed by exposure at set time periods are used to quantify esophageal emptying by various indices. High-frequency intraluminal US demonstrates thickening of the esophageal muscle layers and increased cross-sectional area in patients with achalasia. Achalasia is treated by either pharmacologic or surgical methods. Pharmacologic treatments predominantly act on the lower esophageal sphincter by causing muscular relaxation, thus decreasing sphincter pressure. These include calcium channel blockers, isosorbide, and local botulinum injections. Mechanical treatments disrupt the muscular sphincter by either forced dilatation or myotomy, destroying its ability to contract effectively. Imaging studies after the intervention are helpful to detect postprocedure complications like perforation after dilatation, reflux esophagitis, and subsequent stricture formation after myotomy.

PEARLS

- Achalasia is a primary motility disorder of the esophagus characterized by aperistalsis and lower esophageal sphincter dysfunction, probably secondary to decreasing myenteric ganglia cells in Auerbach plexus and degenerative changes in the vagal trunk.

- Manometry is the most sensitive diagnostic test. Timed barium swallow and radionuclide studies allow evaluation and quantification of esophageal emptying for purposes of comparison in pre- and post-treatment findings.

- Radiographically, absent primary peristalsis and a dilated esophagus with smooth, symmetric, tapered narrowing at the esophagogastric region giving the appearance of "bird-beak" deformity are the best diagnostic signs.

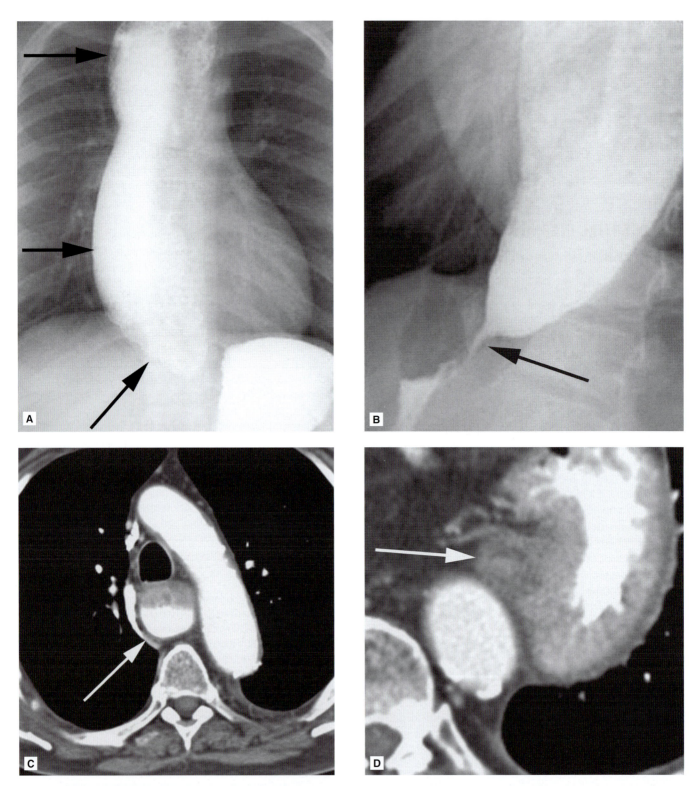

1. A. Frontal view obtained during a barium-swallow examination reveals a diffusely distended esophagus (arrows) in a patient with achalasia. **B.** Smoothly tapered appearance of the distal esophagus (arrow) giving the typical "bird-beak" appearance in a patient with achalasia. **C.** Axial, contrast-enhanced CT image reveals a diffusely distended esophagus (arrow) in a patient with achalasia. **D.** Axial, contrast-enhanced CT image reveals narrowing at the level of the esophagogastric junction (arrow) in a patient with achalasia.

PRESENTATION

The most common esophageal symptoms in patients with scleroderma are heartburn, regurgitation, and dysphagia.

FINDINGS

The classic imaging findings of esophageal involvement in cases of scleroderma are mild-to-moderate dilatation of the esophagus with a distal fusiform stricture and decreased or absent peristalsis. In addition, pulmonary changes in the form of interstitial fibrosis may be identified.

DIFFERENTIAL DIAGNOSIS

- Esophagitis with peptic stricture

- Achalasia

- Esophageal carcinoma

- Postvagotomy changes and fundoplication

COMMENTS

Scleroderma, also known as systemic sclerosis, is a multisystem disease of unknown etiology that affects the connective tissues of small blood vessels, skin, and internal organs. It is characterized by alterations of the microvasculature, disturbances of the immune system, and massive deposition of collagen and other matrix substances in the connective tissue. Systemic sclerosis is divided into two subgroups: diffuse systemic sclerosis and limited systemic sclerosis (CREST syndrome: Calcinosis, Raynaud phenomenon, Esophageal dysfunction, Sclerodactyly, and Telangiectasias). The diffuse form progresses rapidly and affects large areas of the skin and one or more internal organs, frequently the kidneys, esophagus, heart, and lungs. Limited systemic sclerosis is characterized by cutaneous manifestations that mainly affect the hands, arms and face, and minimal visceral involvement.

The esophagus, especially the distal two-thirds is the major site of involvement in the gastrointestinal tract as it is predominantly composed of smooth muscle. Ischemic injury to the neural tissue by either arteriolar changes in the vasa nervorum or compression of nerve fibers by collagen deposits lead to smooth muscle atrophy. Subsequently, there is vascular compromise superimposed on the neural dysfunction along with collagen infiltration that results in smooth muscle fibrosis and, thus, decreased peristalsis and malfunction of the lower esophageal sphincter.

Later in the course of the disease, esophageal injury (from esophagitis) can develop from poor clearance of acid reflux material due to the decreased peristalsis and hypofunctioning lower esophageal sphincter. Chronic, persistent esophageal injury can lead to complications including erosions and bleeding, stricture formation, Barrett metaplasia, and, possibly, adenocarcinoma.

Scleroderma commonly affects African-American women between 30 and 50 years of age. Dysphagia and dyspepsia are the initial symptoms which become progressively worse as esophageal dysfunction progresses. Manometry is the most sensitive test to detect esophageal dysmotility early in the course of the disease. The diagnostic features include decreased or absent lower esophageal sphincter pressure at rest and weak or absent peristalsis in the lower two-thirds of the esophagus. Barium swallow demonstrates normal clearance of contrast in the upper esophagus, which is composed primarily of striated muscle, and retention or slow progression distally, starting at about the level of aortic arch. Some weak peristaltic activity and uncoordinated tertiary contractions may be observed in the lower two-thirds of the esophagus. However, as the disease progresses, these contractions become less frequent and ultimately disappear. Some degree of esophageal dysmotility is found in 80% to 90% of patients with scleroderma. Although the majority of these patients do not complain of esophageal symptoms, they are still at risk for complications resulting from dysmotility. Gastroesophageal reflux is an early and common complication, and is associated with significant morbidity. Chronic acid reflux can lead to esophagitis with erosions and bleeding, stricture formation, Barrett metaplasia, and carcinoma.

PEARLS

- **Scleroderma is a collagen vascular disease that characteristically affects the distal esophagus.**

- **Progressive smooth muscle fibrosis of the esophagus leads to an atonic, dilated distal esophagus with dysfunction of the lower esophageal sphincter.**

- **Gastroesophageal reflux leads to esophageal injury and is associated with significant morbidity from complications, including esophagitis, erosions and bleeding, stricture, Barrett metaplasia, and, possibly, adenocarcinoma.**

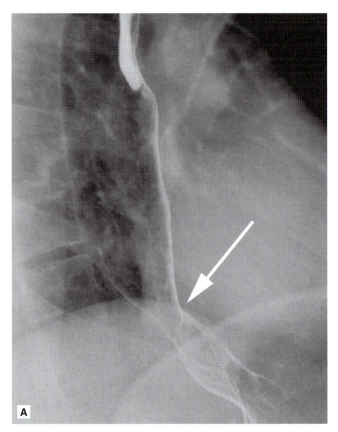

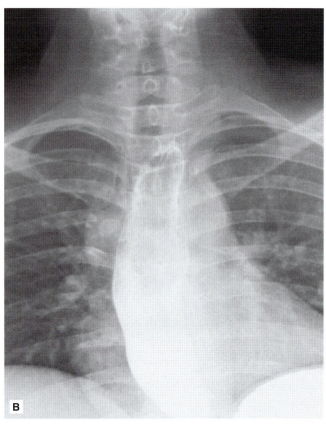

1. A. Oblique view obtained during barium swallow reveals diffuse distension of the distal esophagus with distal narrowing (arrow) secondary to scleroderma. **B.** Frontal view obtained during barium swallow demonstrates moderate dilatation of the esophagus secondary to scleroderma.

PRESENTATION

Esophageal varices present with episodes of hematemesis which may be massive, life threatening or low grade and intermittent bleeding with melena. These patients often have history of cirrhosis and portal hypertension.

FINDINGS

Varices appear as serpiginous filling defects on double-contrast esophagograms. CT demonstrates a thickened, lobulated esophageal wall containing round, tubular, or serpentine structures with homogeneous attenuation which enhance on contrast images.

DIFFERENTIAL DIAGNOSIS

- Esophagitis
- Varicoid esophageal carcinoma

COMMENTS

Varices are formed by alteration in the venous drainage of the esophagus due to either portal hypertension in cases of upstream varices or superior vena cava (SVC) obstruction in cases of downstream varices. Physiologically, the upper cervical esophagus and upper thoracic esophagus are drained by the superior intercostal veins, bronchial veins, inferior thyroid vein, and other mediastinal collaterals; the mid thoracic esophagus is drained by the azygos and hemiazygos veins; and the distal thoracic esophagus is drained by a periesophageal plexus of veins that communicates distally with the coronary vein, which in turn drains into the splenic vein. In portal hypertension, the increased portal venous pressure leads to reversal of venous flow through the coronary vein into the dilated distal esophageal and periesophageal veins that anastomose superiorly with collaterals from the azygos and hemiazygos systems. Thus, portal venous blood drains into the right ventricle through the azygos vein and SVC rather than the inferior vena cava (IVC), ultimately bypassing the obstructed portal system. Because the blood flows upward in dilated distal esophageal veins in portal hypertension, these are called upstream varices.

SVC obstruction leads to reversal of flow in the vein drained by the upper esophagus to bypass the obstruction. If the SVC obstruction occurs above the entry of the azygos vein, venous return from the head and upper extremity reaches the SVC below the obstruction through the azygos vein, and varices are always confined to the upper or mid thoracic esophagus. In cases where the SVC is obstructed at or below the entry of the azygos vein, downhill varices divert the blood into the coronary vein in the distal esophagus, and this blood then drains into the portal vein and IVC. SVC obstruction can be caused by either a benign process like substernal goiter, mediastinal fibrosis, or a malignancy like bronchogenic carcinoma, metastatic tumors, and lymphoma.

The radiographic demonstration of varices requires special attention to fluoroscopic technique, because varices can be easily collapsed with peristalsis, respiration and varying degrees of esophageal distension. Barium esophagogram is usually performed with the patient in a recumbent position, using high-density barium suspension or paste to improve the mucosal coating of barium. Mucosal relief views demonstrate tortuous or serpiginous longitudinal filling defects in the collapsed or partially collapsed esophagus. Peristaltic waves passing through the segment of esophagus containing varices tend to squeeze the blood from the thin-walled varices. As a result, it may take 15 to 30 seconds to refill the varices to be visualized on mucosal relief views. Deep, blocked inspiration, administration of anticholinergic drugs and avoiding swallowing during the study may sometimes provide better visualization of varices. CT demonstrates a thickened esophageal wall with well-defined round, tubular or smooth serpentine structures which enhance to the degree as adjacent veins on postcontrast images. MR depicts multiple areas of flow voids on T1w and T2w images and enhanced varices in portal venous phase of dynamic contrast-enhanced MR. The majority of these patients are asymptomatic until variceal bleeding caused by rupture from inflammation or ulceration occurs. Low-grade intermittent bleeding may present with melena and iron-deficiency anemia. Hematemesis is the usual presentation of upstream varices and is treated by endoscopic ligation or endovascular embolization.

PEARLS

- **Esophageal varices are dilated tortuous submucosal venous plexi; upstream varices are seen in the distal third or half of thoracic esophagus in patients with portal hypertension, whereas downhill varices form in upper or middle third of the esophagus from an occluded SVC.**

- **Esophagogram demonstrates tortuous or serpiginous longitudinal filling defects. CT and MR show a thickened esophagus with well-defined round, tubular, or serpentine structures within the esophageal wall which enhance to the extent of adjacent veins on postcontrast images.**

- **The majority of patients are asymptomatic until variceal rupture with resulting hematemesis, which can be treated with endoscopic ligation or endovascular embolization.**

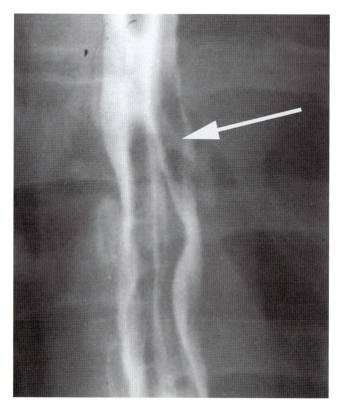

1. Barium study in a patient with SVC occlusion reveals serpiginous filling defects in the mid-esophagus (arrow), in this case of downhill varices.

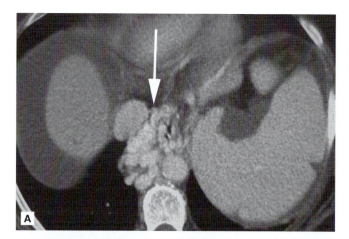

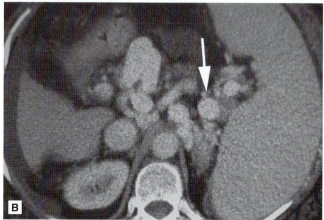

2. A. Axial, contrast-enhanced CT image demonstrates a large amount of enhancing esophageal varices (arrow). Note is made of splenomegaly in this patient with cirrhosis and portal hypertension. **B.** Axial, contrast-enhanced CT image demonstrates large splenic varices (arrow) in this patient with cirrhosis and portal hypertension, also resulting in splenomegaly and esophageal varices.

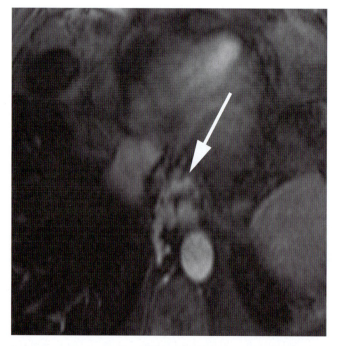

3. Axial, contrast-enhanced MRI image demonstrates tubular, enhancing esophageal varices (arrow) in this patient with cirrhosis and uphill varices.

PRESENTATION

Dysphagia, patients may also present with weight loss.

FINDINGS

The underlying abnormality causing the subjective sensation of dysphagia, the aberrant course of the right subclavian artery, posterior to the esophagus and immediately anterior to cervical vertebral bodies, is readily visualized on cross-sectional imaging.

DIFFERENTIAL DIAGNOSIS

- Foreign body
- Esophageal neoplasm
- Esophageal stricture
- Mediastinal mass

COMMENTS

Dysphagia lusoria is the name given to the clinical scenario whereby an aberrant right subclavian artery (ARSA) results in symptoms of dysphagia. An ARSA is the most common congenital aortic arch anomaly (0.5%-2% of population), with no known genetic link, resulting from involution of embryonic right fourth aortic arch between the right common carotid and right subclavian arteries. In this scenario, the right subclavian artery becomes the last division of a four branch-vessel aortic arch (absent brachiocephalic), which because of this position, originates near the left lung apex. Its origin is often dilated (termed a diverticulum of Kommerell) and its course is posterior to the esophagus and immediately anterior to cervical vertebral bodies. The resultant posterior compression on the esophagus may cause the subjective sensation of dysphagia.

As both nonaneurysmal as well as aneurysmal ARSAs can cause dysphagia, the radiographic findings include subtle mediastinal widening, the presence of an oblique mediastinal edge extending rightward and arising from the aortic arch, the presence of an ill-defined mass in the right medial clavicular area, or evidence of mass effect on the esophagus or trachea. An obliquely oriented impression of the aberrant subclavian artery on the posterior esophagus may be identified at fluoroscopy.

On contrast-enhanced CT, the main challenge in making the diagnosis of ARSA is correctly identifying the anatomical variant. The branching sequence of the aberrant, four-branched aortic arch is as follows from proximal to distal: right common carotid artery, left common carotid artery, left subclavian artery, and right subclavian artery. A diverticulum of Kommerell is the eponym given to a tubular dilation in the origin of the ARSA which may be calcified or seen to contain thrombus. Once recognized, its subsequent course behind the esophagus should be confirmed and described. MR findings are similar to those seen on CT with the distinct advantage of the potential to evaluate this vascular anatomy without ionizing radiation or intravenous contrast in using nonenhanced MRA techniques.

PEARLS

- **Dysphagia lusoria is the name given to the clinical scenario whereby an ARSA results in symptoms of dysphagia.**

- **The course of an ARSA, posterior to the esophagus and immediately anterior to cervical vertebral bodies, results in posterior compression on the esophagus which may cause the subjective sensation of dysphagia.**

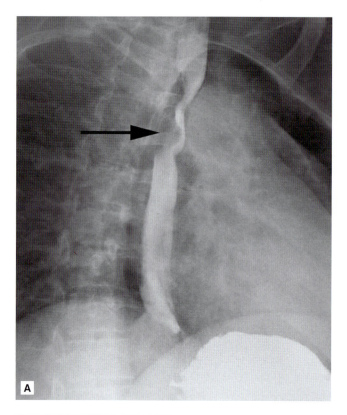

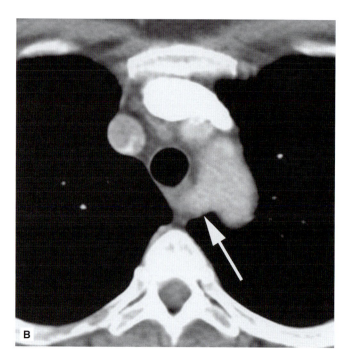

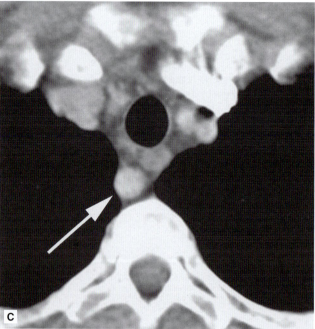

1. A. Fluoroscopic image from a barium-swallow examination demonstrates a focal narrowing of the esophagus (arrow) related to a posterior impression, suggesting the presence of an ARSA in a patient with dysphagia. **B.** Axial, contrast-enhanced CT image demonstrates the origin of an ARSA (arrow), coursing posterior to the esophagus. **C.** Axial, contrast-enhanced CT image demonstrates the course of an ARSA (arrow), posterior to the esophagus, in a patient with dysphagia lusoria.

PRESENTATION

Incidental finding which may be associated with gastro-esophageal reflux and the presence of a hiatal hernia

FINDINGS

Transient, thin, 1- to 2-mm wide striations crossing the entire circumference of the middle and distal thirds of the thoracic esophagus are seen on double-contrast barium esophagography.

DIFFERENTIAL DIAGNOSIS

- Fixed transverse folds of scarring from chronic reflux esophagitis
- Ringed esophagus of idiopathic eosinophilic esophagitis
- *Candida* esophagitis
- Herpes esophagitis
- Caustic esophagitis
- Scleroderma
- Crohn disease

COMMENTS

The presence of multiple fine, transverse folds crossing the entire lumen of the esophagus seen on double-contrast esophagogram is described as "feline esophagus." This appearance is similar to the appearance of folds in the distal esophagus of cats. The folds are seen transiently as 1 to 2 mm wide, linear or with an angular fashion, extending circumferentially around the lumen, especially in the distal esophagus. They appear as a result of transient contractions of the longitudinal fibers of the muscularis mucosa and its overlying loose connective tissue and epithelium. The clinical significance of feline esophagus is not yet established and it is often regarded as a normal variant. Feline esophagus has been observed in patients with gastroesophageal reflux and hiatal hernia; however, the presence of feline esophagus features is not diagnostic of esophagitis.

The fixed transverse folds of chronic esophageal reflux and tertiary esophageal contractions should be differentiated from the transient transverse folds of feline esophagus. Transverse folds seen in some patients with acute and/or chronic reflux esophagitis are persistent folds, 2 to 5 mm wide, along with other signs of reflux and do not involve the entire circumference. Tertiary esophageal contractions are broad transverse bands that appear secondary to nonpropulsive contractions of the muscularis propria.

PEARLS

- Feline esophagus is described as transient, multiple, thin 1- to 2-mm-wide striations crossing the entire circumference of the middle and distal thirds of the thoracic esophagus at double-contrast barium esophagography.

- They appear secondary to contractions of the muscularis mucosa and are considered to be a normal variant. However, they are increasingly seen in patients with gastroesophageal reflux and hiatal hernia.

- On esophagography, feline esophagus should be distinguished from conditions with similar appearance like fixed transverse folds due to scarring from reflux esophagitis, tertiary esophageal contractions, and ringed esophagus of idiopathic eosinophilic esophagitis.

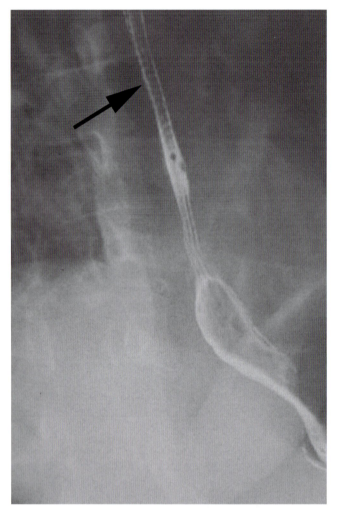

1. Fluoroscopic image during a barium-swallow examination demonstrates multiple, thin striations (arrow) crossing the entire circumference of the middle and distal thirds of the thoracic esophagus which were noted to be transient, consistent with feline esophagus.

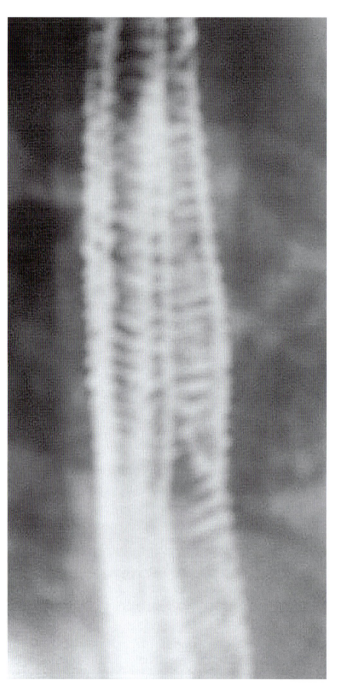

2. Fluoroscopic image during a barium-swallow examination demonstrates multiple, thin striations of the esophagus, noted to be transient, consistent with feline esophagus.

PRESENTATION

The majority of patients are asymptomatic. Marked luminal narrowing or impaction of food above the web causes dysphagia. Patients with Plummer-Vinson syndrome present with iron deficiency anemia, stomatitis, and glossitis.

FINDINGS

Esophagram demonstrates a thin, smooth, shelf-like filing defect along the anterior wall of the cervical esophagus.

DIFFERENTIAL DIAGNOSIS

- Esophageal stricture
- Schatzki ring
- Cricopharyngeal achalasia

COMMENTS

Congenital esophageal webs are smooth, thin mucosal folds situated along the anterior wall of the lower hypopharynx and proximal cervical esophagus, within 2 cm of the pharyngoesophageal junction. They are oriented perpendicular to the esophageal wall, protruding into the lumen, and are mainly composed of lamina propria covered by epithelium. Less frequently, webs can be seen in the distal esophagus and associated with gastroesophageal reflux. Diseases affecting mucosal membranes like pemphigoid or epidermolysis bullosa are known to be associated with pharyngeal or cervical webs. An entity called Plummer-Vinson or Paterson-Kelly syndrome describes an association between cervical esophageal web, iron deficiency anemia, and pharyngeal or esophageal carcinoma. However, some authors consider this association is mere coincidence and, thus, its true existence has remained controversial.

On barium studies, esophageal webs appear as a 1- to 2-mm wide, shelf-like filling defect along the anterior wall of the hypopharynx or cervical esophagus. The webs usually protrude perpendicularly into the esophageal lumen, compromising the luminal diameter. They are best seen in the lateral projection when the barium-filled esophagus is maximally distended. Occasionally, webs can be seen as circumferential ring-like shelves in the cervical esophagus. Dynamic examination may show spurting of the liquid bolus of barium through the ring with dilatation of the esophagus or pharynx proximal to the web, described as a "jet phenomenon" which suggests partial obstruction. The size of the orifice can be assessed by measuring the width of the jet just below the level of the web.

Congenital esophageal webs should not be mistaken for a prominent cricopharyngeal muscle or a postcricoid defect. The prominent cricopharyngeal muscle appears as a round, broad-based protrusion from the posterior pharyngeal wall at the level of the pharyngoesophageal segment. A postcricoid defect is redundant mucosa in the anterior wall of the hypopharynx at the level of the cricoid cartilage.

Patients with a transverse esophageal web are usually asymptomatic, although occasionally they may have food impaction (eg, unchewed meat). Circumferential webs are more likely to cause dysphagia due to a compromised lumen. Balloon dilatation under fluoroscopic guidance is a highly effective technique for treating symptomatic cases. Refractory cases are treated with surgical exploration or endoscopic correction.

PEARLS

- A web is a thin, shelf-like mucosal fold projecting into the lumen, most frequently from the anterior wall of the proximal cervical esophagus.

- Cine-fluoroscopic imaging during swallowing of a large bolus of barium in the lateral projection is the best view for demonstrating the web. Liquid barium shows a jet phenomenon by spurts through the ring.

- Plummer-Vinson syndrome is reported to be associated with esophageal webs. However, insufficient scientific data suggest this may be a coincidental association.

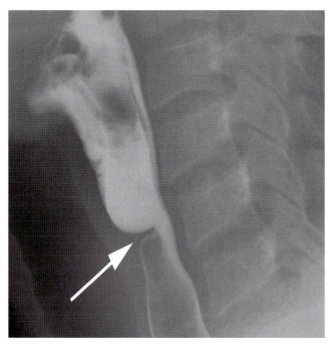

1. Lateral projection during barium-swallow examination reveals a shelf-like filling defect along the anterior cervical esophagus (arrow), consistent with an esophageal web.

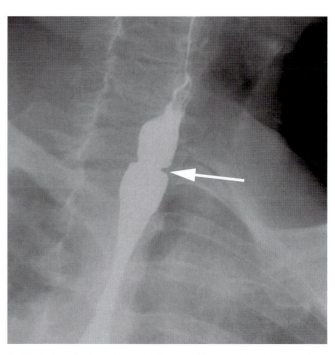

2. Frontal projection during barium-swallow examination reveals a perpendicular, shelf-like filling defect along the cervical esophagus (arrow), consistent with an esophageal web.

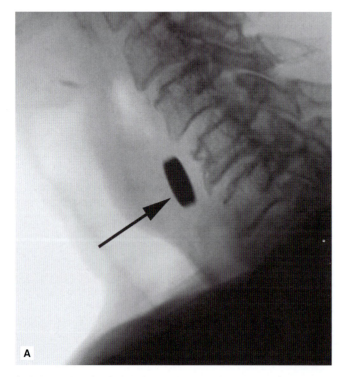

A

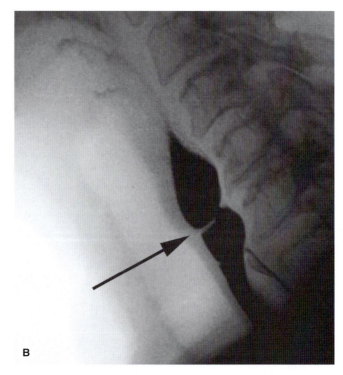

B

3. A. Lateral projection during barium-swallow examination reveals a barium pill (arrow) which was not seen to pass beyond the cervical esophagus. B. Lateral projection during barium-swallow examination reveals the cause of the obstruction of the passage of the barium pill, a narrowing of the cervical esophagus (arrow) consistent with an esophageal web.

PRESENTATION

Patients with Schatzki ring usually experience episodic dysphagia for solids. They are also at risk for impaction above the ring, especially when an unchewed piece of meat is swallowed, which is described as "steak house syndrome."

FINDINGS

Single-contrast barium studies demonstrate a thin, web-like or annular constriction at the gastroesophageal junction above a hiatal hernia.

DIFFERENTIAL DIAGNOSIS

- Muscular or contractile or "A" ring
- Esophageal web
- Annular peptic stricture
- Localized esophageal cancer

COMMENTS

A Schatzki ring is a smooth, concentric narrowing of the distal esophagus located a few centimeters above the diaphragm that marks the junction between the esophageal and gastric mucosa. The causes leading to the development of a Schatzki ring are unclear; some investigators believe that the origin is congenital, while others believe that it forms as a result of scarring from chronic reflux esophagitis. In either case, there is controversy, as the late presentation of symptoms cannot explain a congenital theory and the lesser frequency of reflux seen in these patients weakens the argument of an acquired etiology. Schatzki rings are usually seen in middle-aged patients. The majority of patients are asymptomatic with episodic nonprogressive dysphagia for solids. Impaction of a food bolus (frequently unchewed meat) at or above the level of the ring usually initiates the symptom, often known as "steak house syndrome." The severity of the symptoms is based on the size of the ring. All lower esophageal rings measuring 13 mm or less in diameter cause dysphagia, whereas rings larger than 20 mm are rarely symptomatic. Intermittent history of dysphagia is noted in rings of 13 to 20 mm in diameter, and the severity of dysphagia in these patients depends on the size of the food bolus. A Schatzki ring is frequently associated with a hiatal hernia, and the ring lies above the hernia.

The most valuable investigations performed when a Schatzki ring is suspected at the barium swallow and endoscopy. The single-contrast barium swallow demonstrates a thin, annular narrowing at the lower end of the esophageal vestibule. The ring forms at or just below the squamocolumnar mucosal junction, and demarcates the lower end of the esophageal vestibule and its union with the stomach. Successful radiographic demonstration of the ring depends on the adequate distension of the esophagogastric region and on its location in relation to the esophageal hiatus. Single-contrast studies with a large bolus of barium to distend the distal esophagus beyond the diameter of the ring and with the patient in a prone, right anterior oblique position, preferably performing a Valsalva maneuver, may make the ring more conspicuous. It is also better visualized when the ring is located above the esophageal hiatus, as occurs with hiatal hernias. The ring may be obscured by the overlapping convex surfaces of the distal esophagus and proximal end of hernia in the prone position. This potential pitfall can be avoided by obtaining additional prone views with underdistension of the hiatal hernia. A Schatzki ring should be differentiated from muscular rings, annular peptic strictures, esophageal webs, and esophageal cancer, all of which may have similar imaging findings. Muscular rings represent focal muscular hypertrophy at the tubulovestibular junction, which is entirely covered with squamous epithelium. On barium esophagram, a muscular ring appears as a broad, smooth annular narrowing at the upper end of the esophageal vestibule. Peptic strictures are classically oriented in a vertical fashion. However, in less than 20% of cases, they may be annular and mimic a lower esophageal ring. On imaging, the annular peptic stricture is thick, irregular and asymmetric, with other signs of chronic reflux, such as mucosal thickening and serration. Episodes of dysphagia may be relieved as the impacted food passes through the ring. Proper chewing and adequate consumption of water may improve the symptoms in mild cases. Refractory cases are managed by intervention.

PEARLS

- Schatzki ring is a thin circumferential ingrowth of mucosa at the squamocolumnar junction between the esophagus and the stomach.

- Compromised luminal caliber to 13 mm or less may result in intermittent dysphagia for solids or an episode of acute esophageal food impaction.

- The single-contrast barium swallows with adequate distension of the distal esophagus by various maneuvers is the best radiologic study.

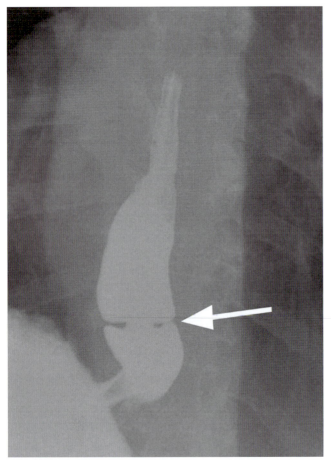

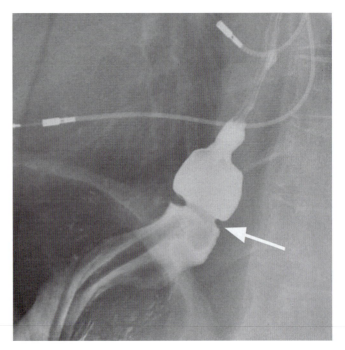

2. Single-contrast image from a barium swallow demonstrates an annular narrowing of the lower end of the esophageal vestibule (arrow) consistent with a Schatzki ring.

1. Single-contrast image from a barium swallow reveals a thin, annular narrowing in the distal esophagus (arrow) consistent with a Schatzki ring.

PRESENTATION

Clinical presentation varies widely and may include oropharyngeal, retrosternal, epigastric pain, dysphagia, odynophagia, hypersalivation, vomiting, hematemesis, abdominal pain, and peritoneal symptoms.

FINDINGS

The typical findings on a barium examination in the acute period after caustic ingestion include gastric and esophageal wall thickening and ulceration as well as contrast extravasation in the setting of perforation.

DIFFERENTIAL DIAGNOSIS

- Esophagitis
- Gastritis
- Trauma
- Esophageal or gastric perforation
- Malignancy

COMMENTS

Caustic ingestion is typically the result of ingestion of either strong alkali or strongly acidic substances which can be found in household cleaners or everyday items such as batteries. Caustic ingestions can rapidly cause severe esophageal or gastric injury depending on the properties, volume, and concentration of the ingested substance. Most toxic ingestions occur in children and are usually accidental; vomiting often occurs before a significant amount of the substance is ingested. Suicidal or psychotic patients or those with a history of substance abuse comprise the majority of the remaining cases of caustic ingestions.

The site of injury due to caustic ingestion will often depend on the type of material which was ingested. The ingestion of alkali tends to affect the esophagus and mediastinum more often than the stomach. Conversely, ingestion of an acidic substance tends to affect the stomach and duodenum more often than the esophagus. However, it should be noted that both substances can affect any portion of the esophagogastric region. Contact of the corrosive substance with the mucosa of the esophagus or upper gastrointestinal (GI) tract results in severe inflammation with mucosal and submucosal edema, ulcer formation, and hemorrhage. The damage can eventually involve the entire thickness of wall and lead to perforation. In addition, as acids typically affect the stomach, as the acid descends toward the pylorus, it can induce contraction and spasm of the pylorus and prevent the toxic substance from further traveling into the duodenum, resulting in a gastric outlet obstruction. It should be noted that induction of a gastric outlet obstruction can be seen after ingestion of alkali as well. Depending on the depth and extent of wall injury from a caustic agent, these patients are prone to development of stricture formation after the initial injury. In addition, patients with a history of caustic ingestion are known to have a significantly higher incidence of squamous cell carcinoma of the esophagus compared to the general population.

As better and more precise techniques in upper endoscopy have evolved, such as fiberoptic endoscopy, the role of radiology in the initial evaluation of caustic ingestion has decreased. However, chest radiography and barium examinations still play a complimentary role in the evaluation of these patients. In addition, radiology examinations are often useful in patients who are not candidates for upper endoscopy and in the evaluation of the long-term complications of caustic ingestion. Chest radiography may demonstrate widening of the mediastinal contours secondary to esophageal and mediastinal inflammation as well as pneumomediastinum and pleural effusion depending on the degree of injury. The typical findings on a barium examination in the acute period include gastric and esophageal wall thickening and ulceration as well as contrast extravasation in the setting of perforation. Intramural contrast pooling and intramural gas can be identified depending on the depth of injury and in the setting of ulceration. Esophageal dilatation with intraluminal gas and fluid levels can be seen which may indicate esophageal atony, possibly secondary to muscular damage. The pylorus can be evaluated to ensure the flow of contrast into the duodenum and for gastric outlet obstruction. In addition, one can evaluate for signs of aspiration and contrast in the tracheobronchial tree. During subsequent evaluations, barium examinations can demonstrate stricture formation, outlet obstructions, and motility abnormalities. Stricture formations due to caustic ingestion can be single, multiple, or diffuse in nature and can be seen on barium examinations. While stricture formation and wall thickening can raise the possibility of dysplastic change, at this time, upper endoscopy is the primary tool used for the evaluation of possible malignancy. In addition to barium examinations, CT may be utilized in the evaluation of caustic ingestion injuries both in the acute setting as well as the subsequent evaluation to assess for complications. On CT, esophageal and gastric edema may be readily identified, including signs of complicating perforation such as extraluminal fluid or air. In addition, evaluating for normal mucosal enhancement or lack thereof, to suggest mural necrosis, may be performed using CT.

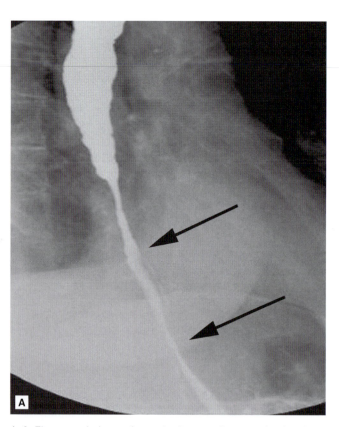

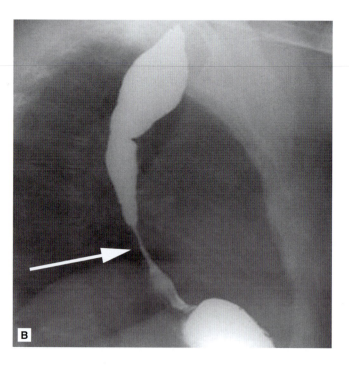

1. A. Fluoroscopic image from a barium-swallow examination demonstrates a chronic esophageal stricture related to caustic injection (arrows). **B.** Fluoroscopic image from a barium-swallow examination demonstrates a severe, chronic stricture of the esophagus related to prior caustic injection (arrow).

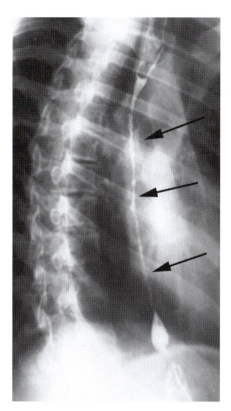

2. Fluoroscopic image from a barium-swallow examination demonstrates a sever, diffuse, chronic esophageal stricture related to prior caustic injection (arrows).

CHAPTER 6

GASTRODUODENAL

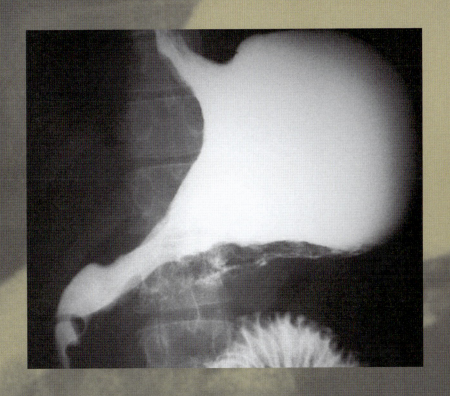

GASTRIC NEOPLASMS

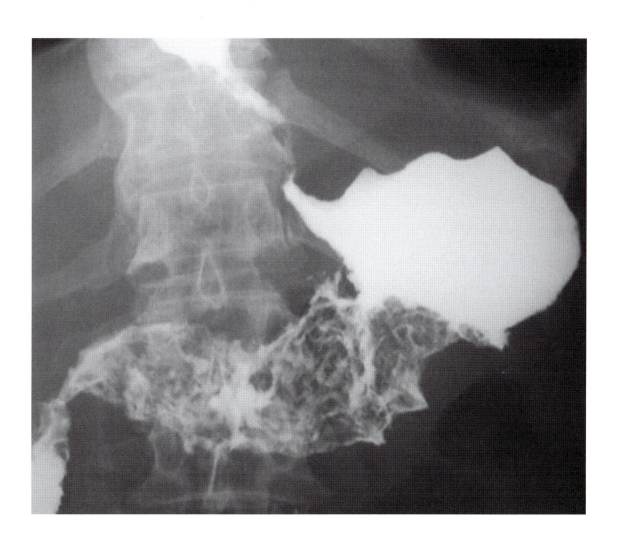

PRESENTATION

Patients typically present with nausea, vomiting, anorexia, and weight loss. Gastric outlet obstruction and gastrointestinal bleeding are less common complications of gastric cancer.

FINDINGS

The appearance gastric carcinomas on computed tomography (CT) parallels the gross pathological types and includes well-circumscribed polypoid tumors, ulcerated tumors with infiltrative margins as well as linitis plastica.

DIFFERENTIAL DIAGNOSIS

- Gastric lymphoma
- Pancreatic carcinoma
- Duodenal carcinoma

COMMENTS

The incidence of gastric cancer varies considerably between different parts of the world, but this tumor remains as a significant cause of death worldwide. Prognosis depends directly on the stage of disease: the 5-year survival varies between 7% and 27% in patients with advanced disease and 85% and 95% in patients with early gastric cancer. Surgery is the first line of therapy and, thus, early detection and accurate preoperative staging are critical for adequate patient care and improving prognosis.

The overwhelming majority of cases of gastric carcinoma are comprised of adenocarcinomas which may be subclassified based on histologic descriptions including tubular, papillary, mucinous, or signet-ring cells, and undifferentiated types. Early gastric cancer is defined as a tumor confined to the mucosa and submucosa while advanced gastric carcinoma is a tumor which has penetrated the muscularis propria. Unfortunately, early gastric carcinoma often produces no specific symptoms when it is superficial and potentially surgically curable. Patients with more advanced disease have nonspecific gastrointestinal complaints, such as dyspepsia. Anorexia and weight loss are common presenting symptoms; other symptoms include nausea, vomiting, and early satiety from gastric outlet obstruction, hematemesis, and melena. Carcinoembryonic antigen (CEA) and cancer antigen 19-9 (CA 19-9) serum levels may be elevated in patients with advanced gastric cancer.

Endoscopy is the most sensitive and specific diagnostic method in patients suspected of having gastric cancer. It allows direct visualization of tumor location, determines extent of mucosal involvement, and provides a means for biopsy (or cytologic brushings) for tissue diagnosis. Double-contrast barium examinations are also useful for demonstrating the luminal and wall changes of gastric cancer: early carcinomas appear as slightly elevated intraluminal lesions or shallow ulcerations, whereas advanced carcinomas appear as filling defects caused by polypoid masses or as irregular, deep ulcers.

CT detects up to 90% of advanced gastric adenocarcinomas. However, the detection rate for earlier-stage tumors is much lower, as the stomach is often incompletely distended. Improved detection rates with thin section multidetector computed tomography (MDCT) and multiplanar reformations have been reported. Gastric distention with a neutral contrast agent (such as water) facilitates evaluation of potential wall abnormalities. The appearance on CT of gastric carcinomas parallels the gross pathological types and includes well-circumscribed polypoid tumors, ulcerated tumors with infiltrative margins and linitis plastica. The main use of CT, however, is for initial staging to determine the optimal therapy, and for follow-up of patients after respective surgery or during treatment with chemotherapy.

Uptake of fluorodeoxyglucose (FDG) on positron emission tomography (PET) imaging of gastric cancer varies with the histologic type: mucinous adenocarcinoma, signet ring cell carcinoma, and poorly differentiated adenocarcinoma tend to show significantly lower FDG uptake than other histologies. Nonetheless, FDG-PET is a valuable tool for staging and follow-up of gastric carcinoma. However, suboptimal detection of peritoneal metastases is a known limitation of FDG-PET.

PEARLS

- Although the incidence of gastric carcinoma is decreasing in many parts of the world, this tumor remains as a significant cause of death from cancer.

- Survival in gastric cancer is determined primarily by the stage of the tumor at presentation; early cancer is a tumor confined to the mucosa and submucosa and advanced carcinoma is a tumor which has penetrated the muscularis propria.

- The main use of CT in gastric cancer imaging is for initial staging for follow-up of patients after respective surgery or during treatment with chemotherapy.

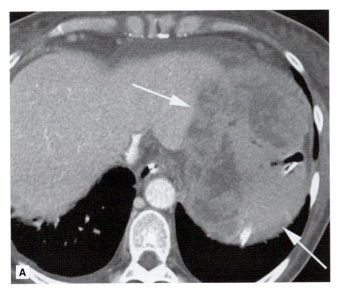

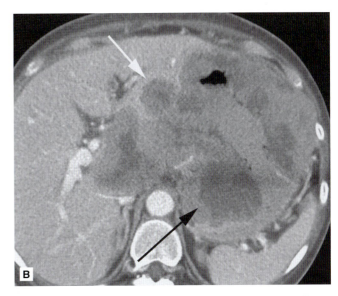

1. A. Axial, contrast-enhanced CT image demonstrates a large, lobulated gastric carcinoma (arrows) in the left upper quadrant. Note direct invasion of the left lobe of the liver. **B.** Axial, contrast-enhanced CT image demonstrates a large, lobulated gastric carcinoma (arrows) in the left abdomen with local invasion of the left and right lobes of the liver.

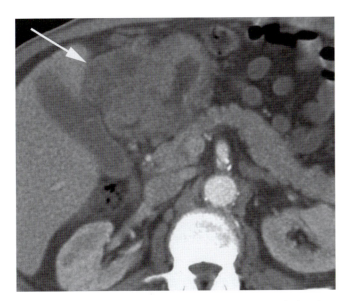

2. Axial, contrast-enhanced CT image demonstrates a lobulated gastric carcinoma in the distal stomach (arrow).

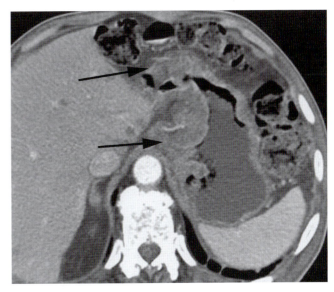

3. Axial, contrast-enhanced CT image demonstrates irregular thickening of the lesser curve of the stomach related to a gastric carcinoma (arrows). Note several small, distant metastases in the liver parenchyma.

PRESENTATION

Patients often present with nausea, abdominal pain, weight loss, and early satiety

FINDINGS

Narrowed, rigid appearance of the stomach with absence of peristalsis and diffuse, circumferential thickening of the wall on cross-sectional imaging

DIFFERENTIAL DIAGNOSIS

- Gastric sarcoidosis
- Caustic gastritis
- Amyloidosis
- Crohn disease

COMMENTS

Linitis plastica or leather bottle stomach, also known as Brinton disease is typically used to describe the morphologic appearance of a narrowed, rigid stomach resulting from primary infiltrative gastric carcinoma or metastatic disease to the stomach. Gastric linitis plastica is a feature of infiltrative gastric carcinoma in which infiltrative, poorly characterized tumor cells, spreading predominately in the submucosa, invoke a marked desmoplastic response, resulting in narrowing and rigidity of the stomach. The prognosis of these tumors, also known as scirrhous gastric carcinomas, is poor secondary to the advanced disease often encountered at presentation, including the presence of peritoneal dissemination and lymph node metastasis. Also, a high incidence of peritoneal and retroperitoneal recurrence has been reported, even after curative operative intervention. In addition to primary tumors, metastatic tumors to the stomach may result in an infiltrating, linitis plastica type appearance; this pattern is commonly described in cases of breast cancer metastases but has been reported in a variety of primary tumors, including lymphoma. Finally, diffusely infiltrating primary carcinomas as well as metastases may result in a linitus plastica type appearance in other portions of the gastrointestinal tract, in addition to the stomach, including the esophagus, small and large bowel.

On barium studies, gastric linitis plastica demonstrates a narrowed, rigid appearance with loss of expected peristalsis and pliability and an absence or distortion of the normal mucosal fold pattern. On CT, diffuse, circumferential thickening with homogeneous enhancement of the stomach with loss of mucosal fold pattern has been described. Also, while atypical, in cases of scirrhous gastric carcinomas, a target sign appearance with stratification of the bowel wall and relatively hyperattenuating inner and outer layers and a hypoattenuating intervening layer has been described. On CT, evidence of advanced disease such as intra-abdominal lymphadenopathy, malignant ascites, as well as omental and peritoneal neoplastic involvement may be seen given a high incidence of advanced disease at the time of presentation. Delayed-phase contrast-enhanced CT has been reported to increase the visualization of fibrosis associated with the infiltrative tumors resulting in a linitis plastica appearance. In the small and large bowel, smoothly tapering strictures have been described on barium studies. On CT, the target appearance has also been described in cases of linitis plastica in patients with scirrhous metastases to the rectum. Finally, bowel obstruction related to the narrowing and rigidity associated with scirrhous carcinomas may be identified on imaging in cases of linitis plastica of the gastrointestinal (GI) tract.

PEARLS

- Gastric linitis plastica typically results from scirrhous gastric carcinoma but a linitis plastica appearance may be seen secondary to infiltrative metastatic disease.

- Advanced disease is often seen at presentation in patients with gastric linitis plastica related to a primary gastric tumor.

- The term linitis plastica may also be used to describe scirrhous tumors of portions of the GI tract other than the stomach.

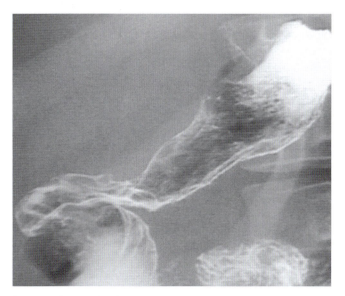

1. Upper GI examination demonstrates narrowing and rigidity of the stomach in a patient with scirrhous gastric carcinoma.

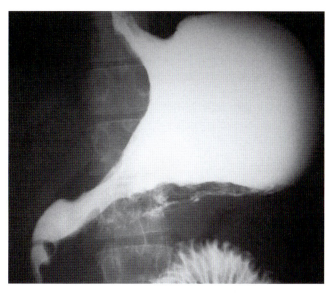

2. Upper GI examination demonstrates narrowing and rigidity of the distal portion stomach with irregular, thickened folds in a patient with scirrhous gastric carcinoma.

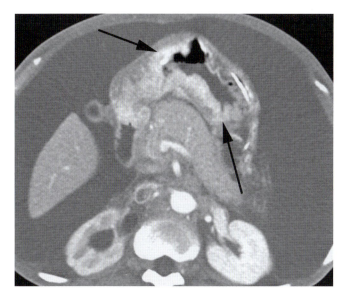

3. Axial, enhanced CT image demonstrates enhancing, irregular thickening of the stomach wall (arrows). Note the presence of malignant ascites in this patient, a common finding as patients with linitis plastica have a high incidence of advanced disease at presentation.

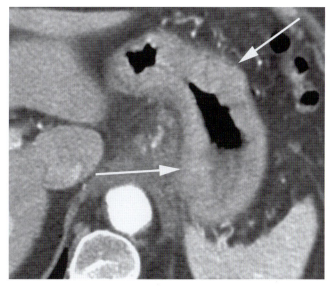

4. Axial, enhanced CT image demonstrates diffuse, circumferential thickening of the stomach (arrows) which appears narrow and rigid in a patient with scirrhous gastric carcinoma.

PRESENTATION

Often, patients may be asymptomatic and a gastrointestinal stromal tumor (GIST) may be incidentally detected. Alternatively, patients may present with abdominal pain, nausea, vomiting, and weight loss. Less commonly, patients may present with anemia from occult blood loss or frank gastrointestinal hemorrhage.

FINDINGS

GISTs often appear as large exophytic masses with peripheral enhancement. Central ulcerations and calcification are also frequently identified upon imaging.

DIFFERENTIAL DIAGNOSIS

- Other mesenchymal neoplasms (true leiomyomas, leiomyosarcomas, schwannomas, neurofibromas)
- Neuroendocrine tumors
- Adenocarcinoma
- Lymphoma

COMMENTS

Although rare, GISTs are the most common mesenchymal tumors of the gastrointestinal tract. GISTs arise from the interstitial cells of Cajal (intestinal pacemaker) and almost always express c-KIT (CD117), a specific tyrosine kinase growth factor; this helps differentiate GISTs from true leiomyomas. The median age at presentation ranges from 55 to 65 years; GISTs show no gender predilection. When GISTs occur in young adults and children, they may be associated with a syndrome such as neurofibromatosis type 1, familial GIST, or the Carney triad (gastric GIST, extra-adrenal paraganglioma, and pulmonary chondroma). Seventy percent of GISTs are located in the stomach, 20% to 30% in the small bowel, and 7% in the anus or rectum. Rarely, GISTs may occur in the esophagus, but leiomyomas are far more common in this anatomic location. GISTs also occur rarely as primary colonic tumors.

The most common clinical manifestation of symptomatic GISTs in the stomach, small intestine, colon, and anorectum is gastrointestinal bleeding from mucosal ulceration. Patients may present with hematemesis, melena, hematochezia, or signs and symptoms of chronic anemia caused by occult bleeding. Other signs and symptoms include nausea, vomiting, abdominal pain, weight loss, abdominal distention, and intestinal obstruction. Occasionally, small asymptomatic GISTs are discovered incidentally during a radiological evaluation or surgical procedure performed for other reasons.

Because GISTs usually involve the outer muscular layer, they have a propensity for exophytic growth. Therefore, the most common appearance is that of a mass arising from the intestinal wall and projecting into the abdominal cavity. Mucosal ulceration is seen on the luminal surface of the tumor in up to 50% of cases. GISTs range in size from several millimeters to greater than 30 cm. They are typically well-circumscribed masses that compress adjacent tissues and lack a true capsule. Cut sections of resected specimens have a pink, tan, or gray surface. Focal areas of hemorrhage, cystic degeneration, and necrosis may occur, particularly in large lesions.

GISTs can be classified histologically on the basis of the predominant cell morphology present: spindle cell, epithelioid or mixed. The spindle cell morphology is present in 70% of GISTs, 20% have a predominance of the epithelioid cell morphology and 10% are the mixed cell type. Immunophenotyping is essential to differentiate GISTs from other mesenchymal tumors. The CD117 (c-KIT) is positive in nearly 100% of tumors and CD34 is positive in approximately 70% to 80% of tumors.

Abdominal radiography may show a nonspecific soft tissue mass indenting or displacing the gastric or intestinal air. Rarely, calcifications may be visible on abdominal radiographs. On barium studies, GISTs have the classic features of submucosal masses, similar to other mesenchymal tumors. At contrast-enhanced CT, GISTs appear as large exophytic masses with peripheral enhancement. The mass is heterogeneous, but the predominant attenuation is similar to that of muscle. Central ulceration is commonly found with barium examinations or CT. Magnetic resonance (MR) imaging features of GISTs are variable. The degree of necrosis and hemorrhage present greatly affects the pattern of signal intensity on the various sequences. The solid components of the tumor are typically low signal intensity on T1-weighted images, high signal intensity on T2-weighted images, and enhance avidly after administration of intravenous contrast. Positron emission tomography (PET) performed with fluorodeoxyglucose (FDG) has high sensitivity for the detection of GISTs; however, glucose uptake in tumors with extensive necrosis or myxoid degeneration may not be sufficient to allow their detection.

Surgery is the treatment of choice for GISTs. However, in more advanced stages of disease, patients may be treated initially with a tyrosine kinase inhibitor such as imatinib mesylate. Treatment in many cases has produced a good response and prolonged survival. CT, MRI, and PET can be used to monitor the effects of treatment.

PEARLS

- GISTs are the most common mesenchymal tumors of the gastrointestinal tract, arise from interstitial cells of Cajal (intestinal pacemaker), and almost always express a specific tyrosine kinase growth factor receptor known as c-KIT (CD117).

- At contrast-enhanced CT, GISTs appear as large exophytic masses with peripheral enhancement.

- FDG-PET has high sensitivity for the detection of GISTs; however, tumors with extensive necrosis or myxoid degeneration may not demonstrate uptake of glucose.

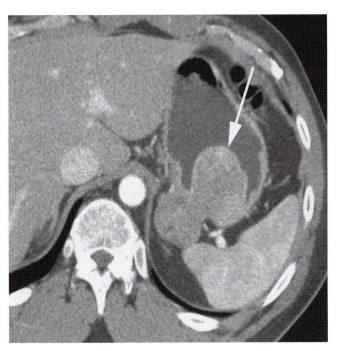

1. Axial, contrast-enhanced CT image demonstrates a large, bilobed soft tissue mass (arrow) projecting both exophytically as well as into the stomach lumen which was found to be a gastric GIST.

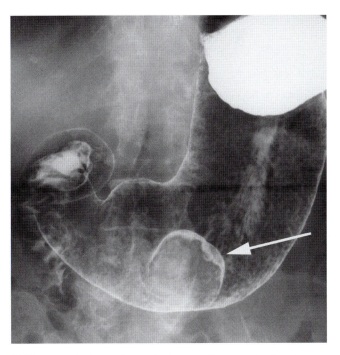

2. Fluoroscopic image from a barium-swallow examination demonstrates a round, well-circumscribed gastric GIST (arrow) projecting into the stomach lumen.

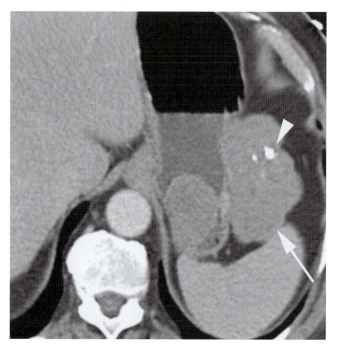

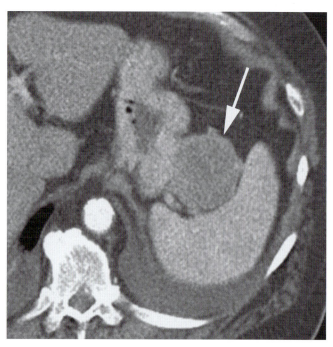

3. Axial, contrast-enhanced CT image demonstrates a lobulated soft tissue mass (arrow) with a large exophytic component containing calcification (arrowhead), typical features of a GIST.

4. Axial, contrast-enhanced CT image demonstrates an exophytic soft tissue mass (arrow) exhibiting typical imaging features of a GIST.

PRESENTATION

Patients typically present with epigastric pain, nausea, vomiting as well as anorexia, and weight loss. Less common presentations include a palpable abdominal mass, anorexia, and weight loss.

FINDINGS

Abnormal gastric wall thickening with relative preservation of fat planes, lack of invasion of surrounding structures, transpyloric spread of the tumor, bulky lymph nodes, and lymphadenopathy below the renal hila all suggest lymphoma over gastric carcinoma.

DIFFERENTIAL DIAGNOSIS

- Gastric carcinoma
- Pancreatic carcinoma
- Duodenal carcinoma

COMMENTS

The stomach is the most common site for involvement with primary lymphoma in the gastrointestinal tract (60%-75%), followed by the small bowel, ileocecal region, and rectum. Gastric lymphoma accounts for 3% to 7% of all malignant tumors of the stomach. The decrease in the incidence of gastric carcinoma in recent years coincides with an increase in the incidence of primary gastric lymphoma. *Helicobacter pylori* plays a role in the development of most mucosa-associated lymphoid tissue (MALT) lymphomas and diffuse large B-cell lymphomas (DLBCLs). However, the exact mechanism is not been fully understood. Chronic inflammation may enhance the probability of malignant transformation in response to *H pylori* infection.

The age at presentation of most gastric lymphoma patients is over 50 years, with a relative predilection for men. Clinical symptoms of gastric lymphoma are nonspecific and indistinguishable from other benign and malignant conditions. The most common complaints are epigastric pain, weight loss, nausea, and vomiting. Occasionally, an abdominal mass is palpable. Palpable lymphadenopathy is rare and patients often have no physical signs. Perforation, bleeding, and obstruction are rare complications. Unlike nodal lymphoma, B-type constitutional symptoms are not common. Although all histological kinds of nodal lymphoma can arise from the stomach, the majority of them are of the B-cell origin and MALT lymphoma and DLBCL account for over 90% of cases. MALT lymphoma comprises up to 50% of all primary lymphomas of the stomach.

Endoscopy cannot reliably distinguish gastric lymphoma from the more common gastric carcinoma. The three main patterns that can be recognized at endoscopy include ulceration, diffuse infiltration, and polypoid mass. Endoscopic ultrasonography (EUS) is used to assess the extent of the lesion and the depth of invasion. Lesions are usually hypoechoic, although few cases of hyperechoic tumors have been reported. Infiltrative carcinoma tends to have a vertical pattern of growth in the gastric wall, while lymphoma tends to show mainly a horizontal extension and more involvement of perigastric lymph nodes. EUS is highly accurate in detecting the depth of lymphomatous infiltration and the presence of perigastric lymph nodes, thus providing additional information for treatment planning, and can differentiate lymphoma from carcinoma both in early stage and in advanced stage.

Radiographic patterns of gastric lymphoma observed in double-contrast upper gastrointestinal (UGI) studies include ulcers, polypoid masses, thickened folds, mucosal nodularity, or infiltrating lesions.

Preservation of gastric distensibility and pliability, despite extensive infiltration and gastric fold thickening, is a finding suggestive of lymphoma. On CT images, the severity of gastric wall thickening can serve as an indication of the grade of lymphoma. In low-grade lymphoma, the thickening of gastric wall is lesser than on high-grade lymphoma. Preservation fat planes and lack of invasion of surrounding structures suggests lymphoma over gastric carcinoma. Transpyloric spread of the tumor, bulky lymph nodes and lymphadenopathy below the renal hila are also more suggestive of lymphoma than carcinoma. The patterns of gastric involvement observed can be segmental or diffuse infiltration as well as localized and polypoid. Tumor infiltration is usually homogeneous although areas of low attenuation may be present in larger tumors.

MRI features of gastric lymphoma include irregularly thickened mucosal folds, extensive submucosal infiltration, annular constricting lesion, exophytic masses, and mesenteric or retroperitoneal lymphadenopathy. The tumors are usually homogeneous on T1-weighted images and intermediate in signal intensity on T2-weighted images. Enhancement with contrast material is usually mild to moderate. Use of FDG-PET/CT in diagnosis or follow-up of gastric lymphoma is challenging due to the physiological FDG activity in the wall of the stomach and the variability in the degree of uptake in various histologic subtypes.

PEARLS

- The stomach is the site of the gastrointestinal tract most commonly involved with lymphoma, followed by the small bowel, ileocecal region, and rectum.

- *H pylori* plays a role in the development of most MALT lymphomas and DLBCLs.

- Radiological examinations (CT, MR, UGI series) help establish the diagnosis and determine the extent of the lesions.

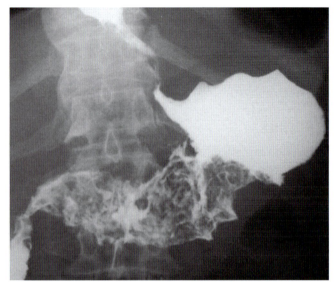

1. Fluoroscopic image from a barium-swallow examination reveals a diffusely narrowing gastric lumen with a highly irregular, ulcerated, nodular mucosal pattern.

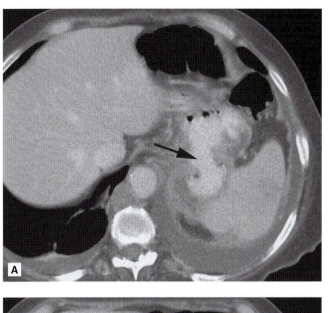

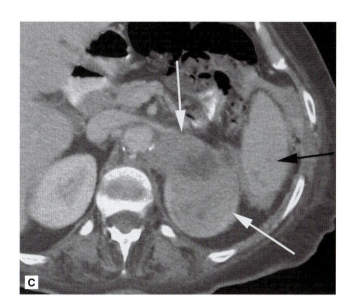

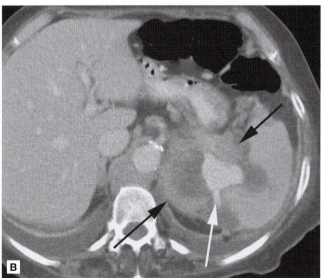

2. A. Axial, contrast-enhanced CT image demonstrates a large gastric ulceration (arrow) related to gastric lymphoma. Note involvement of the spleen in this case. **B.** Axial, contrast-enhanced CT image demonstrates marked circumferential gastric wall thickening (black arrows) with a single ulceration (white arrow) clearly identified in a patient with gastric lymphoma. **C.** Axial, contrast-enhanced CT image demonstrates an infiltrating renal mass (white arrows) and splenic involvement (black arrow) secondary to gastric lymphoma.

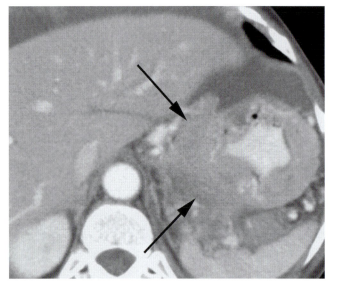

3. Axial, contrast-enhanced CT image demonstrates diffuse, circumferential gastric wall thickening (arrows) secondary to gastric lymphoma.

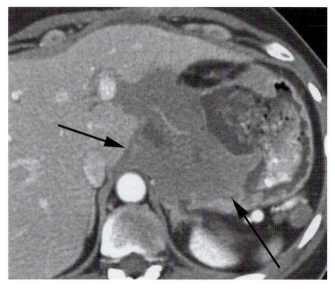

4. Axial contrast-enhanced CT shows a large, exophytic infiltrating (arrows) ulcerated gastric mass infiltrating the gastrohepatic ligament.

PRESENTATION

Although typically incidental and asymptomatic, patients may present with abdominal pain, signs and symptoms of upper gastrointestinal bleeding, iron deficiency anemia, and rarely, gastric outlet obstruction.

FINDINGS

The location of the polyp is a significant determinant of appearance on barium examinations: polyps located dependently appear as filling defects whereas polyps located along the nondependent surface appear as rings with a dense, barium-lined edge.

DIFFERENTIAL DIAGNOSIS

- Gastric bezoars
- Gastrointestinal stromal tumors (GISTs)
- Gastric lymphoma
- Gastric carcinoma
- Carcinoid

COMMENTS

A variety of polyps and polypoid lesions may be found in the gastric wall. Classic epithelial polyps may be hyperplastic, fundic gland, or adenomatous. Other types of polypoid lesions include carcinoids, xanthomas, proliferation of lymphoid tissue, GISTs, leiomyomas, and inflammatory fibroid polyps.

Gastric polyps are typically incidental findings on upper endoscopy performed for an unrelated indication; only rarely do they cause symptoms or other clinical signs. Nonetheless, their discovery can be important since some types of polyps have malignant potential. Fundic gland polyps are the most common type detected by endoscopy. These polyps may occur sporadically or in association with proton pump inhibitor therapy or adenomatous polyposis syndrome. Hyperplastic polyps arise most frequently in patients with an inflamed and often atrophic gastric mucosa and occur most commonly in the antrum. Adenomatous polyps may occur sporadically or as part of the familial adenomatous polyposis syndrome. Sporadic gastric adenomatous polyps may be one of the possible steps in the development of gastric adenocarcinoma. Hamartomatous polyps are found in juvenile polyposis, Cronkite-Canada syndrome, Peutz-Jegher syndrome, and Cowden disease.

The appearance of gastric polyps on barium studies varies with the exact location of the lesion and with the angle formed by the lesion and the x-ray beam. Polyps located in the dependent wall of the stomach appear as filling defects in the pool of contrast. Larger lesions (2-6 cm in size) have a lobulated surface or may be pedunculated. Polyps located in the nondependent surface appear as ring shadows etched in white because of barium trapped between the edge of the polyp and adjacent mucosa. On double-contrast examinations, polypoid lesions may have a reticular surface caused by barium trapped in the interstices of the lesion. On CT, when visible, polyps are typically enhancing, soft tissue attenuating lesions, the characteristic appearance of which is determined by the underlying etiology.

PEARLS

- Fundic gland polyps are currently the most common type of polyp detected and are associated with chronic use of proton pump inhibitors.

- Gastric polyps are typically found incidentally on endoscopy or upper gastrointestinal tract examinations with barium.

- On barium examinations, polyps located in the dependent wall of the stomach appear as filling defects whereas polyps located in the nondependent surface appear as rings with a dense edge caused barium trapped between the polyp and adjacent mucosa.

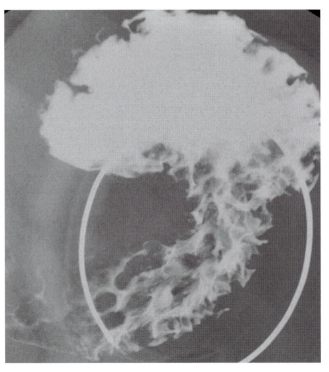

1. Fluoroscopic image from an upper GI examination demonstrates numerous polypoid filling defects, predominately along the nondependent portions of the stomach in a patient with postinflammatory polyposis secondary to Crohn disease.

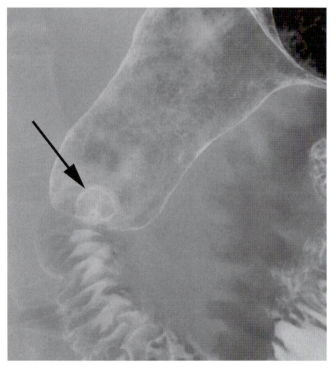

2. Fluoroscopic image from an upper GI examination demonstrates a rounded filling defect in the distal stomach (arrow) in a patient found to have an adenomatous polyp.

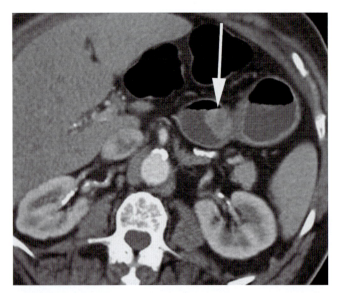

3. Axial, contrast-enhanced CT image demonstrates an enhancing soft tissue–attenuating filling defect in the stomach (arrow) in a patient found to have an adenomatous polyp.

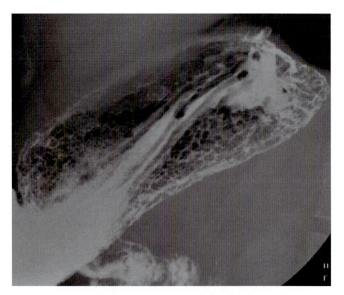

4. Fluoroscopic image from an upper GI examination demonstrates numerous small, rounded filling defects, determined to be hamartomatous polyps in a patient with Peutz-Jegher syndrome.

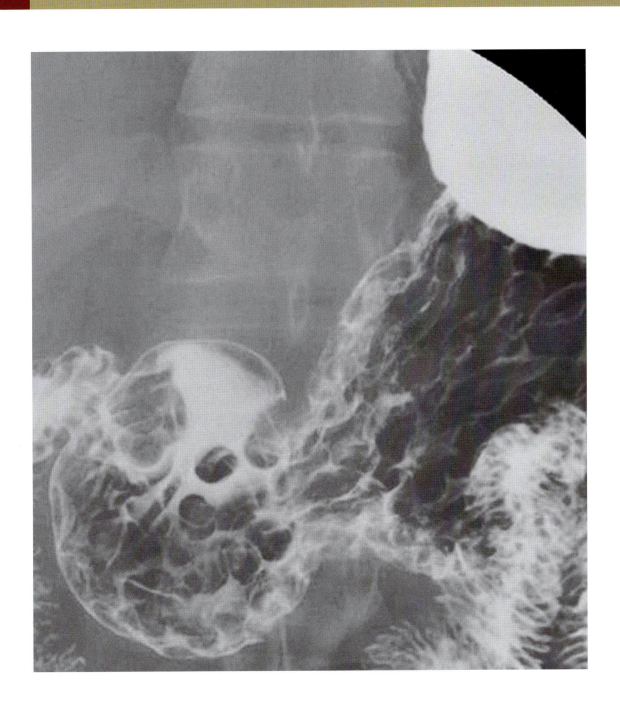

PRESENTATION

Peptic ulcers typically cause dyspepsia with epigastric burning pain.

FINDINGS

Double-contrast barium studies demonstrate a sharply defined focal barium collection projecting beyond the expected confines of the inner margin of the stomach on profile views and smooth uniform folds radiating to the edge of the ulcer crater represented by a focal collection of barium on en face views.

DIFFERENTIAL DIAGNOSIS

- Gastritis
- Malignant gastric ulcer
- Gastric metastasis
- Lymphoma

COMMENTS

Peptic ulcers are focal defects in the gastric or duodenal mucosa which extend into the submucosa or deeper. They are caused by an imbalance between the action of peptic acid and mucosal barriers. A variety of factors may contribute to the development of peptic ulcer disease. Although it is now recognized that the large majority of duodenal and gastric ulcers are caused by *Helicobacter pylori* infection and/or *nonsteroidal anti-inflammatory drug* (NSAID) use, the final common pathway to ulcer formation is peptic acid injury of the gastroduodenal mucosal barrier. *H pylori* predisposes to ulceration, both by acid hypersecretion and by compromise of mucosal defense mechanisms. NSAID use can lead to peptic ulcer disease predominantly by compromise of mucosal defenses. A variety of other diseases are known to cause peptic ulcer, including Zollinger-Ellison syndrome (gastrinoma), antral G-cell hyperfunction and/or hyperplasia, systemic mastocytosis, trauma, burns, and major physiological stress. Other causative agents include drugs (all NSAIDs, aspirin, and cocaine), smoking, alcohol, and psychological stress.

Clinical manifestations of peptic ulcer disease range from silent, asymptomatic disease to severe abdominal pain with bleeding. Peptic ulcers typically cause dyspepsia with epigastric burning pain, and are relieved with antacid therapies. Patients with duodenal ulcers usually experience pain 2 to 3 hours after a meal and at night. The pain of gastric ulcer more commonly occurs with eating and is less likely to awaken the patient at night. Other signs and symptoms include nausea, bloating, weight loss, stool positive for occult blood,

and anemia. Duodenal ulcer is about twice as common in men compared to women, but the incidence of gastric ulcer is similar in men and women. The most common complications of peptic ulcer disease are bleeding, perforation, and obstruction. In the stomach, most benign ulcers are noted in the antrum and lesser curvature, at the junction of the body and antrum. The majority of duodenal ulcers develop in the bulb or pyloric channel. Gastric ulcers often occur later in life with a peak incidence in the sixth decade. Patients with duodenal ulcers tend to have a younger age of onset, often between 30 and 55 years of age on average.

Diagnosis is usually made by upper gastrointestinal (GI) barium studies or endoscopy. Double-contrast barium studies and, to a lesser extent, compression views in the single-contrast examinations are best to demonstrate gastric ulcers. On the en face view, the ulcer projects as a round or oval collection of barium that is more dense than the barium or air-barium mixture covering the surrounding gastric mucosa. On profile view, the ulcer appears as a conical or button-shaped projection of barium beyond the lumen of the stomach due to ulcer excavation in the wall of the stomach. Majority of benign ulcers demonstrate a thick (2-4 mm) smooth rim of lucency, representing edema at the base of the ulcer termed the ulcer collar. When the edema increases, it forms a symmetrical gentle ridge around the ulcer, termed as ulcer mound. Other specific features of benign ulcers are the presence of uniform radiating mucosal folds extending to the edge of crater and thin sharply demarcated lucent line at the base of the ulcer on profile view, called Hampton line. This line represents the preserved overhanging mucosa of benign ulcers. Most benign gastric ulcers detected on double-contrast barium studies are 5 to 10 mm in size. "Giant" ulcers (> 3 cm) are almost always benign but have a higher rate of complications of bleeding or perforation. CT has limited value in early assessment; however, CT with oral contrast may helpful in evaluation of complications.

PEARLS

- Peptic ulcers are focal defects in the gastric or duodenal mucosa, most commonly caused by *H pylori* and NSIAD drugs.

- Barium studies demonstrate a well-defined barium collection and folds radiating to edge of ulcer crater, typically seen on lesser curvature and/or posterior wall of antrum or body.

- Demonstration of Hampton line, ulcer mound, and ulcer collar on profile view of double-contrast studies suggests benign nature of the ulcer.

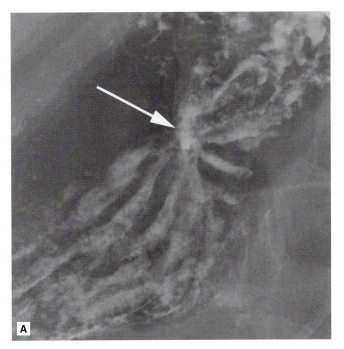

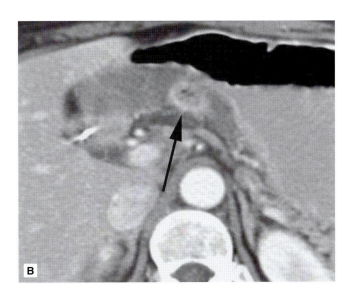

1. A. Upper GI study demonstrates a well-defined collection of barium (arrow) with thickened gastric folds radiating to the edge of the peptic ulcer crater. **B.** Axial, contrast-enhanced CT image reveals a thickened stomach with a focal defect (arrow) secondary to a peptic ulcer.

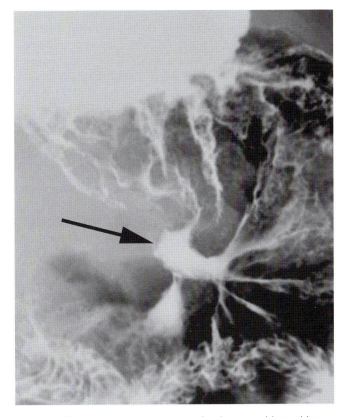

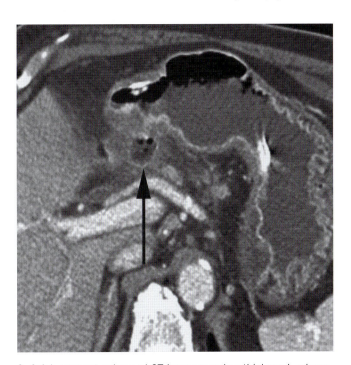

3. Axial, contrast-enhanced CT image reveals a thickened, edematous stomach with a focal defect (arrow) secondary to a peptic ulcer.

2. Upper GI study demonstrates a peptic ulcer as evidenced by a well-defined collection of barium (arrow) extending beyond the lumen of the stomach with thickened, radiating gastric folds.

PRESENTATION

Patients usually present with epigastric pain, reflux, and diarrhea.

FINDINGS

Barium studies demonstrate numerous markedly thickened gastric folds and multiple ulcers.

DIFFERENTIAL DIAGNOSIS

- Peptic ulcer disease
- *Helicobacter pylori* gastritis
- Gastric carcinoma
- Gastric metastases and lymphoma
- Extrinsic inflammation
- Other gastritides

COMMENTS

Zollinger-Ellison syndrome (ZES) is characterized by peptic ulcers and diarrhea secondary to gastric acid hypersecretion due to unregulated gastrin release from non–B islet cell endocrine tumor (gastrinoma). ZES is a rare cause of peptic ulcer disease and accounts for only 0.1% to 1% of ulcers. Men are affected slightly more often than women, with a ratio of 3:2. The majority of gastrinomas are sporadic. However, approximately 25% of ZES patients have gastrinomas as part of the inherited multiple endocrine neoplasia syndrome type 1 (MEN1). Patients with ZES most often present with symptoms arising from excessive gastric acid secretion and only late in the disease course a small percentage of patients show symptoms caused by the gastrinoma itself. The unregulated gastrin production from the causes of parietal cell hyperplasia leading to increased maximal acid output. High serum gastrin levels stimulate the growth of the gastric mucosa, resulting in large gastric folds with not only parietal cell hyperplasia but also proliferation of gastric enterochromaffin-like cells (ECL), which secrete histamine. The increased gastric acid output leads to peptic ulcer diathesis, erosive esophagitis, and diarrhea. Gastrinomas are usually located in the gastrinoma triangle, bounded by the junction of the cystic duct with the common bile duct superiorly, the junction of the second and third portions of duodenum inferiorly, and the junction of the body and head of pancreas medially. These tumors can be difficult to find, especially when they are multifocal. Metastatic disease most often involves the liver and is the usual cause of death.

Gastric acid hypersecretion is responsible for the signs and symptoms observed in patients with ZES. Peptic ulcer is the most common clinical manifestation, occurring in more than 90% of gastrinoma patients. Gastric ulcers in ZES may be indistinguishable from peptic ulcer disease. However, certain characteristics such as ulcers in unusual locations (second portion of the duodenum and beyond), ulcers refractory to standard medical therapy, ulcer recurrence after acid-reducing surgery, ulcers presenting with frank complications (bleeding, obstruction, and perforation), or ulcers in the absence of *H pylori* or nonsteroidal anti-inflammatory drug (NSAID) ingestion raise a suspicion of gastrinoma. Esophageal symptoms ranging from mild esophagitis to frank ulceration with stricture and Barrett mucosa are found in up to 70% of cases. Diarrhea is the next most common clinical manifestation and is found in up to 50% of patients.

The diagnosis of ZES is based on finding an elevated fasting serum gastrin level associated with gastric acid hypersecretion. A variety of provocative tests are also used for the diagnosis, in which tumors are stimulated to produce gastrin by the infusion of secretin, calcium, or other substances. Imaging plays a major role in localization of the tumor after biochemical diagnosis. The main role of imaging is to localize lesions, to identify multiple lesions if present, and to find hepatic or other metastases that may affect the choice of management. Multiple imaging tests using cross-sectional and functional imaging may be required, since no single test is sensitive for both the primary lesion and metastatic disease. Barium studies are of value in the initial stages, when patients present with extensive intractable ulcers or reflux symptoms. These images reveal markedly thickened gastric folds, particularly in the fundus and body, with excessive fluid in the stomach, duodenum, and proximal jejunum. In addition, thickened folds may be found in the duodenum and jejunum as well. Double-contrast studies demonstrate peptic and duodenal ulcers as round or ovoid collections of barium surrounded by a thin or thick radiolucent rim suggestive of edematous mucosa and radiating folds. The majority are found in the stomach or duodenal bulb, but can be seen in the postbulbar duodenum and proximal jejunum as well. Presence of one or more ulcers beyond the ampulla of Vater is highly suggestive of ZES, as isolated peptic ulcers are rarely seen in the third or fourth portions of the duodenum. On CT and MR, there is marked diffuse thickening and inflammation of the stomach and duodenum. The stomach usually contains a large volume of fluid due to hypersecretion, which may dilute the oral contrast. Arterial and portal venous phase images can demonstrate the small pancreatic or peripancreatic tumors and hepatic metastases. Gastrinomas express somatostatin receptors that bind octreotide, and this can be used for tumor imaging. Most gastrinomas can now be localized through the use of somatostatin receptor scintigraphy (SRS) with 111-Indium pentetreotide (OctreoScan) and single photon emission computed tomography. SRS is extremely sensitive for diagnosing primary and metastatic liver lesions as well as bone metastases in affected patients. Endoscopic US is also useful for preoperative tumor localization and staging in ZES patients, especially for tumors in the head and body of the pancreas. In difficult cases of localization, portal venous sampling and selective intra-arterial injection of secretin combined with venous sampling may be helpful.

PEARLS

- ZES is defined as severe peptic ulcer disease and diarrhea secondary to gastric acid hypersecretion due to unregulated gastrin release from a non–B islet cell endocrine tumor (gastrinoma).

- Gastrinomas may be single or multiple, typically seen in the gastrinoma triangle, bounded by the junction of the cystic duct with the common bile duct superiorly, the junction of the second and third portions of the duodenum inferiorly, and the junction of the body and head of the pancreas medially.

- Radiologically, a hypervascular pancreatic mass is noted, with numerous peptic ulcers and thickened gastric, duodenal, and jejunal folds.

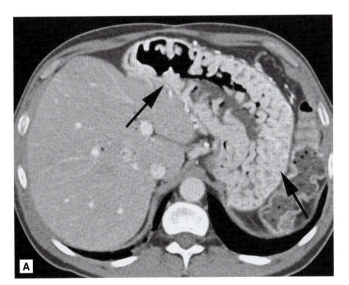

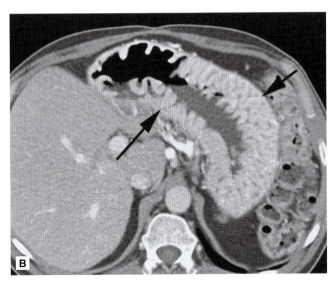

1. A. Axial, contrast-enhanced CT image reveals diffuse thickening of the gastric folds (arrows) related to ZES. **B.** Axial, contrast-enhanced CT image reveals a fluid-filled, thickened stomach (arrows) related to ZES.

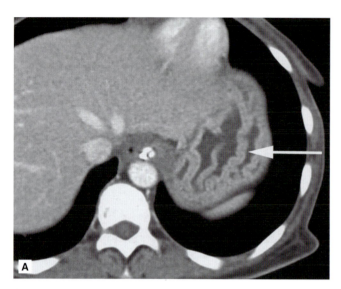

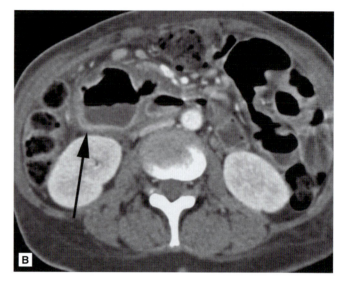

2. A. Axial, contrast-enhanced CT image reveals thickened gastric folds (arrow) related to ZES. **B.** Axial, contrast-enhanced CT image reveals a thickened, fluid-filled duodenum (arrow) related to ZES.

PRESENTATION

Patients often present with abdominal pain, nausea, vomiting, anorexia, and weight loss.

FINDINGS

The inflammatory phase is characterized by enlarged gastric folds and ulcerations while the stenotic or cicatricial phase is characterized by tubular, funnel-shaped narrowing of the distal antrum, pylorus and duodenal bulb.

DIFFERENTIAL DIAGNOSIS

- Gastric lymphoma
- Gastric adenocarcinoma
- Gastroduodenal tuberculosis
- Eosinophilic gastroenteritis

COMMENTS

Crohn disease is a chronic inflammatory disease that can involve any part of the gastrointestinal tract from mouth to the anus. The majority of patients have multiple foci of involvement, such that isolated gastric Crohn disease is a very rare entity, accounting for less than 0.7% of all patients. The diagnosis of Crohn disease is made based on a combination of typical clinical, laboratory, endoscopic, and pathological findings. The diagnosis of gastric involvement is relatively straightforward when patients with known Crohn disease present with clinical and/or endoscopic evidence of gastric involvement. However, the diagnosis is more difficult to establish in patients with atypical presentations, as occurs in the presence of isolated gastroduodenal disease. In this scenario, other possible etiologies must be systematically ruled out in order to establish the correct diagnosis. These may include *Helicobacter pylori* infection, tuberculosis, chronic treatment with nonsteroidal anti-inflammatory drugs (NSAIDs), eosinophilic gastritis, sarcoidosis, collagen vascular disease, and lymphoma, among others.

Endoscopically, gastric Crohn disease manifests with mucosal edema, focal or diffuse redness, nodular lesions or erosions and ulcers, especially in the distal antrum. The histologic hallmark is the presence of noncaseating granulomas, but these are seen in only approximately 10% of cases.

Radiological examinations acquired during the nonstenotic or inflammatory phase demonstrate hypertrophy of the mucosal folds. A cobblestone appearance is frequently identified, with multiple small ulcerations. The stomach demonstrates decreased peristaltic activity with retained secretions and delayed emptying. The stenotic or cicatricial phase is characterized by tubular, funnel-shaped narrowing of the distal antrum, often involving the pylorus and duodenal bulb as well. This appearance has been referred to as a "pseudopost Billroth I deformity." Complete obstruction of the gastric outlet may occur as a complication of either the acute inflammatory or the stenotic phase.

PEARLS

- **Isolated gastric Crohn disease is a very rare entity, accounting for less than 0.7% of all cases of gastrointestinal Crohn disease.**

- **The inflammatory phase is characterized by enlarged gastric folds and multiple small ulcerations.**

- **The stenotic or cicatricial phase is characterized by tubular, funnel-shaped narrowing of the distal antrum, pylorus and duodenal bulb, an appearance that has been referred to as a pseudopost Billroth I deformity.**

- **Complete obstruction of the gastric outlet may be associated with either the acute inflammatory or the stenotic phase.**

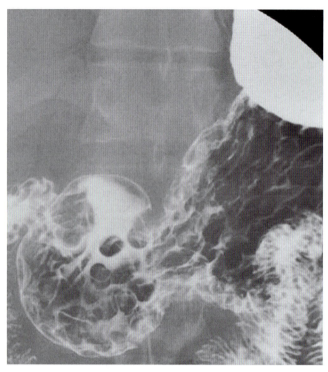

1. Fluoroscopic image during a barium-swallow examination demonstrates thickened gastric folds as well as the presence of numerous post-inflammatory pseudopolyps in a patient with gastric Crohn disease.

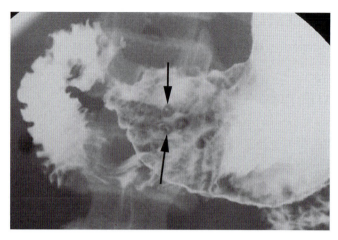

2. Fluoroscopic image during a barium-swallow examination demonstrates the presence of numerous small apthoid ulcerations (arrows) consistent with the inflammatory phase of gastric Crohn disease.

PRESENTATION

Patients with gastritis may be asymptomatic, have mild abdominal discomfort or present with sudden onset of epigastric pain, nausea, and vomiting.

FINDINGS

Barium studies demonstrate thickened, lobulated gastric folds in the antrum and body.

DIFFERENTIAL DIAGNOSIS

- Gastric carcinoma
- Zollinger-Ellison syndrome
- Pancreatitis
- Menetrier disease
- Gastric metastases
- Lymphoma

COMMENTS

Gastritis is defined as inflammation of the gastric mucosa. More than 80% of cases of gastritis diagnosed on histology are caused by *Helicobacter pylori* infection. Other causes include autoimmune gastritis, drugs, allergy, Crohn, sarcoid, vasculitis, and radiation, as well as other bacteria, viruses, or fungi. Gastritis is classified based on the time course (acute vs chronic), histologic features, and anatomic distribution or proposed pathogenic mechanism. However, there is poor correlation between the histologic findings of gastritis, the clinical picture of abdominal pain or dyspepsia, and endoscopic findings noted on gross inspection of the gastric mucosa.

H pylori gastritis is by far the most frequent and important form of gastritis. *H pylori* survives in the acidic gastric environment by creating an alkaline microenvironment through conversion of urea into ammonia. The toxins released by the organism damage the mucosa and causes gastritis. More virulent strains can induce more severe mucosal damage and risk of subsequent development of ulcer, gastric cancer, atrophic gastritis, mucosa-associated lymphoid tissue lymphoma (MALToma), and possibly nonulcer dyspepsia. Acute infection can be asymptomatic or present with sudden onset of epigastric pain, nausea, and vomiting. *H pylori* gastritis may be manifested on double-contrast barium studies by thickened scalloped folds that have a longitudinal or transverse orientation and enlarged areae gastricae, predominantly in the gastric antrum or body. Endoscopy with biopsy is usually performed to confirm the diagnosis as these radiographic findings are nonspecific and may be caused by a variety of inflammatory or neoplastic conditions.

Non–*H pylori* gastritis usually manifests as erosive gastritis with epithelial defects confined within the muscularis mucosa. Erosive gastritis may be asymptomatic or present with vague upper abdominal symptoms such as dyspepsia, epigastric discomfort, or upper gastrointestinal bleeding. Double-contrast barium studies demonstrate mainly two types of erosions. The most common type is the aphoid, or "varioliform," erosion in which punctate or slit-like collections of barium representing the epithelial defects are surrounded by radiolucent halos of edematous, elevated mucosa. Varioliform erosions are often aligned along rugal folds and seen in the gastric antrum. Incomplete or flat erosions are epithelial defects without elevation of the surrounding mucosa. They appear radiographically as linear streaks or dots of barium.

Aspirin and other nonsteroidal anti-inflammatory drugs (NSAIDs) may produce distinctive linear or serpiginous erosions that tend to be clustered in the surfaces of the stomach which come in contact with dissolving drugs, and are more frequently found in the body of the stomach, at or near the greater curvature.

Antral gastritis is associated with alcohol, tobacco, coffee, and *H pylori* infection. Barium studies demonstrate mucosal corrugation of the lesser curvature, thickened scalloped longitudinal folds, and spasm or decreased distensibility of the antrum.

Atrophic gastritis is associated with pernicious anemia, which is a megaloblastic anemia caused by decreased synthesis of intrinsic factor and subsequent malabsorption of vitamin B_{12}. Barium studies show a narrowed, tubular stomach with decreased or absent mucosal folds, predominantly in the body and fundus.

The most common CT finding in patients with gastritis is thickening of the gastric folds. In severe cases, the gastric wall appears stratified due to extensive submucosal edema and mucosal hyperenhancement. This striated appearance helps to distinguish gastritis from gastric cancer.

PEARLS

- **Though etiologic factors of gastritis are broad and heterogeneous, *H pylori* is the major cause.**

- **Barium studies demonstrate thickened scalloped folds that have a longitudinal or transverse orientation and enlarged areae gastricae, predominantly in the gastric antrum or body.**

- **Non–*H pylori* gastritis may show linear, varioliform, or flat erosions with or without thickened folds.**

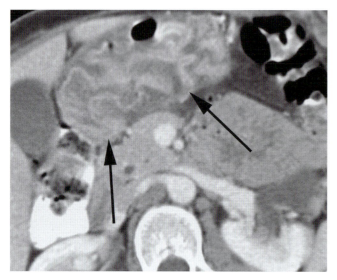

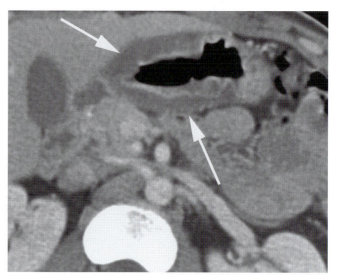

1. Axial, contrast-enhanced CT image demonstrates thickening of the gastric folds and a stratified appearance of the stomach wall related to extensive submucosal edema (arrows) secondary to gastritis.

2. Axial, contrast-enhanced CT image demonstrates a stratified, thickened stomach (arrows) secondary to gastritis.

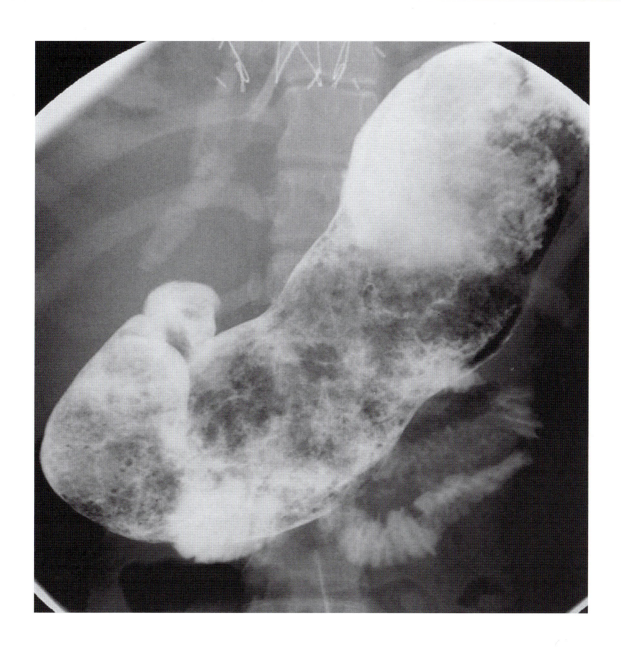

PRESENTATION

Patients with gastric diverticula are often asymptomatic, although they may complain of dyspepsia, vomiting, and abdominal pain. Occasionally, they may present uncommon complications such as ulceration, perforation, haemorrhage, torsion, and malignancy.

FINDINGS

Typically seen as barium-filled outpouchings with air-fluid levels arising from the posterior wall or lesser curvature of the stomach, near the gastroesophageal junction.

DIFFERENTIAL DIAGNOSIS

- Adrenal mass
- Abscess
- Pancreatic mass
- Splenic mass

COMMENTS

Gastric diverticula are rare. Patients are often asymptomatic, and the diagnosis is made incidentally on an imaging study, or they may present with vague and nonspecific upper abdominal symptoms. Gastric diverticula are usually diagnosed in middle-aged individuals, with equal distribution between men and women. Few cases have been reported in children and adolescents as well. Gastric diverticula are usually single, measuring 1 to 3 cm in diameter, although cases have been reported with multiple and large diverticula. Depending on the histology of their wall, they are divided into true diverticula and pseudodiverticula. True diverticula contain all layers (mucosa, submucosa, muscularis, serosa); they constitute about 75% all gastric diverticula. Pseudodiverticula are also known as partial or intramural gastric diverticula. They are often found in the antrum or greater curvature and are typically formed by a projection of the mucosa of the stomach through the muscularis, due to a widening of the space separating the longitudinal muscle fibers. They are almost always seen in association with other gastrointestinal abnormalities such as peptic ulcer disease, malignancy, pancreatitis, or gastric outlet obstruction. Surgical procedures such as the

Roux-en-Y gastric bypass can predispose the stomach to the formation of gastric diverticula.

Gastric diverticula are commonly diagnosed incidentally by radiological or endoscopic examinations. Reported prevalence ranges from 0.04% in barium meal radiographs to 0.01% to 0.11% at endoscopy. Prompt diagnosis is very important given the risk for severe complications including perforation, hemorrhage, and cancer formation within a diverticulum. A barium meal examination is the preferred radiological study. The barium examination demonstrates the diverticula as a contrast-filled outpouching with an air-fluid level along the posterior wall or the lesser sac, near the gastroesophageal junction and can be best demonstrated on the lateral projection. In up to 8% of cases, visualization of the diverticulum may be difficult despite examining in multiple projections. This may be explained by a narrow neck that prevents the diverticulum to fill with contrast. In such cases, gastroscopy may be helpful. Pooling of barium inside an intramural diverticulum may mimic a gastric ulcer. On CT, a typical gastric diverticulum may appear as a soft tissue mass in the left suprarenal location, which may mistake them for other abdominal pathology, such as adrenal tumors or adenopathy. When suspected, prone images help confirm the diagnosis by showing the air-filled diverticulum. There is no specific treatment required for an asymptomatic diverticulum. Surgical resection is recommended when the diverticulum is large, symptomatic or complicated by bleeding, perforation, or malignancy.

PEARLS

- Gastric diverticula are outpouchings from the wall of the stomach, commonly occurring near the gastroesophageal junction along the lesser curvature or posterior wall.

- The majority are true diverticula, composed of all the layers of gastric wall, whereas partial or intramural diverticula are seen along the greater curvature and are associated with other conditions.

- Juxtacardiac diverticula are often mistaken for left adrenal pathology on CT. However, barium studies and prone images may avoid this pitfall.

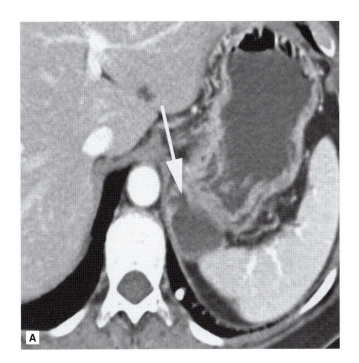

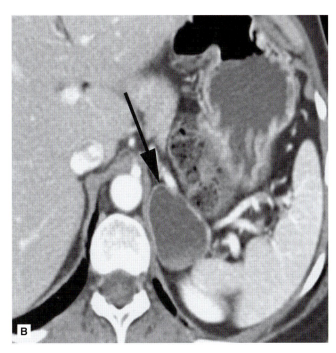

1. Axial contrast-enhanced CT images (**A**, **B**) demonstrate a fluid filled structure emanating from the gastric fundus posteriorly (arrow). Note how it can mimic adrenal pathology.

PRESENTATION

The majority of duodenal diverticula are asymptomatic. However, they may become symptomatic when complicated by diverticulitis, perforation, upper gastrointestinal (GI) bleeding, gastric outlet obstruction, and pancreatico-biliary disease.

FINDINGS

The upper GI series typically demonstrates a true duodenal diverticulum as a smooth, rounded outpouching arising from the medial wall of the descending duodenum in the periampullary region, whereas an intraluminal diverticulum appears as a barium-filled globular structure of variable length, originating in the second portion of the duodenum, with its fundus extending into the third portion and outlined by a thin, radiolucent line.

DIFFERENTIAL DIAGNOSIS

- Pancreatic head pseudocyst
- Cystic pancreatic tumor
- Peripancreatic fluid collection
- Hypermetabolic mass
- Distal common bile duct stone
- Perforated duodenal ulcer

COMMENTS

Duodenal diverticula are the most common acquired diverticula of the small bowel and the second most common site for diverticulum formation after the colon. There are two main types: extraluminal or intraluminal. Extraluminal duodenal diverticula are usually noted incidentally in about 4% to 6% of upper GI series and in about 25% of endoscopic studies performed for an unrelated problem. They are acquired lesions and form as a result of herniation of the mucosal and submucosal layers through a defect in the muscularis. Thus, they are considered true diverticula as they are comprised of all the three GI tract layers. They usually develop in an area of duodenal wall where a blood vessel penetrates the muscularis or where the dorsal and ventral pancreases fuse in embryologic development. More than 70% are located in the periampullary region (within a 2-cm radius of the ampulla) and protrude from the medial wall of the duodenum. Occasionally, they are found in the

third or fourth portions of the duodenum and also along the lateral wall.

Radiologically, they are diagnosed on upper GI series as a smooth, round, or ovoid outpouching arising from the medial border of the descending duodenum. CT and MRI demonstrate air or a combination of air and inside the diverticulum in close relationship with the duodenum. A fluid-distended juxtapapillary diverticulum may resemble a cystic neoplasm of the pancreas on CT. Extraluminal duodenal diverticula are relatively common, but they are often asymptomatic unless associated with complications like diverticulitis, perforation, upper GI bleeding, gastric outlet obstruction, common bile duct stones, and pancreaticobiliary disease. Duodenal diverticulitis presents with pain in the upper abdomen, often radiating to the back and may have signs and symptoms of sepsis if perforated. The abdominal radiograph may demonstrate focal retroperitoneal gas adjacent to the duodenum and the upper pole of the right kidney as duodenal diverticula are located in the retroperitoneum. CT may reveal extravasation of contrast, thickening of the duodenal wall, retroperitoneal air, phlegmon, or abscess. Dieulafoy-like lesions or ulcers within diverticula may cause massive upper GI bleeding which usually requires a tagged red blood cell scintigram or angiography or endoscopy for localization and treatment. Diverticula may also be present at the level of the ampulla of Vater which may produce partial or complete mechanical obstruction of the common bile duct and pancreatic duct as they enter the duodenum. These patients are at increased risk for biliary obstruction, bile duct stones, cholangitis, and pancreatitis.

An intraluminal duodenal diverticulum is a single saccular structure that arises from the second portion of the duodenum. They originate from a congenital duodenal web or diaphragm. Over time, intraluminal mechanical forces such as duodenal peristalsis act on the duodenal web or diaphragm and gradually elongates as far distally as the fourth portion of the duodenum, inside the lumen. Therefore, both sides of the diverticulum are lined by duodenal mucosa. There is often a second opening located eccentrically in the sac. Duodenal diverticula are far less common than extraluminal diverticula. An intraluminal diverticulum is asymptomatic until the development of duodenal obstruction. The upper GI series demonstrates a barium-filled globular structure of variable length, originating in the second portion of the duodenum, with its fundus extending into the third portion, and outlined by a thin, radiolucent line. CT reveals a ring-like soft tissue density in the lumen of the second portion of the duodenum, containing oral contrast and a small amount of air.

PEARLS

- Extraluminal duodenal diverticula are acquired lesions with herniation of mucosa and submucosa through a muscular defect. Intraluminal duodenal diverticula originate from congenital web or diaphragm.

- Approximately 70% of extraluminal diverticula are located within 2 cm of the ampulla and appear as a smooth, rounded outpouching from the medial border of the descending duodenum on upper GI series.

- On barium studies, intraluminal duodenal diverticula (or windsock diverticula) appear as barium-filled globular structures of variable length, originating in the second portion of the duodenum, with its fundus extending into the third portion, and outlined by a thin, radiolucent line.

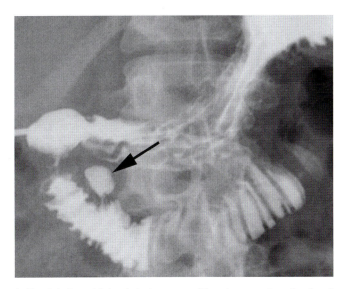

1. Frontal view obtained during upper GI series reveals a duodenal diverticulum extending from the medial wall of the second portion of the duodenum (arrow).

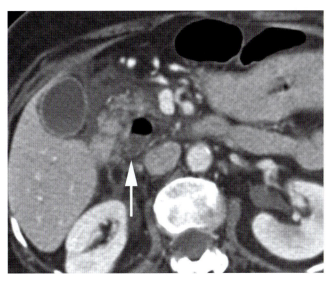

2. Axial contrast-enhanced CT image reveals a duodenal diverticulum (arrow) with surrounding inflammatory stranding secondary to duodenal diverticulitis.

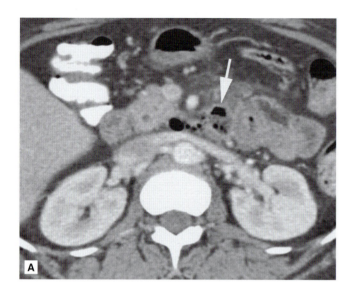

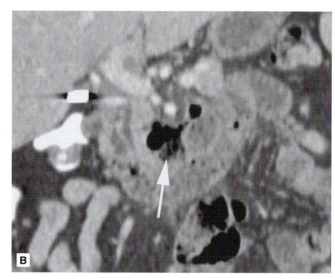

3. A. Axial contrast-enhanced CT image reveals a duodenal diverticulum (arrow) with surrounding inflammatory stranding and extraluminal air secondary to perforation related to duodenal diverticulitis. **B.** Coronal contrast-enhanced CT image demonstrates free air and inflammation surrounding a duodenal diverticulum (arrow), consistent with perforated duodenal diverticulitis.

PRESENTATION

Patients present with epigastric pain, at times accompanied by nausea, vomiting, anorexia, peripheral edema, and weight loss.

FINDINGS

Double-contrast barium studies demonstrate grossly thickened, lobulated folds in the gastric fundus and body, with relative sparing of the antrum. CT scans show a markedly thickened gastric wall with giant heaped-up folds protruding into the lumen.

DIFFERENTIAL DIAGNOSIS

- *Helicobacter pylori* gastritis
- Gastric carcinoma and gastric metastases
- Lymphoid hyperplasia and lymphoma
- Zollinger-Ellison syndrome
- Gastric varices
- Other various types of gastritis

COMMENTS

Ménétrier disease is a rare condition characterized by large, tortuous gastric mucosal folds, hypochlorhydria, and hypoproteinemia. The mucosal folds in Ménétrier disease are often most prominent in the body and fundus. The etiology of this unusual clinical entity is unknown. However, histologically, most of the chief and parietal cells are replaced with massive foveolar hyperplasia (hyperplasia of surface and glandular mucus cells). This hyperplasia leads to prominent folds in the fundus and body, predominantly along the greater curvature. Based on the time of diagnosis, 20% to 100% of patients develop a protein-losing gastropathy accompanied by hypoalbuminemia and edema.

Gastric acid secretion is usually reduced or absent because of the replacement of the parietal cells.

Ménétrier disease is seen in older male patients. Patients present with epigastric pain, at times accompanied by nausea, vomiting, anorexia, peripheral edema, and weight loss. Radiologically, the double-contrast barium meal series demonstrates grossly thickened, lobulated folds in the gastric fundus and body with relative sparing of the antrum. Abnormal folds across the greater curvature are usually thickest and longest among all the folds seen in the stomach. The disease can also affect only a focal area of the stomach and mimic polypoid carcinoma. CT scans again show a markedly thickened gastric wall with giant heaped-up folds protruding into the lumen. Diagnosis is usually confirmed by endoscopic biopsy.

The differential diagnosis of large gastric folds includes a long list of benign and malignant conditions; however, none of them has the degree of fold thickening seen in Ménétrier disease. Clinical history and presentation may provide additional information, apart from imaging, to differentiate these conditions form Ménétrier disease.

PEARLS

- **Ménétrier disease is a rare condition characterized by large, tortuous gastric mucosal folds, hypochlorhydria, and hypoproteinemia.**

- **Double-contrast barium studies demonstrate grossly thickened, lobulated folds in the gastric fundus and body, with relative sparing of the antrum. CT scans show a markedly thickened gastric wall with giant heaped-up folds protruding into the lumen.**

- **None of the other conditions associated with thickened gastric folds have the degree of fold thickness seen in Ménétrier disease.**

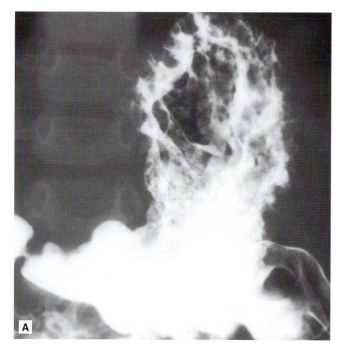

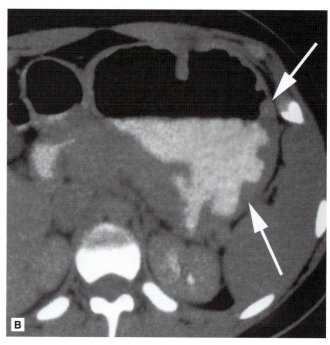

1. A. Upper gastrointestinal (GI) study demonstrates marked thickening of the gastric folds with relative sparing of the antrum related to Ménétrier disease. **B.** Axial CT image reveals marked thickening of the gastric folds (arrows) related to Ménétrier disease.

PRESENTATION

The majority of patients have vague symptoms of epigastric discomfort and pain. They may also complain of nausea, bloating, early satiety, halitosis, and weight loss.

FINDINGS

Upper gastrointestinal (GI) series may demonstrate a conglomerate mass of debris with a mottled appearance. CT may show a heterogeneous intraluminal mass floating at the air-fluid interface with a mottled gas pattern.

DIFFERENTIAL DIAGNOSIS

- Gastric carcinoma
- Intramural mass
- Postprandial food

COMMENTS

Bezoar is an intragastric mass of undigested material derived from ingested matter. They are seen anywhere in the GI tract, but most commonly in the stomach. A variety of bezoars are described in the literature. However, the most frequently encountered types are phytobezoars, trichobezoars, tricophytobezoars, and pharmacobezoars. Phytobezoars are most common, and are made up of undigested vegetable or fruit matter. They typically develop in patients who eat foods containing large amounts of insoluble and indigestible fibers, especially unripe persimmons. The fruit pulp of persimmons forms a coagulum when mixed with gastric acid, which then attracts other ingested material to develop the bezoar. Trichobezoars are composed of matted hair and are classically seen in young women with schizophrenia or other psychiatric disorders who have the habit of chewing their hairs and cloths. Bezoars composed of both vegetable and hair components are called tricophytobezoars. Medication bezoars can result from fiber-containing medications, resin-water formulas, or extended-release medications. Patients with gastroparesis, prior gastric surgery, or outlet obstruction from any other reason are at increased risk for development of bezoars.

The majority of patients have vague symptoms of epigastric discomfort and pain. They may also have nausea, bloating, early satiety, halitosis, and weight loss. Bezoars can cause crampy epigastric pain and a sense of fullness or heaviness in the upper abdomen, and can progress to mechanical obstruction. Phytobezoars can induce peptic ulcers by abrasion and pressure necrosis which can cause bleeding or gastric outlet obstruction.

Abdominal radiographs may demonstrate a mottled soft tissue density in the stomach, at the air-fluid interface. Upper GI barium series may show a filling defect with smooth layering of barium on it or a conglomerate mass of debris with a mottled appearance from barium filling the interstices of the bezoar. Unlike mass lesions of the gastric wall, a bezoar moves freely with changes in patient position. Impacted bezoars may cause gastric outlet obstruction. They appear as a well-defined, low-density, intraluminal mass with mottled air lucencies on CT and do not enhance on postcontrast images.

PEARLS

- Bezoar is an intragastric mass of undigested material derived from ingested matter, the most frequently encountered are phytobezoars, trichobezoars, tricophytobezoars, and pharmacobezoars.

- Abdominal radiographs may demonstrate a mottled density in the stomach and an upper GI barium series may show a filling defect or a conglomerate mass of debris with a mottled appearance.

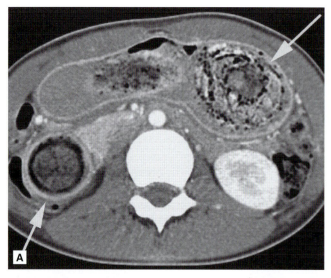

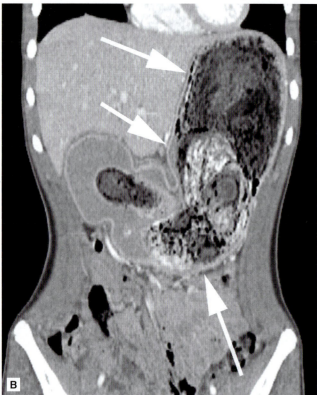

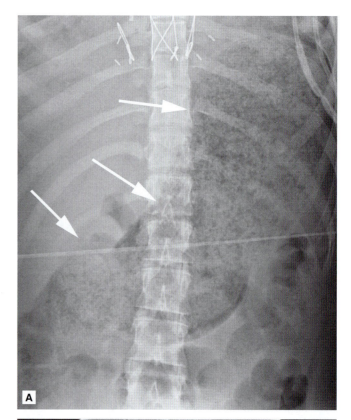

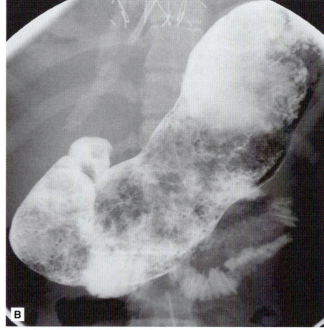

1. A. Axial, contrast-enhanced CT image demonstrates a large, mottled-appearing filling defect within a distended stomach secondary to a phytobezoar (arrows). **B.** Coronal, contrast-enhanced CT image reveals a large, mottled-appearing filling defect (arrows) resulting in gastric distension, the imaging features of which are typical of a bezoar, in this case, a phytobezoar.

2. A. Frontal abdominal radiograph demonstrates a markedly distended, debris-filled stomach (arrows). **B.** Fluoroscopic image acquired during an upper GI series demonstrates a large filling defect within the stomach with barium filling the interstices of the bezoar. In this case, the patient recently underwent surgery and developed a large bezoar secondary to a postoperative functional ileus.

PRESENTATION

Gastric volvulus causes severe pain in the upper abdomen or lower chest.

FINDINGS

Barium upper gastrointestinal (GI) radiographs show an inverted stomach above the diaphragm with the greater curvature situated above the lesser curvature, cardia, and pylorus.

DIFFERENTIAL DIAGNOSIS

- Hiatal hernia
- Postoperative stomach
- Cup-spill stomach

COMMENTS

Gastric volvulus is a twisted stomach on its axis. In healthy individuals, the stomach is fixed in its position by various structures such as the gastrohepatic and gastrosplenic ligaments, omentum, and diaphragm. The distal stomach is immobile as a result of the retroperitoneal attachment of duodenum. Any loss of integrity of these ligaments, in particular the gastrosplenic ligament or fixation of an otherwise mobile stomach to a specific point by focal adhesions or a gastric tumor can lead to volvulus. The majority occur above the diaphragm in association with a paraesophageal or mixed diaphragmatic hernia with proximal migration of the stomach into the thorax.

Volvulus occurs along the stomach's longitudinal axis (organoaxial) in about two-thirds of cases and along the vertical axis (mesenteroaxial) in one-third of cases. The axis of rotation of organoaxial volvulus usually passes through the gastroesophageal and gastropyloric junctions. This leads to either anterior-superior rotation of the greater curvature, antrum and fundus or anterior-superior rotation of the antrum, and posterior-inferior rotation of the fundus along this axis. It is usually associated with a diaphragmatic hernia. In mesenteroaxial volvulus, the stomach turns on its short axis, running across from the middle of the lesser curvature to the greater curvature with the antrum twisting anteriorly and superiorly. This line corresponds to the axis of the mesenteric attachments of the greater and lesser omentum. This type of volvulus gives the appearance of an "upside-down stomach" with the distal antrum and pylorus occupying a position cranial to the fundus and proximal stomach. Mesenteroaxial volvulus is usually partial (< 180 degrees), recurrent, and may be associated with diaphragmatic rupture.

Acute gastric volvulus causes sudden severe pain in the upper abdomen or lower chest. Vascular compromise can lead to stomach infarction and is a surgical emergency. It is clinically diagnosed by noting the combination of severe epigastric pain, unproductive retching, and inability to pass a nasogastric tube. Chronic gastric volvulus is associated with mild and nonspecific symptoms such as dysphagia, epigastric discomfort or fullness, bloating, and heartburn, particularly after meals. Upright plain films of the abdomen on clinical suspicion reveal a double air-fluid stomach in the chest or upper abdomen with associated elevation of the diaphragm. The diagnosis can be confirmed by barium contrast studies or upper GI endoscopy. Barium studies show a flipped stomach in the thorax with the greater curvature lying above the level or to the right of the lesser curvature, the pylorus above or the same level of the cardia, and downward pointing of the pylorus and duodenum. Gastric volvulus is recognized incidentally on CT examinations as an enlarged, twisted stomach with an area of torsion along with other abnormalities of diaphragm or upper abdomen if any present.

Complications are mainly from luminal obstruction and vascular occlusion. Bowel obstruction depends on the degree of torsion; less than 180 degrees of twisting may not occlude the vasculature, whereas twisting beyond 180 degrees invariably causes complete obstruction and leads to strangulation, necrosis, perforation, and shock.

PEARLS

- Gastric volvulus is a twisting of the stomach on its own axis, usually associated with a diaphragmatic defect. In an organoaxial volvulus the stomach rotates horizontally along the pylorus-to-gastroesophageal junction axis and in a mesenteroaxial volvulus the stomach rotates vertically on an axis parallel to the gastrohepatic ligament.

- Barium upper GI series demonstrate an inverted intrathoracic stomach with the greater curvature lying above the level or to the right of the lesser curvature, the pylorus above or the same level of the cardia, and downward pointing of the pylorus and duodenum.

- Gastric volvulus may be asymptomatic or produce only mild symptoms or may present as an acute surgical emergency due to impending strangulation and ischemic necrosis.

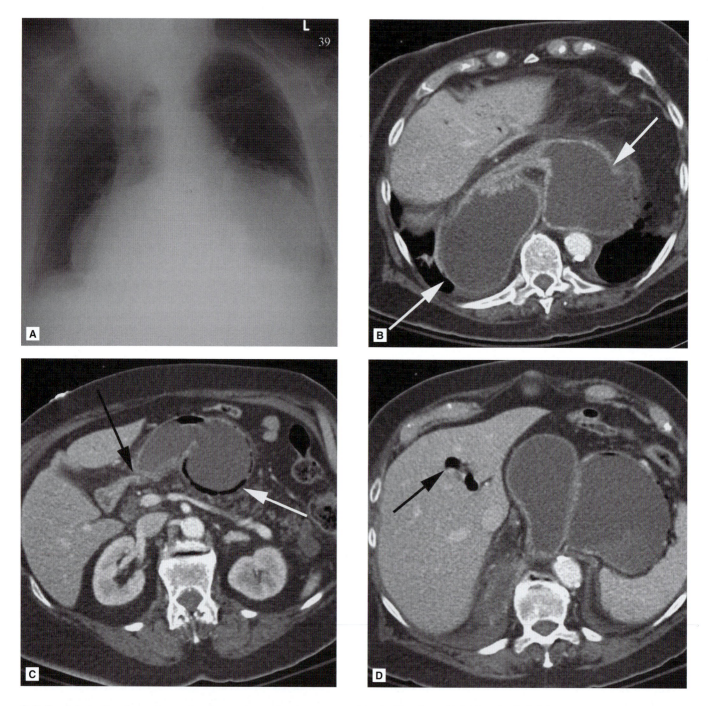

1. A. Frontal chest radiograph reveals a large retrocardiac lucency consistent with a large hiatal hernia. **B.** Axial, contrast-enhanced CT image demonstrates an intrathoracic location of the majority of the stomach (arrows) in this case of organoaxial volvulus. **C.** Axial, contrast-enhanced CT image demonstrates an area of visible twisting (black arrow) of the distal stomach in this organoaxial volvulus with complications of ischemia and pneumatosis noted (white arrow). **D.** Axial, contrast-enhanced CT image demonstrates portal venous gas (arrow) related to ischemia of the stomach secondary to organoaxial volvulus. **E.** Coronal, contrast-enhanced CT image demonstrates an intrathoracic location of the majority of the stomach in this case of organoaxial volvulus.

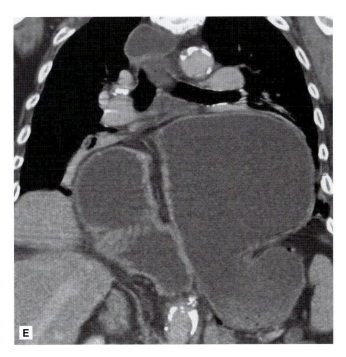

1. (*continued*)

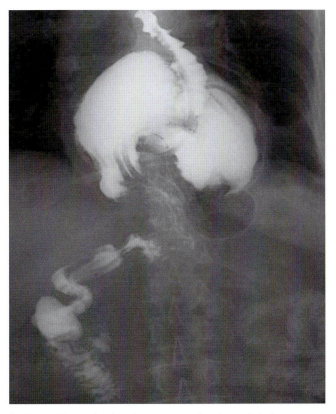

2. Upper GI examination demonstrates the stomach to have assumed an intrathoracic location in this case of organoaxial volvulus.

PRESENTATION

Patients typically present with nausea, vomiting, and abdominal pain.

FINDINGS

Rigler triad in which an ectopic gallstone is seen in the stomach or duodenum along with pneumobilia and gastric outlet obstruction is diagnostic of Bouveret syndrome.

DIFFERENTIAL DIAGNOSIS

- Gastric and duodenal tumors
- Perforated peptic ulcer disease
- Pancreatitis
- Malignant fistulas

COMMENTS

Cholecystoenteric fistulas occur in less than 1% of patients with gallstones. The majority (60%-70%) are cholecystoduodenal fistulas, but cholecystocolic, cholecystogastric, and choledochoduodenal fistulas can also occur. Large stones passing through the fistula may cause intestinal obstruction, especially in the terminal ileum. Gallstone-induced ileus (obstruction) is a rare complication of cholelithiasis, and gastric outlet obstruction is even more rare. Bouveret syndrome refers to gastric outlet obstruction produced by a gallstone impacted in the distal stomach or proximal duodenum. The condition was described by Leon Bouveret in 1896 and occurs most commonly in elderly women (mean age nearly 70 years).

A duodenal location accounts for only 2% to 3% of cases of gastrointestinal (GI) obstruction caused by an obstructing gallstone. The presenting symptoms are variable and nonspecific but often include nausea, vomiting, and epigastric pain. A small minority of patients may present with GI bleeding secondary to duodenal mucosal erosions or arterial erosion. Laboratory study results can suggest an obstructive biliary pattern, with increased bilirubin and elevated alkaline phosphatase levels.

Early diagnosis is important because mortality is high (reportedly exceeding 30%) given the advanced age of the typical patient, along with other comorbidities and their impact on the risks associated with surgical intervention. In approximately 30% to 35% of patients, the diagnosis may be suggested on the basis of the clinical presentation and the presence of Rigler triad which includes evidence of a bowel obstruction, pneumobilia, and an ectopic gallstone.

On CT, pneumobilia and an ectopically located gallstone in the distal stomach or duodenum are clearly identified, as it is the gastric dilatation. A potential pitfall on CT related to the fact that the offending gallstone (which is usually located in the duodenum) may isoattenuating to bile and fluid in 15% to 20% of cases and thus difficult to detect directly. In some cases, the fistula itself may be visible if the tract fills with positive oral contrast or gas. A useful secondary sign in diagnosing Bouveret syndrome on CT is the identification of positive oral contrast material within the gallbladder. MR cholangiopancreatography may be useful for confirming the diagnosis of Bouveret syndrome, especially in the setting of isoattenuating stones.

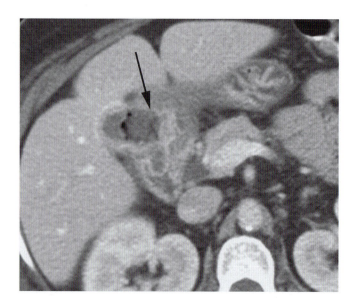

1. Axial, contrast-enhanced CT demonstrates a relatively isoattenuating, air-containing gallstone (arrow), eroding through a cholecystoduodenal fistula.

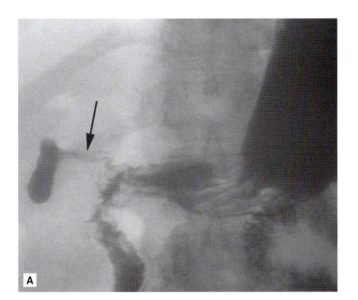

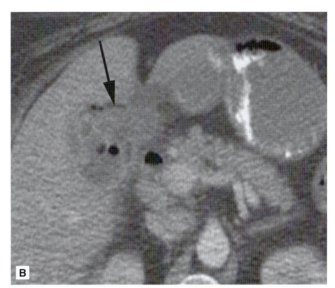

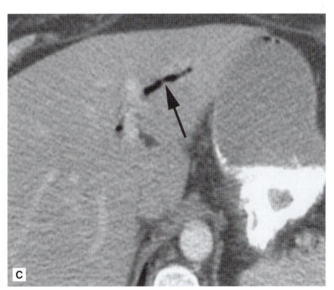

2. **A.** Fluoroscopic image acquired during an upper GI examination reveals direct evidence of a cholecystoduodenal fistula (arrow). **B.** Axial, contrast-enhanced CT image reveals the suggestion of direct evidence of a cholecystoduodenal fistula (arrow) though the offending stone was difficult to visualize directly on CT in this case of Bouveret syndrome. **C.** Axial, contrast-enhanced CT image reveals the presence of pneumobilia (arrow) and moderate gastric distention, two components of Rigler triad, in this patient with Bouveret syndrome.

PRESENTATION

The majority of patients with type I and III hiatal hernia are asymptomatic or have mild reflux symptoms, while most patients with type II hiatal hernias are symptomatic, with nonspecific complaints other than reflux such as epigastric pain, dysphagia, and postprandial fullness.

FINDINGS

Upper gastrointestinal (GI) barium studies demonstrate fixed or transient intrathoracic displacement of the gastroesophageal junction and/or stomach.

DIFFERENTIAL DIAGNOSIS

• Epiphrenic diverticulum

• Phrenic diverticulum

• Postoperative changes

COMMENTS

Hiatal hernia is transdiaphragmatic migration of intra-abdominal contents through the enlarged esophageal hiatus. It is the most common type of diaphragmatic hernia and is usually caused by an enlargement of the esophageal hiatus due to developmental defects or acquired from increased intra-abdominal pressure and depletion of elastic fibers in the phrenoesophageal membrane with aging. Hiatal hernias are classified based on the location of the gastroesophageal junction and the hernia sac content. Type I or sliding hiatal hernias are the most common type and are characterized by upward migration of the gastroesophageal junction into the posterior mediastinum. Type II or paraesophageal hernias are the least common type of hiatal hernia. They are characterized by an upward displacement of the fundus of the stomach with a normally positioned intra-abdominal gastroesophageal junction. Type III hiatal hernias are a combination of type 1 and II, characterized by cephalad displacement of both the gastroesophageal junction and a portion of the fundus and body of the stomach into the chest in a manner that the normal relation between fundus and gastroesophageal junction is maintained. Type IV hernias are basically type III hernias in which other viscera such as the colon or spleen are migrated into the hernia sac. These are quite uncommon.

Hiatal hernias are more common in women and the incidence increases with age. Most type I or sliding hiatal hernias are asymptomatic and found incidentally when an upper GI barium study or an endoscopy is performed for other reasons. More than 90% are associated with gastroesophageal reflux disease. Type II or paraesophageal hiatal hernias cause nonspecific symptoms such as epigastric pain, dysphagia, postprandial fullness, chest pain, shortness of breath, or palpitations. Paraesophageal hernias can present with complications from mediastinal compression, acute gastric volvulus, incarceration, or strangulation. The gastric mucosa over the ridge of the hiatus is prone to suffering repeated injury leading to development of ulcers, known as "riding ulcers."

Radiologically, sliding hernias are best demonstrated on prone images of a single-contrast barium esophagram. The lower esophageal mucosal ring demarcates the anatomic location of the gastroesophageal junction; a sliding hiatal hernia is diagnosed when this ring is noted to lie 2 cm or more above the diaphragmatic hiatus. On double-contrast images, gastric folds within the hernia sac are seen 2 cm or more above the diaphragmatic esophageal hiatus. However, double-contrast images with the patient in the upright position are far less sensitive than the single-contrast study with the patient prone. This is due to reduction of the hernia into the abdomen and lack of adequate distension of the lower esophagus. Double-contrast images are helpful in assessing the mucosa in moderate-to-large size hiatal hernias for ulcers, neoplasm, or other abnormalities. A paraesophageal hernia is suspected on chest radiographs when a retrocardiac air bubble with or without an air-fluid level is present, particularly on the lateral view. Confirmation can be obtained with a barium swallow which shows a portion of the stomach in the thorax along with the gastroesophageal junction depending on the type of hiatal hernia. Sometimes, there may be organoaxial rotation of the herniated portion of fundus. Paraesophageal hernias should be distinguished from a parahiatal hernia in which the fundus herniates through a diaphragmatic defect separate from the hiatus. Paraesophageal hiatal hernias are incidentally diagnosed on CT scans of the chest or upper abdomen. In general, CT scans are of little value in the diagnosis or evaluation of a hiatal hernia.

PEARLS

• **Esophageal hiatal hernia is the most common diaphragmatic hernia, usually asymptomatic and diagnosed incidentally on barium study, endoscopy, or CT scan.**

• **Type I hiatal hernias are often associated with gastroesophageal reflux disease and paraesophageal hiatal hernias can present with gastric volvulus.**

• **Upper GI barium series with the patient in a prone position is the best study to demonstrate a hiatal hernia, with proximal migration of the gastroesophageal junction and/or a portion of the stomach.**

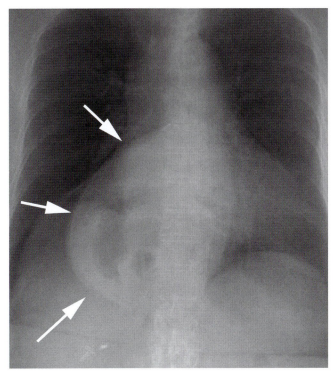

1. Frontal chest radiograph reveals a large retrocardiac opacity (arrows) with a central lucency suggesting air, in this case representing a large type I hiatal hernia.

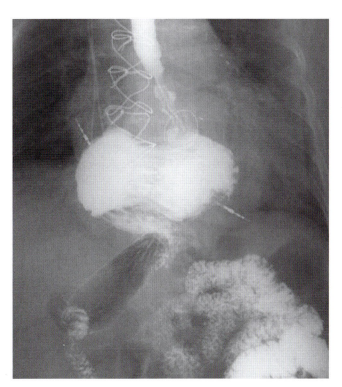

2. Upper GI series in a patient with a large type I hiatal hernia reveals the majority of the stomach within the thorax.

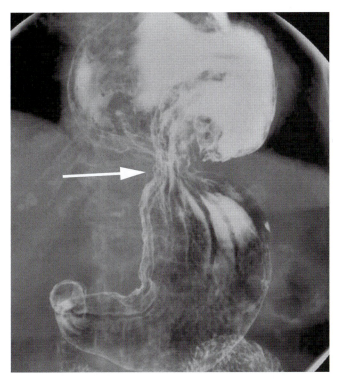

3. Upper GI series demonstrates a large hiatal hernia with the majority of the stomach in the thorax that save for the gastric antrum and pylorus which course through the esophageal hiatus (arrow) and extend into the abdomen.

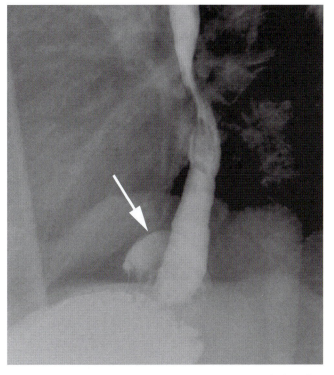

4. Upper GI series demonstrates a paraesophageal herniation of a small portion of the gastric fundus (arrow), a type II hiatal hernia.

PRESENTATION

Patients typically present with nausea, vomiting, and abdominal pain and may report anorexia and weight loss.

FINDINGS

Imaging studies demonstrate the presence of a significantly dilated stomach with retained fluid or food content; differentiation between benign malignant causes of gastric outlet obstruction is based on evidence of a mass lesion or by demonstration of inflammatory disease in local vicinity.

DIFFERENTIAL DIAGNOSIS

- Small bowel obstruction
- Gastric carcinoma
- Pancreatic carcinoma
- Duodenal carcinoma
- Pancreatitis

COMMENTS

Gastric outlet obstruction is a common clinical manifestation in patients with benign and malignant diseases of the distal stomach, duodenum, and pancreatic area. The most common causes of malignant gastroduodenal obstruction are gastric and pancreatic carcinoma. Other causes include lymphoma, ampullary carcinoma, biliary tract cancer, metastases to the duodenum or proximal jejunum, peptic ulcer disease, and extrinsic compression. Less frequently, the condition is caused by mural infiltration or spasm resulting from inflammatory disorders such as severe pancreatitis or cholecystitis. Antral narrowing may also be caused by fibrous scarring after ingestion of corrosive agent.

The typical presentation of patients with gastric outlet obstruction includes nausea, vomiting, malnutrition, and dehydration. Although affected patients are usually able to eat, they soon develop recurrent episodes of debilitating emesis, eventually developing what has been termed "food fear." Gastroduodenal obstruction severely limits the quality of life.

All imaging studies demonstrate the presence of a significantly dilated stomach with retained fluid/food residue. Differentiation between obstructive and nonobstructive causes of gastric dilatation and delayed emptying (gastroparesis) can be difficult on the basis of imaging studies alone and relies mostly on identifying an intrinsic or extrinsic cause of obstruction. Differentiation between a benign and a malignant cause of gastric outlet obstruction is based on evidence of a mass in the region of the gastric outlet or by demonstration of inflammatory disease in the vicinity of those structures.

Surgical gastrojejunostomy is the traditional palliative treatment for gastric outlet obstruction but is associated with a high complication rate, and delayed gastric emptying is a frequent problem. Gastroduodenal stent placement is a very safe and effective palliation method in patients with unresectable malignant tumors causing gastric outlet obstruction, with adequate palliation of symptoms achieved in most cases.

PEARLS

- Gastric outlet obstruction is a common clinical manifestation in patients with benign and malignant diseases affecting the upper gastrointestinal tract.

- The main radiological manifestation is a markedly dilated stomach which could be accompanied by a mass lesion in patients with malignant obstruction.

- Gastroduodenal stent placement is a very safe and effective palliation method in patients with unresectable malignant tumors causing gastric outlet obstruction.

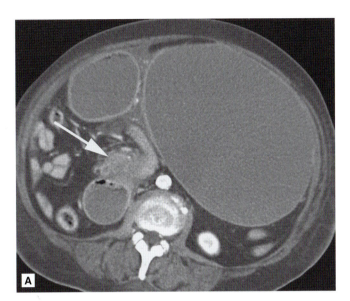

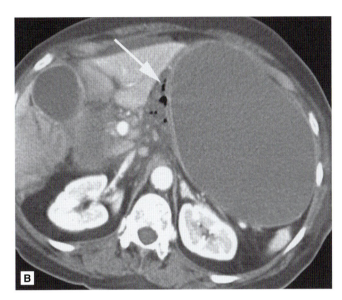

1. **A.** Axial, contrast-enhanced CT image demonstrates marked distention of the stomach related to an obstructing pancreatic carcinoma (arrow). **B.** Axial, contrast-enhanced CT image demonstrates marked distention of the stomach with adjacent extraluminal gas and fluid (arrow) consistent with perforation related to the obstruction by the pancreatic carcinoma.

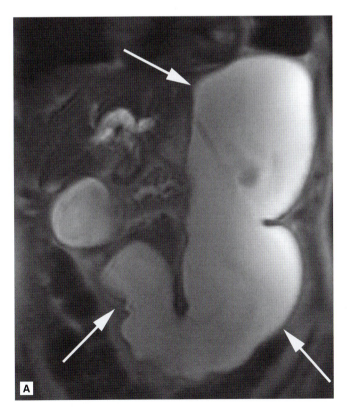

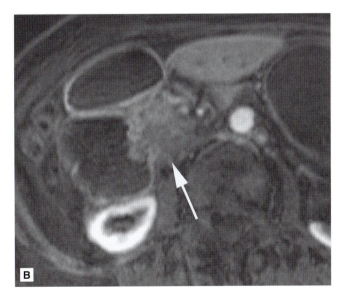

2. **A.** Coronal, T2-weighed MRI image demonstrates marked distention of a fluid-filled stomach (arrows). Also note the telltale findings of biliary and pancreatic ductal dilatation. **B.** Axial, contrast-enhanced MRI image demonstrates marked distention of the stomach and proximal duodenum related to an obstructing pancreatic carcinoma (arrow).

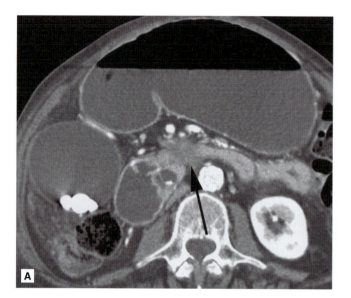

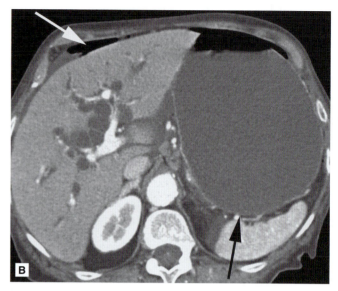

3. A. Axial, contrast-enhanced CT image demonstrates marked distention of the stomach and proximal duodenum related to a large, obstructing pancreatic carcinoma (arrow). **B.** Axial, contrast-enhanced CT image demonstrates marked distention of the stomach (black arrow) with gross free intraperitoneal air (white arrow) related to perforation of the stomach. Also note marked intrahepatic biliary dilatation related to the obstructing pancreatic neoplasm.

CHAPTER 7

SMALL BOWEL

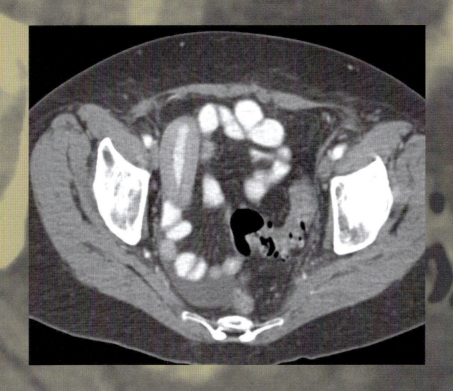

SMALL BOWEL NEOPLASMS

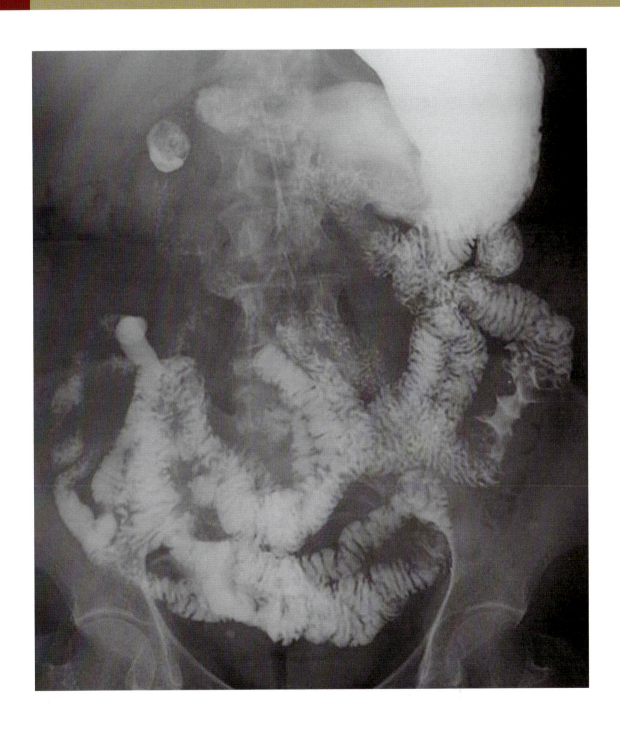

PRESENTATION

While the findings of hereditary polyposis may be identified due to screening, patients may present with abdominal pain or other manifestations of their particular syndrome such as cutaneous findings.

FINDINGS

A double-contrast barium study demonstrates multiple radiolucent filling defects of various sizes throughout the small intestine.

DIFFERENTIAL DIAGNOSIS

- Familial adenomatous polyposis
- Brunner gland hyperplasia (hamartoma)
- Lymphoid follicle hyperplasia
- Metastases and lymphoma (gastrointestinal tract)

COMMENTS

Small intestine polyps occur as a part of hereditary and nonhereditary polyposis syndromes. Several hereditary polyposis syndromes have been described that are characterized by multiple hamartomatous polyps of the gastrointestinal tract. These include Peutz-Jeghers syndrome (PJS), juvenile polyposis syndrome, phosphatase and tensin homolog (PTEN), hamartoma tumor syndromes (Cowden syndrome and Bannayan-Riley-Ruvalcaba syndrome), and other rare syndromes like hereditary mixed polyposis syndrome, intestinal ganglioneuromatosis and neurofibromatosis, Devon family syndrome, basal cell nevus syndrome. Nonhereditary polyposis syndromes include Cronkhite-Canada syndrome, hyperplastic polyposis syndrome, and nodular lymphoid hyperplasia. Many of these syndromes are associated with an increased risk of colorectal cancer. Although the pathophysiology of the transformation of a polyp into carcinoma is not well understood, it is postulated that changes that affect the lamina propria are responsible for this change and is known as "landscaper phenomenon." Patients with PJS have hamartomatous polyps throughout the gastrointestinal tract and present with abdominal pain, stool that is positive for occult blood, obstruction, or intussusception. On clinical examination, these patients demonstrate mucocutaneous melanin deposits. PJS is associated with an increased

risk for developing gastrointestinal cancers (colon, small intestine, stomach, pancreas), breast cancer, and sex cord tumors. Cowden syndrome is characterized by juvenile polyps in the gastrointestinal tract, skin lesions (trichilemmomas), macrocephaly, and increased risk for breast and thyroid cancers. A juvenile polyp is a hamartomatous non-neoplastic polyp characterized by dilated, cystic spaces lined by columnar epithelium with an inflammatory lamina propria. The syndrome may present in a severe form in infancy, may be limited to the colon, or may involve the stomach and intestines. Patients develop multiple polyps, which may obstruct or bleed, but the chief concern is the associated colorectal cancer risk. Cronkhite-Canada syndrome is characterized by the presence of diffuse gastrointestinal polyposis, dystrophic changes in the fingernails, alopecia, cutaneous hyperpigmentation, diarrhea, weight loss, abdominal pain, and complications of malnutrition. Gastrointestinal polyps are found from the stomach to the rectum.

The diagnosis is made using either small bowel follow-through examinations or endoscopy. On barium studies, radiolucent filling defects are noted in the intestine. Morphologically, these polyps can be sessile or pedunculated. The size of the polyps varies from small to medium to large. Large polyps usually have lobulated surfaces. PJS affects the stomach to the rectum, with a jejunal and ileal predominance. Polyps are typically broad based and appear in clusters or carpeting the bowel mucosa.

PEARLS

- Small intestinal polyposis is a spectrum of familial and nonfamilial syndromes that are characterized by the presence of intestinal polyps. The most common syndromes include PJS and juvenile polyposis.

- Polyps typically affect jejunal and ileal loops with higher frequency than the remainder of the gut. Many of these syndromes are associated with an increased risk of colorectal and other gastrointestinal tract cancers.

- The diagnosis is usually made on capsule endoscopy or small bowel follow-through. Barium studies typically demonstrate multiple radiolucent filling defects either in clusters or carpeting the involved gut.

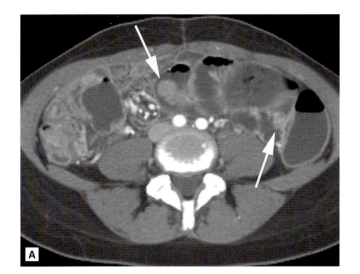

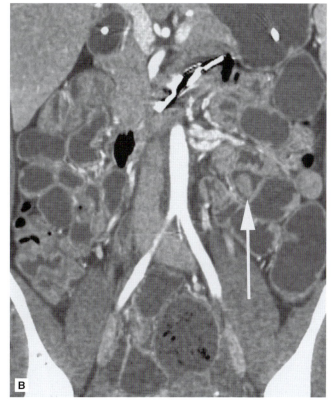

1. A. Axial, contrast-enhanced computed tomography (CT) reveals multiple enhancing polyps in the small bowel (arrows) in a patient with PJS. **B.** Coronal, contrast-enhanced CT reveals an enhancing polyp in the small bowel (arrow) in a patient with PJS.

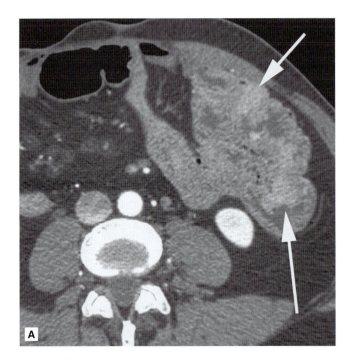

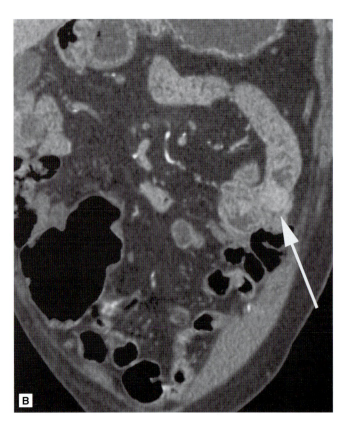

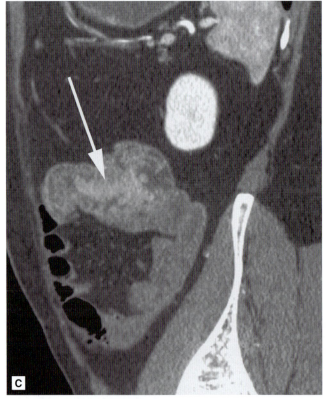

2. A. Axial, contrast-enhanced CT reveals multiple enhancing polyps in the small bowel (arrows) in a patient with PJS. **B.** Sagittal, contrast-enhanced CT reveals multiple enhancing polyps in the small bowel (arrow) in a patient with PJS. **C.** Sagittal, contrast-enhanced CT reveals multiple enhancing polyps in the small bowel (arrow) in a patient with PJS.

PRESENTATION

Most common symptoms are abdominal pain, weight loss, anemia, nausea, and vomiting.

FINDINGS

Small bowel enteroclysis shows an infiltrating annular or polypoid lesion. CT demonstrates annular, discrete nodular or ulcerative lesions within the small intestinal wall.

DIFFERENTIAL DIAGNOSIS

- Lymphoma
- Leiomyosarcoma
- Metastases
- Carcinoid tumor
- Crohn disease

COMMENTS

Adenocarcinomas constitute nearly half of the malignant tumors of the small intestine. Peak incidence occurs in the seventh decade of life, with a slight male predominance. Most of these tumors are located in the duodenum and proximal jejunum. Adenocarcinoma developing in association with Crohn disease tends to occur at a somewhat younger age, and the majority of these tumors arise in the ileum. Risk factors for adenocarcinoma of the small bowel include adenomatous polyps, polyposis syndromes, celiac disease, Crohn disease, and a family history of hereditary nonpolyposis colorectal cancer (HNPCC). The clinical presentation of these tumors depends on their location.

Adenocarcinoma arises from the glandular epithelium. These tumors tend to grow into the lumen, but they can also grow through the submucosa and muscularis layers, often becoming large before the diagnosis is made. Most neoplasms of the small intestine are not associated with symptoms and are diagnosed either late in their course or incidentally at imaging performed for other indications. Periampullary tumors present with obstructive jaundice, bleeding, or duodenal obstruction. Adenocarcinomas in the jejunum and ileum most commonly present with abdominal pain and weight loss due to obstruction. If a lesion becomes large enough, patients can present with cramping periumbilical pain, bloating, nausea, and vomiting resulting from mechanical small bowel obstruction. Gastrointestinal bleeding, usually chronic, is another common symptom of carcinoma of the small intestine.

On imaging, small bowel adenocarcinoma may demonstrate various morphologic features, ranging from infiltrative to polypoidal to ulcerative. Plain abdominal radiographs are rarely useful for localization of small intestinal tumors, but they may be helpful clinically in the setting of a suspected intestinal obstruction or perforation. In patients who present with jaundice, ultrasound (US), abdominal CT, or magnetic resonance cholangiopancreatography (MRCP) may demonstrate the duodenal mass and site of biliary obstruction. On small intestinal follow-through, adenocarcinomas of small intestine can have a varied appearance: annular constricting lesion, a filling defect, a polypoid and/or ulcerated mass, or a combination of the above. Infiltrative growth presents as circumferential narrowing with mucosal destruction and shouldering of the margins or as an apple core lesion. Small bowel enteroclysis has more sensitivity and specificity than small intestinal follow-through in detecting small bowel lesions. Contrast-enhanced CT demonstrates mural thickening, compromising the lumen either concentrically or asymmetrically. Polypoidal lesions may show uniform or heterogeneous enhancement. Advanced disease demonstrates mesenteric infiltration, lymphadenopathy, vascular invasion, and distant metastases to the liver, peritoneum, or ovaries. CT enteroclysis distends the small intestinal loops homogeneously, which helps to demonstrate the wall thickening and subtle mural and extramural abnormalities.

PEARLS

- Adenocarcinoma is the most common malignant neoplasm of the small intestine and is usually a solitary lesion mostly located in the proximal small intestine, usually the duodenum.

- CT demonstrates an annular or plaque-like polypoid lesion with compromised luminal diameter, either concentrically or asymmetrically.

- Localized tumors are treated with curative surgical resection. Mesenteric infiltration with lymph node metastases, distant metastases, carcinomatosis, and vascular invasion are poor prognostic indicators.

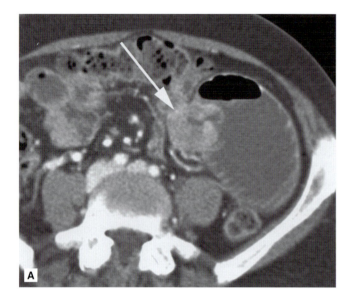

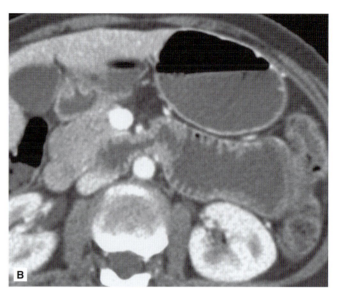

1. A. Axial, contrast-enhanced CT reveals an irregularly enhancing, obstructing adenocarcinoma in the ileum (arrow). **B.** Axial, contrast-enhanced CT reveals distention of the duodenum and stomach related to the obstruction due to the small bowel adenocarcinoma of the ileum more distally.

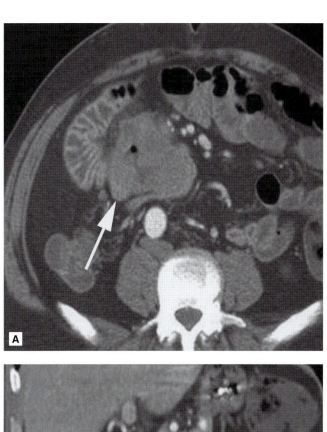

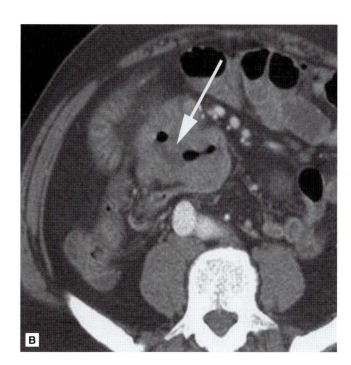

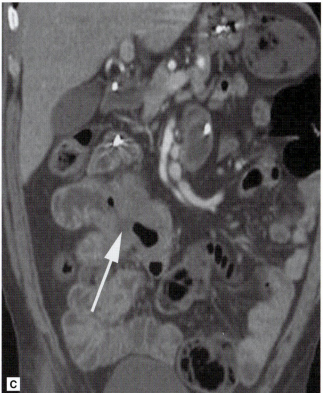

2. A and **B.** Axial, contrast-enhanced CT reveals a large, irregular mass lesion in the distal ileum (arrow) in this case of small bowel adeno-carcinoma. **C.** Coronal, contrast-enhanced CT reveals a large, irregular mass lesion in the distal ileum (arrow) in this case of small bowel adenocarcinoma.

PRESENTATION

Small bowel carcinoid usually presents with pain and/or obstruction. Carcinoid syndrome patients present with episodes of flushing, secretory diarrhea, abdominal pain, telangiectasia, wheezing, and valvular heart disease.

FINDINGS

On CT, an enhancing lesion in the distal ileum with mesenteric infiltration and distant metastases, often to the liver, may be identified in cases of gastrointestinal (GI) carcinoid.

DIFFERENTIAL DIAGNOSIS

- Small bowel carcinoma
- Small bowel metastases and lymphoma
- Fibrosing mesenteritis
- Desmoid tumor
- Intramural hematoma

COMMENTS

Carcinoids are indolent malignant neuroendocrine tumors that arise from the enterochromaffin cells at the base of the crypts of Lieberkuhn. Although the majority of carcinoids originate in the gastrointestinal tract, a small percentage of primary carcinoid tumors occur in the bronchus or lung. Other sites, such as the ovaries, testicles, pancreas, and kidneys are far less common. Within the gastrointestinal tract, carcinoids are most often identified in the appendix, followed by the small bowel. In the small intestine, carcinoids almost always occur within the last 2 ft of the ileum. In one-third of cases, carcinoids of the small bowel are multicentric and associated with other primary malignancies, most frequently of the breast and colon. Carcinoid tumors have a variable malignant potential and are composed of multipotential cells with the ability to secrete numerous humoral agents, the most prominent of which are serotonin and substance P. A few patients with malignant carcinoids develop carcinoid syndrome, which is characterized by episodic attacks of cutaneous flushing, bronchospasm, diarrhea, and vasomotor collapse.

The most common presenting symptom for patients with small bowel carcinoid is abdominal pain. As carcinoids grow, tumors may serve as a lead point for intussusceptions, which give rise to intermittent symptoms and signs of obstruction.

Diagnosis is made based on the imaging finding, elevated 5-hydroxyindoleacetic acid (5-HIAA) and direct visualization.

Small carcinoids are rarely detected on routine small bowel examination. Most carcinoids tend to grow extraluminally, infiltrating the bowel wall, lymphatic channels, and eventually grow into the regional lymph nodes and mesentery. Local release of serotonin leads to hypertrophic muscular thickening and an intense desmoplastic response. As a result, the mesentery of the small bowel becomes fibrotic and foreshortened, leading to kinking of the bowel and intussusception and bowel obstruction or even intestinal ischemia as a result of sclerosis of the mesenteric blood vessels. These findings are readily identified on contrast-enhanced CT, especially when a neutral oral contrast agent is administered. Barium radiographic studies of the small bowel may exhibit submucosal lesions and multiple filling defects as a result of kinking and fibrosis of the bowel. CT demonstrates single or multiple submucosal enhancing lesions with bowel wall thickening and mesenteric desmoplastic changes. As the tumor progresses, mesenteric extension appears as ill-defined, heterogeneous spiculated masses with a stellate pattern and areas of calcification. CT also helps demonstrate multifocal disease and metastases. The liver is the most common site of metastatic disease. These lesions are best seen in the arterial phase given their commonly identified early arterial enhancement. Angiography of infiltrative carcinoid demonstrates a stellate arterial configuration at the tumor periphery, poor-to-moderate accumulation of contrast within the tumor, nonfilling of major draining veins, and irregular narrowing of mesenteric artery branches. However, angiography is not a routine choice of investigation when carcinoid demonstrates typical features on cross-sectional imaging. Indium-111 (^{111}In) octreotide or somatostatin receptor scintigraphy is helpful to localize the tumor and to evaluate the extent of metastatic disease, with high sensitivity and specificity.

PEARLS

- Carcinoid tumor is a primary malignant neoplasm of small bowel that arises from enterochromaffin cells of Kulchitsky and secrets serotonin and substance P.

- Contrast-enhanced CT with negative intraluminal contrast demonstrates solitary well or ill-defined enhancing lesion in the distal ileum with mesenteric infiltration and distant metastases, often to the liver.

- Elevated 5-HIAA levels and In-111 octreotide or somatostatin receptor scintigraphy have greater sensitivity and specificity for the diagnosis of carcinoid tumor.

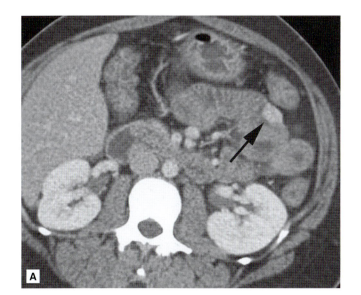

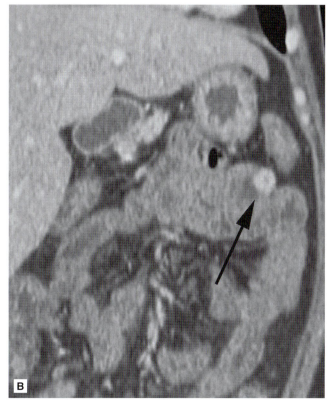

1. A. Axial, arterial phase, contrast-enhanced CT image reveals a focal, arterially enhancing carcinoid in the jejunum (arrow). **B.** Coronal, arterial phase, contrast-enhanced CT image reveals a focal, arterially enhancing carcinoid in the jejunum (arrow).

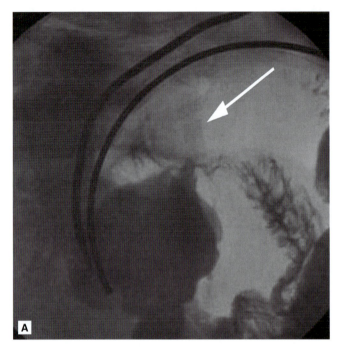
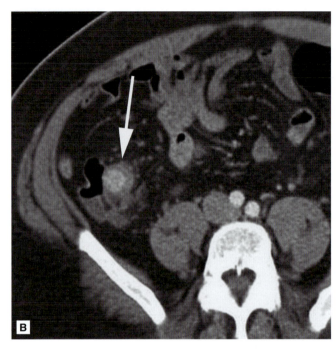

2. A. Spot compression view during barium study reveals a nonspecific filling defect in the cecum (arrow). **B.** Axial, arterial phase, contrast-enhanced CT image reveals a focal, arterially enhancing carcinoid in the cecum corresponding to the filling defect seen during the barium study (arrow).

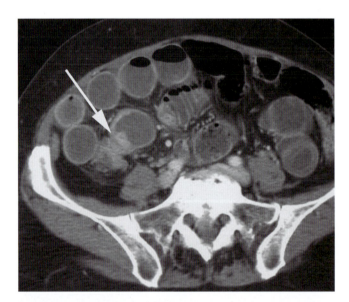

3. Axial, contrast-enhanced CT image reveals an irregular enhancing mass in the terminal ileum (arrow), in this case representing a carcinoid tumor, with proximal small bowel obstruction as evidenced by distention of proximal loops of small bowel, well seen on this image.

PRESENTATION

Abdominal pain and tenderness, fatigue, malaise, diarrhea, and obstruction

FINDINGS

CT demonstrates circumferential thickening of the small bowel wall or a polypoid mass with mild enhancement. The mesenteric form shows multiple soft tissue mass lesions in the mesentery with conglomerate mesenteric and retroperitoneal lymphadenopathy.

DIFFERENTIAL DIAGNOSIS

- Small bowel carcinoma
- Metastasis
- Hemorrhage
- Vasculitis of the small intestine
- Crohn disease
- Whipple disease
- Opportunistic infection

COMMENTS

Lymphoma represents about one-fifth of primary small intestinal malignancies. The stomach is the most common site of gastrointestinal lymphoma, followed by the small bowel and then the colon. Small bowel lymphoma occurs most commonly in the fifth to sixth decade of life, with a slight male predominance, and can be multifocal in some patients. These tumors arise from lymphoid tissue in the intestinal wall. The distal or terminal ileum is the most commonly involved site because of the greatest concentration of gut-associated lymphoid tissue in that particular segment of the small bowel, the exception being in the setting of celiac disease, when proximal lymphomas are more common. Most primary lesions are non-Hodgkin B-cell lymphomas with intermediate or high-grade features. There is an increased incidence of small intestinal lymphoma in patients with malabsorptive or inflammatory conditions such as celiac sprue or Crohn disease and patients who are immunosuppressed either because of therapeutic suppression (post-transplant lymphoproliferative disease) or diseases of immunologic function (AIDS, systemic lupus erythematosus, agammaglobulinemia).

Patients with small bowel lymphoma typically present with abdominal pain, fatigue, malaise, and weight loss. In primary intestinal lymphoma, fever, night sweats, and superficial lymphadenopathy are characteristically absent. An abdominal mass is present in about one-third of patients. Approximately 25% of the patients present with a complication of their lymphoma such as intussusception, obstruction, perforation, or hemorrhage. Mediterranean lymphoma is a variant more commonly seen in underdeveloped countries which affects young adults and presents with diarrhea, steatorrhea, and colicky pain. The entire small bowel is diffusely involved and the prognosis is poor due to progressive malnutrition and transformation to a disseminated aggressive lymphoma.

The diagnosis of small bowel lymphoma is usually made by small bowel follow-through studies or CT scanning. On imaging, primary intestinal lymphoma appears as either a polypoid or an exophytic ulcerated lesion or diffusely infiltrative mass. Small bowel contrast studies characteristically demonstrate luminal narrowing with mucosal destruction, occasional shouldering of the margins and stricture formation, broad-based ulceration, cavitation, thickening of the valvulae conniventes, discrete intraluminal filling defects, and an extraluminal mass. The polypoid or nodular forms demonstrate multiple mucosal or submucosal nodules or masses throughout the involved segments. Occasionally, extensive lymphomatous invasion of the muscle layers and neural plexi causes focal aneurysmal dilatation of bowel. Consequently, the CT or MR appearances of intestinal lymphoma are variable and may be classified as infiltrative, polypoid, nodular, aneurysmal, ulcerative, constrictive, and mesenteric forms. Contrast-enhanced CT images of circumferential infiltrative lymphoma demonstrate a sausage-shaped soft tissue mass with mild enhancement. Advanced cases demonstrate luminal narrowing, stricture formation, and aneurysmal dilatation. Mesenteric involvement may be in the form of a large lobulated soft tissue mass lesion displacing the bowel loops or conglomerate mesenteric and retroperitoneal lymphadenopathy with mesenteric fat stranding. The "sandwich-like" complex is observed when enlarged, confluent mesenteric lymph nodes encase and surround the enlarged mesenteric vessels.

PEARLS

- Small intestinal lymphoma is the second most common site of involvement of gastrointestinal lymphoma, the distal ileum being the most common site.

- Intestinal lymphoma shows variable morphology and is described as infiltrative, polypoid, nodular, aneurysmal, ulcerative, constrictive, and mesenteric lymphoma.

- Imaging demonstrates either circumferential thickening of the intestinal wall in the form of sausage or multiple mucosal or submucosal nodules. A conglomerate of enlarged mesenteric and retroperitoneal lymph nodes is commonly seen in mesenteric lymphoma.

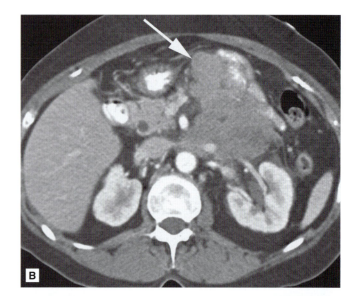

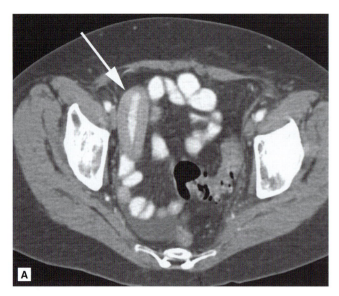

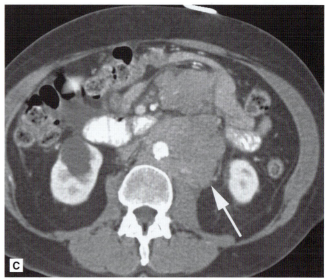

1. A. Axial, contrast-enhanced CT reveals smooth thickening of the distal ileum (arrow) in a case of small bowel lymphoma. **B.** Axial, contrast-enhanced CT reveals a nodal mass in the retroperitoneum and small bowel mesentery (arrow). **C.** Axial, contrast-enhanced CT reveals nodal masses in the retroperitoneum and small bowel mesentery (arrow) in this case of lymphoma.

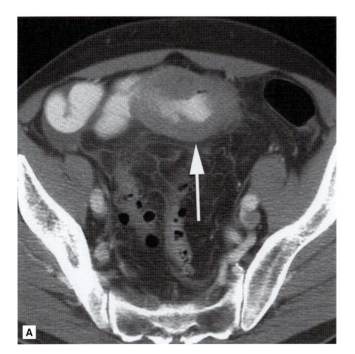

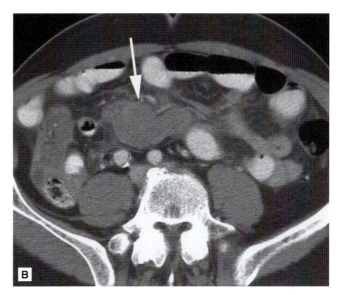

2. A. Axial, contrast-enhanced CT reveals smooth thickening and aneurysmal dilatation of the distal ileum (arrow) in a case of small bowel lymphoma. **B.** Axial, contrast-enhanced CT reveals a nodal mass in the small bowel mesentery (arrow) in this case of lymphoma.

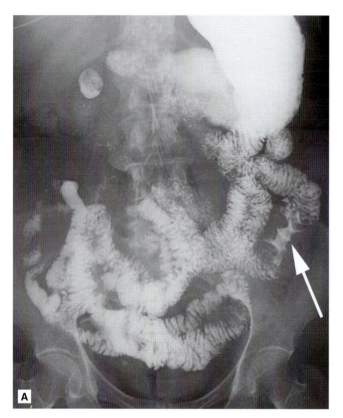

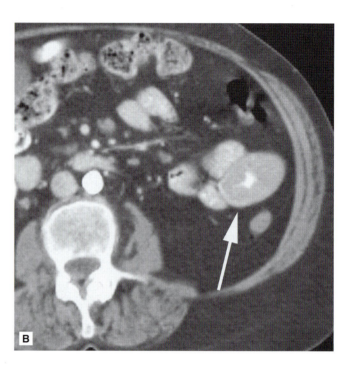

3. A. Small bowel follow-through reveals a short segment of narrowing of the jejunum (arrow) in this case of small bowl lymphoma. **B.** Axial, contrast-enhanced CT reveals smooth thickening of the jejunum (arrow) corresponding to the abnormality found on small bowel follow-through in a case of small bowel lymphoma.

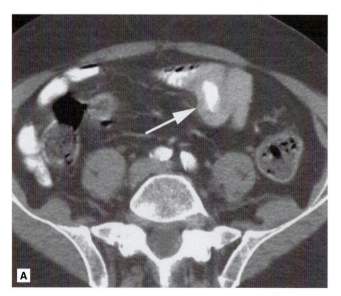

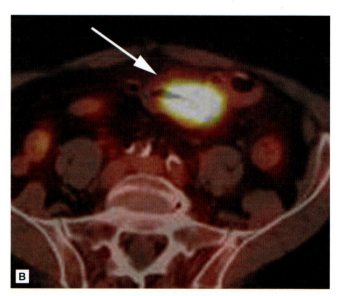

4. A. Axial, contrast-enhanced CT reveals smooth thickening of the ileum (arrow) in a case of small bowel lymphoma. **B.** Positron emission tomography (PET)/CT image reveals marked fluorodeoxyglucose (FDG) avidity of the lesion in the ileum (arrow) in this case of small bowel lymphoma.

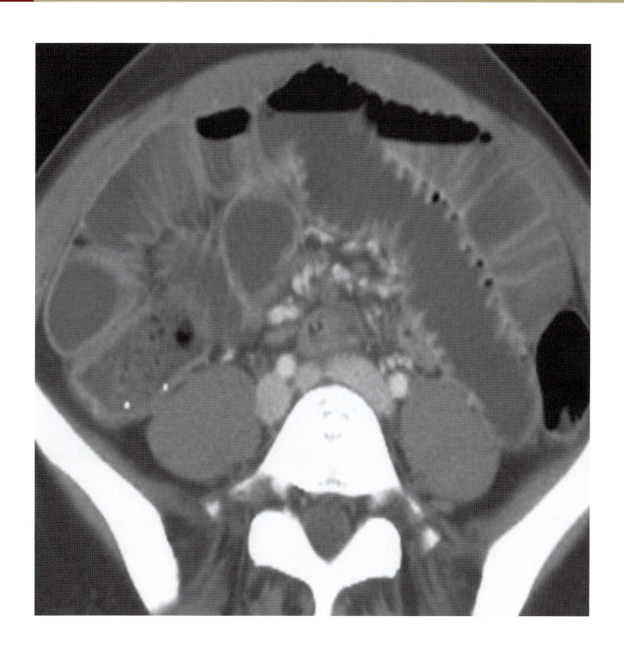

PRESENTATION

Varies between vague intermittent abdominal pain and acute abdomen with nausea, vomiting, leukocytosis, and fever

FINDINGS

CT of jejunoileal diverticulitis typically demonstrates multiple diverticula with surrounding inflammatory changes and often an adjacent mass containing gas and/or feces-like material. Wall thickening of the involved segment of bowel and edema in the surrounding tissues, including fat and fascial layers, are also common.

DIFFERENTIAL DIAGNOSIS

• Inflammatory bowel disease

• Enteritis

• Appendicitis

• Small bowel malignancy

COMMENTS

Small bowel diverticulitis is defined as inflammation or infection (or both), associated with jejunal or ileal diverticula. Diverticular disease of the small intestine is relatively common. Small bowel diverticula may occur in any portion of the small intestine and they may present as either true or false diverticula. A true diverticulum contains all layers of the intestinal wall and is usually congenital. False diverticula are the more common of the two and result from the herniation of the mucosa and submucosa through the muscular layer of the bowel wall, where blood vessels penetrate it at the mesenteric site and are usually acquired defects. False diverticula are thought to be secondary to abnormalities of the myenteric plexus with consequent motor dysfunctions. These motility disorders vary in severity and magnitude from localized dysmotility to universal jejunoileal dyskinesia resulting in increased intraluminal pressure and, ultimately, herniation of the mucosa and submucosa through the muscular wall of the small bowel. Duodenal diverticula are the most common acquired diverticula of the small bowel, and Meckel diverticulum is the most common true congenital diverticulum of the small bowel. The acquired form of small bowel diverticulosis is a disease of advanced age, with a peak during the sixth and seventh decades of life. Its distribution along the small bowel decreases from proximal to distal. Thus, jejunal

diverticula are more common and are larger than those occurring in the ileum.

Most jejunoileal diverticula are asymptomatic but can cause clinical symptoms due to complications such as acute diverticulitis, hemorrhage, intestinal obstruction, contained perforation with interloop abscess, pneumoperitoneum, and megaloblastic anemia due to vitamin B_{12} malabsorption secondary to chronic stasis and bacterial overgrowth within the diverticula. Unlike colonic diverticula, jejunoileal diverticula are an uncommon site of inflammation, possibly due to their larger size and better intraluminal flow of the relatively sterile, liquid content of the distal small intestine.

Jejunoileal diverticula are usually identified with small bowel follow-through, enteroclysis or CT as saccular outpouchings filled with air or oral contrast material–located structure adjacent to the mesenteric side of the proximal small bowel. Diverticulitis shows elongated, deformed, irregular diverticula with narrowed adjacent loops of small bowel due to localized inflammation, edema, and spasm on barium studies. In acute diverticulitis, CT demonstrates peridiverticular inflammation, edema, hemorrhage, or abscess with mesenteric fat. In advanced cases, CT demonstrates an inflammatory mass with displacement of bowel loops, thickened bowel wall, obstruction, abscesses, perforation with peritonitis, fistula and sinus tracts. Diverticulitis of the terminal ileum is a rare entity and is commonly seen near the ileocecal valve, which often mimics appendicitis.

PEARLS

• Jejunoileal diverticulosis is thought to be a motor dysfunction of the smooth muscle or the myenteric plexus, resulting in herniation of the mucosa and submucosa through the weakest portion of the bowel wall.

• Small bowel follow-through, CT or enteroclysis demonstrate irregular diverticula with partial adjacent bowel obstruction, an omental mass displacing the small bowel loops or leakage of barium into adjacent mesenteric abscess.

• CT of jejunoileal diverticulitis demonstrates irregular diverticula with a surrounding inflammatory mass that contains gas and/or feces-like material, wall thickening of the involved segment of bowel, and edema or inflammation of the surrounding tissues including fat and fascial layers.

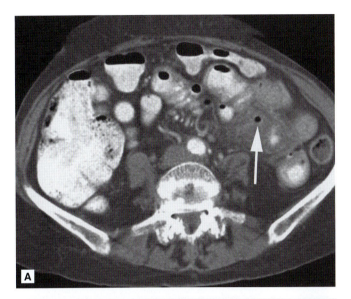

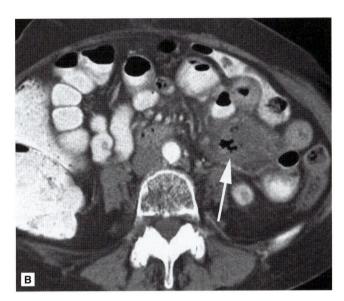

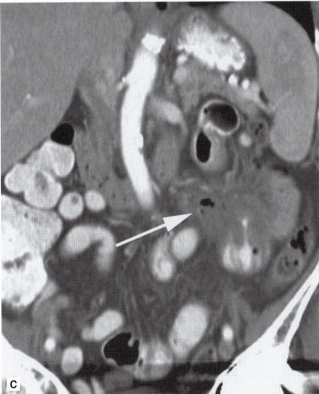

1. A. Axial, contrast-enhanced CT reveals a diverticulum of the ileum (arrow) with significant surrounding inflammation in a case of small bowel diverticulitis. **B.** Axial, contrast-enhanced CT reveals a diverticulum of the ileum (arrow) with surrounding inflammatory stranding in a case of small bowel diverticulitis. **C.** Coronal, contrast-enhanced CT reveals a diverticulum of the ileum (arrow) with significant surrounding inflammation and thickening of adjacent small bowel loops in a case of small bowel diverticulitis.

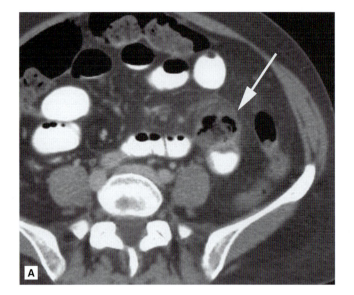

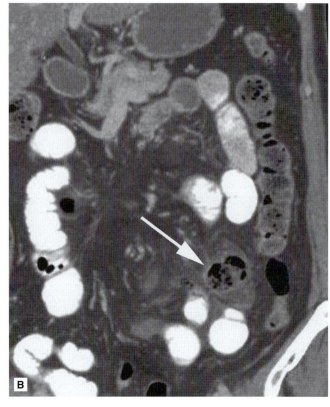

2. A. Axial, contrast-enhanced CT reveals a diverticulum of the ileum (arrow) with surrounding inflammation in a case of small bowel diverticulitis. **B.** Coronal, contrast-enhanced CT reveals a diverticulum of the ileum (arrow) with surrounding inflammation in a case of small bowel diverticulitis.

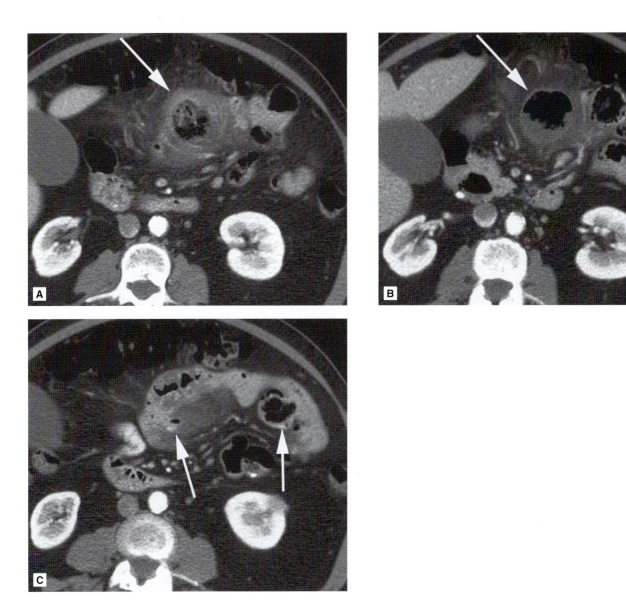

3. A. Axial, contrast-enhanced CT reveals a large diverticulum of the ileum (arrow) with surrounding inflammation in a case of small bowel diverticulitis. **B.** Axial, contrast-enhanced CT reveals an additional large diverticulum of the ileum (arrow) with surrounding inflammation in a case of small bowel diverticulitis. **C.** Axial, contrast-enhanced CT reveals a multiple diverticula of the ileum (arrows) with surrounding inflammation in a case of small bowel diverticulitis.

PRESENTATION

The most common clinical presentation is acute abdominal pain, which mimics appendicitis.

FINDINGS

The diagnosis of Meckel diverticulitis is made on contrast-enhanced CT as a thick-walled, fluid-filled tubular mass adjacent to a distal ileal loop or arising from the antimesenteric border of a loop of distal ileum, with surrounding inflammatory changes in the mesentery.

DIFFERENTIAL DIAGNOSIS

- Appendicitis
- Crohn disease
- Mesenteric adenitis
- Cecal diverticulitis

COMMENTS

Meckel diverticulitis is acute inflammation of a Meckel diverticulum, which is the most commonly encountered congenital anomaly of the small intestine, occurring in about 2% of the population. A Meckel diverticulum is located on the antimesenteric border, within 45 to 60 cm of the ileocecal valve, and is due to persistence of the omphalomesenteric or vitelline duct. An equal incidence is found among men and women. Meckel diverticulum may persist in different forms, ranging from a small bump that may be easily missed to a long projection that communicates with the umbilicus by a persistent fibrous cord or, much less commonly, a patent fistula. The usual manifestation is a relatively wide-mouth diverticulum measuring about 5 cm in length, with a diameter of up to 2 cm. Cells lining the vitelline duct are pluripotent; therefore, it is not uncommon to find heterotopic tissue within a Meckel diverticulum, the most common of which is gastric mucosa; less commonly, these diverticula may harbour pancreatic or colonic mucosa.

Most Meckel diverticula are entirely benign and are incidentally discovered during autopsy, laparotomy, or barium studies. The most common clinical presentation of a Meckel diverticulum is gastrointestinal bleeding, which occurs in up to 50% of patients who present with complications; hemorrhage is the most common symptomatic presentation in children aged 2 years or younger. Another common presenting symptom of Meckel diverticulum is intestinal obstruction; it may be caused by strangulation of bowel, intussusception, volvulus, incarceration of the diverticulum in a Littre hernia, or tumors originating in the diverticulum.

Meckel diverticulitis is the most common complication in adults (~ 25% of patients). Affected patients present with acute abdominal pain, which may mimic the symptoms of acute appendicitis. The inflammation usually results from the effect of peptic acids produced by ectopic gastric mucosa on the surrounding ileal mucosa or from obstruction of lumen by enteroliths or a phytobezoar. On imaging, a Meckel diverticulum appears as a blind-ending outpouching arising from the antimesenteric side of the terminal ileum. Inflammation makes it readily visible as a thick-walled, fluid-filled tubular mass or soft tissue mass with an air-fluid level in the mid-abdomen, adherent to the wall of the distal ileum, and with surrounding inflammatory changes in the mesentery.

PEARLS

- Meckel diverticulitis is the most common complication of a Meckel diverticulum; patients typically present with acute abdominal pain.

- Meckel diverticulum is a true diverticulum of congenital origin and develops from a persistent omphalomesenteric or vitelline duct.

- An inflamed Meckel diverticulum can be easily identified on CT as a thick-walled, fluid-filled tubular mass or a soft tissue mass with an air-fluid level in the mid-abdomen, adherent to the wall of the distal ileum and with surrounding inflammatory changes.

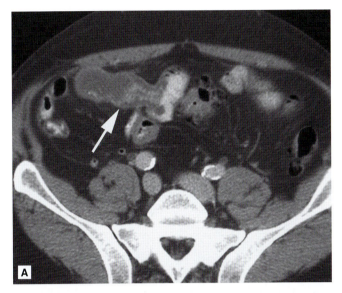

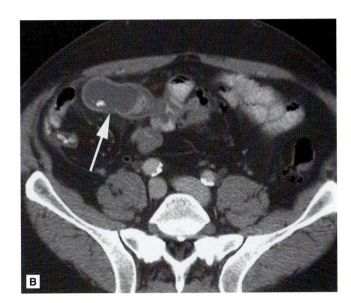

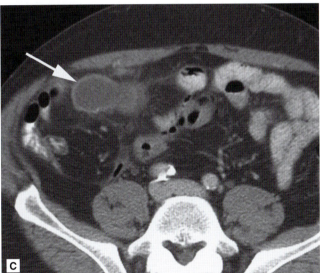

1. A. Axial, contrast-enhanced CT reveals a fluid-filled tubular mass (arrow) emanating from the distal ileum in a case of Meckel diverticulitis. **B.** Axial, contrast-enhanced CT reveals a fluid-filled, thick-walled tubular mass (arrow) emanating from the distal ileum in a case of Meckel diverticulitis. An enterolith is identified within the lumen of the diverticulum. **C.** Axial, contrast-enhanced CT reveals a fluid-filled tubular mass (arrow) with surrounding inflammation in a case of Meckel diverticulitis.

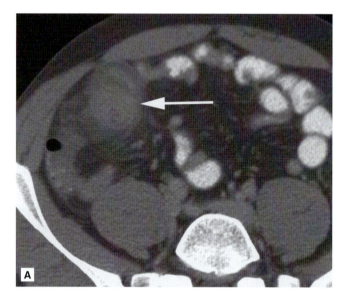

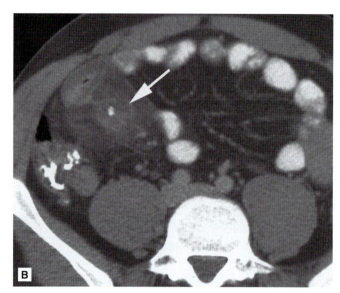

2. A. Axial, contrast-enhanced CT reveals a rounded mass in the right lower quadrant with surrounding inflammation (arrow) in this case of Meckel diverticulitis. **B.** Axial, contrast-enhanced CT reveals a rounded mass in the right lower quadrant containing an enterolith with surrounding inflammation (arrow), including the adjacent ileum, in this case of Meckel diverticulitis.

PRESENTATION

Abdominal pain, diarrhea, fever, nausea, and vomiting

FINDINGS

Barium studies demonstrate mucosal ulcerations, nodules, and luminal narrowing from thickened bowel wall. CT demonstrates thickened bowel wall and lymphadenopathy.

DIFFERENTIAL DIAGNOSIS

- Crohn disease
- Small bowel lymphoma

COMMENTS

Small bowel infection and enteritis can be caused by viral pathogens, bacteria, protozoa, or fungus. Infectious enteritis is one of the most frequent causes of morbidity worldwide. Major causes are salmonellosis, shigellosis, and infections due to *Yersinia enterocolitica, Staphylococcus, Escherichia coli, Yersinia paratuberculosis, Clostridium difficile,* and *Campylobacter jejuni.*

Salmonella and *Shigella* infections result in an acute terminal ileitis. *Giardia lamblia* and *Strongyloides stercoralis* infect the proximal bowel, while *Y enterocolitica* and *Mycobacterium tuberculosis* involve the terminal ileum and can mimic Crohn disease. *Yersinia* infection presents with marked mural thickening of the terminal ileum and colon accompanied by mesenteric lymphadenopathy. Several pathogens in the small bowel are associated with AIDS; these include *Mycobacterium avium-intracellulare* complex (MAC), cytomegalovirus (CMV), and *Cryptosporidium parvum.* MAC usually involves the colon and causes bulky, low-density lymphadenopathy. CMV results in mural thickening and can involve the entire gastrointestinal (GI) tract with skip lesions. The submucosal hemorrhage seen in CMV is secondary to submucosal venous thrombosis.

Enteric infections result in gastroenteritis occurring 6 to 48 hours after ingestion of contaminated food or water. The most common symptoms are abdominal pain, diarrhea, fever, nausea, and vomiting. The combination of fever and fecal leukocytes or erythrocytes suggests an inflammatory cause of the diarrhea, but the definite diagnosis is based on culture or demonstration of specific organisms on stained fecal smears. Thus, the role of imaging in the diagnosis of infectious enteritis is limited. Imaging features of enteritis caused by *C jejuni, E coli,* and *C difficile* are often nonspecific; barium studies show mucosal ulcerations with edematous bowel wall, while CT reveals ileal or cecal wall thickening and enlarged mesenteric lymph nodes. *Salmonella* and *Shigella* infections result in an acute terminal ileitis. Small bowel follow-through examinations in these patients show terminal ileal ulcers, irregular narrowing of the lumen, and thickened folds. CT reveals a circumferential, homogeneous thickening of the terminal ileum and mild colonic wall thickening. *Yersinia enterocolitis* is an acute, self-limiting enteritis with symptoms referable to the right lower quadrant mimicking appendicitis or acute Crohn disease. Imaging shows increased number of thickened, tortuous mucosal folds in the terminal ileum with typical small, discrete nodular filling defects of lymphoid hyperplasia and mesenteric adenopathy. Occasionally, *Y enterocolitis* presents with small bowel intussusception, presumably secondary to enlarged mesenteric nodes. *G lamblia*, a flagellate protozoan parasite of the upper small intestine, is commonly associated with diarrhea in the tropics. *Giardia* can be found in the stool or duodenal aspirate. Barium studies in giardiasis demonstrate irregularly thickened valvulae conniventes, predominantly in the duodenum and proximal jejunum. *S stercoralis* affecting the small intestine causes abdominal pain, vomiting, diarrhea, and weight loss. Small bowel contrast studies demonstrate delay in the passage of barium and thickening or absence of the valvulae conniventes in the duodenum and proximal jejunum. In advanced cases, a rigid "pipe-stem" stenosis with irregular narrowing may be seen. Ascariasis is most commonly seen in developing countries. Affected individuals may be symptomatic depending on the worm load. Bowel obstruction, perforation, and peritonitis are usually seen in heavily infested children. Worms filling the gut can be easily imaged on abdominal radiographs, US, and barium studies. CT demonstrates worms as a long, thin, tubular soft tissue structures coiled in the small bowel. Intestinal tuberculosis classically presents with abdominal pain, fever, weight loss, diarrhea, and intestinal obstruction. The terminal ileum and ileocecal junction are commonly involved segments of small bowel. Radiologically, the terminal ileum shows discrete, transverse ulcers with a funnel-shaped, contracted cecum. CT demonstrates diffuse mural thickening, multiple enlarged lymph nodes with central necrosis and ascites.

- Enteritis can be caused by viral pathogens, bacteria, protozoa, or fungal infections. Major causes are salmonellosis, shigellosis, and infection due to *Y enterocolitica*, *Staphylococcus*, *E coli*, *C difficile*, and *C jejuni*.

- Imaging plays a limited role in the diagnosis of specific pathogens in infectious enteritis. The definitive diagnosis is made with cultures or demonstration of specific organisms on stained fecal smears.

- Most of the cases show nonspecific bowel wall thickening, nodules, and mesenteric lymphadenopathy on imaging.

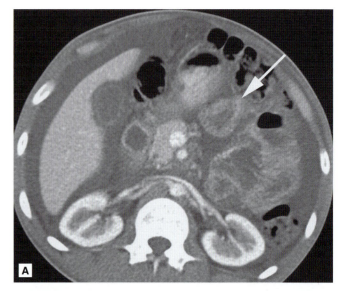

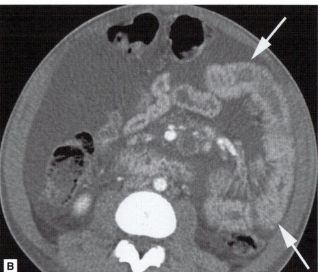

1. A. Axial, contrast-enhanced CT image reveals thickened, hyperenhancing jejunum (arrow) with ascites in this case of CMV enteritis. **B.** Axial, contrast-enhanced CT image reveals diffuse thickening and hyperenhancement of the jejunum (arrows) with ascites in this case of CMV enteritis.

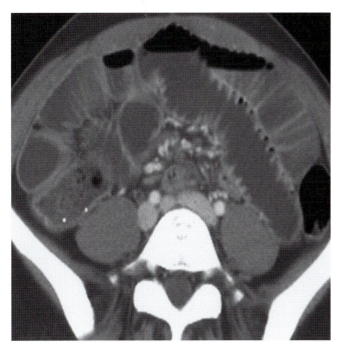

2. Axial, contrast-enhanced CT image reveals fluid-filled small bowel loops with mucosal hyperenhancement in this case of *C jejuni* infection.

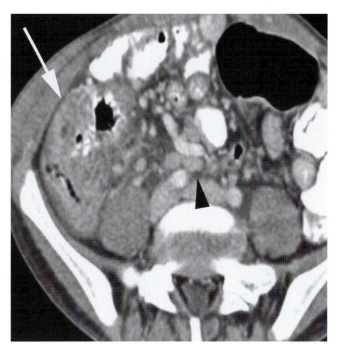

3. Axial, contrast-enhanced CT image reveals marked ileocecal thickening (arrow) with prominent mesenteric lymph nodes (arrowhead).

PRESENTATION

Patients may remain asymptomatic or present with abdominal pain, nausea, and vomiting.

FINDINGS

Plain radiographs of the abdomen demonstrate foreign bodies in the intestine with or without signs of perforation or obstruction. CT demonstrates foreign body in the small intestine and the level of obstruction or other complications such as perforation or abscess formation.

DIFFERENTIAL DIAGNOSIS

- Small bowel obstruction
- Paralytic ileus
- Perforation

COMMENTS

Small bowel foreign bodies are rare, because of impaction of the majority of the ingested foreign bodies in the pharynx or upper gastrointestinal tract. Ingested foreign bodies which escape the anatomic narrowing in the upper tract will progress through the gastrointestinal tract uneventfully. However, objects with sharp edges are more prone to impaction at areas of physiological narrowing in the lower tract such as the ileocecal valve and terminal ileum. Various types of foreign bodies have been described to lodge in the small bowel; bone and food boluses are most common. Others include bezoars, batteries, safety pins, magnets, doll's heads, and snail's shells. Ingested foreign bodies are commonly seen in infants and children. Among adults, accidental swallowing of foreign bodies such as dentures and toothpicks is well known. Psychiatric patients are vulnerable to foreign body ingestion. Prisoners and drug smugglers may deliberately swallow objects to conceal from legal authorities. Most nondigestible substances pass readily through the small bowel without any complications. Pre-existing pathology such as polyps or strictures may cause impaction of the foreign bodies, leading to obstruction. Sharp foreign bodies may perforate the bowel wall and initiate local inflammation, abscess, and peritonitis.

Foreign bodies in the small bowel are often asymptomatic. However, they may cause symptoms due to obstruction, perforation, or abscess formation. From a radiological perspective, these ingested foreign bodies fall under four main groups: (1) opaque foreign bodies, for example, metallic objects; (2) semiopaque foreign bodies like bone fragments and any other substances containing calcium; (3) nonopaque foreign bodies; and (4) translucent foreign bodies such as fatty masses. Abdominal radiograph usually demonstrate radio-opaque and semiradio-opaque foreign bodies. Positive contrast such as barium may be required to demonstrate nonopaque or translucent foreign bodies. Plain radiographs may also demonstrate gaseous distension of the small bowel, with signs of obstruction. CT is a better tool to localize any foreign body and to identify the level of impaction. In addition, CT readily demonstrates any associated complications.

PEARLS

- **Small bowel foreign bodies are one of the rare causes of small bowel obstruction and are usually caused by accidental ingestion.**

- **Plain radiograph is often sufficient for the diagnosis and monitoring. CT may be required to assess complications and sometimes localize the foreign body itself.**

- **Sharp foreign bodies may perforate and initiate local inflammation and abscess formation.**

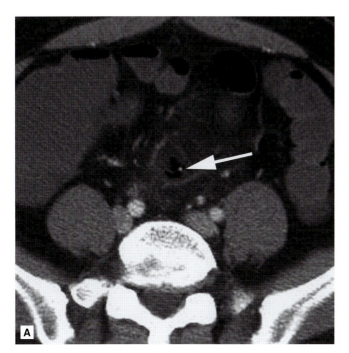

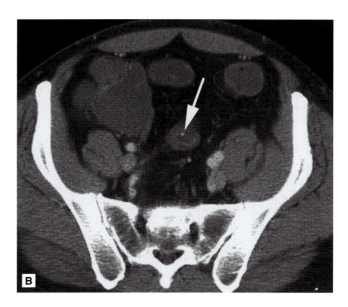

1. A. Axial, contrast-enhanced CT image demonstrates a small degree of free air with central focus of hyperattenuation (arrow) representing a toothpick causing small bowel perforation. **B.** Axial, contrast-enhanced CT image demonstrates a linear hyperattenuating structure within the lumen of the ileum (arrow), adjacent to the area of free air, representing a toothpick causing small bowel perforation.

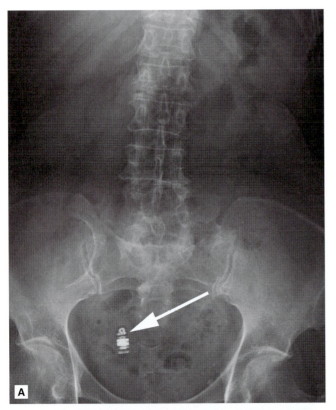

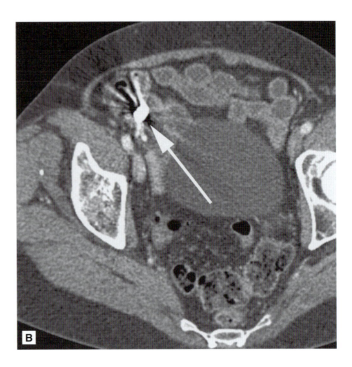

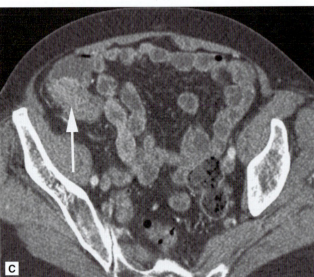

2. A. Frontal abdominal radiograph reveals a metallic structure within the right lower quadrant (arrow) representing a capsule endoscope. **B.** Axial, contrast-enhanced CT image demonstrates a metallic structure within the lumen of the distal small bowel representing a retained capsule endoscope (arrow). **C.** Axial, contrast-enhanced CT image demonstrates a cecal mass (arrow) causing retention of the capsule endoscope within the terminal ileum.

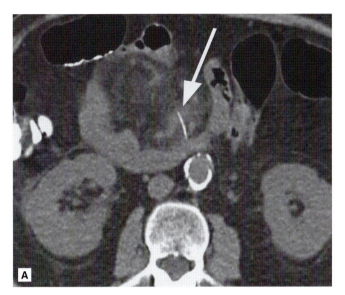

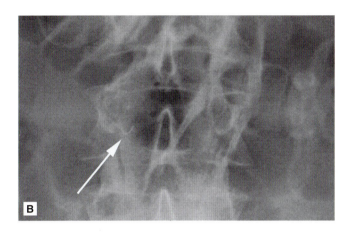

3. A and **B.** Axial, contrast-enhanced CT image demonstrates a curvilinear, hyperattenuating structure located at the root of the mesentery with surrounding inflammation (arrow) noted to be a curvilinear metallic structure on plain film representing a wire which had perforated the duodenum.

PRESENTATION

Patients present with watery diarrhea, nausea, vomiting, and abdominal cramping after high-dose radiation treatment.

FINDINGS

Small bowel follow-through or CT examinations demonstrate thickened bowel loops with decreased luminal diameter. In advanced stages, thickened bowel loops progress to multiple strictures, fibrosis, and intestinal obstruction.

DIFFERENTIAL DIAGNOSIS

- Crohn disease
- Ischemic enteritis
- Metastases
- Lymphoma

COMMENTS

Radiation enteritis is the primary treatment-limiting toxicity in the radiation treatment of abdominal and pelvic malignancies. The small intestinal epithelium may suffer severe, acute, and chronic deleterious effects during radiation treatment of malignancies of the stomach, pancreas, rectum, and anus, as well as during treatment of gynecologic malignancies. The amount of radiation is directly related with the probability of developing radiation enteritis. Serious late complications are unusual if the total radiation dose is less than 4000 cGy; morbidity risk increases with dosages exceeding 5000 cGy. The epithelium of the gastrointestinal tract has a high proliferative rate, making it susceptible to radiation- and chemotherapy-induced mucositis. The intestinal lining is normally replaced every 3 to 5 days, reflecting this high cellular turnover rate. Irradiation of intestinal mucosa primarily affects the clonogenic intestinal stem cells within the crypts of Lieberkuhn. Stem cell damage, either as a primary result of radiation damage or as a result of radiation-induced microvascular damage, leads to a decrease in cellular reserves for the intestinal villi, resulting in mucosal denudement, shortened villi, and decreased absorptive area, with associated intestinal inflammation and edema. Histologic changes are seen within hours of irradiation. Within the first few weeks, an infiltration of leukocytes with crypt abscesses and ulcerations can be seen. As a result of radiation injury, absorption of fats, carbohydrates, proteins, bile salts, and vitamin B_{12} are impaired, with associated loss of water, electrolytes, and protein. Patients usually develop diarrhea, flatulence, and distention as a result of the altered bacterial environment inside the gut due to impaired ileal bile salt absorption and impaired digestion of lactose. The late effects of radiation injury are the result of damage to the small submucosal blood vessels, with a progressive obliterative arteritis and submucosal fibrosis, eventually resulting in thrombosis and vascular insufficiency. This injury may produce necrosis and perforation of the involved intestine but, more commonly, it leads to stricture formation with symptoms of obstruction or small bowel fistulas.

Patients with acute radiation enteritis experience diarrhea, abdominal cramping or pain, nausea and vomiting, anorexia, and malaise. Radiation enteritis can be acute (< 2 months after treatment), subacute (2-12 months after treatment), or chronic (12 months after treatment). The small bowel follow-through examination in the acute stage demonstrates shallow ulcerations of the mucosa and decreased luminal diameter of bowel secondary to submucosal thickening (edema). The subacute and chronic stages of radiation enteritis demonstrate thickened valvulae conniventes and intestinal wall with straightening of folds and nodular filling defects which separate the bowel loops. Advanced cases demonstrate single or multiple strictures, small bowel obstruction with dilatation of proximal bowel loops, adhesions, sinus tracts, and fistulas. CT is superior for demonstration of acute and chronic changes, especially thickened bowel wall and surrounding fibrosis.

PEARLS

- **Radiation enteritis is the radiation-induced damage to the gastrointestinal tract after radiation therapy to the abdomen. The ileum is the most sensitive and commonly involved segment of small bowel.**

- **Endarteritis with vascular occlusion and bowel ischemia plays a central role in the pathogenesis of radiation enteritis.**

- **Acute injury demonstrates diffuse bowel wall edema with shallow mucosal ulcers and bowel spasm. Chronic stages show thickened bowel due to submucosal edema and fibrosis, with straightening of folds, multiple strictures, adhesions, sinus tracts, and fistulas.**

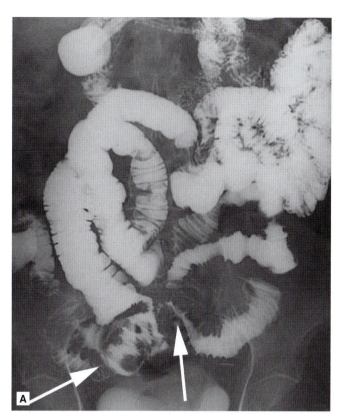

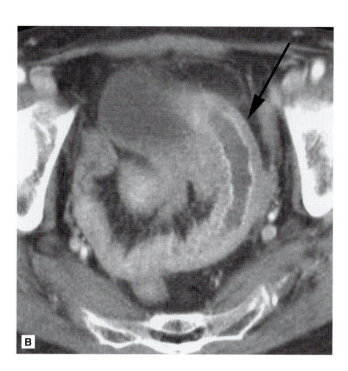

1. A. Small bowel follow-through reveals narrow, angulated loops of small bowel in the pelvis (arrows) secondary to radiation enteritis. **B.** Axial, contrast-enhanced CT demonstrates marked thickening and mucosal hyperenhancement of the small bowel (arrow) in the pelvis secondary to radiation enteritis.

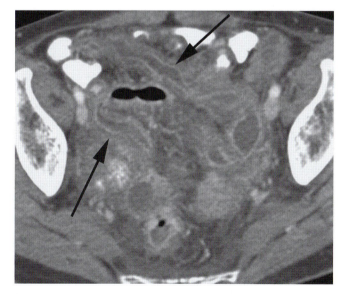

2. Axial, contrast-enhanced CT demonstrates thickening, irregular-appearing loops of small bowel with mucosal hyperenhancement (arrows) in the pelvis secondary to radiation enteritis.

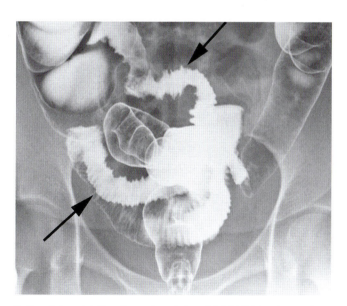

3. Small bowel follow-through reveals mild fold thickening and decreased caliber of small bowel loops in the pelvis (arrows) related to radiation.

PRESENTATION

Most common symptoms of Crohn disease are abdominal pain, diarrhea, and weight loss.

FINDINGS

CT enterography demonstrates thickened bowel wall with mural hyperenhancement, increased density of perienteric fat, segmental dilatation of the vasa recta in the involved intestinal loop, perienteric abscess, fistula, sinus tracts, and strictures.

DIFFERENTIAL DIAGNOSIS

- Ulcerative colitis
- Infection
- Ischemia
- Radiation enteritis
- Metastases and lymphoma
- Mesenteric adenitis

COMMENTS

Crohn disease is a chronic, idiopathic inflammatory disease with a predilection to affect the distal ileum, although any part of the alimentary tract can be involved. This disease is characterized by sustained inflammation secondary to failure of the immune system to control or downregulate an inappropriate inflammatory process in the intestinal mucosa. The exact etiology of Crohn disease is not known, and the possible causes for the disease have been the subject of many theories and much speculation. The earliest manifestation of Crohn disease is the development of small mucosal ulcers, known as aphthous ulcers. They usually develop over microscopic lymphoid aggregates. As the disease progresses, the aphthous ulcers enlarge and become stellate. The ulcerations coalesce to form longitudinal mucosal ulcerations. In Crohn disease of the small bowel, these linear ulcerations almost always occur along the mesenteric aspect of the bowel wall. Further progression of disease leads to a serpiginous network of thin, linear ulcerations that surround islands of edematous mucosa; these produce the classic "cobblestone" appearance. Mucosal ulcerations penetrate through the submucosa and coalesce to form intramural channels. Subsequently, they can penetrate through the bowel wall and produce abscesses, fistulae, or sinuses. The pathological hallmark of Crohn disease is focal, transmural inflammation of the

intestine. The inflammation also involves the mesentery and regional lymph nodes, leading to massively thickened mesentery and lymphadenopathy. Fatty tissue commonly develops from the mesentery and extends over the serosal surface of the small bowel resulting in a phenomenon known as "creeping fat." During early or acute intestinal inflammation, the bowel wall is hyperemic. As the inflammation progresses, fibrotic scarring develops, and the bowel becomes thickened and leathery which decreased caliber and stricture formation. The disease tends to be discontinuous and segmental, affecting isolated segments of the gastrointestinal tract. Disease of the terminal ileum with or without some involvement of the cecum is the most common pattern.

Clinical features are highly variable among individual patients and depend on the segments of the gastrointestinal tract, are predominantly affected, the intensity of inflammation, and the presence or absence of specific complications. However, the most common symptoms of Crohn disease are abdominal pain, diarrhea, and weight loss.

Diagnosis is always based on a complete assessment of the clinical presentation with confirmatory findings derived from radiographic, endoscopic, and, in most cases, pathological tests. Barium studies are especially useful to delineate typical early findings and late transmural complications of Crohn disease. These include aphthous ulcers, a coarse villus mucosal pattern, and thickened folds. Submucosal edema may be evident as thickening or flattening of the valvulae conniventes, whereas transmural edema manifests as increased separation between bowel loops. Ulcers most often occur on the mesenteric border, with consequent pseudosacculation of the antimesenteric border because of shortening of the mesenteric side. Later findings include a cobblestone appearance resulting from edema and inflammation of relatively spared islands of mucosa separated by intersecting longitudinal and transverse ulceration. Advanced stages demonstrate adhesions, fistulae, sinus tracts, and fixed strictures. CT enterography in the acute phase demonstrates thickened bowel wall with mural hyperenhancement ("target" appearance), increased attenuation of perienteric fat, and segmental dilatation of the vasa recta in the involved intestinal loop ("comb" sign). Features of the chronic stage include homogeneous hyperenhancement of the thickened bowel wall, perienteric abscess, fistula, sinus tracts, and mesenteric thickening from chronic inflammation. Thickened bowel with mural hyperenhancement (target appearance), perienteric fat stranding, and dilated vasa recta (comb sign) are often well correlated with endoscopic evidence of Crohn disease activity. Accuracy of MR enterography approximates that of CT enterography for identification of activity in Crohn disease of the large and small bowel.

PEARLS

- Crohn disease is a chronic, idiopathic, relapsing inflammatory disease which predominantly affects the distal ileum and proximal colon.

- Aphthous ulcer and focal, transmural inflammation of the intestine are the pathological hallmarks of Crohn disease, which can be recognized by barium studies and CT and MR enterography for proper diagnosis.

- CT enterography findings such as thickened bowel wall with mural hyperenhancement (target appearance), perienteric fat stranding, and dilated vasa recta (comb sign) can accurately identify disease activity, which can also monitored accurately with MR enterography.

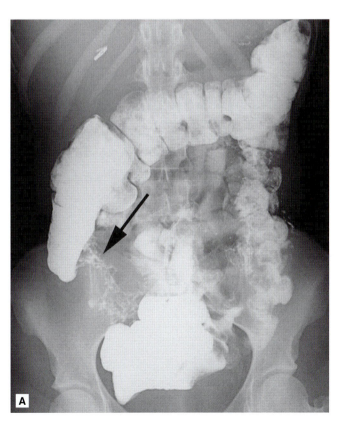

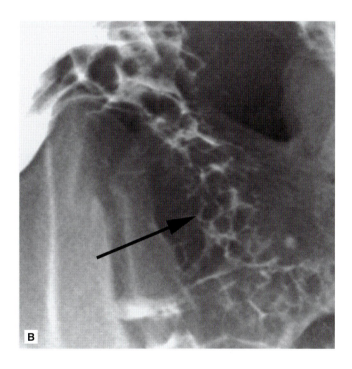

1. **A.** Spot film acquired during small bowel follow-through reveals thickening and separation of the terminal ileum (arrow). **B.** Magnified spot film acquired during small bowel follow-through reveals marked thickening of the terminal ileum (arrow).

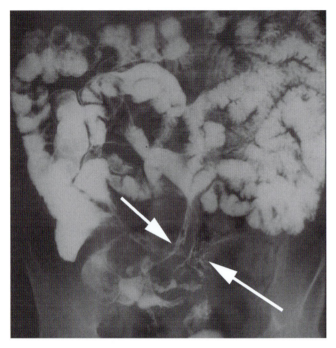

2. Spot film acquired during small bowel follow-through reveals complex, enteroenteric fistulae (arrows) within the mid-pelvis.

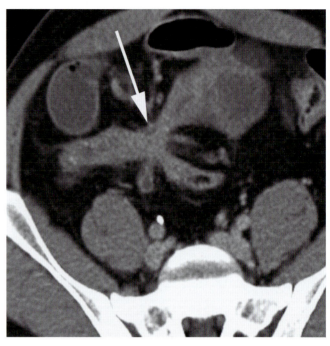

3. Axial, contrast-enhanced CT image reveals several enteroenteric fistulae (arrow) involving the distal small bowel.

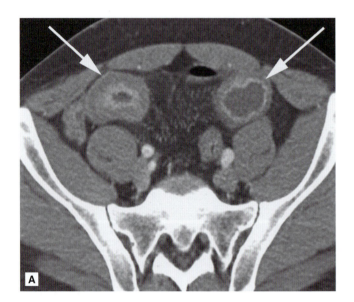

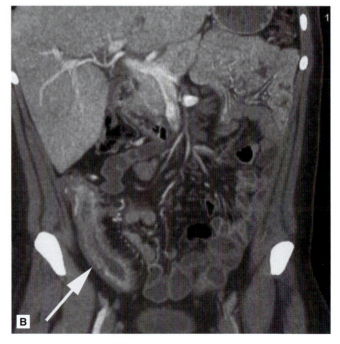

4. A. Axial, contrast-enhanced CT image reveals thickening and mucosal hyperenhancement of the terminal ileum (arrows) along with dilation of the surrounding vasa recta. **B.** Coronal, contrast-enhanced CT image reveals thickening and mucosal hyperenhancement of the terminal ileum (arrow) along with dilation of the surrounding vasa recta, typical findings in Crohn disease.

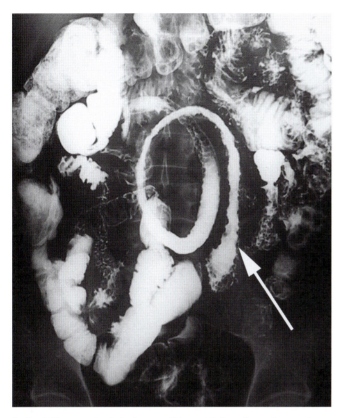

5. Spot film acquired during small bowel follow-through reveals a long segment of structuring involving the small bowel (arrow) with separation from the adjacent, normal-appearing small bowel.

PRESENTATION

Diarrhea due to malabsorption and subsequent weight loss

FINDINGS

Small bowel follow-through demonstrates altered bowel transit times, decreased number of jejunal folds, increased number of ileal folds, thickened bowel wall, loss of valvulae conniventes. CT demonstrates thickened, fluid-filled, dilated bowel loops and mesenteric lymphadenopathy.

DIFFERENTIAL DIAGNOSIS

- Crohn disease
- Whipple disease
- Opportunistic infection
- Ischemia
- Cystic fibrosis
- Immunologic disorders

COMMENTS

Celiac disease is the most common cause of small intestinal malabsorption. It is caused by intolerance to ingested wheat gluten or related proteins from rye and barley, which induces chronic inflammatory changes and small intestinal injury resulting in malabsorption of various nutrients. Celiac disease affects the mucosa of the small intestine; the submucosa, muscularis propria, and serosa usually are not involved. The hallmark of this disease is villus atrophy of the small intestinal mucosa. Prompt clinical and histologic improvement follow strict adherence to a gluten-free diet. Clinical and histologic relapse occur when gluten is reintroduced in the diet. In individuals with celiac disease, alcohol-soluble protein components of wheat gluten (gliadins) peptides are presented by the antigen-presenting cells in association with human leukocyte antigen (HLA) DQ2 or DQ8. The gluten antigen is presented to cytotoxic T cells, initiating activation and production of lymphocytes, which are responsible for releasing cytokines. Cytokines produce an immune response with hyperplasia of the mucosal crypts followed by atrophy of the small intestinal villi, which produces the clinical symptoms. The damaged mucosa triggers the release of tissue transglutaminase (tTG), a cytosolic enzyme that deamidates gluten and catalyzes deamidation of gluten which in turn augments the gluten presentation by HLA DQ2 or DQ8. In addition, released cytokines increase the expression of HLA DQ2 on small intestine epithelia, allowing increased antigen presentation to sensitized lymphocytes.

Celiac disease classically presents with diarrhea due to malabsorption and subsequent weight loss. The diarrhea is associated with bloating, borborygmi, and relatively little pain. Other symptoms include indigestion, fatigue, iron deficiency, peripheral neuropathy, ataxia, infertility, aphthous ulcerations of the mouth, sore tongue, generalized weakness, and arthritis. In severe cases, vitamin deficiency syndromes may occur. Dermatitis herpetiformis is a blistering skin disease characterized by pruritic, papulovesicular skin lesion, that is considered a manifestation of celiac disease.

Serology (immunoglobulin A [Ig A] endomysial antibody, Ig A tTG antibody) and small intestinal biopsy are the most reliable diagnostic tests for celiac disease. Radiological studies of the small intestine seldom are required in evaluating patients with suspected celiac disease; however, they are most useful in suggesting diagnoses other than celiac disease. Small bowel follow-through can be normal in moderate disease or may show changes in the proximal jejunum. Patients with celiac disease have altered transit times and nonpropulsive peristalsis due to motor abnormalities of gut. Barium studies demonstrate thickened mucosal folds, straightening of the valvulae conniventes, decreased jejunal folds with decreased interspaces and increased ileal folds, especially in the distal ileum. This entire pattern is called "jejunoileal fold reversal." Advanced cases with villous atrophy demonstrate a mosaic pattern of bowel opacification and loss of mucosal folds and valvulae conniventes in the jejunum (known as "moulage" sign). Excessive secretion of fluid into the proximal small intestine, coupled with defective absorption of intraluminal contents, causes dilution, flocculation, segmentation, and clumping of barium. US may demonstrate fluid-filled, thickened, dilated small bowel with disordered motility. CT demonstrates abnormal bowel (mild wall thickening, increased fluid content) along with other diagnostic clues to the presence of celiac disease such as splenic atrophy, ascites, and mesenteric lymphadenopathy, which may contain central cavitation.

PEARLS

- Celiac disease is a chronic inflammatory condition associated with small intestinal injury induced by gluten exposure and results in malabsorption of different nutrients.

- Serology (Ig A endomysial antibody, Ig A tTG antibody) and small intestinal biopsy are the most reliable diagnostic tests for celiac disease. Villus atrophy of the small intestinal mucosa is the key finding on biopsy.

- Barium studies demonstrate a reversed jejunoileal fold pattern, loss of valvulae conniventes, complete loss of jejunal folds, and mosaic opacification of bowel.

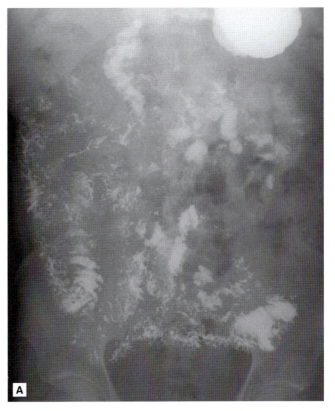

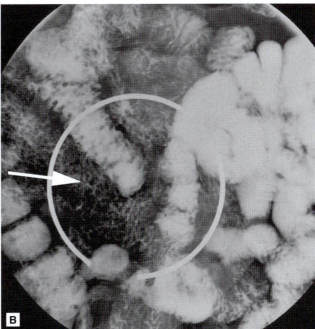

1. A. Spot film from small bowel follow-through reveals nodular fold thickening of the jejunum with flocculation of the orally administered contrast. **B.** Magnified spot film from small bowel follow-through reveals nodular fold thickening of the jejunum (arrow).

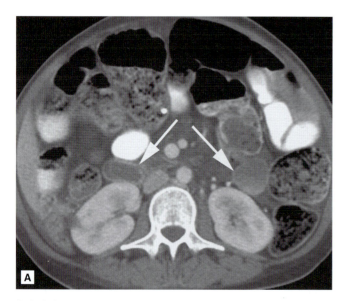

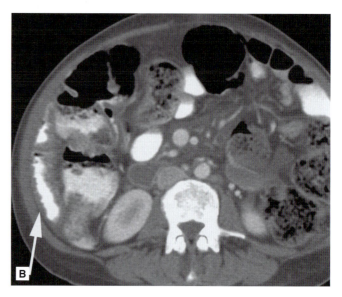

2. A. Axial, contrast-enhanced CT image reveals fluid-filled loops of small bowel causing dilution of the orally administered contrast (arrows). **B.** Axial, contrast-enhanced CT image reveals mild thickening (arrow) as well as fluid distention of small bowel loops.

PRESENTATION

The main clinical symptoms are chronic diarrhea, weight loss, abdominal pain, polyarthralgias, and lymphadenopathy.

FINDINGS

CT typically demonstrates thickened mucosal folds.

DIFFERENTIAL DIAGNOSIS

- Opportunistic infection in AIDS
- Dysgammaglobulinemia
- Non-Hodgkin lymphoma

COMMENTS

Whipple disease is a rare chronic bacterial infection, caused by *Tropheryma whippelii* and involves multiple systems. This disease occurs mainly in middle-aged individuals (mean age at diagnosis about 50 years) and is about eight times more in men than in women. Mode of transmission of bacteria, source of infection, and the sequence of events leading to bacterial multiplication and pathological changes are unclear. Once *T whippelii* has been acquired, it usually affects the proximal small intestine where the bacteria invade the mucosa. Bacteria are thought to spread via lymphatics into mesenteric and mediastinal lymph nodes and into the systemic circulation. Fluorescence imaging indicates that most viable bacteria are extracellular and located just below the epithelial basement membrane in the lamina propria. Patients with Whipple disease express a large variety of immune dysfunction or response.

As Whipple disease is a systemic process that affects multiple organs, clinical manifestations are varied. Gastrointestinal symptoms are reported most commonly, which include chronic diarrhea, weight loss, abdominal pain, and lymphadenopathy. The main underlying mechanism producing intestinal symptoms is bacterial and macrophage-predominant inflammatory cell infiltration of the small intestinal mucosa and obstruction of mesenteric lymph nodes. In some cases, symptoms of nondestructive polyarticular, migratory arthritis precede the gastrointestinal manifestations by several years.

Small bowel barium examinations reveal findings such as micronodules, prominent and edematous duodenal and jejunal folds, and intestinal dilatation. CT demonstrates thickened, edematous small bowel folds, especially in the proximal small bowel and low-density lymphadenopathy. Intra- and extraperitoneal lymphadenopathy with central low density is characteristic of Whipple disease. However, this finding may be seen with other infectious processes such as tuberculosis and with diffuse neoplasms. Diagnosis is usually made by intestinal biopsy showing periodic acid-Schiff (PAS)–positive material in involved histiocytes.

PEARLS

- **Whipple disease is a rare, systemic disorder caused by a rod-shaped gram-positive aerobic bacillus, called *T whippelii*.**

- **The gastrointestinal tract is the most common system affected in majority of the patients.**

- **CT demonstrates thickened edematous bowel with micronodularity and low-density abdominal lymphadenopathy.**

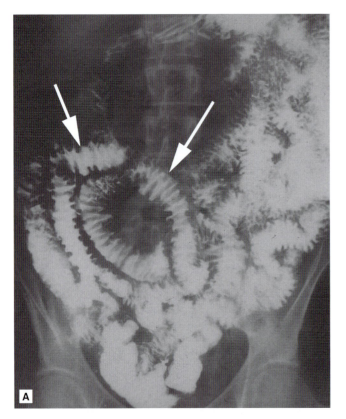

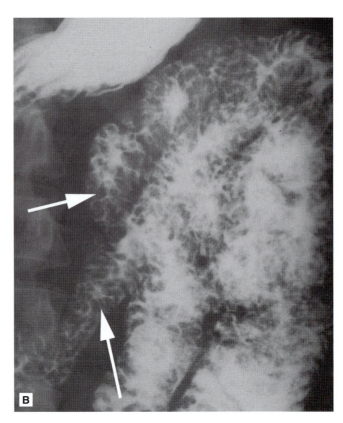

1. A. Spot film acquired during a small bowel follow-through demonstrates irregularly thickened loops of small bowel in a patient with Whipple disease (arrows). **B.** Nodular thickening of the small bowel wall is well seen on this spot film acquired during a small bowel follow-through in a patient with Whipple disease (arrows).

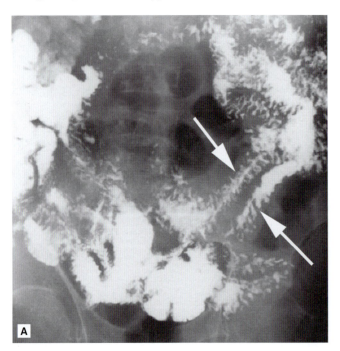

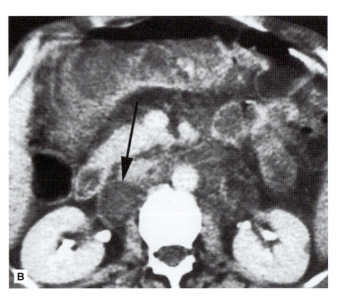

2. A. Spot film acquired during a small bowel follow-through demonstrates diffuse, irregular thickening of the small bowel in a patient with Whipple disease (arrows). **B.** Axial, contrast-enhanced CT reveals low-attenuating retroperitoneal lymph nodes (arrow), a characteristic feature of Whipple disease.

PRESENTATION

Nausea, vomiting, diarrhea, abdominal pain, hepatomegaly, portal hypertension, splenomegaly, and ascites

FINDINGS

Small bowel barium studies demonstrate duodenal ulcers, mucosal nodules, bull's-eye lesions resembling metastases, edema, thickened folds, and thickened bowel wall. CT demonstrates hepatosplenomegaly, lymphadenopathy, and bone lesions.

DIFFERENTIAL DIAGNOSIS

- Small bowel metastasis
- Lymphoma
- Carcinoid syndrome
- Zollinger-Ellison syndrome
- Celiac sprue
- Whipple disease

COMMENTS

Systemic mastocytosis is a clonal disorder of the mast cell progenitor, characterized by a dense infiltrate of mast cells in extracutaneous tissue such as bone marrow, spleen, liver, lymph nodes, and gastrointestinal tract. It is associated with somatic gain-in-function mutation in the *c-kit* gene. Systemic mastocytosis may present with or without dermatologic manifestations. Systemic mastocytosis is typically diagnosed in adults and has a slight preponderance in men. Symptoms in mastocytosis are caused by biological mediators like histamine and prostaglandins (eg, PGD$_2$) released from mast cells and/or the infiltration of neoplastic mast cells in various organs. These substances act both at the local site of infiltration and at distal sites. Skin and bone marrow are the most common sites of involvement. However, the gastrointestinal tract is involved in a majority of patients. Gastrointestinal symptoms include nausea, vomiting, diarrhea, and abdominal pain. Mast cell–mediated fibrotic changes occur in the liver, spleen, and bone marrow and manifest as hepatomegaly, portal hypertension, splenomegaly, and ascites. Fibrosis does not involve the gastrointestinal tissue or skin. These symptoms can be aggravated by consumption of alcohol, aspirin, anticholinergics, nonsteroidal anti-inflammatory drugs (NSAIDs), contrast media, and exposure to heat. Hyperhistaminemia produces gastric hypersecretion which causes gastritis and peptic ulcer in the upper gastrointestinal tract. In the lower gastrointestinal tract, mast cell mediators cause increased motility, which manifests as diarrhoea and abdominal pain. Morphologic changes in the absorptive mucosa lead to malabsorption, which can also cause secondary nutritional insufficiency and osteomalacia.

Barium-contrast studies demonstrate multiple ulcers in gastric and duodenal mucosa, nodular mucosal pattern (some of these nodules with central collections of barium that resemble bull's-eye lesions), thickened valvulae conniventes, and bowel wall. CT demonstrates fluid-filled thickened bowel loops, abdominal lymphadenopathy, hepatosplenomegaly and other signs of portal hypertension. The hallmark of bone marrow involvement is the combination of osteolytic and sclerotic lesions.

PEARLS

- Systemic mastocytosis is characterized by an abnormal proliferation of mast cells and infiltration of various structures. The skin and bone marrow are the more frequently involved structures.

- Diagnosis is usually made on the basis of clinical findings and laboratory evidence of elevated histamine and tryptase levels and bone marrow biopsy.

- The stomach and small bowel are the most common sites of involvement.

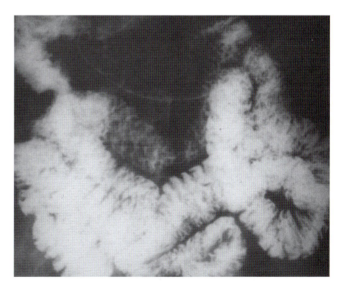

1. Spot film obtained during small bowel follow-through study demonstrates diffuse small bowel wall fold thickening in a patient with mastocytosis.

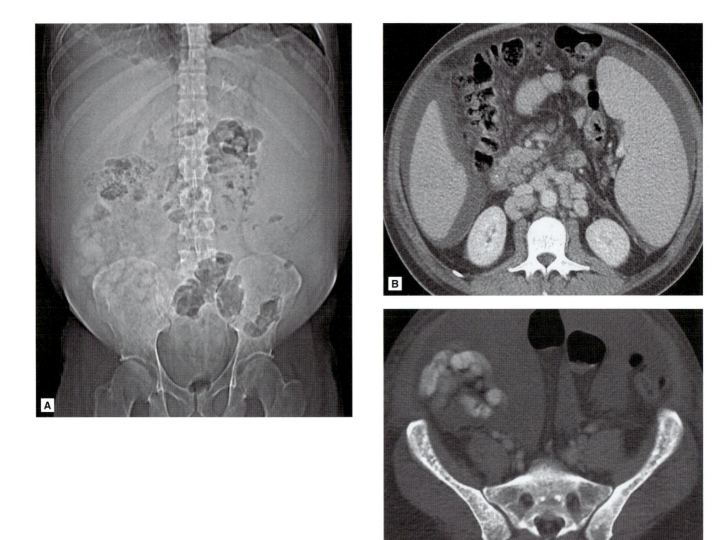

2. A. Scout topogram reveals displacement of the bowel medially secondary to marked enlargement of the liver and spleen in a patient with mastocytosis. **B.** Axial, contrast-enhanced CT image reveals hepatosplenomegaly and ascites, findings associated with mastocytosis. **C.** Axial CT image demonstrates the typical features of bone involvement with mastocytosis, the presence of osteolytic and sclerotic lesions.

PRESENTATION

Patients with gastrointestinal (GI) manifestations of scleroderma may present with abdominal pain, dysphagia, nausea, vomiting, diarrhea, or constipation.

FINDINGS

On imaging, including barium examinations and CT, distended loops of small bowel with a "hide-bound" appearance are typically seen.

DIFFERENTIAL DIAGNOSIS

- Mechanical small bowel obstruction
- Celica disease
- Functional ileus (postsurgical, etc)

COMMENTS

Scleroderma, also known as systemic sclerosis, represents a systemic connective tissue disease which manifests as widespread tissue fibrosis and occlusion of microvasculature as well as chronic inflammation in a number of organ systems. Scleroderma affects the skin and may involve the respiratory tract, the most common cause of morbidity and mortality, renal, cardiovascular, GI, and genitourinary systems. The peak age of onset of scleroderma is 30 to 50 years and the risk is reported to be up to 9 times higher in women than men. While the underlying causes of this heterogeneous group of diseases remain unclear, both genetic contributions and environmental exposures have been implicated in some studies.

GI involvement is reported in up to 90% of patients with scleroderma, most frequently affecting the esophagus. In the case of the small bowel, involvement is reported in approximately half of patients with systemic sclerosis. In the GI tract, smooth muscle atrophy and abnormal collagen deposition lead to abnormal function. In the small bowel, this abnormal function typically manifests as hypomotility with resultant stasis and bowel dilatation. This may result in abdominal pain, distention, and food intolerance. Other complications related to small bowel involvement by systemic sclerosis include malabsorption related to bacterial overgrowth which results from altered motility of the small bowel.

On imaging, the so-called hide-bound appearance of the small bowl is typical in patients with scleroderma. The hide-bound appearance refers to dilated small bowel with an abnormally narrow separation of the valvulae conniventes, which are of normal thickness, secondary to contraction of the longitudinal smooth muscle. This is in contradistinction to the separation of the valvulae conniventes which typically occurs with luminal distention related to other etiologies, such as true mechanical obstruction. The hide-bound appearance of the small bowel is reported to be most prominent in the jejunum and proximal ileum. While classically described on barium studies, the hide-bound appearance of the small bowel in systemic sclerosis may also be readily identified on CT. In addition, given the altered motility of the small bowel in patients with scleroderma, intussusceptions are seen more frequently in this patient population and may be readily identified on imaging. Finally, while more commonly seen in the colon, pseudosacculations may be identified along the antimesenteric aspect of the small bowel in patients with systemic sclerosis.

PEARLS

- Hide-bound appearance of the small bowel is useful in distinguishing scleroderma from other causes of small bowel distention such as mechanical obstruction.

- Small bowel intussusceptions are seen more frequently in patients with scleroderma.

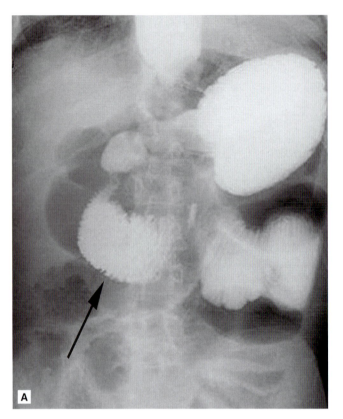

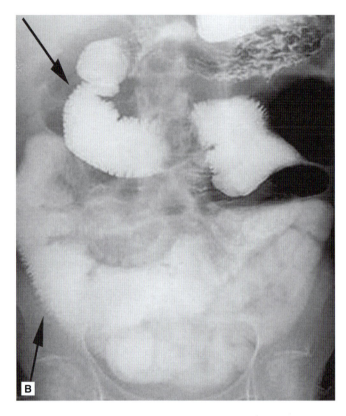

1. A. Fluoroscopic image from an upper GI series demonstrates dilated small bowel with hide-bound appearance (arrow) in which relative crowding of the valvulae conniventes is seen. **B.** Fluoroscopic image from an upper GI series demonstrates diffusely dilated small bowel with a hide-bound appearance (arrows) in which an abnormally narrow separation of the valvulae conniventes is seen.

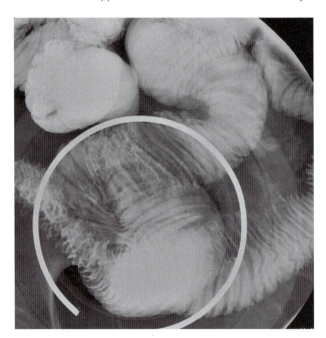

2. Spot compression image from an upper GI series demonstrates the characteristic hide-bound appearance of the small bowel, useful in distinguishing scleroderma from other causes of small bowel distention.

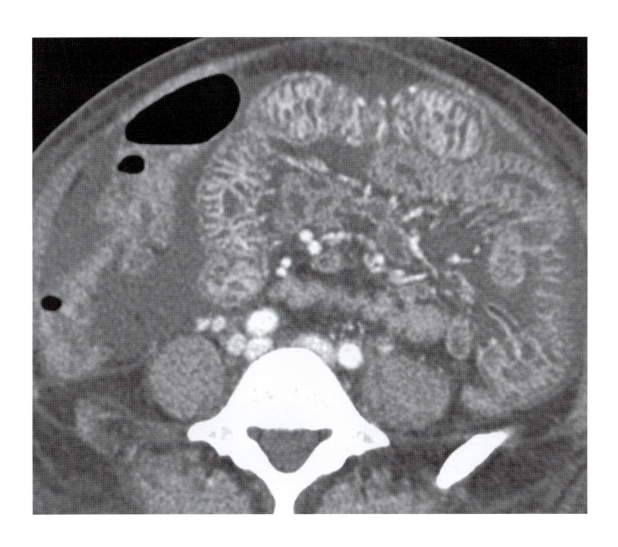

PRESENTATION

Sudden onset of abdominal pain, diarrhea, vomiting, and abdominal distension

FINDINGS

CT demonstrates bowel wall thickening, mural hyperemia or decreased enhancement, intramural hemorrhage, abnormally dilated bowel loops, pneumatosis intestinalis, and portomesenteric venous gas and filling defects suggestive of thromboembolic disease in the mesenteric vessels.

DIFFERENTIAL DIAGNOSIS

• Shock bowel

• Crohn disease

• Fibrosing mesenteritis

• Carcinoid tumor

COMMENTS

Small bowel ischemia can be classified as acute or chronic and of venous or arterial origin. Acute bowel ischemia is more common than the chronic type, and arterial disease is more common than venous disease. Acute bowel ischemia develops from inadequate blood flow to all or part of the small intestine and can also involve the right half of the colon because of their shared blood supply from the superior mesenteric artery. Main pathophysiologic mechanisms leading to acute small bowel ischemia include arterial embolus, arterial thrombosis, vasospasm (also known as nonocclusive mesenteric ischemia, or NOMI), and venous thrombosis. Emboli are the most common cause of acute bowel ischemia in more than half of the affected population. The heart remains the leading source; most often from left atrial or ventricular thrombi or valvular lesions. Most emboli tend to occlude the branch points in the mid to distal superior mesenteric artery, usually distal to the origin of the middle colic artery. In contrast, acute occlusions from thrombosis tend to occur in the proximal mesenteric arteries, near their origins. NOMI is usually seen in critically ill patients who are receiving vasopressor agents and is the result of vasospasm. Mesenteric venous thrombosis can be primary without any etiologic factors or secondary to heritable or acquired coagulation disorder. The final end result of ischemic injury from various causes is similar: a spectrum of bowel damage that ranges from transient alteration of bowel function to transmural gangrene. Intestinal mucosal sloughing can occur within 3 hours of onset and full-thickness intestinal infarction by 6 hours. In contrast, atherosclerotic lesions in the main mesenteric arteries lead to inadequate blood flow to the intestine to support the normal functional demands and results in chronic mesenteric arterial ischemia. Bowel ischemia can also be caused by bowel obstruction, neoplasms, vasculitis, abdominal inflammatory conditions, trauma, chemotherapy, radiation, and corrosive injury.

Clinical manifestations of acute bowel ischemia include abdominal pain, nausea, vomiting, and abdominal distension. Chronic mesenteric ischemia presents with insidious postprandial abdominal pain and weight loss.

Findings of bowel ischemia on abdominal radiographs include dilated bowel loops, bowel wall thickening, submucosal focal mural thickening, intramural pneumatosis and mesenteric or portal vein gas. CT is more sensitive for demonstrating bowel wall changes and vascular abnormalities. CT features of bowel ischemia include occluded mesenteric arteries, mesenteric or portal vein thrombosis, bowel dilatation, engorgement of mesenteric veins and mesenteric edema, intramural gas, mesenteric or portal vein gas, lack of bowel enhancement, increased enhancement of thickened bowel wall, and infarction of other abdominal organs. Angiography may demonstrate arterial or venous occlusion or vasospasm with diminished flow in nonocclusive ischemia.

PEARLS

• Small bowel ischemia can be caused by various conditions such as arterial occlusion, venous occlusion, strangulating obstruction, and hypoperfusion associated with nonocclusive vascular disease and other bowel pathology.

• Regardless of the etiology of bowel ischemia, the end result is bowel damage. CT can demonstrate early nonspecific bowel thickening to late bowel necrosis from bowel ischemia with more sensitivity and specificity.

• Pneumatosis and portomesenteric gas occur secondary to mucosal injury, but this is not always due to infarction. Lack of bowel enhancement and filling defects within mesenteric vessels almost always represent bowel ischemia.

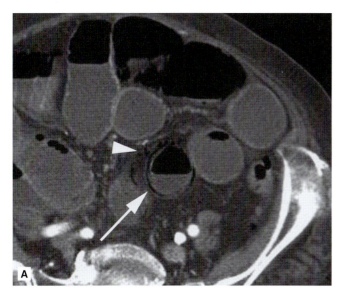

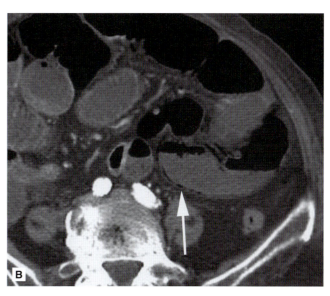

1. A. Axial, contrast-enhanced CT demonstrates small bowel pneumatosis (arrow) and mesenteric venous gas (arrowhead). Of note, there is decreased mucosal enhancement of the involved segment of small bowel, a highly specific feature of ischemia. **B.** Axial, contrast-enhanced CT demonstrates small bowel pneumatosis (arrow) and decreased mucosal enhancement of the involved segment of small bowel.

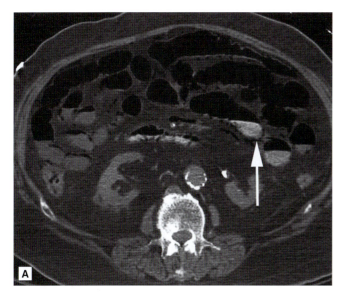

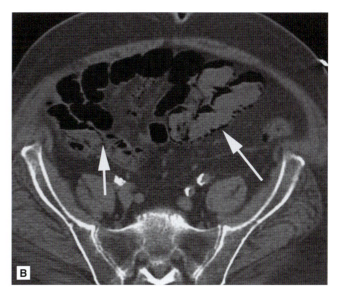

2. A. Axial CT image demonstrates diffuse small bowel pneumatosis (arrow). **B.** Axial CT image demonstrates diffuse small bowel pneumatosis (arrows). **C.** Coronal CT image demonstrates diffuse small bowel pneumatosis (white arrow), mesenteric venous gas within the superior mesenteric vein (SMV) (arrowhead) and portal venous gas (black arrow). **D.** Axial CT image demonstrates extensive portal venous gas. **E.** Axial CT image demonstrates air within the SMV (arrow) and diffuse small bowel pneumatosis. **F.** Axial CT image demonstrates air throughout the mesenteric and portal venous vasculature as well as pneumatosis within the gallbladder wall (arrow). **G.** Axial CT image demonstrates pneumatosis involving the stomach (arrows) in a patient with extensive small bowel ischemia, gastric and gallbladder ischemia.

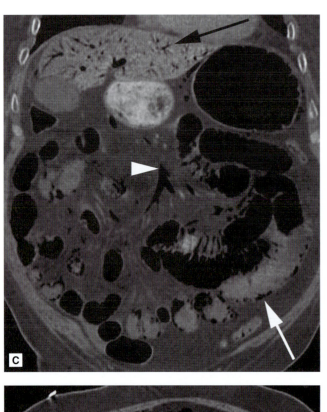

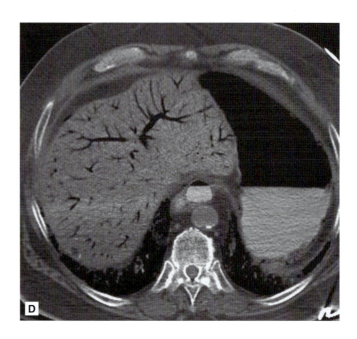

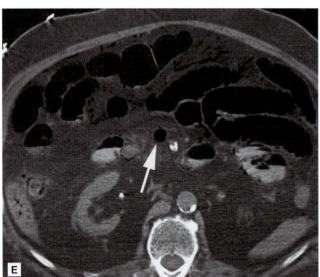

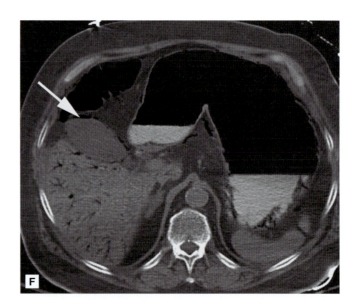

2. (*continued*)

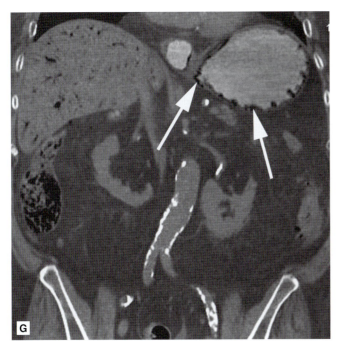

2. (*continued*)

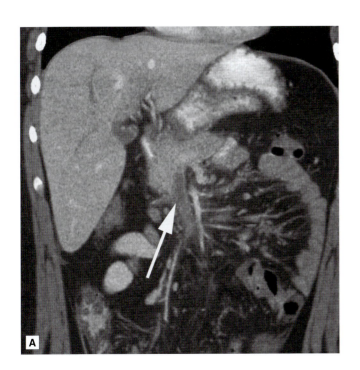

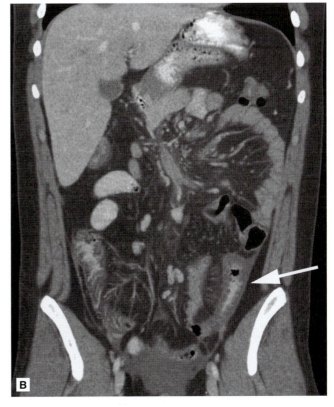

3. A. Axial, contrast-enhanced CT image reveals a large thrombus within the SMV (arrow). **B.** Axial, contrast-enhanced CT image demonstrates thickening of a focal segment of small bowel (arrow) secondary to ischemia resulting from the SMV thrombosis.

PRESENTATION

Depending on the cause, patients may be asymptomatic, present with nonspecific abdominal pain and distension, or may be acutely ill with melena, fever, vomiting, and diarrhea.

FINDINGS

CT demonstrates intramural band-like or linear densities in the affected bowel loop or entire intestine. Similar findings may be found on abdominal radiographs.

DIFFERENTIAL DIAGNOSIS

- Bowel necrosis
- Postendoscopy with polypectomy
- Postsurgical, medication-induced, autoimmune disease
- Pulmonary disease

COMMENTS

Pneumatosis intestinalis is an uncommon condition in which gas is found in a linear or cystic form in the submucosa or subserosa and, rarely, the muscularis layer of the bowel wall. Size of air collections varies from microscopic to several centimeters in diameter. Pneumatosis intestinalis is classified as either primary or secondary. Primary pneumatosis intestinalis is idiopathic and usually involves the colon in the adult population. Approximately less than one-fifth of cases of pneumatosis intestinalis are of the primary type. Secondary pneumatosis intestinalis usually involves the small bowel, especially jejunal loops, and is associated with bowel necrosis (from various causes: ischemic, inflammatory, obstructive, or infectious conditions of the intestine), chronic obstructive pulmonary diseases (COPDs), immunocompromised states (AIDS, post-transplant patients), and postendoscopy. A number of theories have been proposed to explain the pathophysiology of pneumatosis intestinalis of which mechanical, mucosal damage, bacterial and pulmonary theories appear to be most promising. The most common and most emergent life-threatening cause of intramural bowel gas is due to bowel ischemia and infarction, caused by necrotizing enterocolitis, neutropenic colitis, volvulus, or sepsis. Pneumatosis intestinalis secondary to mucosal disruption presumably due to overdistension of the bowel can also be caused by ulcerations, erosions, or trauma. Pneumatosis intestinalis in AIDS and immunosuppressive states is secondary to increased mucosal permeability. In COPD, severe cough leads to alveolar rupture resulting in the dissection of air into the mediastinum, which can then track through the diaphragm, along the major vessels and in the root of the mesentery into the bowel wall.

Symptoms are nonspecific and include abdominal pain, abdominal distension, diarrhea, mucus in stools, nausea, vomiting, and weight loss. In pneumatosis associated with other disorders, the symptoms may be those of the associated diseases. Complications caused by pneumatosis intestinalis occur infrequently, and include volvulus, intestinal obstruction, hemorrhage, and intestinal perforation.

The diagnosis can made with plain abdominal radiographs which may show pneumatosis intestinalis as radiolucent areas within the bowel wall. These radiolucencies may be linear or curvilinear or appear as grape-like clusters or tiny bubbles and must be differentiated from intraluminal intestinal gas. CT demonstrates band-like or linear distribution of air in the affected bowel wall. Pneumatosis typically disappears once blood flow to the affected segment is improved in cases of pneumatosis intestinalis secondary to transient ischemia of bowel without signs of bowel necrosis or other signs of peritoneal irritation.

PEARLS

- Pneumatosis intestinalis is a nonspecific finding, and can be found in benign conditions of the bowel or life-threatening bowel ischemia.

- Although the diagnosis can be made on plain abdominal radiographs, CT has more sensitivity and at the same time allows assessment of any underlying bowel pathology.

- No treatment is necessary if the finding is isolated finding. Otherwise, treatment is directed at the underlying cause of the pneumatosis.

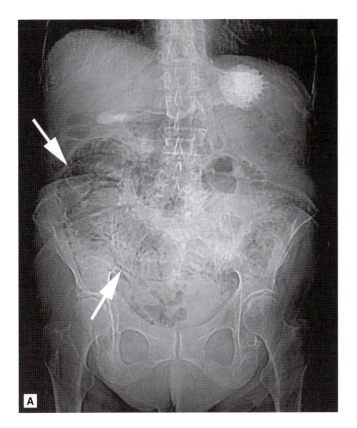

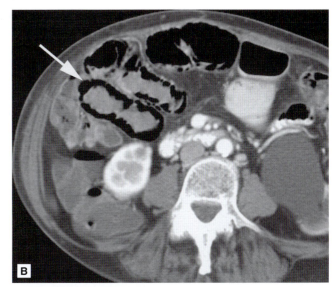

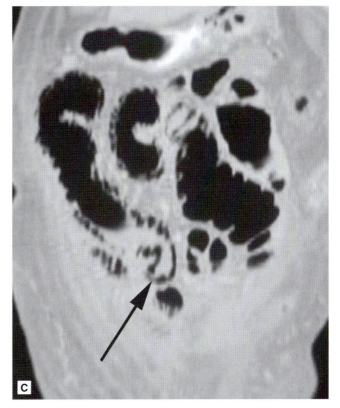

1. A. Abdominal radiograph reveals mottled lucencies within the bowel in the right lower quadrant (arrows), suspicious features for pneumatosis. **B.** Axial, contrast-enhanced CT image reveals extensive pneumatosis within bowel loops in the right lower quadrant (arrow). **C.** Coronal CT image reveals extensive pneumatosis within bowel loops in the right lower quadrant (arrow).

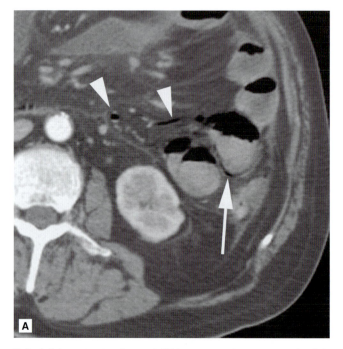

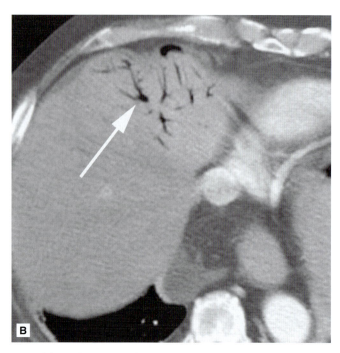

2. A. Axial, contrast-enhanced CT image reveals pneumatosis of the small bowel (arrow) extending into adjacent mesenteric veins (arrowheads). **B.** Axial, contrast-enhanced CT image reveals portal venous gas (arrow), a common feature in cases of pneumatosis.

PRESENTATION

Fever, abdominal pain, nausea, vomiting, diarrhea or constipation, and weight loss

FINDINGS

CT demonstrates findings of mesenteric arteritis, aneurysms, thromboembolism, focal or diffuse bowel wall thickening, dilated bowel, abnormal bowel wall enhancement, ascites, and lymphadenopathy.

DIFFERENTIAL DIAGNOSIS

- Crohn disease
- Small bowel obstruction
- Ischemic enteritis
- Shock bowel

COMMENTS

Vasculitis is the inflammation and necrosis of the wall of the blood vessels. Based on the size of the affected blood vessel, vasculitis can be classified into large vessel vasculitis such as giant cell arteritis and Takayasu arteritis that affect the aorta and its major branches, medium vessel vasculitis such as polyarteritis nodosa and Kawasaki disease that affect the visceral arteries and their branches and small vessel vasculitis such as Wegener granulomatosis, Churg-Strauss syndrome, microscopic polyangiitis, Henoch-Schonlein syndrome, systemic lupus erythematosus, rheumatoid vasculitis, and Behcet syndrome which involve the arterioles, venules, and capillaries. Gastrointestinal manifestations of vasculitis include abdominal pain, nausea, vomiting, diarrhea, and bleeding. Diffuse involvement of the mesenteric vasculature by vasculitis affects the small or large bowel and may produce a variety of complications including intestinal ischemia, hemorrhage, ileus, ulceration, infarction, and perforation.

There is significant overlap in the imaging features of the various vasculitis. Takayasu arteritis is predominantly seen in young women and classically involves the aortic arch but can also affect the abdominal aorta and mesenteric branches.

Conventional or CT angiograms demonstrate diffuse wall thickening and stenosis of the mesenteric arteries. Polyarteritis nodosa can affect medium-sized vessels such as the mesenteric and renal arteries leading to the formation of aneurysms typically at branch points. Henoch-Schonlein purpura is a vasculitis of small vessels and bowel is predominantly affected as a part of systemic disease. CT demonstrates wall thickening, luminal narrowing, fold thickening, and ulcerations. Systemic lupus erythematosus is a multisystem autoimmune disorder affecting small vessels. Antiphospholipid syndrome is seen in patients with lupus and predisposes to the development of mesenteric arterial or venous thrombosis, which subsequently leads to bowel ischemia. CT features of bowel ischemia include bowel thickening, edema, intramural hemorrhage, altered bowel wall enhancement, pneumatosis, and mesenteric venous gas. Behcet disease is a nonspecific necrotizing vasculitis characterized by orogenital ulcers and ocular inflammation, with gastrointestinal tract involvement occurring in less than half of the patients. The disease predominantly affects the terminal ileum in the form of large, deeply penetrating ulcers of the submucosa, muscular layer, or the entire wall. Thus, intestinal Behcet disease mimics Crohn disease on small bowel series and CT. The affected bowel demonstrates concentric bowel wall thickening or a polypoid mass with intense contrast enhancement on CT.

PEARLS

- Vasculitis is often a systemic disease with inflammation and necrosis of blood vessels resulting in ischemic changes in the end organs.

- Diffuse or focal involvement of gastrointestinal tract is often part of systemic manifestations leading to mesenteric ischemia, submucosal edema and hemorrhage, and bowel perforation.

- Radiological findings of various vasculitis often overlap significantly. Therefore, vasculitis should be suspected whenever mesenteric ischemic changes occur in younger patients.

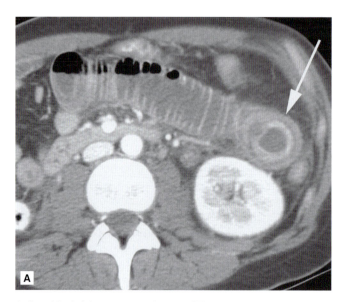
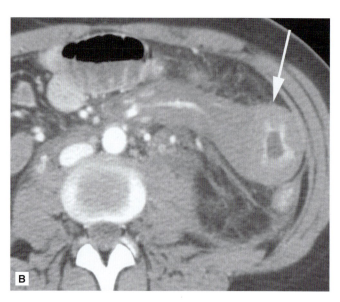

1. A and **B.** Axial, contrast-enhanced CT reveals marked submucosal edema on the small bowel of a patient with Henoch-Schonlein purpura (arrow).

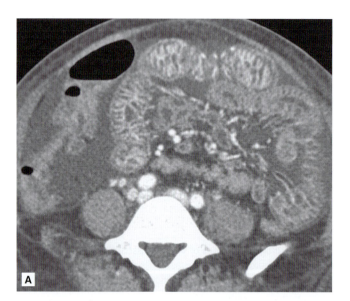
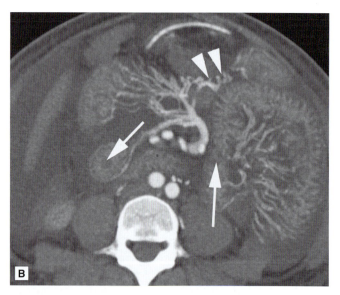

2. A. Axial, contrast-enhanced CT reveals bowel mucosal hyperenhancement and wall edema in a patient with systemic lupus erythematosus. **B.** Axial, contrast-enhanced CT reveals small bowel wall thickening (arrows) and a corkscrew appearance of the small vessels of the mesenteric vasculature (arrowheads) in a patient with systemic lupus erythematosus.

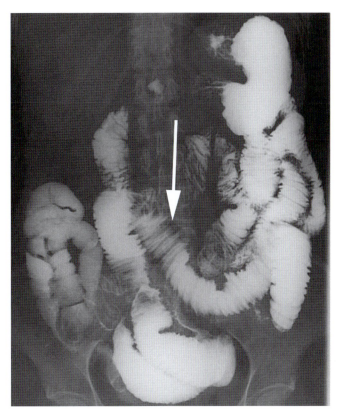

3. Spot film acquired during small bowel follow-through demonstrates regular small bowel fold thickening (arrow) in a patient with systemic lupus erythematosus.

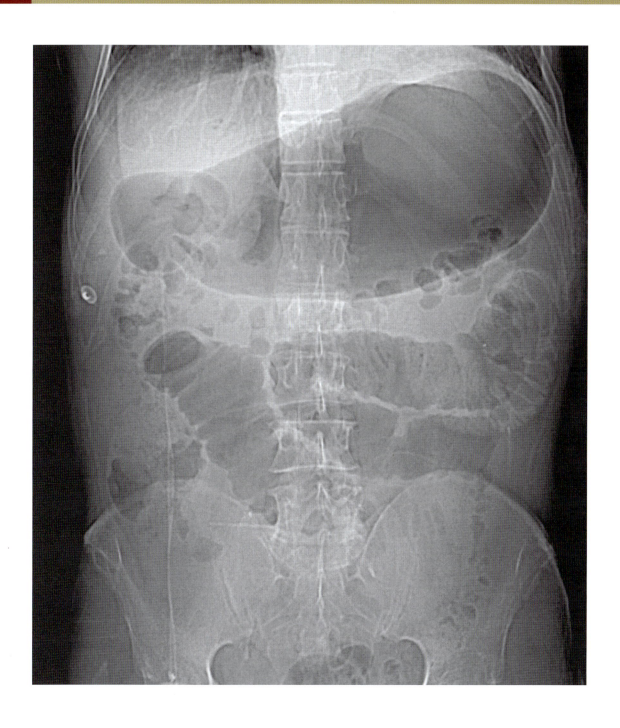

PRESENTATION

Pain, vomiting, constipation, fever, abdominal distention, tenderness, and guarding

FINDINGS

CT demonstrates a discrete transition zone with dilation of bowel proximally, decompression of bowel distally, intra-luminal contrast that does not pass beyond the transition zone, and a colon containing little gas or fluid.

DIFFERENTIAL DIAGNOSIS

- Paralytic ileus
- Aerophagia
- Ascites
- Cystic fibrosis

COMMENTS

Mechanical small bowel obstruction is the most frequently seen disorder of the small intestine. A wide range of etiologies have been identified, but intra-abdominal adhesions related to prior surgery is the leading cause of obstruction in majority of series. Other common etiologies include hernias, Crohn disease, and primary intestinal neoplasms. Obstruction can be simple or strangulated; in a simple obstruction, the intestinal lumen is partially or completely occluded without compromise of the intestinal blood flow. In strangulated obstruction, blood flow to the obstructed segment is compromised leading to tissue necrosis and gangrene. The etiologies of mechanical intestinal obstruction are classified based on the anatomic relationship of the obstructing lesion to the intestinal wall: (1) intralumi-nal causes such as foreign bodies, gallstones, inspissated intestinal contents; (2) intramural causes such as tumors, hematoma, and strictures related to inflammatory bowel disease; (3) extrinsic causes such as adhesions, hernias, or carcinomatosis. Based on the pattern of obstruction, they can be open-looped or closed-loop obstructions. An open-looped obstruction occurs when intestinal flow is blocked but proximal decompression is possible whereas in closed-loop obstruction, inflow and outflow from the loop are both blocked. This obstruction leads to accumulation of gas and secretions within the loop thus compromising the macrovascular perfusion of the intestine leading to intestinal ischemia and, ultimately, necrosis.

The clinical manifestations of small bowel obstruction are colicky abdominal pain, nausea, vomiting, obstipation, abdominal distention, and hyperactive bowel sounds. The prime role of imaging studies is to confirm the diagnosis of bowel obstruction, identify the site of obstruction and the lesion responsible for the obstruction, and to assess development of complications. The abdominal radiograph demonstrates dilated small bowel loops (> 3 cm in diameter), air-fluid levels (upright films), and a paucity of air in the colon. Bowel distension and air-fluid level may be absent on the abdominal radiograph in spite of bowel obstruction if the obstruction is located in the proximal small bowel and in cases of closed-loop obstruction where bowel is filled with only fluid without gas. CT has higher sensitivity and specificity in the detection of small bowel obstruction. CT demonstrates a discrete transition zone with dilation of bowel proximally, decompression of bowel distally, intra-luminal contrast that does not pass beyond the transition zone, and a colon containing little gas or fluid. Severity of the obstruction can be estimated grossly by the degree of proximal bowel dilation and distal bowel collapse. A greater than 50% difference in caliber between the proximal dilated bowel and the distal collapsed bowel is suggestive of high-grade obstruction. Closed-loop obstruction is seen as a U-shaped or C-shaped dilated bowel loop with a radial distribution of mesenteric vessels converging toward the point of obstruction. Strangulation is diagnosed by identifying thickening of the bowel wall, pneumatosis intestinalis, portal venous gas, mesenteric haziness, and a poorly enhancing diseased segment of bowel. CT can also precisely demonstrate extrinsic causes of bowel obstruction.

PEARLS

- Intra-abdominal adhesions related to prior surgery is the leading cause of obstruction in majority of the cases of small bowel obstruction followed by hernias, inflammatory bowel disease, and primary neoplasms.

- The main goals of imaging are to confirm the diagnosis of bowel obstruction, identify the site of obstruction and the lesion responsible for the obstruction, and assess nature and complications of obstruction.

- Although the abdominal radiograph is often the first radiological study performed, CT is the best modality to obtain all the relevant information necessary for decision making and planning operative therapy when indicated.

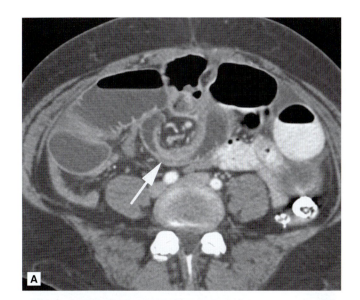

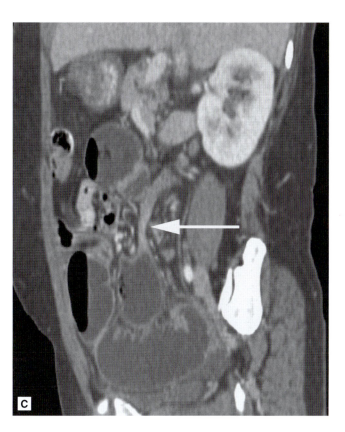

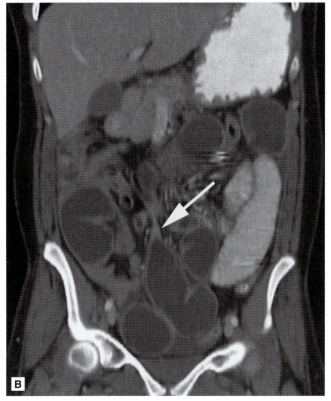

1. A. Axial, contrast-enhanced CT reveals abnormally dilated, fluid-filled loops of small bowel proximal to a clearly identified transition point (arrow) in a patient with mechanical small obstruction related to adhesive disease. **B.** Coronal, contrast-enhanced CT demonstrates a transition point (arrow) immediately distal to dilated, fluid-filled loops of small bowel. **C.** Sagittal, contrast-enhanced CT reveals a transition point (arrow) in a patient with an uncomplicated small bowel obstruction.

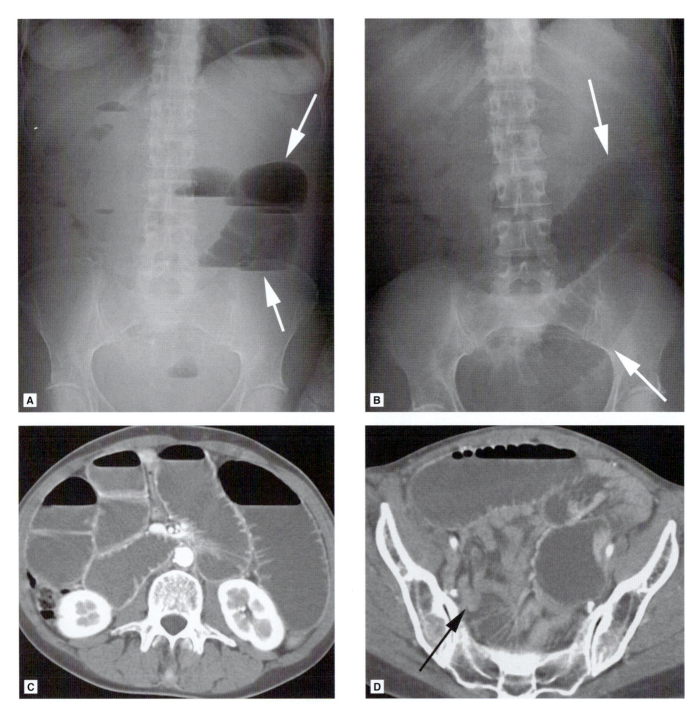

2. A. Upright abdominal radiograph demonstrates distended loops of small bowel (arrows) with multiple air-fluid levels in the leftward aspect of the abdomen. **B.** Supine abdominal radiograph reveals significant distention of a segment of small bowel (arrows) with relative paucity of gas within the colon, findings consistent with a mechanical small bowel obstruction. **C.** Axial, contrast-enhanced CT reveals diffusely distended loops of small bowel; of note, normal mucosal enhancement is seen throughout. **D.** Axial, contrast-enhanced CT reveals normal, collapsed small bowel loops (arrow) within the pelvis, consistent with a mechanical small bowel obstruction.

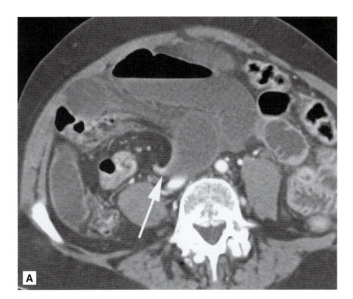

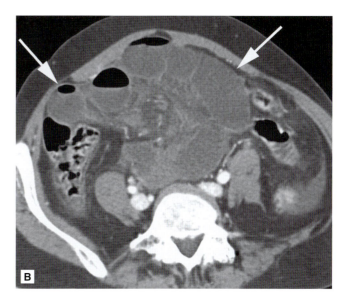

3. A. Axial, contrast-enhanced CT reveals a focal, C-shaped region of dilated loops of small bowel with one transition point clearly identified (arrow) in a patient with a closed-loop obstruction. **B.** Axial, contrast-enhanced CT reveals a focal, C-shaped region of dilated loops of small bowel with mesenteric edema (arrows), findings typically seen in cases of closed-loop obstruction.

PRESENTATION

Recurrent right upper quadrant pain, nausea, vomiting, and other signs of bowel obstruction

FINDINGS

CT demonstrates a calcified ectopic gallstone, air in the biliary tree, dilated bowel loops, and a cholecystoenteric fistula.

DIFFERENTIAL DIAGNOSIS

- Dropped gallstone
- Small bowel obstruction secondary to adhesions
- Intussusception
- Small bowel tumor
- Pseudo-obstruction

COMMENTS

Gallstone ileus is a rare type of intestinal obstruction caused by a gallstone or gallstones within the lumen of the bowel. This complication of gallstone cholecystitis is more common in the elderly women, with most patients presenting in the seventh or eighth decades of life. Nausea, vomiting, abdominal pain, and other signs and symptoms of intestinal obstruction are the most common presenting clinical symptoms of patients with gallstone ileus. The pathophysiology of gallstone ileus is initiated by inflammation of the gallbladder wall caused by a gallstone obstructing the cystic duct. The Inflamed gallbladder may become adherent to the adjacent duodenum or, less frequently, stomach, common bile duct, or colon. A cholecystoenteric fistula is then be formed between the adjacent viscus with ischemic necrosis and erosion of the gallbladder wall from an impacted gallstone. When gallstones large enough to cause obstruction enter the bowel via a cholecystoenteric fistula, they travel through the intestinal tract and produce intermittent obstruction, with relapsing and recurrent symptoms. The culprit gallstone will then be passed spontaneously in the majority of cases. However, stones with a diameter larger than 2.5 cm may become impacted. The terminal ileum and ileocecal valve are the most frequent sites of obstruction, but other obstruction locations, including the duodenum, jejunum, and colon are also possible.

Abdominal radiographs will demonstrate evidence of intestinal obstruction with pneumobilia or a calcified stone distant from the gallbladder. CT demonstrates a calcified ectopic gallstone, dilated bowel loops, air in the biliary tree, and, possibly, a cholecystoenteric fistula. CT also has the added advantage of locating the exact site of stone impaction and obstruction which can be used for preoperative planning. The classic radiological features of gallstone ileus including pneumobilia, intestinal obstruction, and aberrant intraluminal gallstone location are known as Rigler triad.

PEARLS

- Gallstone ileus is a rare complication of gallstone cholecystitis and causes intestinal obstruction due to impaction of a gallstone or gallstones within the lumen of the bowel.

- Obstruction occurs more often with stones larger than 2.5 cm and at the terminal ileum.

- The classic radiological features of gallstone ileus include pneumobilia, intestinal obstruction, aberrant gallstone location, and a change in the location of a previously observed stone.

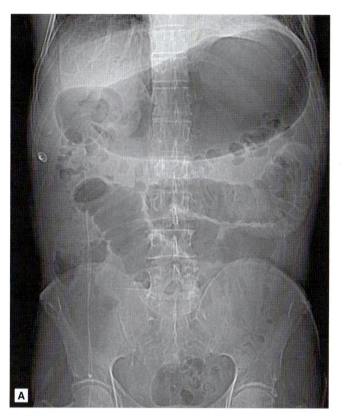

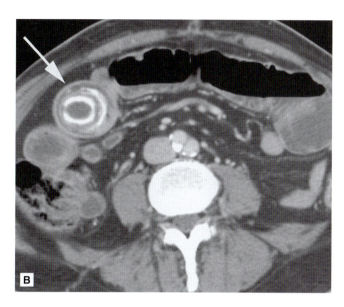

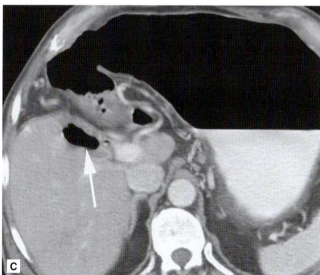

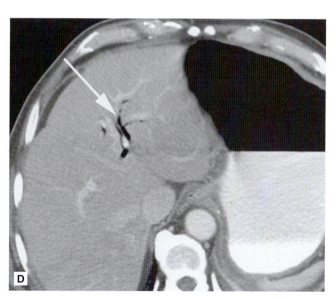

1. A. Scout topogram image reveals several loops of moderately distended small bowel within the mid-abdomen. **B.** Axial, contrast-enhanced CT image reveals a lamellated gallstone within the distal ileum (arrow) causing a mechanical small bowel obstruction. **C.** Axial, contrast-enhanced CT image reveals air within the gallbladder lumen (arrow). **D.** Axial, contrast-enhanced CT image reveals pneumobilia (arrow), a classic feature associated with gallstone ileus.

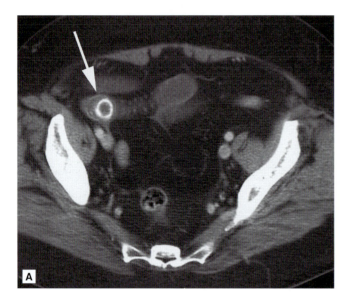

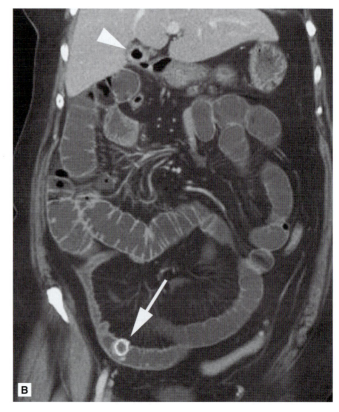

2. A. Axial, contrast-enhanced CT image reveals a calcified gallstone within the distal ileum (arrow) causing a mechanical small bowel obstruction. **B.** Coronal, contrast-enhanced CT image reveals a calcified gallstone within the distal ileum (arrow) causing a mechanical small bowel obstruction. Air within the gallbladder lumen is also noted (arrowhead).

PRESENTATION

Vague abdominal pain which can be acute, intermittent or chronic; vomiting; red blood in stool

FINDINGS

CT demonstrates bowel-within-bowel appearance with a target- or sausage-shaped mass.

DIFFERENTIAL DIAGNOSIS

- Metastases and lymphoma
- Primary bowel tumor
- Serosal endometrial implant
- Meckel diverticulum

COMMENTS

An intussusception represents invagination of a proximal segment of a bowel (intussusceptum) into the lumen of the immediately distal segment (intussuscipiens). When compared to childhood intussusception, adult intussusceptions are rare and the majority of them have a lead point. An intussusception results in obstruction and ischemic injury to the intussuscepting segment. Four common types of intussusception are recognized: ileoileal (enteric), ileocolic, ileocecal, and colonic. Most intussusceptions in the small intestine are secondary to benign neoplasms (polyps, lipoma, leiomyolipoma, hemangioma, neurofibroma), adhesions, Meckel diverticulum, lymphoid hyperplasia, adenitis, trauma, celiac disease, intestinal duplication, and malignant lesions such as lymphoma or metastases. Intussusceptions occur when a mass in the bowel is pulled forward by normal peristalsis, with resultant invagination o the involved wall. Intussusceptions may also be caused by functional disturbances of the intestine without a gross mural abnormality. Patients with AIDS are more prone to develop intussusceptions because of the association of AIDS with a variety of infectious and neoplastic conditions of the bowel. Intussusception seen following abdominal surgery may be due to adhesions, intestinal dysmotility, submucosal bowel edema, anatomic suture lines, and long intestinal tubes. Small bowel intussusception may be transient, a phenomenon that is more commonly seen in the proximal small bowel associated with celiac disease, Crohn disease, malabsorption syndromes, and intestinal tumors. The clinical findings are variable. Most patients are present with intermittent, subacute, or chronic abdominal symptoms. Abdominal pain is the most common, symptom followed by nausea. It presents acutely as intestinal obstruction. The classic triad includes abdominal pain, palpable sausage-shaped mass, and heme-positive stools.

The abdominal radiograph is usually the first diagnostic imaging modality and shows signs of intestinal obstruction and some clues regarding the site of obstruction. Barium studies can help identify the site and common causes of intussusceptions, especially in chronic cases. The barium meal follow-through typically shows a "stacked coins" or "coiled spring" appearance which represents the barium-filled intestinal folds of the intussuscipiens. Barium studies are absolutely contraindicated in cases of bowel perforation or ischemia. US may demonstrate a "target" or "doughnut" sign on transverse views and a "pseudokidney sign" on longitudinal views. Abdominal CT is the most useful tool for the diagnosis of intussusception and for distinguishing between lead point intussusception secondary to bowel pathology and transient intussusception without any lead point. CT characteristically demonstrates a target- or sausage-shaped mass in the early stages with a bowel-within-bowel configuration, with or without adjacent mesenteric fat and vessels. In the later stages, longitudinal compression and venous congestion in the intussusceptum give a layering effect to the entire mass.

PEARLS

- Adult small intestinal intussusception is a rare entity when compared to the pediatric population and is often associated with small bowel pathology such as benign bowel tumors.

- Ileoileal intussusceptions is the most common type and presents with vague abdominal symptoms.

- CT is the most useful imaging modality for the diagnosis of intussusception and identifying the lead point. CT typically demonstrates a bowel-within-bowel appearance.

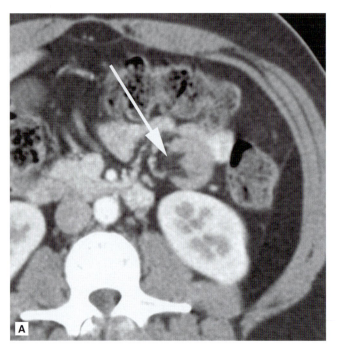
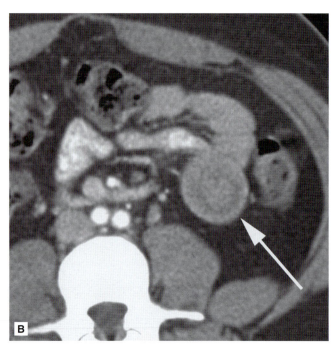

1. A. Axial, contrast-enhanced CT image reveals extension of the mesenteric fat and vessels into a small bowel loop (arrow). **B.** Axial, contrast-enhanced CT image reveals a classic bowel-within-bowel appearance of a small bowel intussusception (arrow).

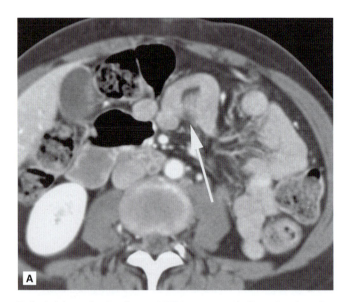
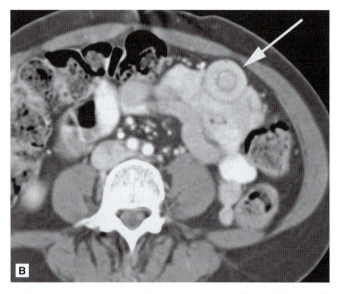

2. A. Axial, contrast-enhanced CT image reveals the extension of mesenteric fat and vessels into an adjacent loop of small bowel (arrow). **B.** Axial, contrast-enhanced CT image reveals a bowel-within-bowel appearance of a small bowel intussusception (arrow).

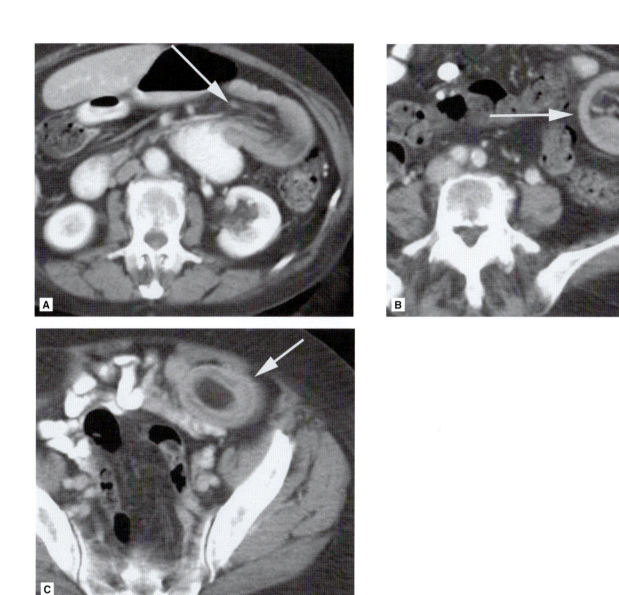

3. A. Axial, contrast-enhanced CT image reveals extension of a large portion of mesenteric fat and vessels into a small bowel loop (arrow). **B.** Axial, contrast-enhanced CT image reveals a large intussusception with the intussuscipiens containing bowel as well as a large portion of mesenteric fat (arrow). **C.** Axial, contrast-enhanced CT image reveals a large portion of mesenteric fat contained within the intussuscipiens (arrow).

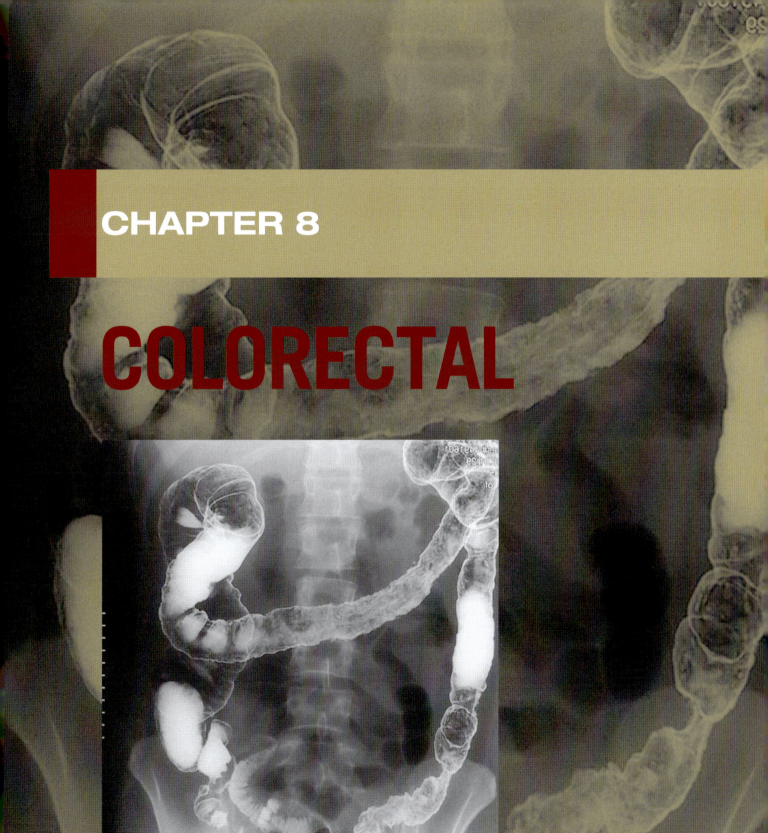

CHAPTER 8

COLORECTAL

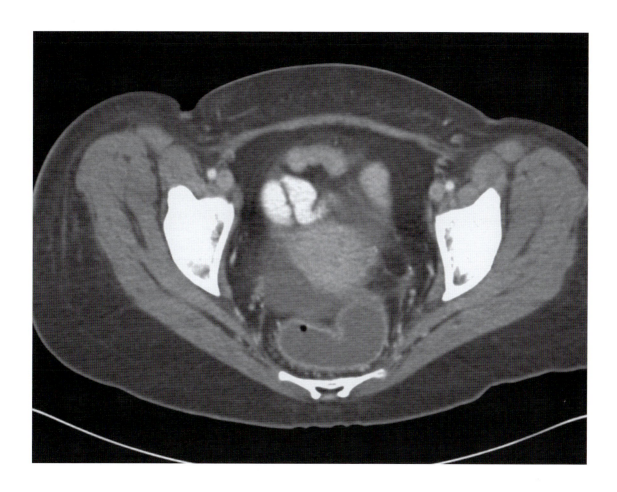

PRESENTATION

Patients usually present with left lower quadrant pain and tenderness with or without fever. In addition, some patients also have a palpable mass and altered bowel movements.

FINDINGS

CT demonstrates colonic wall thickening, fat stranding, and thickening of the mesentery adjacent to the site of diverticulitis. Advanced cases also show pericolic abscess, fistulae, and sinus tracts.

DIFFERENTIAL DIAGNOSIS

- Colon carcinoma
- Radiation colitis
- Ischemic colitis
- Pseudomembranous colitis

COMMENTS

Diverticulitis refers to inflammation or infection associated with a diverticulum. It is estimated to affect up to one-fourth of the population with diverticulosis. Diverticular disease is the most common pathological process affecting the colon in the general population. The sigmoid colon is the most commonly affected segment of the colon in more than 90% of the population. Diverticula typically develop at points of weakness in the bowel wall, usually corresponding to the areas at which the vasa recta penetrate the circular muscle layer of the bowel. Obstruction of the neck of the diverticulum by stool, inflammation, or food particles results in perforation. Macroscopic or microscopic perforation of a diverticulum leads to contamination, inflammation, and infection in the peridiverticular and pericolic regions. This leads to a spectrum of diseases ranging from mild uncomplicated diverticulitis to perforation and diffuse peritonitis.

Patients with acute diverticulitis typically present with left lower quadrant abdominal pain, fever, and lower abdominal tenderness. Nausea, vomiting, diarrhea, constipation, dysuria, and urinary frequency are less common symptoms. Few patients may present with a lower abdominal mass, tachycardia, and elevated white blood cell count with leftward shift. Location of the abdominal pain and tenderness can vary depending on the segment of the colon that is inflamed.

An upright chest film, together with upright and supine abdominal films may be abnormal in up to 50% of patients, with abnormal findings such as pneumoperitoneum, bowel dilatation from obstruction or ileus, or a soft tissue density suggesting an abscess. Barium enema using water-soluble contrast demonstrates extravasation of contrast material with or without an abscess cavity, an intramural sinus tract, or a fistula. Computed tomography (CT) is the most appropriate test for the diagnosis of acute diverticulitis and has the ability to image mural and extraluminal disease and to direct therapy with percutaneous drainage of abscesses. CT features of acute diverticulitis include the presence of diverticula with fat stranding, thickening of the colonic wall, and formation of abscesses. Complications such as perforation and colovesical fistula are better evaluated with CT. An abscess appears as a low-attenuation mass (fluid density) with central air or air-fluid levels and surrounding inflammatory changes. Sigmoid diverticulitis tends to form colovesical fistulas in the left posterolateral aspect of the urinary bladder. CT demonstrates air within the bladder and thickening of the bladder wall, adjacent to a diseased segment of bowel. Colon cancer is one of the important differentials to be considered in the setting of acute diverticulitis. Imaging features of colon cancer and diverticulitis are indistinguishable in many patients. Fluid in the root of the sigmoid mesentery and engorgement of adjacent sigmoid mesenteric vasculature favor the diagnosis of diverticulitis, whereas the presence of a large inflammatory mass, bowel obstruction, and pericolic lymph nodes more likely represents colon cancer rather than diverticulitis.

PEARLS

- Inflammation of diverticula occurs in up to one-fourth of the population with diverticulosis. Microperforation from an occluded diverticular neck is the initiating event of the disease process.

- CT demonstrates diverticulosis with long-segment colonic wall thickening, pericolonic mesenteric fat stranding, and vessel engorgement.

- Colon cancer mimics the imaging appearance of diverticulitis; presence of a large inflammatory mass, bowel obstruction, and pericolonic lymph nodes should raise suspicion for colon cancer rather than diverticulitis.

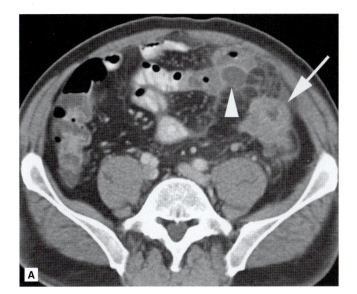

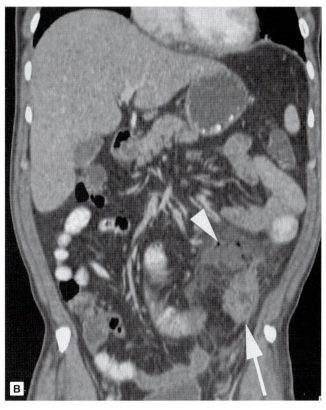

1. A. Axial, contrast-enhanced CT image demonstrates circumferential thickening of the descending colon (arrow) as well as a diverticular abscess (arrowhead). **B.** Coronal, contrast-enhanced CT image demonstrates circumferential thickening of the descending colon (arrow), pericolonic fat stranding, as well as a diverticular abscess (arrowhead).

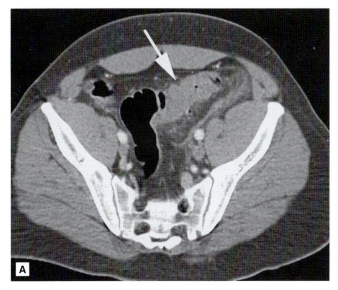

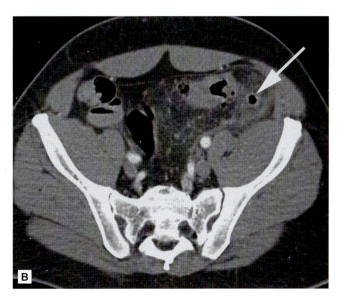

2. A. Axial, contrast-enhanced CT image demonstrates circumferential thickening of the sigmoid colon (arrow) with surrounding fat stranding consistent with acute diverticulitis. **B.** Axial, contrast-enhanced CT image demonstrates direct visualization of an inflamed diverticulum (arrow), as evidenced by marked surrounding fat stranding, in a case of acute sigmoid diverticulitis. **C.** Axial, contrast-enhanced CT image demonstrates circumferential thickening of the sigmoid colon (arrow), which is seen to normalize more distally, in this case of acute diverticulitis.

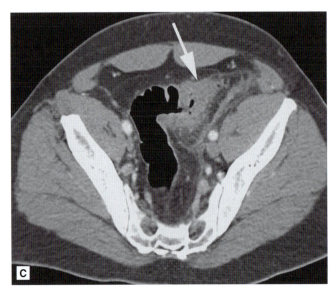

2. (*Continued*)

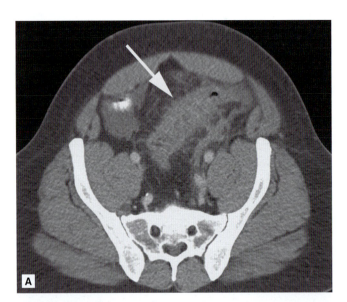

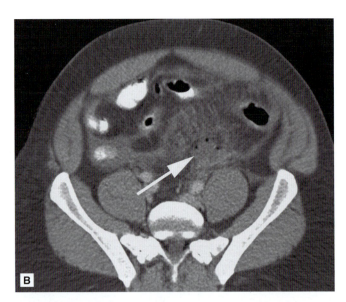

3. A. Axial, contrast-enhanced CT image reveals thickening of the sigmoid colon (arrow) with surrounding pericolonic fat stranding. **B.** Axial, contrast-enhanced CT image reveals a small diverticular abscess (arrow) adjacent to the sigmoid colon in the pelvis.

PRESENTATION

Continuous abdominal pain occurs for several days in an area corresponding to the contour of the colon. Constitutional symptoms such as nausea, vomiting, and anorexia are less frequent. Localized tenderness over the site of inflammation is common and is often associated with marked rebound tenderness without rigidity.

FINDINGS

CT demonstrates oval-shaped fat-density appendages in the pericolonic area, with surrounding inflammatory and edematous changes.

DIFFERENTIAL DIAGNOSIS

- Diverticulitis
- Acute omental infarction
- Sclerosing mesenteritis
- Primary or metastatic tumor involvement of the mesocolon

COMMENTS

Epiploic appendagitis represents primary inflammation of the colonic epiploic appendages. Epiploic (or omental) appendages arise from the serosal surface of the colon and are composed of adipose tissue and blood vessels. Epiploic appendagitis usually results from infarction of the colonic appendages secondary to torsion and inflammation. Other causes include incarcerated hernia, intestinal obstruction, and intraperitoneal loose body. In decreasing order of frequency, the most common sites of acute epiploic appendagitis are areas around the sigmoid colon, the descending colon, and the right hemicolon. Acute epiploic appendagitis is associated with obesity, hernias, and unusually extreme exercise. An acute episode of epiploic appendagitis is self-limited in the majority of patients. Complications are occasionally seen in acute epiploic appendagitis and include adhesions, bowel obstruction, intussusception, intraperitoneal loose body, peritonitis, and intra-abdominal abscesses.

Patients with epiploic appendagitis present with acute lower quadrant abdominal pain localized to the involved segment of the colon. Constitutional symptoms such as nausea, vomiting, and anorexia are less frequent. Patients usually have a normal white blood cell count and body temperature.

Epiploic appendagitis is predominantly diagnosed on cross-sectional imaging. CT demonstrates an oval fat-density lesion adjacent to anterior wall of colon with surrounding signs of inflammation and edema. In addition, a central area of high attenuation due to venous thrombosis, if present, increases the diagnostic specificity. Progression of inflammation leads to thickening of the colonic wall and parietal peritoneum. Intestinal obstruction and abscess formation are very rare complications. Targeted ultrasonography (US) in the area of pain and tenderness may show an oval noncompressible hyperechoic focus, adjacent to the colon, without central blood flow. T1- and T2-weighted magnetic resonance (MR) images show an oval lesion with fat-signal and surrounding inflammation and peripheral rim enhancement.

PEARLS

- Epiploic appendagitis is a self-limiting inflammation of the colonic epiploic appendages, which most commonly involves the rectosigmoid colon and which clinically presents with acute lower abdominal pain.

- CT demonstrates a round, fatty lesion in the pericolonic region with a hyperdense rim and peripheral enhancement.

- Cross-sectional images such as CT plays important role in differentiating various etiologies which may mimic epiploic appendagitis.

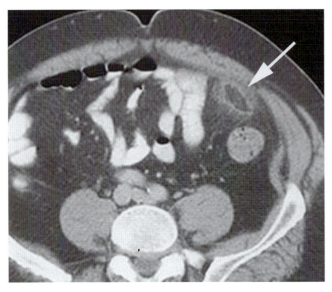

1. Axial, contrast-enhanced CT image demonstrates an ovoid, fat-attenuating lesion (arrow) surrounded by inflammatory stranding in the left lower quadrant, the imaging features of which are highly suggestive of epiploic appendagitis.

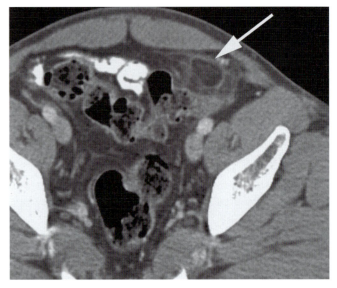

3. Axial, contrast-enhanced CT image reveals an ovoid, fat-attenuating lesion (arrow) with surrounding inflammatory stranding adjacent to the sigmoid colon, findings consistent with epiploic appendagitis.

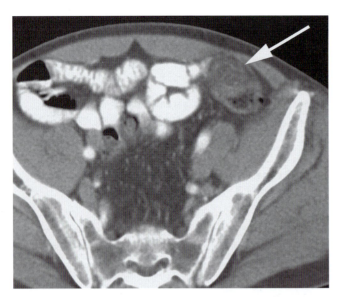

2. Axial, contrast-enhanced CT image demonstrates an inflamed, ovoid, fat-attenuating lesion (arrow) abutting the descending colon in a case of epiploic appendagitis.

PRESENTATION

Typically presents with periumbilical pain that migrates to the right lower quadrant, followed by anorexia and nausea.

FINDINGS

CT demonstrates a distended appendix of greater than 7 mm in diameter and circumferential wall thickening, which may give the appearance of a halo or target. Advanced cases also show periappendiceal fat stranding, edema, peritoneal fluid, phlegmon, or a periappendiceal abscess.

DIFFERENTIAL DIAGNOSIS

Differential diagnoses are considered if the abnormal appendix is not directly visualized, and include the following:

- Crohn disease
- Cecal diverticulitis
- Ileal diverticulitis
- Perforated cecal or appendiceal carcinoma
- Pelvic inflammatory disease

COMMENTS

Inflammation of the appendix is initiated by obstruction of the lumen by various etiologies such as inspissated stool (fecalith or appendicolith), lymphoid hyperplasia, vegetable matter or seeds, parasites, or a neoplasm. The lumen of the appendix is small in relation to its length, and this configuration may predispose to closed-loop obstruction. Obstruction of the appendiceal lumen leads to progressive accumulation of secretions which cause intraluminal distention and increased wall pressure. Luminal distention produces the visceral pain sensation experienced by the patient as periumbilical pain. Overgrowth of bacteria within the lumen and distension of the lumen can cause impairment of lymphatic and venous drainage, leading to mucosal ischemia. These findings in combination promote a localized inflammatory process that may progress to gangrene and perforation. Inflammation of the adjacent peritoneum gives rise to localized pain in the right lower quadrant. Although there is considerable variability, perforation typically occurs after at least 48 hours from the onset of symptoms and is accompanied by an abscess cavity walled-off by the small intestine and omentum. Rarely, free perforation of the appendix into the peritoneal cavity occurs that may be accompanied by peritonitis and septic shock and can be complicated by the subsequent formation of multiple intraperitoneal abscesses.

The plain abdominal radiograph may demonstrate the appendicolith, which is suggestive of appendicitis in the right clinical setting. However, US is often the first imaging study obtained to evaluate for possible appendicitis. US has about 85% specificity and up to 90% sensitivity for diagnosing appendicitis. In acute appendicitis, US demonstrates a thick-walled, noncompressible, blind-ending tubular structure in the right lower quadrant measuring 7 mm or more in anteroposterior diameter, with or without an appendicolith. The appearance on cross-sectional images is referred to as a target lesion. More advanced cases may demonstrate periappendiceal fluid or a mass lesion. The appendix is difficult to assess by US in the presence of gas-distend bowel and obesity. A negative or inconclusive examination should be followed by a CT study. Contrast-enhanced CT has a sensitivity, specificity, and accuracy of more than 95% in the diagnosis of acute appendicitis. On CT, the abnormal appendix presents as a slightly distended, circumferentially thickened fluid-filled structure approximately 0.5 to 2 cm in diameter with peripheral enhancement and linear fat stranding in the adjacent mesoappendix suggestive of periappendiceal inflammation. The diagnosis of acute appendicitis on noncontrast CT scans requires the detection of a thickened appendix with associated inflammatory changes in the periappendiceal fat or abnormal thickening of the right lateroconal fascia, with or without a calcified appendicolith. The combination of right lower quadrant inflammation, phlegmon, and an abscess adjacent to the cecum is suggestive but not diagnostic of appendicitis. CT is the optimal imaging modality to assess intra-abdominal complication of appendicitis. Finally, in cases of suspected appendicitis in pregnant patients, noncontrast MRI is being successfully applied.

PEARLS

- Inflammation of the appendix is caused by luminal obstruction, often by a fecalith or appendicolith leading to an enlarged, thickened appendix which can be easily imaged with cross-sectional modalities.

- US is often the first test obtained and demonstrates a thick-walled, noncompressible, blind-ending tubular structure in the right lower quadrant, measuring 7 mm or more in anteroposterior diameter with or without an appendicolith.

- A negative or inconclusive US is usually followed by a contrast-enhanced CT if the clinical suspicion remains high for appendicitis and imaging confirmation is required. Noncontrast MRI is valuable in pregnant woman with abdominal pain suspicious for appendicitis.

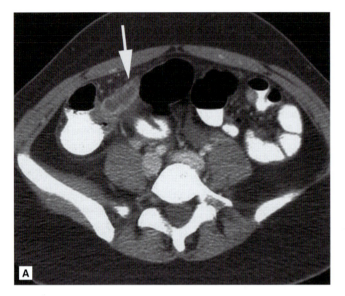
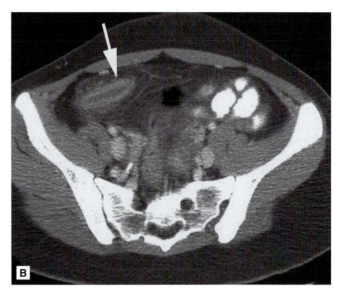

1. **A.** Axial, contrast-enhanced CT image demonstrates an abnormally dilated, fluid-filled appendix (arrow). Note the secondary finding of inflammation of the cecum at the base of the appendix. **B.** Axial, contrast-enhanced CT image demonstrates an abnormally dilated, fluid-filled appendix with periappendiceal stranding (arrow), consistent with acute appendicitis.

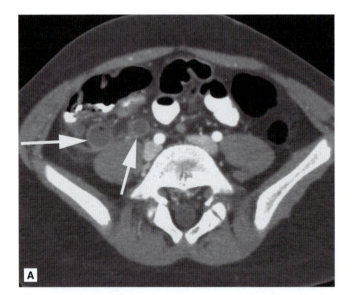
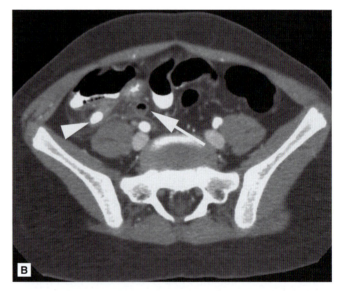

2. **A.** Axial, contrast-enhanced CT image demonstrates a dilated, fluid-filled appendix with periappendiceal stranding (arrows). **B.** Axial, contrast-enhanced CT image demonstrates an appendicolith (arrowhead) at the base of an abnormally distended appendix. Note the presence of air within the distal aspect of the appendix (arrow), a finding which may be seen in cases of acute appendicitis.

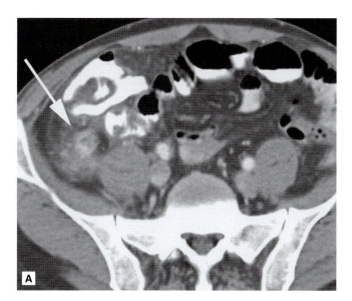

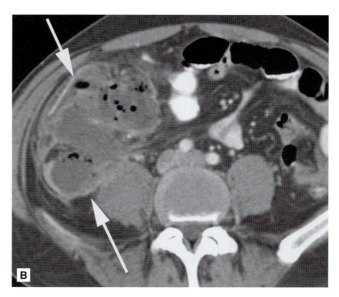

3. A. Axial, contrast-enhanced CT image demonstrates an enlarged appendix (arrow) with surrounding stranding and phlegmon. **B.** Axial, contrast-enhanced CT image demonstrates a large abscess (abscess) in the right lower quadrant secondary to perforation in a case of acute appendicitis (arrows).

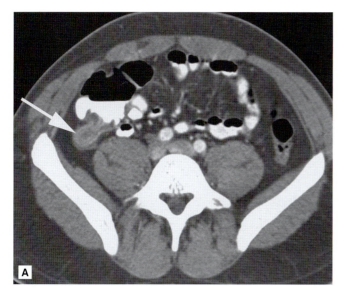

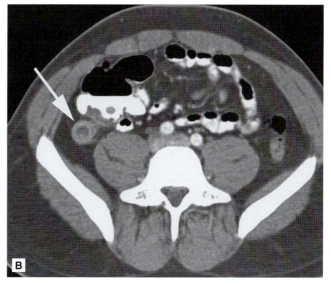

4. A. Axial, contrast-enhanced CT image demonstrates an enlarged appendix (arrow) in a case of acute appendicitis. Again, inflammation of the cecum at the base of the appendix is seen, a secondary sign in cases of acute appendicitis. **B.** Axial, contrast-enhanced CT image demonstrates an enlarged appendix (arrow) with surrounding stranding; inflammation of the cecum is again seen. **C.** Coronal, contrast-enhanced CT image demonstrates an abnormally dilated, fluid-filled appendix (arrow) with mild surrounding stranding in a case of acute appendicitis.

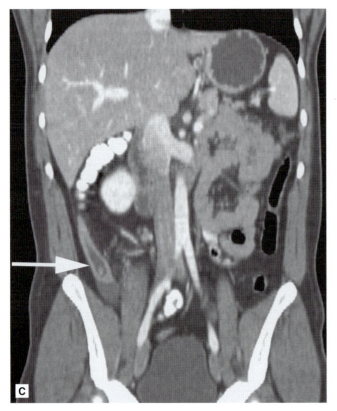

4. (*Continued*)

PRESENTATION

Patients commonly present with colicky abdominal pain, distention, as well as nausea and vomiting.

FINDINGS

On CT, in cases of cecal volvulus, the cecum is abnormally positioned in the upper-, mid-, and left-abdomen and can be traced back to the level of the volvulus, which appears as an area of swirling of the bowel and its mesentery.

DIFFERENTIAL DIAGNOSIS

- Ileus
- Small bowel obstruction
- Sigmoid volvulus
- Intestinal malrotation

COMMENTS

Cecal volvulus represents torsion of the cecum about its own mesentery, a condition responsible for approximately 1% of acute intestinal obstructions and for 25% to 40% of all cases of colonic volvulus. Hypermobility of the proximal colon leading to volvulus is caused by an abnormal peritoneal fixation. A cecal volvulus may occur if there is an additional insult such as scarring, adhesions, or an abdominal mass that serves as a fulcrum for the colon to rotate. Factors that predispose to dilatation of the right colon, such as pregnancy and recent colonoscopy, may also promote a cecal volvulus. Patients with cecal volvulus present with colicky abdominal pain, nausea, vomiting, and obstipation.

The classic findings on abdominal radiographs are signs of bowel obstruction and presence of a focal round loop of markedly air-distended bowel with haustral markings directed toward the left upper quadrant. The loop may resemble a coffee bean, which has an appearance similar to that of the well-known radiographic sign of sigmoid volvulus. Although the barium enema examination has a high sensitivity for cecal volvulus, it has largely been replaced by CT in the acute setting. At barium enema, the distal colon appears decompressed, and there is a beak-like tapering at the level of the volvulus. At CT, the cecum is located abnormally positioned in the upper-, mid-, and left-abdomen and can be traced back to the level of the volvulus, which appears as an area of swirling of the bowel and its mesentery (the "whirl" sign).

Complications of cecal volvulus include closed-loop bowel obstruction and vascular compromise, which can lead to gangrene, perforation, and death. Thus, a clinical suspicion should lead promptly to a CT examination for a timely diagnosis and surgical intervention in order to prevent these sequelae. Imaging plays a central role in delineating the level and cause of bowel obstruction and may demonstrate findings that constitute the definitive evidence of cecal volvulus.

PEARLS

- Cecal volvulus accounts for 1% of acute intestinal obstructions and for 25% to 40% of colonic volvulus cases.

- Abdominal radiographs demonstrate a markedly distended cecum directed toward the left upper quadrant.

- CT is highly accurate and is currently the preferred method for diagnosis of cecal volvulus in the acute setting.

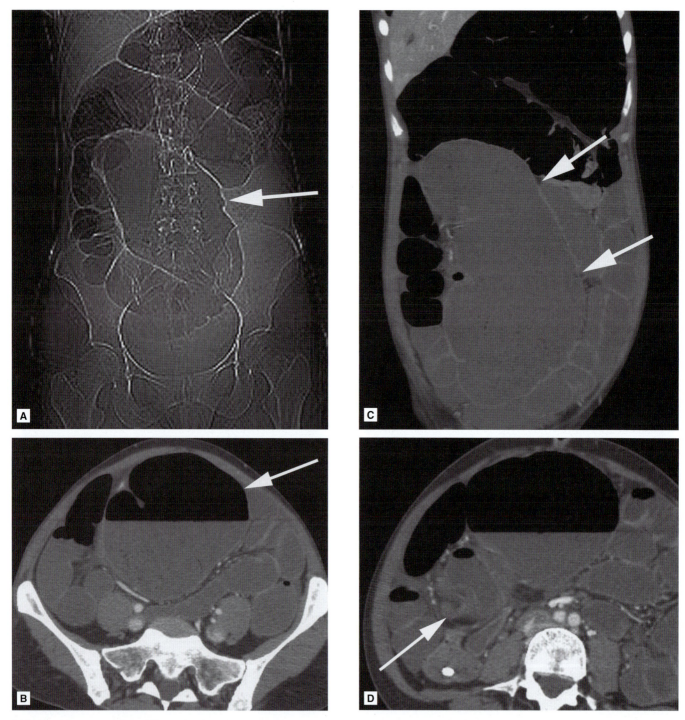

1. A. Scout tomogram from CT examination demonstrates a markedly distended loop of bowel in the mid-abdomen (arrow). **B.** Axial, contrast-enhanced CT image demonstrates a focal, dilated fluid- and air-filled loop of bowel in the mid-pelvis (arrow). **C.** Coronal, contrast-enhanced CT image demonstrates a markedly distended cecum (arrows) projecting out of the right lower quadrant in a patient with cecal volvulus. **D.** Axial, contrast-enhanced CT image demonstrates a narrowed, twisted-appearing portion of the cecum (arrow), confirming a diagnosis of cecal volvulus.

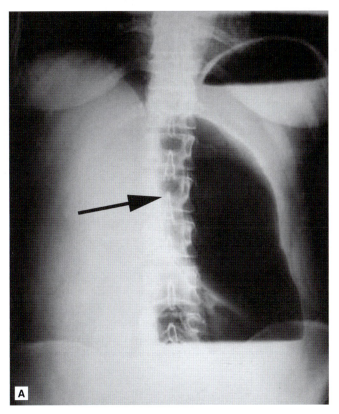

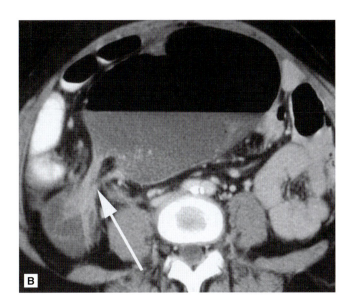

2. A. Abdominal radiograph displays a classic feature of a cecal volvulus, the presence of a markedly distended loop of bowel directed toward the left upper quadrant (arrow). **B.** Axial, contrast-enhanced CT image demonstrates a narrowed, twisted-appearing portion of the cecum (arrow), confirming a diagnosis of cecal volvulus.

PRESENTATION

Patients with typhlitis are typically profoundly neutropenic and present clinically with fever, abdominal pain, nausea, and diarrhea.

FINDINGS

CT demonstrates circumferential bowel wall thickening and edema involving the cecum and ascending colon, with adjacent mesenteric fat stranding and thickening.

DIFFERENTIAL DIAGNOSIS

- Diverticulitis
- Appendiciti
- Pseudomembranous colitis

COMMENTS

Typhlitis, also known as neutropenic colitis, is an infection of the cecum and ascending colon caused by enteric pathogens and occurs primarily in patients with neutropenia or severe immunosuppression. It is most commonly seen in patients with acute leukemia receiving chemotherapy but also occurs in the setting of AIDS, aplastic anemia, multiple myeloma, and bone marrow transplantation. In the setting of neutropenia and compromised immune system, bacteria, viruses, and fungi penetrate the damaged cecal mucosa. These organisms can proliferate and produce edema and inflammation involving the cecum, ascending colon, and, occasionally, the ileum. Without appropriate therapy, the inflammation can advance further to cause transmural necrosis, perforation, and death. The pathophysiologic mechanism causing the condition is not known, but it is probably due to a combination of ischemia, infection (especially with cytomegalovirus), mucosal hemorrhage, and perhaps neoplastic infiltration.

Patients usually present with fever, abdominal pain, nausea, and diarrhea. Early diagnosis and aggressive treatment with antibiotics and fluids are required to prevent transmural necrosis and perforation. Surgical resection is indicated in patients with complications such as transmural necrosis, intramural perforation, abscess, uncontrolled sepsis, and gastrointestinal hemorrhage.

CT is the study of choice in suspected typhlitis. CT demonstrates circumferential mural thickening of the cecum and ascending colon, low-density areas within the colonic wall secondary to edema, pericolonic inflammation and fluid, and, in severe cases, pneumatosis. In addition, inflammatory changes are also noted in the adjacent mesenteric fat. Clinically, CT is used to monitor the decrease in mural thickness with therapy and to detect subtle pneumoperitoneum in cases of silent perforation or necrosis. Direct visualization and barium enema are contraindicated in these critically ill patients due to the risk of bowel perforation. US may be useful in selected cases. Typical US findings include a hypoechoic or hyperechoic thickened wall of the cecum and ascending colon. Complications such as abscess or fluid collections can be imaged bedside using US.

PEARLS

- Typhlitis is an inflammatory or necrotizing colitis involving the cecum and ascending colon in neutropenic or immunosuppressed patients.

- CT demonstrates diffuse mural thickening of the cecum and ascending colon with pericolonic inflammation.

- Early diagnosis and treatment are essential to improve prognosis and CT is often used to monitor the response of the disease.

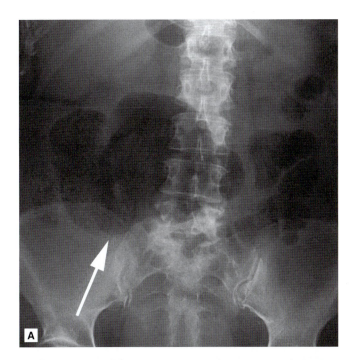

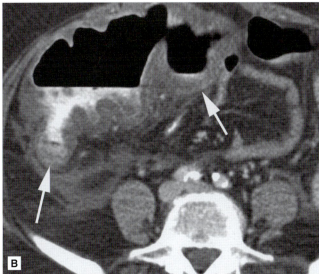

1. A. Abdominal radiograph demonstrates marked distention of the cecum (arrow). **B.** Axial, contrast-enhanced CT image reveals a thickening and distension of the cecum (arrows) as well as surrounding inflammatory stranding in a patient with typhlitis.

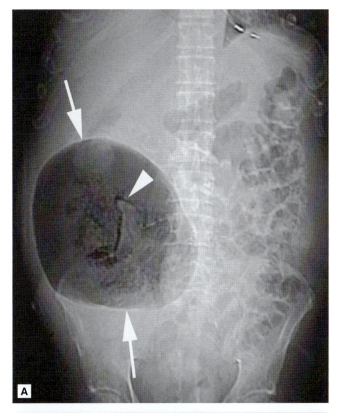

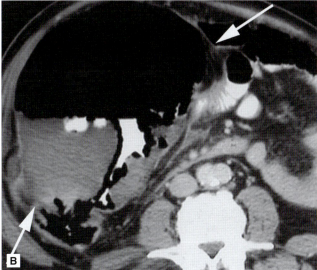

2. A. Abdominal radiograph demonstrates marked distention of the cecum (arrows) with mottled lucencies in the right lower quadrant (arrowhead) suggesting pneumatosis. **B.** Axial, contrast-enhanced CT image reveals distention of the cecum (arrows) with pneumatosis identified within the wall, a known finding in cases of severe typhlitis. **C.** Coronal, contrast-enhanced CT image reveals pneumatosis within the wall of the cecum (arrow) in a case of typhlitis.

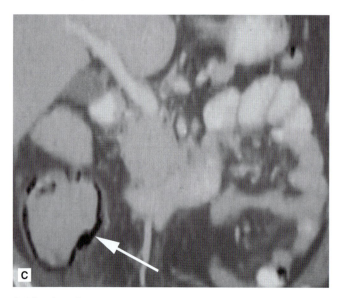

2. (*Continued*)

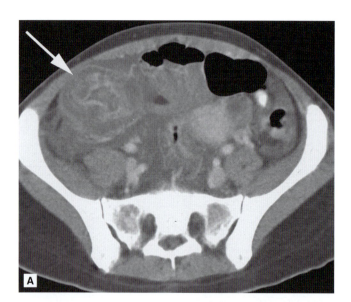

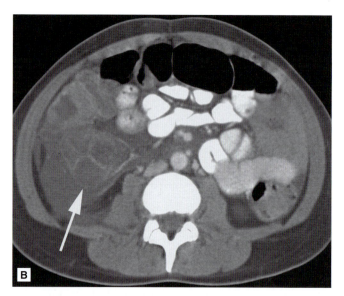

3. A. Axial, contrast-enhanced CT reveals a markedly edematous, thickened cecum (arrow) with surrounding stranding and free intraperitoneal fluid. **B.** Axial, contrast-enhanced CT reveals inflammation and thickening in a patient with neutropenic colitis extending to the ascending colon (arrow).

PRESENTATION

Patients are typically very ill, presenting with abdominal pain, distention, and tenderness as well as tachycardia, fever, anemia, and leukocytosis. Presentation may also include altered mental status, dehydration, or hypotension.

FINDINGS

Nonobstructive dilatation of the colon greater than 6 cm and clinical signs of toxicity

DIFFERENTIAL DIAGNOSIS

- Mechanical obstruction
- Ogilvie syndrome
- Paralytic ileus
- Colonic volvulus

COMMENTS

Toxic megacolon, or acute toxic colitis along with dilatation of the colon, is defined as dilatation of the colon greater than 6 cm in patients with clinical signs of toxicity. It is important to keep in mind that acute toxic colitis in the absence of distention as well as megacolon without toxicity may also occur. In toxic colitis, inflammation is not limited to the mucosa as in uncomplicated colitis, but extends into the smooth muscle layers and serosa. It is hypothesized that the generation of increased amounts of nitric oxide secondary to inflammation inhibits smooth muscle tone and results in the distention seen in toxic megacolon. Toxic megacolon has been described as a complication of various infectious colitides such as *Clostridium difficile* colitis, inflammatory bowel disease, ischemic colitis, colonic volvulus, and radiation colitis. Iatrogenic factors which have been implicated in the development of toxic megacolon include drugs such as narcotics, chemotherapeutics, and anticholinergics as well as procedures including colonoscopy and barium enema. Currently, the most common cause of toxic megacolon is *C difficile* colitis.

In patients with clinical signs consistent with toxic colitis, an abdominal radiograph demonstrating distention of the colon, whether it be segmental or total, exceeding 6 cm is diagnostic. The ascending and transverse colon have been found to be the segments most commonly affected. As colonic distention exceeding 6 cm may be seen in a variety of condition, other imaging features which are seen in toxic megacolon include markedly edematous haustral folds, or thumbprinting. Nodular masses of inflamed mucosa, termed pseudopolyps, may be seen projecting into the lumen of the abnormal segments of the colon, in between which deep, air-filled crevices may be identified. On CT imaging, distention and marked thickening of the bowel wall may be identified as well as submucosal edema and complications such as abscess formation and free intraperitoneal air related to perforation. In addition, imaging findings of septic thrombophlebitis of the mesenteric and portal venous circulation may be identified on CT.

PEARLS

- Toxic megacolon is a life-threatening condition defined by dilatation of the colon in excess of 6 cm in patients with clinical signs of toxic colitis.

- Abdominal radiographs are useful in diagnosis, evaluating the degree of colonic distention, while CT scans offer improved visualization of potential complications of toxic megacolon.

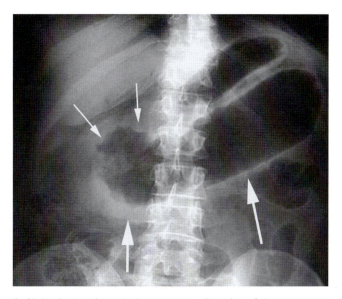

1. Abdominal radiograph demonstrates dilatation of the transverse colon in excess of 6 cm (large arrows) as well as edematous haustral folds (small arrows).

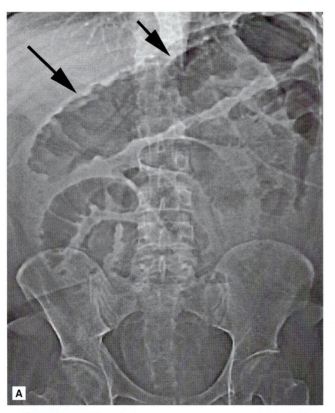

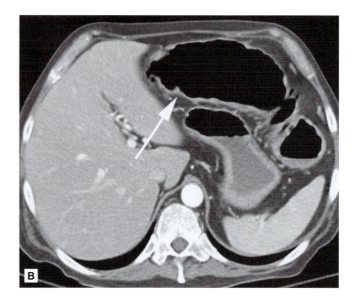

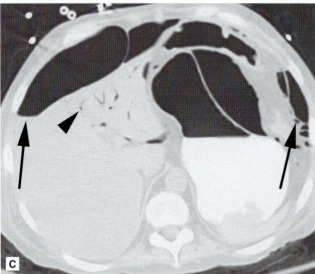

2. A. Scout topogram reveals distention of the transverse colon (arrows) with a mildly thickened, edematous appearance of the haustral folds. **B.** Axial, enhanced CT image demonstrates distention of the transverse colon (arrow) in a patient with toxic megacolon. **C.** Subsequent axial, enhanced CT scan (within 48 hours of image in **B**) demonstrates complications of toxic megacolon including portal venous gas (arrowhead) and free intraperitoneal air (arrows) related to frank perforation of the bowel wall.

PRESENTATION

Typically, patients with Ogilvie syndrome present with abdominal distention and pain, and may have associated with nausea and vomiting.

FINDINGS

Distention of the colon, often with a zone of relative transition to more decompressed bowel in the region of the splenic flexure.

DIFFERENTIAL DIAGNOSIS

- Mechanical obstruction
- Colonic volvulus
- Paralytic ileus

COMMENTS

Ogilvie syndrome, also termed colonic pseudo-obstruction, is a syndrome in which the clinical signs and symptoms are similar to a mechanical obstruction of the colon without an underlying cause of mechanical obstruction. Though no underlying mechanical obstruction exists, pseudo-obstruction can nevertheless cause significant morbidity and mortality with progression to bowel perforation. Alternatively, false diagnosis of mechanical colonic obstructions due to the similar clinical presentation as well as imaging features may lead to inappropriate surgical exploration. It has been suggested that acute and chronic forms of colonic pseudo-obstruction may occur and that the acute form represents a reversible condition associated with major illness or surgery while patients with the chronic form present with repeated episodes related to colonic distention. Patients with the chronic form are felt to be less prone to the complications of pseudo-obstruction such as frank perforation of the colon. While the term Ogilvie syndrome has been applied to both acute and chronic forms of colonic pseudo-obstruction, many authors feel that this term is more appropriately used to describe cases of acute colonic pseudo-obstruction. While not completely understood, the pathogenesis of acute colonic pseudo-obstruction likely results from abnormal autonomic regulation of the motor function of the colon. The most common causes include nonoperative trauma, infection, and cardiac disease.

On imaging, abdominal radiographs demonstrate marked distention of the colon. Barium studies have been used to rule out an underlying obstructing lesion, however, the possibility of pre-existent colonic perforation related to pseudo-obstruction should be considered a contraindication to this study. Thus, the possibility of a pre-existing perforation should be gauged on clinical and imaging grounds prior to performing a barium study. On CT scan, the majority of cases reveal a zone of relative transition to more collapse-appearing bowel in which, by definition, no underlying cause of mechanical obstruction is identified. Often, this transition occurs in the region of the splenic flexure, the region in which the parasympathetic innervation of the colon transitions from the vagal nerve to the sacral nerve, supporting the hypothesis that transient impairment at the sacral plexus results in functional obstruction of the more proximal bowel. As opposed to mechanical obstruction related to an adhesive band in which the zone of transition is relatively narrow, the transition zones in cases of Ogilvie syndrome are somewhat longer. In addition, CT scan is useful for evaluating for possible complications of pseudo-obstruction such as frank perforation as well as for accurately measuring the degree of cecal distention which may be a factor in determining whether surgical decompression is warranted.

PEARLS

- Ogilvie syndrome, also termed colonic pseudo-obstruction, demonstrates marked colonic distention without an underlying mechanical obstruction.

- Transition zones from distended to relatively collapsed distal segments of colon are typically identified, often in the region of the splenic flexure.

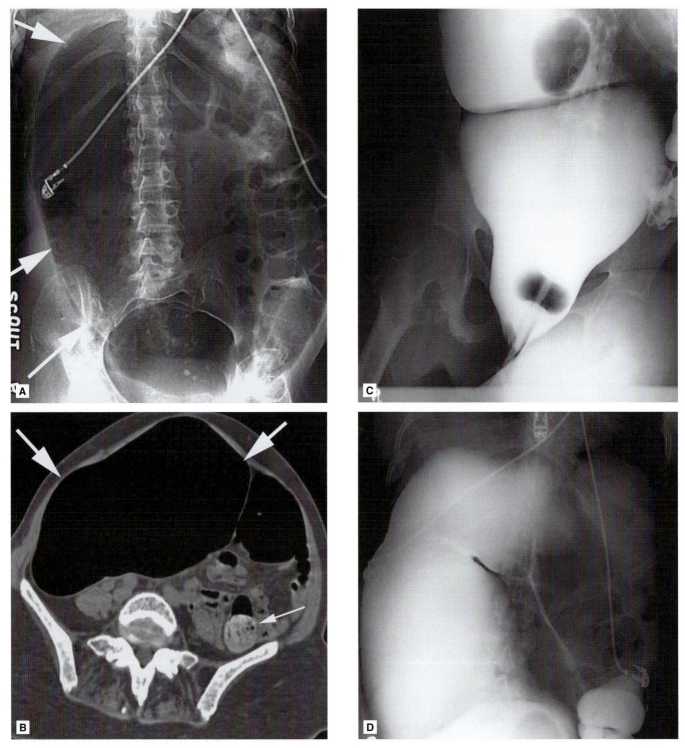

1. A. Abdominal radiograph demonstrates marked colonic distention, predominately involving the right colon (arrows). **B.** Axial, unenhanced CT scan reveals marked distention of the colon (large arrows) with relatively decompression of the descending colon (small arrow), often seen in Ogilvie syndrome. **C.** Fluoroscopic image during barium enema demonstrates no evidence of mechanical obstruction to the passage of contrast. **D.** Fluoroscopic image during barium enema demonstrates no evidence of mechanical obstruction to the passage of contrast with distention again noted to be more prominent in the right colon.

PRESENTATION

Chronic diarrhea, abdominal pain, and weight loss

FINDINGS

Early colonic manifestations identified on double-contrast barium enema are lymphoid follicle hyperplasia and aphthoid ulcerations. Progression of inflammation leads to filiform polyposis and diffuse mural thickening. Thickened bowel wall is noted in Crohn disease on CT and MRI, the appearance of which may be used to differentiate acute inflammation or chronic disease.

DIFFERENTIAL DIAGNOSIS

- Ulcerative colitis
- Infection
- Ischemia
- Radiation enteritis
- Metastases and lymphoma

COMMENTS

Crohn disease is one of the major forms of inflammatory bowel disease. It typically occurs in the second and third decades of life and is equally distributed between genders. There is a fivefold or greater risk among first-degree relatives of diseased individuals.

Although the etiology of Crohn disease remains largely unexplained, recent advances revolve around multiple factors such as genetic predisposition, external environment, intestinal microbial flora, and the immune system. These multifactorial pathogenic mechanisms initiate and maintain the chronic intestinal inflammation. Crohn disease is characterized by aggregation of macrophages that frequently form noncaseating granulomas. Although any site of the gastrointestinal tract may be affected, involvement of the terminal ileum is most common and the earliest mucosal lesions in Crohn disease often appear over Peyer patches. Unlike ulcerative colitis, Crohn disease may be patchy and segmental, and inflammation is typically transmural. In the majority of patients, the disease progresses to a relapsing and chronic disease. The disease affects the small bowel alone in about one-third, the colon alone in one-third, and both the colon and the small bowel in about one-third of cases. Perianal disease is most common when Crohn affects the colon but it may be present with disease in any location or, occasionally, be an isolated manifestation.

Chronic diarrhea, abdominal pain, and weight loss are the most common presenting symptoms of colonic Crohn disease. Blood and/or mucus in the stool are observed in up to one-half of the patients with Crohn colitis, but much less frequently than in ulcerative colitis. Extraintestinal manifestations are more common when Crohn disease affects the colon.

The main aim of the diagnostic test is to establish the diagnosis and distribution of the disease. Colonoscopy with multiple biopsy specimens is a first-line diagnostic test for diagnosing colitis. If colonoscopy is incomplete due to a stricture, then barium enema is the procedure of first choice. CT can show the mucosal pattern and show colitis proximal to a stricture. Early colonic manifestations of Crohn disease consist of lymph follicle prominence and presence of aphthoid ulcers which are readily detected with a double-contrast barium enema. The presence of aphthoid ulcers implies active colitis. Progression of inflammation leads to filiform polyposis and diffuse mural thickening. With advanced disease, the presence of homogeneously thickened bowel wall seen on CT or MR studies generally implies the presence of fibrosis. CT or MR enterography is very reliable in both detecting and evaluating the extent of Crohn disease. In the acute or noncicatrizing phase, CT or MR demonstrate discontinuous asymmetric bowel wall thickening with minimal narrowing. Contrast-enhanced CT reveals mural stratification with the "target" sign, which includes intense enhancement of the inner mucosa, a middle edematous low-attenuation submucosa and outer muscularis propria. In addition, mesenteric fat hypertrophy, prominent vasa recta, and enlarged draining lymph nodes are usually seen as well. In the chronic or cicatrizing phase, CT or MR demonstrate a homogeneously thickened bowel wall with loss of mural stratification and a target sign, which indicate irreversible fibrosis. Crohn proctitis leads to

PEARLS

- **Crohn colitis is a chronic inflammatory bowel disease with multifactorial etiology. It is a transmural disease with segmental or patchy involvement of the colon.**

- **Active disease demonstrates mural stratification with the "target" sign, whereas advanced disease with development of fibrosis demonstrates loss of the target appearance and luminal narrowing and strictures.**

- **Perianal, enteroenteric, and rectovaginal fistulae are known complications of chronic disease. Adenocarcinoma is more likely to develop in diseased segments.**

presacral space widening, mostly secondary to infiltration by fat-containing linear and nodular soft tissue densities. Several complications are known to occur in the chronic phase, which includes fistulae, anal fissures, and colon cancer. Most sinus tracts and fistulae seen in Crohn colitis end blindly or are enteroenteric although, occasionally, rectovaginal fistulas are known to occur. Most urinary tract fistulae involve the bladder. There is an increased incidence of adenocarcinoma in bowel affected by Crohn disease. Typically the interval from initial Crohn diagnosis until detection of cancer is up to 20 years, and these cancers mimic a benign stricture.

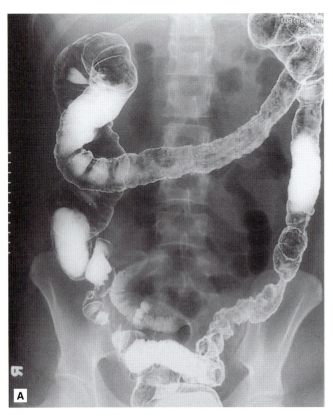

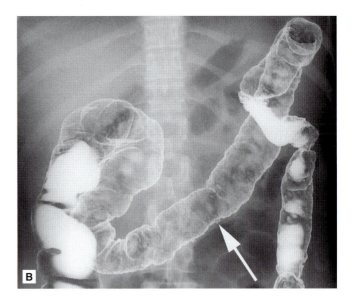

1. A. Double-contrast barium enema demonstrates Crohn involvement of the colon beginning at the level of the transverse colon as evidenced by shaggy, irregular mucosa, areas of luminal narrowing, and the presence of aphthous ulcers. **B.** Double-contrast barium enema in a patient with Crohn disease demonstrates an irregular appearance of the mucosa. An aphthous ulcer is well seen on this image (arrow).

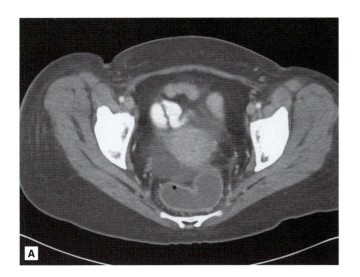

2. A. Axial, contrast-enhanced CT demonstrates diffuse thickening of the rectum as well as prominence of the vasa recta in a patient with Crohn disease. **B.** Axial, contrast-enhanced CT demonstrates diffuse thickening of the colon, prominence of the vasa recta, and pericolonic stranding in a patient with Crohn disease.

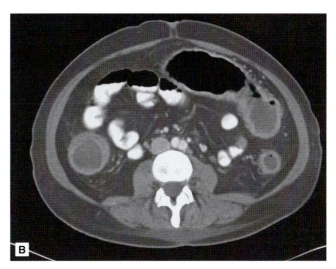

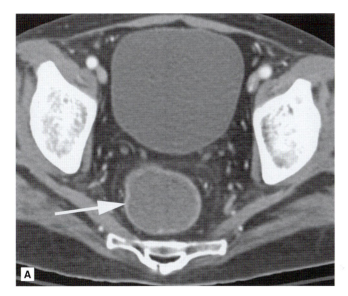

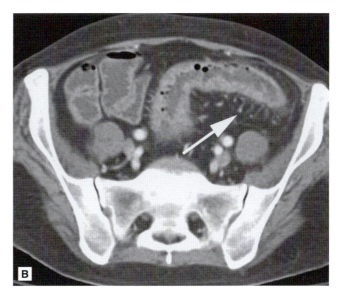

3. A. Axial, contrast-enhanced CT demonstrates diffuse thickening of the rectum (arrow), mild prominence and infiltration of the perirectal fat, and prominence of small perirectal lymph nodes in a patient with Crohn disease. **B.** Axial, contrast-enhanced CT demonstrates thickened, hyperenhancing distal colon and sigmoid (arrow) with prominence of the vasa recta which display the so-called "comb sign" in which the hyperemic vasa recta are aligned as the teeth of a comb. **C.** Axial, contrast-enhanced CT demonstrates irregular thickening of the splenic flexure (arrow) in a patient with Crohn disease.

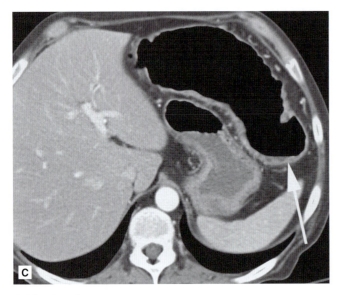

3. (*Continued*)

PRESENTATION

Common symptoms include diarrhea, rectal bleeding, passage of mucus, tenesmus, urgency, and abdominal pain.

FINDINGS

In the acute stage, the double-contrast barium enema demonstrates multiple mucosal ulcerations involving the entire length of the colon with loss of haustral pattern. CT demonstrates targeted appearance or mural stratification. In the chronic stage, the double-contrast enema demonstrates luminal narrowing, with a lead pipe appearance, and findings of backwash ileitis. CT shows enhancement of bowel wall without mural stratification.

DIFFERENTIAL DIAGNOSIS

- Crohn colitis
- Ischemic colitis
- Neutropenic enterocolitis
- Cathartic colon

COMMENTS

Ulcerative colitis (UC) is a chronic idiopathic inflammatory disease of the large bowel. Although the etiology is not completely established, the current hypothesis revolves around genetic susceptibility, host immunity, and environmental factors. Inflammation in UC is typically limited to the mucosa, in contrast to the transmural involvement of Crohn disease. The inflammatory changes typically end at the luminal aspect of the muscularis mucosa. With worsening inflammation, however, the surface epithelial cells become flattened, eventually ulcerate, and can become undermined if the ulcers are deep. At this stage of the disease, some inflammation and vascular congestion may be present in the submucosa, and ulcerations can extend into the muscularis mucosa.

Patients usually present with diarrhea, rectal bleeding, passage of mucus, tenesmus, urgency, and abdominal pain. The disease is most commonly diagnosed in the second and third decades of life and affects predominantly the female population. Rectosigmoid involvement is seen in the majority of patients at the time of initial presentation and not uncommonly progresses to pancolitis. Inflammation is typically most severe in the distal colon and rectum, with less severe in the proximal colon. In contrast to Crohn disease, continuous and symmetrical involvement is the hallmark of UC, with a sharp transition between diseased and uninvolved segments of the colon. Mild disease shows mucosal edema and hyperemia. As disease progresses, the mucosa becomes hemorrhagic, with visible punctate ulcers. These ulcers can enlarge and extend into the lamina propria. They often are irregular in shape with overhanging edges or may be linear along the line of the teniae coli. Epithelial regeneration with recurrent attacks results in the formation of pseudopolyp, which is typical of long-standing UC but which also may be seen in acute disease. In chronic disease, the colon is foreshortened and narrowed, with an atrophic featureless mucosa. Patients with severe disease can develop acute dilatation of the colon, also characterized by thin bowel wall and grossly ulcerated mucosa with only small fragments or islands of mucosa remaining.

Plain abdominal radiography can demonstrate thickened colonic wall and distension of small bowel and the colon. The presence of marked colonic dilatation suggests fulminant colitis or toxic megacolon. Barium enema is less often performed in the current clinical practice dominated by endoscopy and CT for the evaluation of UC. Barium studies are very useful in the evaluation of strictures. The barium enema in the acute stage of disease demonstrates mucosal granularity and ulcers, thickened haustra, and inflammatory polyps. On CT, mural changes produce a "target" or "double-halo" appearance with an inner enhancing ring of mucosa, lamina propria, and hypertrophied muscularis mucosae, surrounded by a low-density ring of submucosa, and then turn by an enhancing ring of muscularis propria. This mural stratification is not specific and can also be seen in Crohn disease, infectious enterocolitis, pseudomembranous colitis, ischemic and radiation enterocoliti, mesenteric venous thrombosis, bowel edema, and graft-versus-host disease. With long-standing disease, the colon becomes a featureless tubular structure due to

PEARLS

- UC is a chronic idiopathic inflammatory disease of the colon that predominantly affects the luminal aspect of the muscularis mucosa.

- CT has demonstrated a high diagnostic yield for detecting disease, complications, and extent. The CT appearance of mural stratification with pericolonic inflammatory is a nonspecific finding.

- UC has higher risk of colorectal carcinoma than Crohn disease. Follow-up imaging should concentrate not only on disease activity but also to recognize intestinal complications and extraintestinal manifestations.

the loss of haustral folds in the ascending and transverse colon. Other chronic changes include foreshortening of the colon, strictures, widening of the presacral space. Local complications of UC include perforation with peritonitis and abscess, toxic megacolon, venous thrombosis, and carcinoma. Extraintestinal manifestations of UC include arthritis, ankylosing spondylitis, erythema nodosum, pyoderma gangrenosum, and primary sclerosing cholangitis.

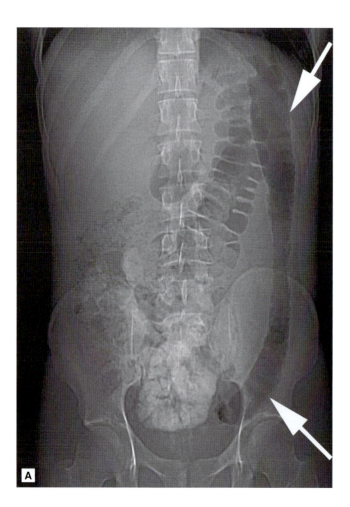

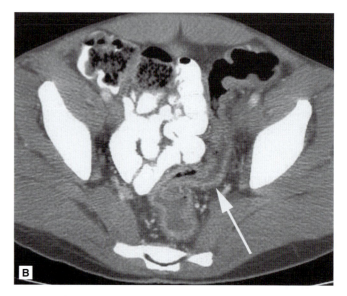

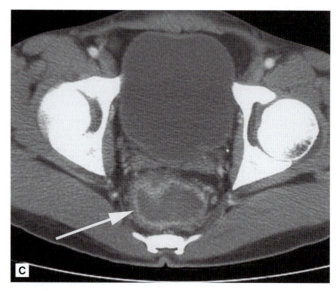

1. A. Frontal scout topogram image reveals a featureless appearance of the descending colon (arrows), the imaging appearance of which is highly suggestive of UC. **B.** Axial, contrast-enhanced CT image reveals thickening and mucosal hyperenhancement of the sigmoid colon (arrow). **C.** Axial, contrast-enhanced CT image reveals thickening and mucosal hyperenhancement extending to the rectum (arrow), in keeping with the continuous bowel involvement of UC.

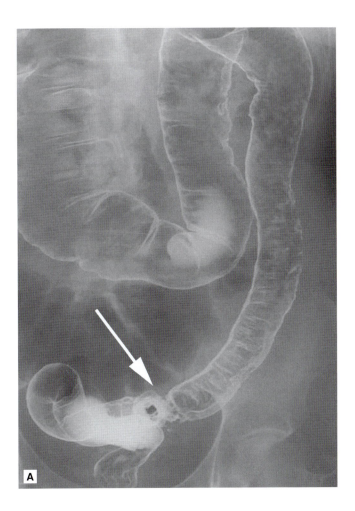

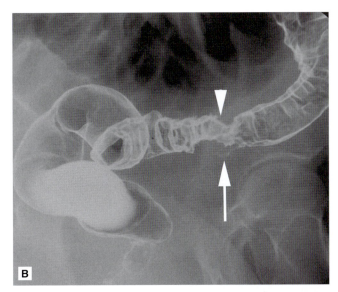

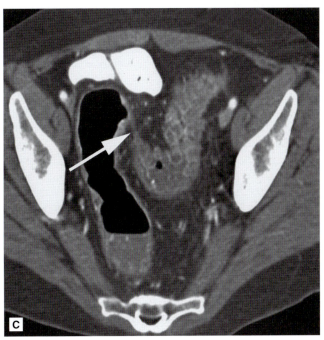

2. A. Frontal image acquired during a double-contrast barium enema reveals the hallmarks of long-standing UC, most obvious in the descending colon, as evidenced by a relatively featureless appearance. In addition, a focal stricture, concerning for a colon carcinoma is identified (arrow). **B.** Frontal image acquired during a double-contrast barium enema reveals irregular thickening of the sigmoid colon suspicious for a colon carcinoma (arrow), the incidence of which is markedly increased in patients with UC. **C.** Axial, contrast-enhanced image reveals narrowing in the sigmoid colon, the etiology of which was found to be an inflammatory stricture related to the patient's UC. Note the inflammation and thickening of the bowel proximal and distal to the stricture.

PRESENTATION

Acute watery or bloody diarrhea, crampy abdominal pain, and tenderness

FINDINGS

CT demonstrates diffuse or focal thickening of colonic wall with mucosal and serosal enhancement.

DIFFERENTIAL DIAGNOSIS

- Pseudomembranous colitis
- Crohn colitis
- Ulcerative colitis
- Ischemic colitis

COMMENTS

There are numerous bacterial, viral, protozoal, and parasitic causes of colitis. The specific etiology depends on the country or region of residence, travel history, and immune status of the patient. Some of the infectious agents are likely to cause recognizable tissue pathology whereas many infectious agents are culture-negative. Common bacteria known to cause colitis include *Campylobacter, Salmonella, Shigella, Yersinia, Escherichia coli, Staphylococcus,* and *Clostridium difficile.* Common viral organisms known to cause colitis include herpes virus, cytomegalovirus (CMV), Norwalk virus, and rotavirus. *Histoplasma* and *Mucor* are the common fungi. *Entamoeba histolytica, Schistosoma, Strongyloides, Trichuris,* and *Anisakis* are known parasites associated with colitis especially in underdeveloped countries.

Campylobacter jejuni is a leading cause of infectious colitis worldwide and has become one of the major causes of infectious diarrhea in the United States. *C jejuni* is a curved, microaerophilic, gram-positive rod. Toxic megacolon resulting from *C jejuni* is rare but has been reported.

Yersinia enterocolitica also can cause enteric infection, typically involving the ileocecal region. It is most commonly seen in infants, young children, and young adults. *Yersinia* enteritis is a self-limiting disease, although patients should be treated with appropriate antibiotics.

Salmonella typhi causes an infectious enterocolitis and is the cause of typhoid fever. Invasion of the mucosa and submucosa of the small bowel and colon leads to an inflammatory reaction and release of an endotoxin from the bacterial cell. Severe septicemia may also occur if the organism enters the bloodstream. Toxic megacolon and intestinal perforation have been reported with *S typhi* infection. Massive lower gastrointestinal bleeding and gangrenous

cholecystitis have also been reported as complications of *Salmonella* infection.

C difficile is a gram-positive, spore-forming anaerobic micro-organism that is related to the bacteria that cause tetanus and botulism. Usually the growth of the active organism is suppressed by the normal bacteria of the colon, but antibiotics that suppress the colonic flora permit overgrowth of *C difficile*, which releases toxins that cause pseudomembranous colitis and diarrhea. *C difficile* produces two toxins (A and B), both of which are important in the pathogenesis of pseudomembranous colitis. *C difficile* colitis typically begins within 4 to 9 days after the initiation of antibiotics, although some patients may not become symptomatic until up to 10 weeks after a course of antibiotics.

Symptoms and findings of infectious colitis are similar to other nonspecific inflammatory diseases of bowel and include bloody diarrhea, abdominal pain, fever, nausea, and vomiting. Patients may also have fever, leukocytosis, and electrolyte abnormalities.

The diagnosis is usually established by demonstrating the organism or toxins in the stool. Proctoscopy or flexible sigmoidoscopy may reveal inflamed mucosa in unclear cases. Imaging is primarily indicated in cases of negative stool tests or failed colonoscopy. Cross-sectional imaging is performed to assess complications. Barium enemas demonstrate diffuse or focal thickening of the colonic wall, with luminal narrowing. Various forms of mucosal ulcers and irregularity may be seen depending on the etiology and severity of disease. Diffuse mucosal granularity and inflammatory polyps seen in chronic disease simulate ulcerative colitis and is difficult to differentiate without biopsy. CT demonstrates mucosal and serosal enhancement of diseased segments, with wall thickening. Depending on the etiology, pericolonic inflammation, enlarged mesenteric lymph nodes, and multiple air-fluid levels may be seen in infectious colitis.

PEARLS

- Infectious colitis is caused by various bacterial, viral, protozoal, and parasitic agents. The specific etiology depends on the country or residence, travel history, and immune status of the patient.

- Diagnosis is usually established by demonstrating the organism or toxins in the stool and by mucosal visualization and sampling.

- Imaging studies are primarily performed in difficult cases and to assess complications such as perforation, abscess, or toxic megacolon. CT of affected segments demonstrate mucosal and serosal enhancement with diffuse mural thickening and pericolonic inflammation.

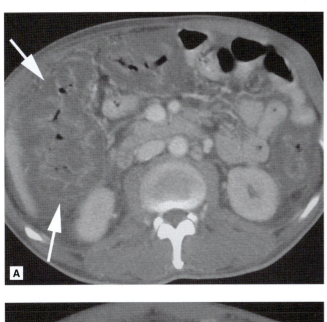

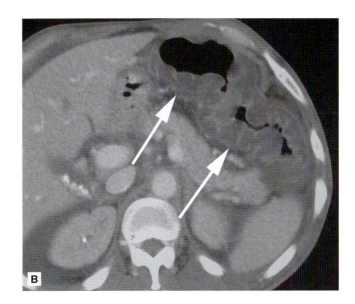

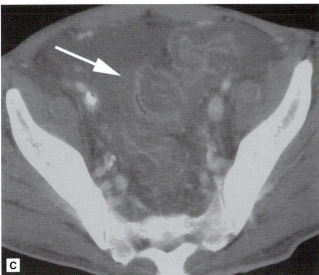

1. A. Axial, contrast-enhanced CT demonstrates marked thickening of the entirety of the colon (arrows) in a patient with *C difficile* colitis. **B.** Axial, contrast-enhanced CT demonstrates marked, edematous thickening of the entirety of the colon (arrows) in a patient with *C difficile* colitis. **C.** Axial, contrast-enhanced CT demonstrates thickening of the entirety of the colon (arrow) in a patient with *C difficile* colitis.

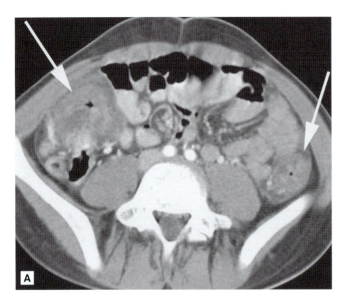

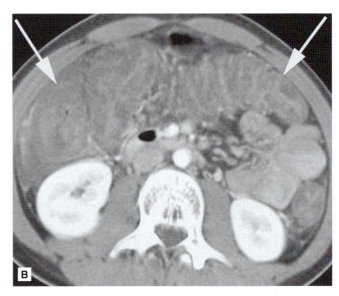

2. A. Axial, contrast-enhanced CT demonstrates thickening the colon (arrows), pericolonic stranding, and associated lymphadenopathy in a patient with *E coli* colitis. **B.** Axial, contrast-enhanced CT demonstrates thickening the colon (arrows) and pericolonic stranding, in a patient with *E coli* colitis.

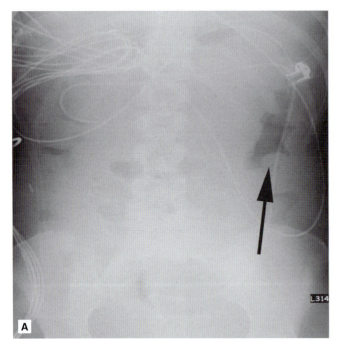

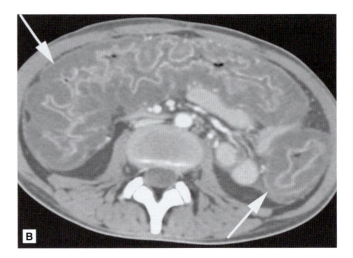

3. A. Abdominal radiograph demonstrates marked thickening of the wall of the colon (arrow) in a patient with *C difficile* colitis. **B.** Axial, contrast-enhanced CT demonstrates marked thickening of the entirety of the colon (arrows) in a patient with *C difficile* colitis.

PRESENTATION

Perirectal pain during defecation, sinus discharge, history of perirectal and perianal abscess.

FINDINGS

MR demonstrates an enhancing tract in the perianal and perirectal region with or without high T2 signal within the tract.

DIFFERENTIAL DIAGNOSIS

- Hidradenitis suppurativa
- Pilonidal sinus
- Inflammation and fistulas associated with inflammatory bowel disease
- Low rectal and anal canal carcinomas

COMMENTS

Perirectal fistulas occur as a complication of a perirectal abscess. Most fistulas derive from sepsis originating in the anal canal glands at the dentate line. The majority of sepsis resolves completely after appropriate treatment with antibiotic or surgical drainage. However, in about one-fourth of patients, the abscess cavity does not heal completely, becoming instead an inflammatory track with a primary opening (internal opening) in the anal crypt at the dentate line and a secondary opening (external opening) in the perianal skin. Other causes of perianal fistulas include Crohn disease, tuberculosis, and trauma during childbirth, pelvic infection, pelvic malignancy, and radiation therapy. The fistulous tracts course through the anatomic plane of least resistance, most commonly along the fascial or fatty planes, especially the intersphincteric space between the internal and the external sphincter into the ischiorectal fascia. In such instances, the tract passes directly to the perineal skin. In some cases, circumferential spread may also occur in the ischiorectal fossa, with the tract passing from one fossa to the contralateral one through the posterior rectum, a fistula known as the horseshoe fistula. The perirectal fistulas are classified into four main categories based on the relation of the fistula to the sphincter muscles, and include intersphincteric, trans-sphincteric, suprasphincteric, and extrasphincteric. Intersphincteric fistula is the most common type and is confined to the intersphincteric plane. The trans-sphincteric fistula traverses the external sphincter to travel through the ischiorectal fossa and end at the perineal skin. The suprasphincteric fistula is rare. It usually tracks upward in the intersphincteric plane before taking a lateral direction over the puborectalis and finally downward through the ischiorectal fossa to the perineal skin. Extrasphincteric fistula is rare and is typically caused by trauma such as a fishbone piercing through the rectal wall, carcinoma or Crohn disease. The fistula tracks from the rectal wall above the levator ani to the perineal skin, completely external to the sphincter complex.

Clinical manifestations of perirectal fistula include perirectal pain and sinus discharge. The majority of patients have a previous history of perirectal abscess and subsequent discharge. On examination, the skin opening is usually identified as a red elevation of granulation tissue with purulent or serosanguineous drainage on compression. The simple or superficial fistula can be easily palpable as an indurated cord but deeper fistulas are usually evaluated by imaging.

Radiological evaluation is crucial in determining the surgical management of perirectal fistulas, which depends on the type of the fistula and presence or absence of an associated abscess. The main aim of the treatment is to eliminate the tract without causing damage to the external sphincter and fecal continence mechanism. Conventional fistulography is the traditional technique to evaluate perirectal fistulas but it fails to provide sufficient anatomic details to plan surgical management. MRI is the study of choice for better fistula mapping and for assessing coexistence of an abscess in the perirectal region. Anatomic details of the sphincter complex, levator ani, and ischiorectal fossae are obtained on the unenhanced T1-weighted images. Fistulous tracts, fluid, and abscess are better seen on T2-weighted and fluid-sensitive images. Dynamic, contrast-enhanced images provide additional sensitivity as the active fistula and abscess cavity demonstrate wall enhancement. Because of inherent high soft tissue resolution, MRI provides information about the relationship of the fistulous tract to the sphincter complex, involvement of sphincter, secondary tracts or ramifications, and abscess.

PEARLS

- Perirectal fistulas are invariably seen as a complication of perirectal abscess and the intersphincteric fistula is the most common type.

- The goal of the surgical management is to prevent damage to the external sphincter and preserve fecal continence.

- Contrast-enhanced MRI is the best imaging test for fistula mapping, assessment of sphincter complex involvement, and complications.

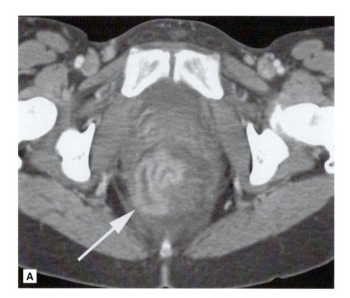

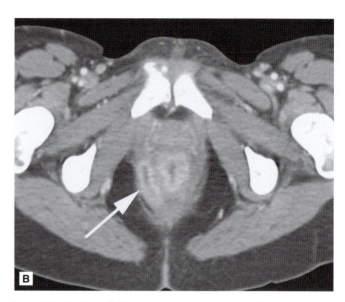

1. A. Axial, contrast-enhanced CT image demonstrates an enhancing, perirectal fistula (arrow). **B.** Axial, contrast-enhanced CT image demonstrates an enhancing, intersphincteric perirectal fistula (arrow) extending inferiorly.

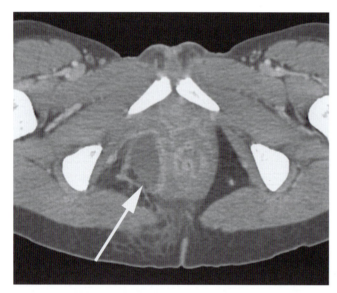

2. Axial, contrast-enhanced CT demonstrates a well-defined, peripherally enhancing perirectal abscess (arrow).

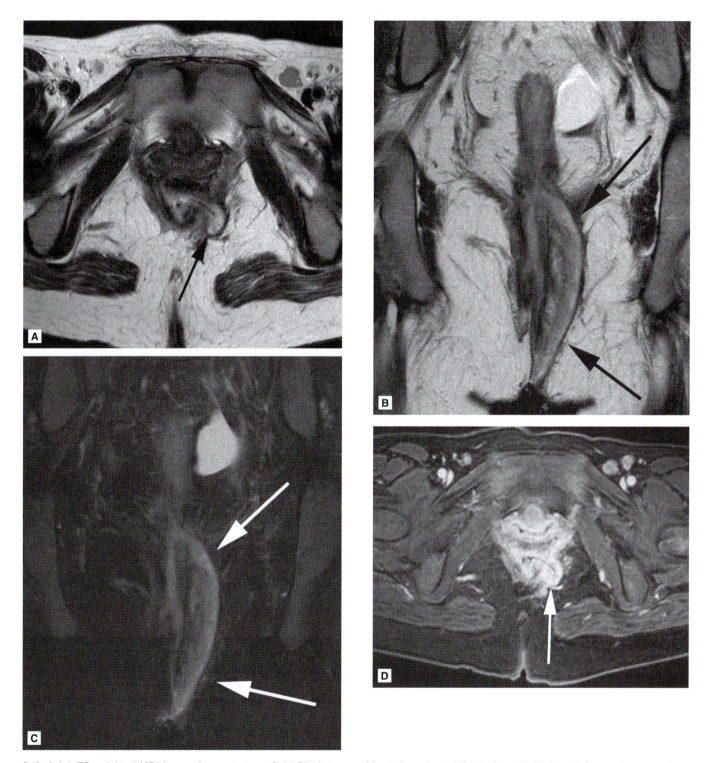

3. A. Axial, T2-weighted MRI image demonstrates a fluid-filled, trans-sphincteric perirectal fistula (arrow) which contains a seton, as evidenced by a central curvilinear hypointense structure. **B.** Coronal, T2-weighted MRI image demonstrates a fluid-filled, trans-sphincteric perirectal fistula (arrows). **C.** Coronal, T2-weighted, fat-suppressed MRI image demonstrates a fluid-filled, trans-sphincteric perirectal fistula (arrows). **D.** Axial, contrast-enhanced MRI image demonstrates avid enhancement of the trans-sphincteric perirectal fistula; seton is again well seen centrally within the fistula (arrow).

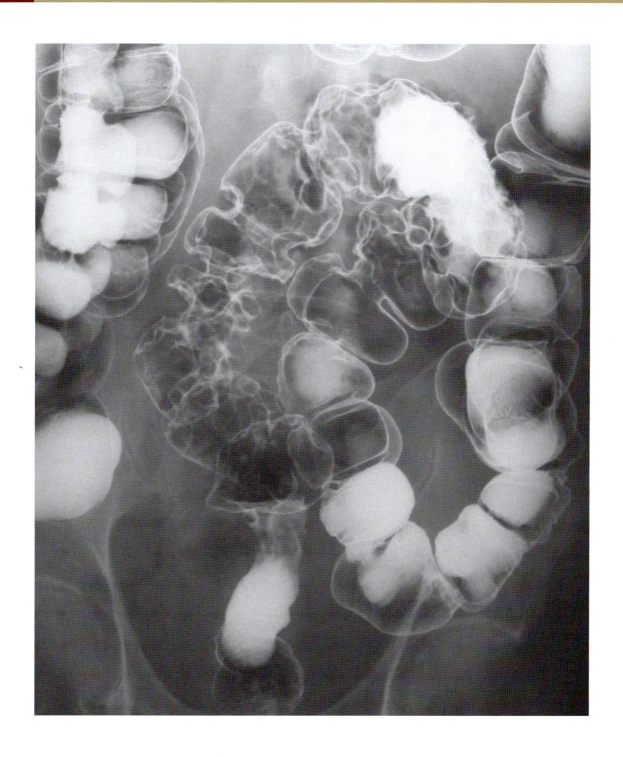

PRESENTATION

Patients classically present with abdominal pain and tenderness, absolute constipation, abdominal distension, and nausea. Vomiting occurs late when distension is severe. In cases of complications related to sigmoid volvulus such as frank perforation, patients may present with shock.

FINDINGS

Plain abdominal radiographs are typically diagnostic and demonstrate an inverted-U appearance of the sigmoid colon, the characteristic "bird-beak" sign, "coffee-bean" sign, loss of haustra, and colonic gaseous distension proximal to the volvulus that may extend to the ileum. On CT, a "whirl" sign caused by twisting of the sigmoid colon and the mesentery may be identified as well as "beaking" that is caused by the rapid tapering of the afferent and efferent limbs of the bowel.

DIFFERENTIAL DIAGNOSIS

- Acute ileus
- Severe constipation
- Ogilvie syndrome
- Other causes of mechanical obstruction, colorectal cancer, stricture
- Giant sigmoid diverticulum

COMMENTS

Sigmoid volvulus is caused by torsion of the sigmoid colon about its mesenteric axis. A rare variant of sigmoid volvulus is termed ilieosigmoid knotting which occurs when a segment of the ileum is wrapped about the sigmoid colon, resulting in obstruction. Sigmoid volvulus represents the majority (60%-75%) of cases of colonic volvulus but is the cause of less than 10% of all cases of intestinal obstruction in the United States. Mortality rates resulting from this condition are high, especially if the presentation is late and complications such as perforation and gangrene occur. Predisposing factors in the onset of sigmoid volvulus which have been reported include a redundant sigmoid colon with a narrow mesenteric attachment, a large distended colon resulting from chronic constipation, a high-fiber diet leading to bulky stools, obtundation from medication, and previous abdominal surgeries. Colonic volvulus is more common in elderly men institutionalized in medical facilities.

Patients present with a sudden onset of severe abdominal pain, vomiting, abdominal distension, and obstipation suggestive of acute or subacute intestinal obstruction. These patients are prone to develop bowel ischemia either by mural ischemia associated with the increased tension of the distended bowel wall or by arterial occlusion caused by torsion of the mesenteric arterial supply; therefore, severe abdominal pain, rebound tenderness, and tachycardia are ominous signs.

Radiological evaluations place a crucial role in the prompt diagnosis and treatment. Plain abdominal radiography is typically diagnostic for sigmoid volvulus. The classic findings include a distended sigmoid colon resulting in the inverted-U appearance, the coffee-bean sign which is formed by the distended colon and a dense white line formed by the apposed colonic wall which points toward the pelvis as well as projection of the distended sigmoid above the transverse colon giving the "northern exposure" sign. In addition, a loss of haustral marking and gaseous distension of the proximal colon that may reach the small bowel with absence of rectal gas in both supine and prone decubitus may be identified. A single-contrast barium or water soluble contrast enema will demonstrate a smoothly tapered narrowing of the rectosigmoid junction, resulting in the characteristic bird-beak or "bird of prey" sign which refers to the tapered appearance of the distal aspect of the volvulus. If the contrast material passes through the obstructed segment, signs of colonic ischemia such as thumbprinting, transverse ridging, and mucosal ulceration may be seen. On CT scan, tight twisting of the sigmoid colon and the mesentery resulting in the so-called whirl sign may be identified as well as tapered narrowing of the afferent and efferent limbs, leading to "beaking." In addition, CT scan may be used to identify complications of sigmoid volvulus such as ischemia or frank perforation.

PEARLS

- Sigmoid volvulus is the most common form of colonic volvulus.

- Patients are usually elderly men and present with abdominal pain and tenderness, distension, absolute constipation, and nausea.

- Plain abdominal radiography is usually diagnostic and demonstrates the characteristic bird-beak sign, inverted-U appearance of the sigmoid colon, coffee-bean sign, loss of haustra, and gaseous distension proximal to the volvulus.

- CT may demonstrate the whirl sign caused by twisting of the sigmoid colon and the mesentery as well as beaking caused by the tapered afferent and efferent limbs.

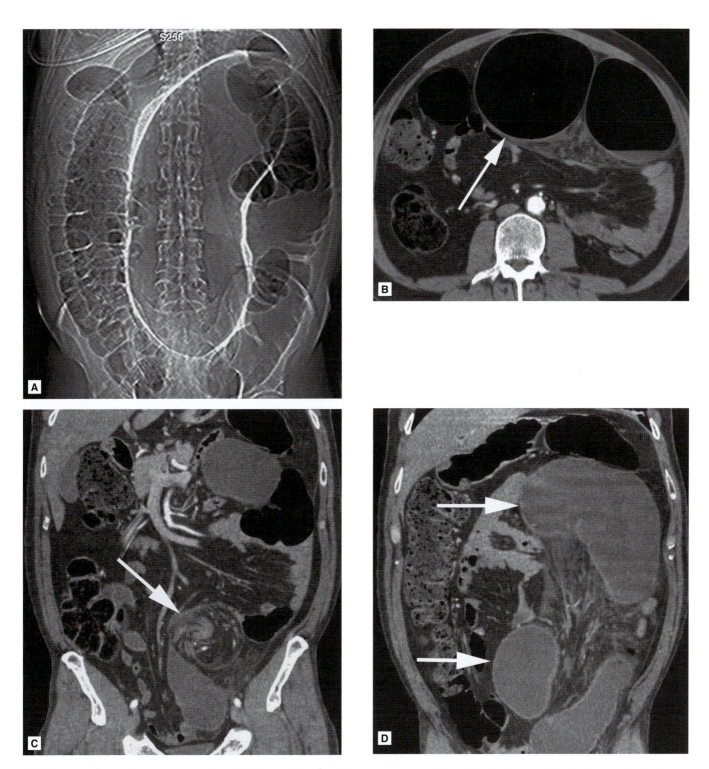

1. A. Scout topogram demonstrates marked dilatation of the sigmoid colon in a case of sigmoid volvulus, resulting in the so-called coffee-bean sign. **B.** Axial, contrast-enhanced CT image demonstrates marked distention of the sigmoid colon in the involved segment (arrow). **C.** Coronal, contrast-enhanced CT image demonstrates the so-called whirl sign resulting from twisting of the sigmoid colon and sigmoid mesocolon (arrow). **D.** Axial, contrast-enhanced CT image demonstrates marked distention of the sigmoid colon in the involved segment (arrows). No complications such as frank perforation as evidenced by free intraperitoneal air or pericolonic fluid collections are identified.

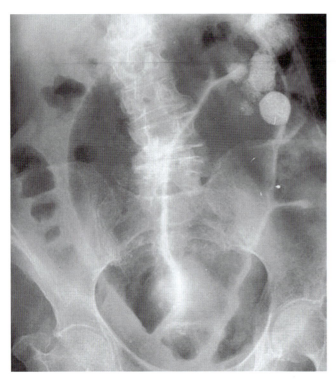

2. Plain abdominal radiograph demonstrates the characteristic coffee-bean sign in a patient with sigmoid volvulus.

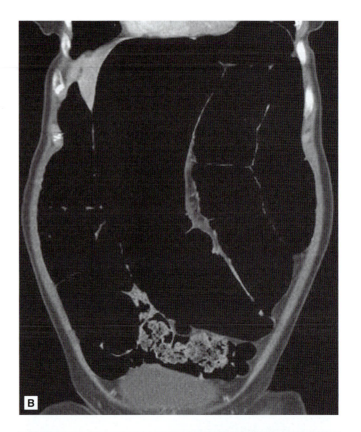

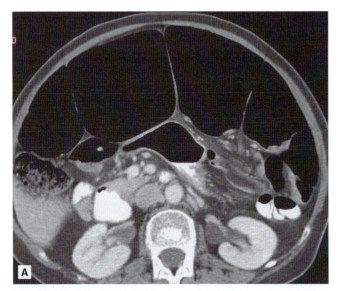

3. A. Axial, contrast-enhanced CT image demonstrates marked distention of the sigmoid colon in the involved segment. **B.** Coronal, contrast-enhanced CT image demonstrates marked gaseous distention of the sigmoid colon throughout the involved segment. **C.** Coronal, contrast-enhanced CT image demonstrates the so-called whirl sign in a case of sigmoid volvulus (arrow).

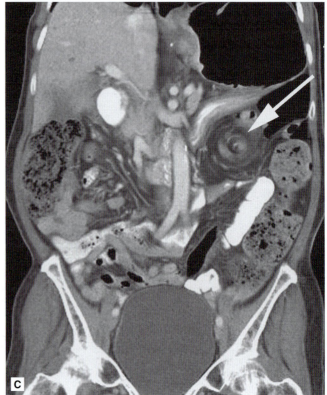

3. (*Continued*)

PRESENTATION

Patients present with acute abdominal pain, nausea, and vomiting in acute intussusception causing bowel obstruction.

FINDINGS

Abdominal CT demonstrates an edematous segment with "bowel within bowel" or "target-like" appearance with or without mesenteric fat and a cross-sectional diameter greater than that of adjacent bowel.

DIFFERENTIAL DIAGNOSIS

- Primary intestinal tumor
- Metastasis
- Lymphoma
- Endometrial implants

COMMENTS

Intussusception is telescopic invagination of bowel loop into the lumen of an adjacent contiguous segment of bowel in the direction of peristalsis. Intussusception can be transient, usually without any lead point or persistent, with a lead point. Transient intussusception is commonly seen in small bowel; however, it is rarely seen in large bowel. The pathophysiology of intussusception is not well understood, especially without a lead point. Dysrhythmic contractions in bowel can predispose the bowel loops to telescope into each other. The presence of pathological lesions within the intestinal wall or lumen such as polyps or mass lesions can act as a lead point and cause intussusception. There are four major forms of intussusception: enteroenteric, ileocolic, ileocecal, and colocolic. The majority involve the small bowel, whereas large bowel intussusception is rare and often associated with malignant lesions like primary tumors and metastatic disease. Large bowel intussusception is often associated with a lead point caused by benign lesions such as lipoma, adenomatous polyp, motility disorders, and postoperative adhesions or malignant lesions such as metastatic disease, primary adenocarcinoma, and lymphoma.

Patients usually present with nausea, vomiting, and crampy abdominal pain secondary to partial bowel obstruction.

Some patients with malignant disease may also present with constipation, melena, weight loss, and a palpable abdominal mass. CT is the modality of choice to evaluate suspected bowel obstruction. The CT appearance of intussusception depends on the etiology and mechanism of development, such as presence of a lead point, the configuration of the lead mass, the degree of bowel wall edema, and the amount of invaginated mesenteric fat and vessels. Typically, abdominal CT reveals a bowel within bowel or a target-like appearance, with or without mesenteric fat or vessels. An intussusception with a lead mass appears as an abnormal target-like lesion with a cross-sectional diameter greater than that of the normal bowel and may be associated with proximal bowel obstruction.

Ileocolic or ileocecal intussusception is often associated with metastatic disease of the distal small bowel. Melanoma metastases are the most common metastatic lesions of bowel which predominantly affect the small intestine, followed by stomach and large bowel. Lipomas are the most common cause of colocolic intussusception, followed by adenomatous polyps. Almost all lipomas occur in the submucosa and are easily detected by radiological tests as fat-containing lesions. Adenocarcinoma is the most common malignant cause associated with colonic intussusception. Patients typically present with symptoms and signs of malignancy rather than those caused by the intussusception itself. CT demonstrates the lead mass within the bowel wall.

PEARLS

- **Intussusception affecting the large bowel is rare when compared to small bowel and is often associated with malignant disease.**

- **Lipoma and adenomatous polyps are the most common benign etiologies and adenocarcinoma is the most common malignant etiology associated with colonic intussusceptions.**

- **CT demonstrates the bowel within bowel or target-like appearance, with or without mesenteric fat and vessels, with a cross-sectional diameter greater than that of adjacent bowel. The proximal bowel is usually dilated secondary to bowel obstruction.**

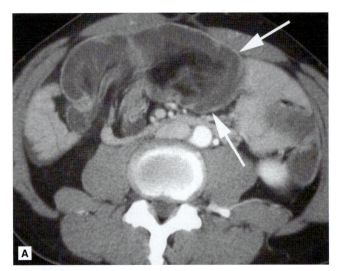

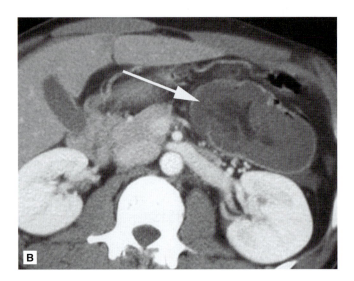

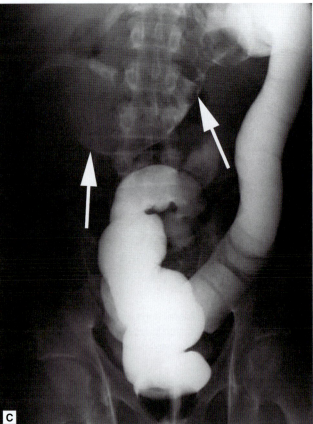

1. A. Axial, contrast-enhanced CT demonstrates a large ileocolic intussusception (arrows) with the mesenteric fat well seen within the intussusception. **B.** Axial, contrast-enhanced CT demonstrates a large ileocolic intussusception (arrow) extending into the transverse colon with the mesenteric fat well seen within the intussusception. **C.** Barium enema demonstrates a large filling defect (arrows) in the right and transverse colon related to a large ileocolic intussusception.

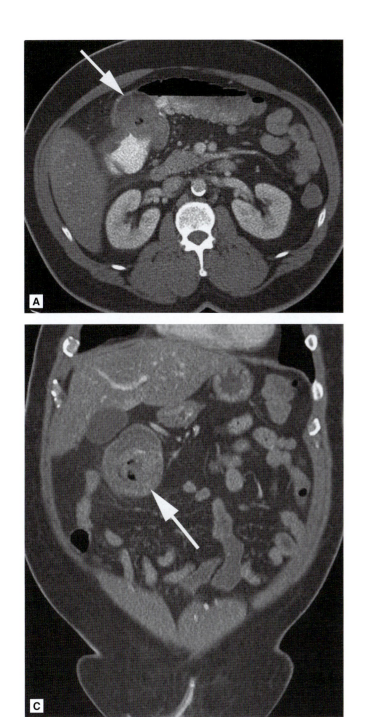

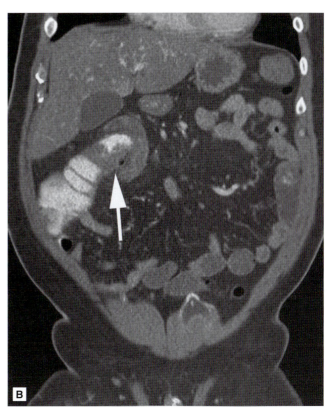

2. A. Axial, contrast-enhanced CT demonstrates a colocolic intussusception (arrow) with a bowel within a bowel appearance well seen on this image. **B.** Axial, contrast-enhanced CT demonstrates a colocolic intussusception related to an underlying malignancy (arrow). **C.** Coronal, contrast-enhanced CT demonstrates a colocolic intussusception (arrow) with a bowel within a bowel appearance well seen on this image.

PRESENTATION

While typically asymptomatic, patients may present with vague right lower quadrant abdominal pain, weight loss, nausea, or vomiting.

FINDINGS

CT examinations reveal a well-defined, cystic mass; calcification may be seen within the wall or lumen of an appendiceal mucocele. A heterogeneous soft tissue component may be identified in cases of mucinous cystadenocarcinoma.

DIFFERENTIAL DIAGNOSIS

- Acute appendicitis
- Appendiceal carcinoma
- Appendiceal lymphoma
- Adnexal cysts
- Mesenteric and omental cysts

COMMENTS

The term appendiceal mucocele is descriptive and refers to the distention of the appendix by mucin-rich fluid. While originally thought to result from chronic appendiceal obstruction, more recent evidence suggests that appendiceal mucoceles are usually caused by mucosal hyperplasia, mucinous cystadenoma, or mucinous cystadenocarcinoma. Rarely, appendiceal mucoceles are caused by chronic obstruction in which case they may be termed retention cysts. The most common cause of appendicular mucoceles is mucinous cystadenomas. The main clinical significance of appendiceal mucoceles lie in their complications; benign or malignant mucoceles may rupture or leak which may lead to pseudomyxoma peritonei which is difficult to treat both medically or surgically and leads to significant morbidity and mortality. Overall, mucoceles are uncommon, being found in approximately 0.2% to 0.3% of appendectomy specimens.

On imaging, the presence of a well-defined mass in the right lower quadrant with curvilinear calcification has been described as a radiographic finding in cases of appendiceal mucoceles. A barium enema examination may demonstrate failure to fill the appendix with barium; in cases of large mucoceles, prominent filling defects may be identified within the cecum along with displacement of the terminal ileum. US may reveal a fluid-filled, cystic mass with a layering appearance, termed the "onion skin" sign, along with calcifications which may be visible in the lumen and appendiceal wall. On CT, a well-defined, fluid-filled lesion with intramural or intraluminal calcification is highly suggestive of an appendiceal mucocele. In cases of cystadenocarcinomas, a heterogeneous soft tissue component with areas of hemorrhage and necrosis may be identified. On MRI, the imaging features are largely determined by the mucin-to-fluid ratio in a mucocele. Mucoceles which have a high-fluid content are hypointense on T1-weighted images and hyperintense on T2-weighted images while mucoceles which are mucin rich are hyperintense on both T1- and T2-weighted images.

PEARLS

- On CT, a well-defined cystic mass with intraluminal or intramural calcification may be identified.

- Visible soft tissue components within an appendiceal mucocele raise the suspicion for an underlying appendiceal cystadenocarcinoma.

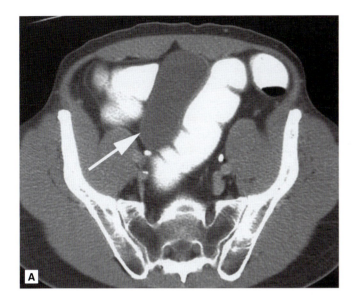

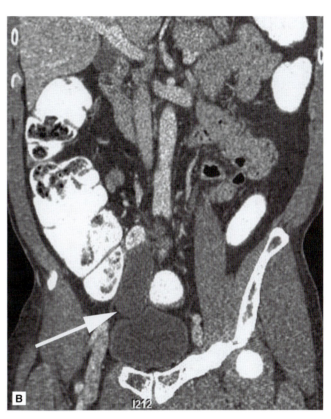

1. A. Axial, enhanced CT image reveals a markedly distended, fluid-filled, appendiceal mucocele in the right lower quadrant (arrow).
B. Coronal, enhanced CT image reveals a markedly distended, fluid-filled, appendiceal mucocele in the right lower quadrant (arrow).

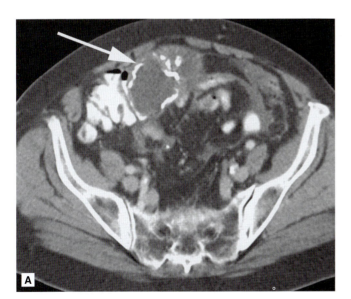

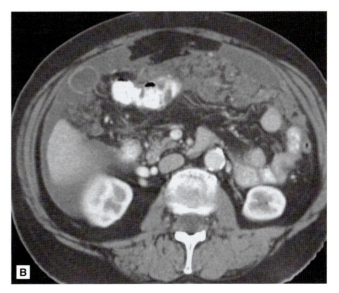

2. A. Axial, enhanced CT image reveals an irregular, fluid-filled appendiceal mucocele (arrow) with typical intraluminal and intramural calcifications. In addition, fluid is seen throughout the peritoneal cavity suggestive of pseudomyxoma peritonei given the presence of a mucocele. **B.** Axial, enhanced CT image reveals fluid and soft tissue nodularity throughout the peritoneal cavity. Given the presence of an appendiceal mucocele, these findings suggest a diagnosis pseudomyxoma peritonei secondary to an underlying mucinous cystadenocarcinoma of the appendix.

PRESENTATION

May be incidental finding in asymptomatic patients. Patients may present with mild gastrointestinal symptoms such as diarrhea or constipation, mucous discharge, and rectal bleeding.

FINDINGS

Clustered, air-filled cystic structures within the colon wall

DIFFERENTIAL DIAGNOSIS

- Imaging pitfall of intraluminal gas bubbles surrounding stool
- Linear pneumatosis intestinalis

COMMENTS

Pneumatosis cystoides coli (PCC) is a descriptive term which represents the presence of numerous submucosal or subserosal gas-filled cyst within the colonic wall and is synonymous with the term pneumatosis cystoides intestinalis (PCI), when limited to the colon. The submucosal cysts are more common in PCC, while the subserosal cysts are more common in the small bowel. Primary PCC is rare and often, an underlying association is identified; PCC is associated with a variety of diseases such as connective tissue disorders, obstructive pulmonary diseases, inflammatory bowel disease, and trauma. Additionally, PCC has been associated with drugs such as corticosteroids, alpha-glucosidase inhibitors, chemotherapy, the ingestion of lactulose and sorbitol, as well as a history of abdominal surgery and colonoscopy. Hypothetical mechanisms for the formation of PCC (and PCI) include the pulmonary theory in which pulmonary diseases result in alveolar rupture with gas eventually tracking through the mesentery into the bowel, the mechanical theory in which increased intraluminal pressure in the bowel results in gas tracking into the bowel wall, and the bacterial theory in which gas-producing bacteria gain entrance to the bowel wall through a mucosal defect.

When air is identified within the bowel wall, the clinical signs and symptoms are critical in determining the clinical significance and whether benign etiologies of PCC should be considered. Several CT features of intramural gas have been evaluated to differentiate benign, self-limited etiologies of pneumatosis from those requiring direct management. Among these, the morphology of the intramural air has been studied and the cystic appearance of PCC has been felt to be more highly correlated with a benign etiology when compared to a linear appearance. Nevertheless, life-threatening etiologies of intramural air may demonstrate the cystic appearance of PCC and, thus, clinical signs and symptoms associated with the patient's presentation and critical in determining appropriate care. On radiographs, bubble-like lucencies may be identified along the periphery of the bowel. On fluoroscopic barium enema studies, bubbly intramural lucencies may also be readily identified. On CT examinations, clusters of rounded or cystic intramural gas-filled structures are seen. On computed tomographic colonography (CTC) examinations, pneumatosis PCC may simulate polyposis though the two-dimensional (2D) CT images readily reveal the gas-filled nature of the cysts.

PEARLS

- PCC is a descriptive term relating to clusters of gas-filled cystic structure on the colon wall.

- While pneumatosis cystoides coli has been shown to correlate more highly with benign etiologies of intramural gas, clinical signs and symptoms are critical in determining appropriate management in patients with this imaging finding.

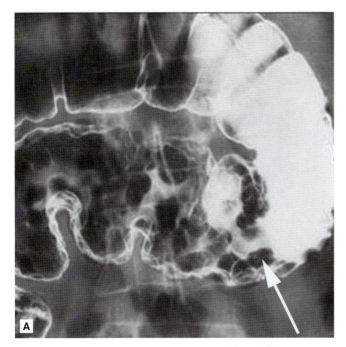

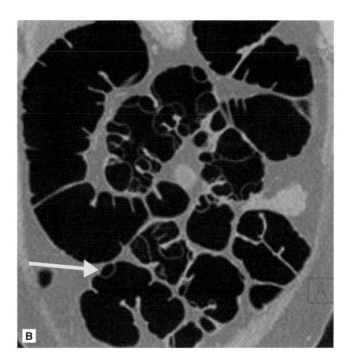

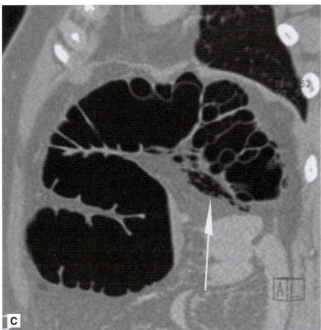

1. A. Fluoroscopic image from barium enema examination reveals cystic lucencies within the colonic wall (arrow). **B.** Fluoroscopic image from barium enema examination reveals bubbly, rounded filling defects within the colonic wall (arrow) is termed pneumatosis cystoides coli. **C.** Sagittal view not only demonstrates the bubbly pneumatosis but shows evidence of extraluminal air from perforation of cyst into the retroperitoneum (arrow).

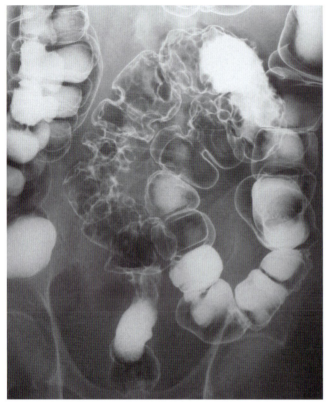

2. A. Coronal CT image demonstrates cystic, air-filled structures throughout the colon wall (arrow).

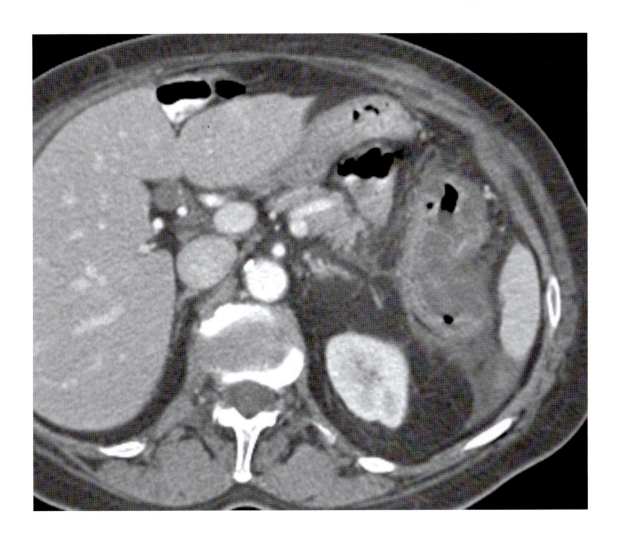

Case 8–16   Iischemic Colitis

PRESENTATION

Patients typically present with the acute onset of mild-to-severe, crampy abdominal pain and tenderness over the affected bowel segment along with diarrhea, nausea, and vomiting. Passage of bright red blood in the stool may follow after the onset of pain within several hours.

FINDINGS

Plain radiography may be normal or demonstrate non-specific ileus, thumbprinting, and loss of haustral markings. On CT, colonic wall thickening, decreased mucosal enhancement, and pneumatosis or air within the mesenteric and portal venous vasculature are seen.

DIFFERENTIAL DIAGNOSIS

- Diverticulitis
- Ulcerative colitis
- Crohn disease
- Pseudomembranous colitis
- Colorectal cancer

COMMENTS

Ischemic colitis is the most common vascular disorder of the gastrointestinal tract and a common cause of colitis in the elderly. While any segment of the colon may be affected, the incidence is higher in so-called watershed areas such as the junction between the distribution of the superior mesenteric artery (SMA) and the inferior mesenteric artery (IMA) in the splenic flexure and the anastomotic plexus of the IMA and hypogastric arterial supply in the rectosigmoid junction. The rectum is relatively protected from ischemic given the presence of excellent collateral blood supply. In younger patients, right-sided ischemia is more common secondary to hemorrhagic shock due to trauma while in elderly patients, left-sided ischemia is more typical secondary to hypoperfusion.

Causes of colonic ischemia include episodes of hypotension and shock, heart failure, atherosclerotic disease, arrhythmias, cardiac or aortic surgery, vasculitis, constipation, colonic obstruction, and some drugs including diuretics, antihypertensive agents, digoxin, and cocaine. In addition, the congenital absence of the marginal artery of Drummond, the anastomosis between the SMA and the IMA, has been reported to result in increased susceptibility to colonic ischemia. The most common mechanism of colonic ischemia is acute, self-limited compromise of colonic blood flow. Depending on the severity of the ischemia, the injury may be confined to the mucosa, involved the submucosa, or may extend transmurally. The mucosa receives most of the colonic blood flow, rendering it most susceptible to damage. Depending on the severity and duration of ischemia, the resultant outcomes include reversible ischemic colitis, chronic ulcerative ischemic colitis, ischemic colonic stricture, or colonic necrosis with perforation and sepsis.

Plain abdominal radiography may be normal or demonstrate a nonspecific ileus in cases of ischemic colitis. In addition, so-called thumbprinting may be identified which is present in 75% of the cases of ischemic colitis and consists of multiple smooth and round filling defects projecting into the colonic lumen representing thickened edematous mucosal folds, mucosal edema, or bleeding. Thumbprinting typically appears during the initial 24 hours of the insult and usually resorbs within 1 week. Other plain radiographic findings of ischemic colitis include loss of haustral folds, pneumatosis, and luminal narrowing.

On CT, which has become the imaging modality of choice for the imaging evaluation of patients with suspected colonic ischemia, common appearances of the involved segments include abnormal thickening of the bowel wall along with pericolonic inflammatory stranding. After reperfusion, the imaging findings evolve and persistent decreased attenuation of the bowel wall related to edema or an increase in attenuation related to intramural hemorrhage may be identified. In cases in which the colonic vasculature remains completely occluded without revascularization, the colonic wall appears thin with an absence of mucosal enhancement. In cases of suspected colonic ischemic, the mesenteric vasculature should be scrutinized to identify any offending thrombi within arteries or veins. While nonspecific, pneumatosis or mesenteric and portal venous air may be identified and, when related to ischemia, suggest frank necrosis.

PEARLS

- Ischemic colitis is the most common vascular disorder of the gastrointestinal tract.

- The most common finding on plain radiography is thumbprinting, described as present in 75% of cases.

- CT has become the imaging modality of choice for ischemic colitis in which bowel wall thickening, edema, decreased enhancement, as well as pneumatosis and portal or mesenteric venous air may be identified.

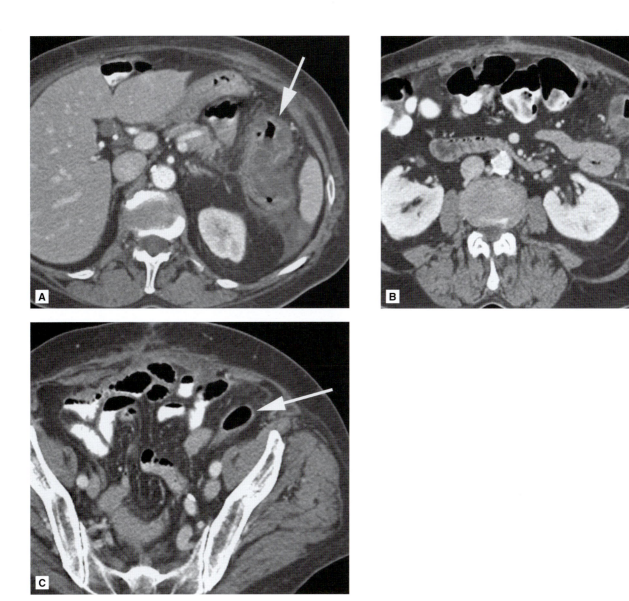

1. A. Axial, contrast-enhanced CT demonstrates abnormally thickened, edematous bowel in the watershed region of the splenic flexure (arrow) related to colonic ischemia. **B.** Axial, contrast-enhanced CT demonstrates abnormally thickened, edematous bowel (arrows) related to colonic ischemia. **C.** A relative normal appearing sigmoid colon is seen (arrow) corresponding to segmental involvement.

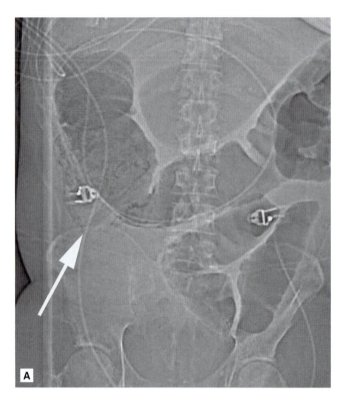

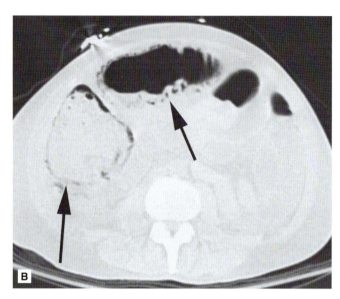

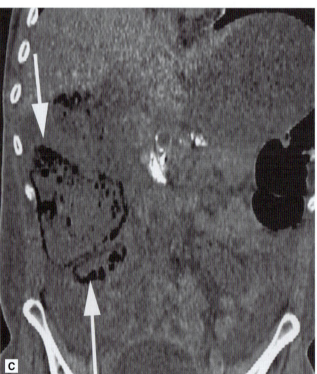

2. A. Scout topogram demonstrates pneumatosis as evidenced by scattered lucencies in the right lower quadrant in the expected location of the cecum and ascending colon (arrow). **B.** Axial CT demonstrates pneumatosis involving the cecum and ascending colon (arrows). While nonspecific, if related to colonic ischemia as in this case, this is an ominous imaging finding suggestive of bowel wall necrosis. **C.** Coronal CT demonstrates pneumatosis involving the cecum and ascending colon (arrows) secondary to colonic ischemia.

COLORECTAL NEOPLASMS

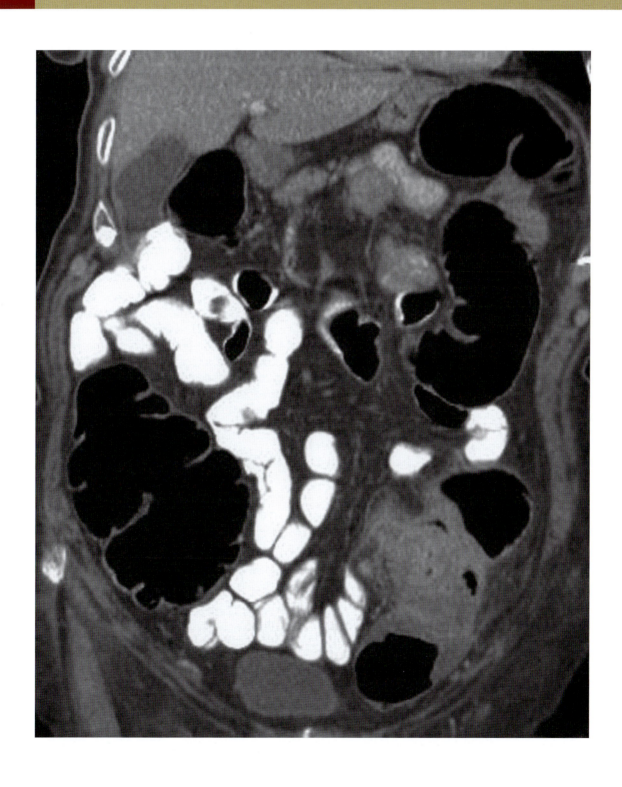

PRESENTATION

While often asymptomatic, patients may present with abdominal pain, gastrointestinal bleeding, or rectal discharge.

FINDINGS

On barium examinations, polyposis syndrome patients have numerous polypoid lesions in the colon, which vary in size and morphology (sessile, flat, or pedunculated).

DIFFERENTIAL DIAGNOSIS

- Inflammatory bowel disease
- Infectious colitis
- Colon cancer

COMMENTS

Familial adenomatous polyposis (FAP) is the most common polyposis syndrome, with a prevalence of approximately 1 in 6000 persons. FAP is characterized by the progressive development of hundreds to thousands of adenomatous polyps in the colon, beginning in the second decade of life. This syndrome carries a 100% risk of developing colorectal cancer at a mean age of 40 years. Patients affected with an attenuated form of the FAP (AFAP) have considerably fewer adenomas (100 or less), but still have a much higher lifetime risk of colorectal cancer (~ 70%). In addition, more than 90% of patients with FAP develop duodenal, ampullary, or periampullary adenomas, and 5% to 10% of them develop duodenal carcinoma by age 60. MUTYH-associated polyposis (MAP) is another autosomal recessive colon cancer syndrome.

Although patients with sporadic hyperplastic polyps in the rectum and sigmoid colon do not have an increased risk of malignant transformation, the hyperplastic polyposis syndrome does confer a higher risk of developing colon cancer. Peutz-Jeghers syndrome is a rare autosomal dominant condition (1 in 150,000) characterized by the pigmented macules on lips, buccal mucosa, hands, and feet and by the development of benign hamartomatous polyps in the gastrointestinal tract. Sporadic juvenile polyps, a type of hamartomatous polyp, are relatively common in the pediatric population and carry little malignant potential. Patients with juvenile polyposis syndrome present with multiple juvenile polyps throughout the gastrointestinal tract. Common symptoms in patients with these syndromes include bleeding, obstruction, and intussusception. It confers a 10% to 38% lifetime risk of colon cancer with an average age of diagnosis at 34 years. Patients affected with hyperplastic or hamartomatous polyposis syndromes have a higher risk of developing colorectal carcinoma than the general population. Effective cancer prevention in affected individuals and family members at risk requires timely recognition of these hereditary syndromes followed by proper genetic testing.

On barium examinations, polyposis syndrome patients have numerous polypoid lesions in the colon, which vary in size and morphology (sessile, flat, or pedunculated). These polyps appear as filling defects in pools of dependent barium or as elevated lesions outlined by a coating of high-density barium on nondependent walls or with double-contrast examinations. However, barium enemas severely underestimate the number of polyps, particularly in young patients whose lesions are often less than 3 mm in diameter. The size of the lesions varies considerably. CT can also demonstrate the innumerable polypoid lesions arising from the wall of the colon. Surgical intervention is necessary once the condition is diagnosed, with continuous surveillance afterward because of the extremely high risk of malignant degeneration of adenomatous polyps and the development of carcinoma. Prophylactic total colectomy is recommended for patients with FAP.

PEARLS

- FAP carries a 100% risk of colorectal cancer. Patients with hyperplastic and hamartomatous polyposis syndromes also have a higher risk of developing colorectal carcinoma.

- More than 90% of patients with FAP will develop duodenal, ampullary, or periampullary adenomas.

- Polyps appear as multiple filling defects in the colon. However, barium enema markedly underestimates the total number of polyps present.

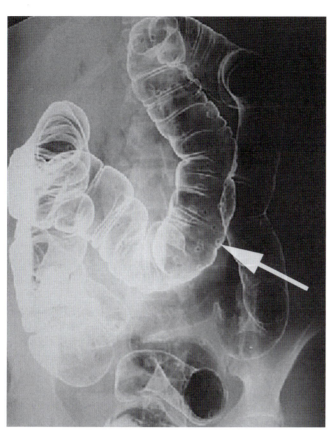

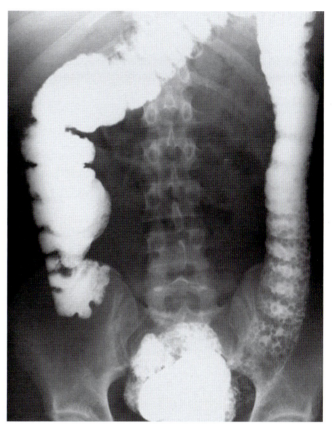

1. Fluoroscopic image from a barium enema examination demonstrates innumerable filling defects within the colon (arrow) in a patient with familial adenomatous polyposis.

2. Fluoroscopic image from a barium enema examination demonstrates innumerable filling defects within the colon, well seen in the descending colon, in a patient with familial adenomatous polyposis.

PRESENTATION

Ranges from asymptomatic to myriad symptoms such as a change in bowel habits, constipation or diarrhea, obstruction, tenesmus, melena, hematochezia, abdominal pain, as well as weight loss of unknown etiology.

FINDINGS

Colorectal cancer or colon cancer may be identified as a filling defect or a short segment of circumferential narrowing resulting in an "apple-core" appearance on a barium enema examination.

An intraluminal soft tissue mass lesion or a short segment of irregular wall thickening may be seen on CT or MRI.

DIFFERENTIAL DIAGNOSIS

- Diverticulosis
- Ischemic colitis
- Infectious or inflammatory colitides

COMMENTS

Colorectal or colon cancer is the most common tumor of the gastrointestinal tract. It is the third most common cancer diagnosed in men and women and is also the second most common cause of cancer-related mortality in the United States. Most colorectal cancers arise from benign adenomatous polyps. More than 95% of colorectal malignancies are adenocarcinomas while squamous cell carcinoma constitutes less than 5% of the cases. Known risk factors of colorectal cancer include benign colonic polyps, family history of colorectal cancer, age above 50, genetic mutation of specific proto-oncogenes and tumor suppressor genes, inflammatory bowel disease, and a diet that is low in fiber and high in lipid and animal protein.

Approximately 70% of colorectal carcinomas arise from benign polyps that undergo malignant transformation, a slow process which requires a period of 7 to 10 years. Thus, screening using barium enema, CT colonography (CTC), or optical colonoscopy allows for the early detection and removal of colonic polyps. Although barium enema is a simple and inexpensive screening tool, it is less sensitive to the detection of small polyps when compared to CTC. In comparison to optical colonoscopy, CTC offers the advantages of being less invasive, not requiring intravenous (IV) sedation, being able to screen the entirety of the colon in cases in which this is technically difficult or impossible using optical colonoscopy, and offers the potential advantage, on a population basis, of an extracolonic evaluation.

The imaging appearance of colorectal cancer is varied and depends significantly on the tumor morphology. On a fluoroscopic-guided double-contrast barium enema, colorectal cancer may appear as circumferential narrowing to yield the apple-core appearance or may appear as a polypoidal or sessile filling defect. On CT, asymmetric bowel wall thickening that is more than 6 mm is considered abnormal and raises the suspicion for possible malignancy. Alternatively, colorectal cancer may appear as a soft tissue mass within the colonic lumen. If the tumor extends beyond the wall of the colon, there may be an irregular appearance of the pericolonic fat which may appear similar to fatty infiltration and stranding. Local invasion of the surrounding structures including the urinary bladder, uterus, or the surrounding bone may be identified at CT. Metastatic lymph nodes and distant metastasis are seen in advanced cases; common locations of distant metastases of colon cancer include the liver while rectal cancer often demonstrates metastases in the lungs and bone. MRI is being increasingly applied to the imaging of rectosigmoid tumors given its relatively fixed position in the pelvis and prognostic information provided by the local disease extent. On T1-weighted images, the tumors are typically iso- or slightly hyperintense to skeletal muscle and on T2-weighted images rectal tumors are typically hyperintense to skeletal muscle. An endorectal coil may be employed to improve MRI image quality. Transrectal ultrasound (TRUS) is also used for rectal cancer imaging as it provides visualization of the different layers of colonic wall and allows for a determination of local tumor stage, similar to MRI. Positron emission tomography (PET)/CT is used in the staging of colorectal cancer and visualization of distant metastasis. It is also used for the detection of postoperative recurrence which might be difficult to detect on CT and MRI, especially in the pelvic region.

PEARLS

- Colorectal cancer is the most common tumor of the gastrointestinal tract.

- Colorectal cancer can present at a very late stage and by a wide range of symptoms, emphasizing the importance of screening.

- The appearance of colorectal cancer varies according to the tumor morphology but commonly leads to narrowing of the bowel lumen.

- There is a role for multiple modalities, including fluoroscopy, US, CT (including PET/CT), and MRI in the screening and disease characterization in colorectal malignancy.

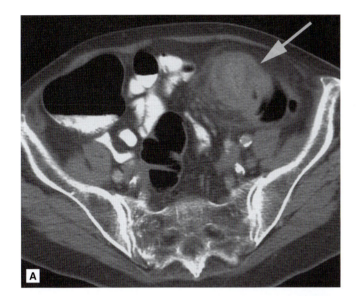

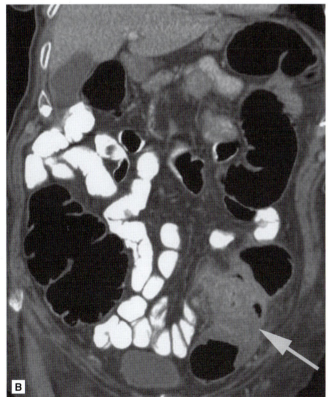

1. **A.** Axial, enhanced CT image demonstrates a short segment of irregular bowel wall thickening in the sigmoid colon (arrow) with adjacent fat stranding, highly suspicious of a primary colonic malignancy. **B.** Coronal, enhanced CT image demonstrates a short segment of irregular colonic wall thickening and resultant luminal narrowing (arrow), highly suspicious for a primary colonic neoplasm.

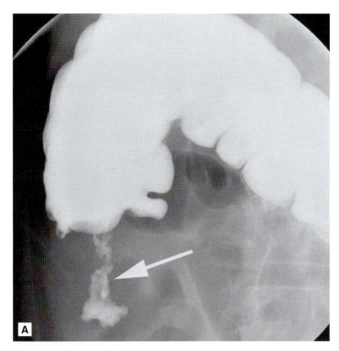

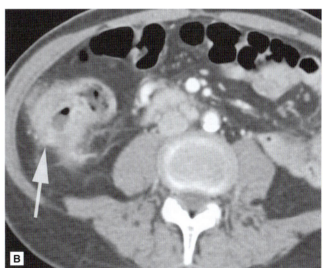

2. **A.** Fluoroscopic image acquired during a barium enema reveals a short segment of irregular narrowing in the ascending colon (arrow) with a classic apple-core appearance of a colorectal malignancy. **B.** Axial, enhanced CT image demonstrates irregular wall thickening in the ascending colon (arrow) corresponding to the abnormality on barium enema. **C.** Axial, contrast-enhanced CT image demonstrates numerous relatively hypoattenuating lesions in the liver (arrow), typical findings of hepatic metastases in this patient with primary colorectal carcinoma. **D.** Image lower in abdomen demonstrates large cecal soft tissue mass corresponding to the primary cecal carcinoma (arrow).

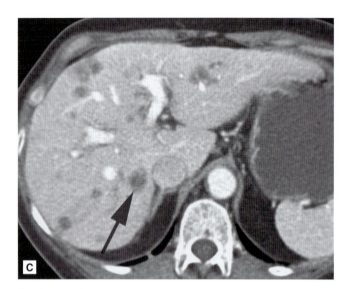

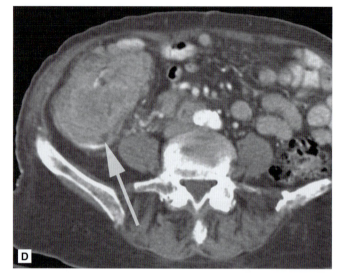

2. (*Continued*)

PRESENTATION

While rectal carcinomas may be incidentally discovered at screening, patients may present with altered bowel habits, rectal pain, or bleeding.

FINDINGS

MRI is widely used for the local staging of rectal cancer given the ability to distinguish between malignant tissue and the muscularis propria, allowing differentiation between T2 and T3 lesions as well as clear, direct delineation of the mesorectal fascia.

DIFFERENTIAL DIAGNOSIS

- Anal cancer
- Ulcerative proctitis
- Crohn proctitis
- Rectal hemorrhoids
- Squamous cell carcinoma (anorectal junction)
- Rectal carcinoid
- Metastatic disease

COMMENTS

Nearly one million patients are diagnosed with colorectal cancers annually in the world and approximately 30% to 40% of them arise in the rectum, defined as the distal margin of the tumor located within 15 cm of the anal verge.

Rectal cancer is palpable via digital rectal examination in 40% to 80% of cases. However, colonoscopy (or sigmoidoscopy) with biopsy is considered as the gold-standard investigation to confirm the diagnosis of rectal cancer and to exclude synchronous lesions. After diagnosis, patients then undergo a variety of staging procedures to assess the extent of locoregional disease and to identify potential sites of distant spread.

Traditional rectal cancer surgery is associated with high rates of local recurrence of 5% to 20%. However, with the combination of high-quality resection using total mesorectal excision along with the use of neoadjuvant and adjuvant treatment (chemotherapy, radiation, or both), there has been a significant reduction in the frequency of local recurrent tumor and a resulting improved survival.

Accurate preoperative staging of rectal cancer is crucial for proper patient selection and planning of surgical treatment. Stage at diagnosis is the strongest predictor for recurrence and prognosis. Thus, results of staging tests help plan correct management options, which usually demand the input of a structured multidisciplinary team.

Preoperative staging of rectal cancer can be divided into local and distant staging. Local staging requires the assessment of mural depth of invasion (T), status of the predicted circumferential resection margin, and the status of perirectal lymph nodes (N). Distant staging assesses for evidence of metastatic disease (M). Currently, several modalities exist for the preoperative staging of rectal cancer. A combination of modalities involving use of CT, MR, and/or endorectal ultrasonography (EUS) is used to precisely assess the extent of spread of rectal cancer. The specific choice of tests performed, however, is influenced by local expertise and availability. Imaging is also crucial for defining radiotherapy fields to avoid unnecessary radiation of adjacent vital structures. MRI is the most widely used technique for the local staging of rectal cancer. The two major advantages of MRI are the ability to distinguish between malignant tissue and the muscularis propria, allowing differentiation between T2 and T3 lesions and clear direct delineation of the mesorectal fascia. However, MR has a tendency for overstaging disease, related to the desmoplastic reaction commonly elicited by rectal tumors, which can cause spiculations in the perirectal fat that may or may not contain viable tumor cells. The majority of rectal carcinomas are hypermetabolic on PET imaging. PET is generally indicated when there is clinical, biochemical, or radiological suspicion of local recurrence or systemic disease.

PEARLS

- Accurate preoperative staging of rectal cancer is mandatory for proper selection of therapeutic options and to improve the chances of survival.

- MR is highly accurate for predicting a clear circumferential resection margin. CT and PET are preferred for regional and distant staging and restaging.

- The combination of mesorectal excision and neoadjuvant or adjuvant chemoradiation has helped reduce the frequency of local tumor recurrence and improve survival rates.

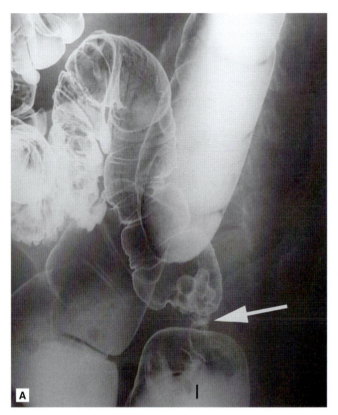

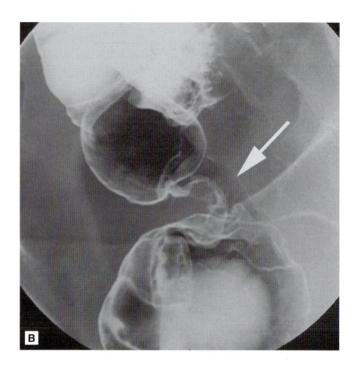

1. A. Fluoroscopic image from barium enema examination demonstrates an irregular, strictured segment of the rectum (arrow), consistent with rectal carcinoma. **B.** Fluoroscopic image from barium enema examination demonstrates a classic "apple-core" appearance of a narrow, irregular stricture (arrow) related to a rectal carcinoma.

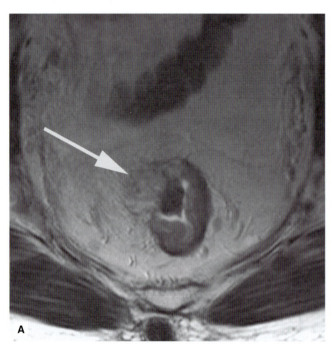

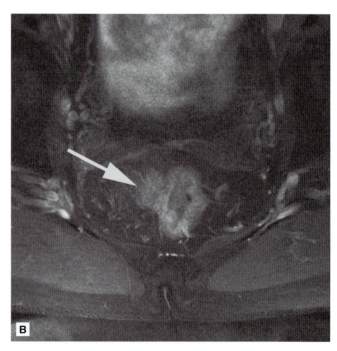

2. A. Axial, T2-weighted MRI image demonstrates a relatively hyperintense mass lesion (arrow) clearly extending into the mesorectal fat. **B.** Axial, contrast-enhanced MRI image demonstrates a rectal tumor (arrow) extending into the mesorectal fat.

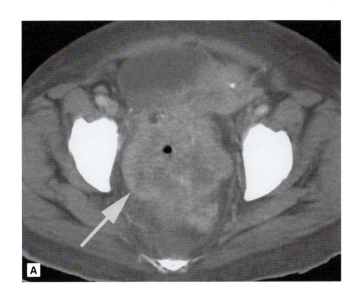

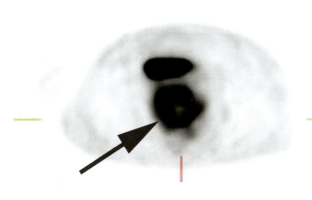

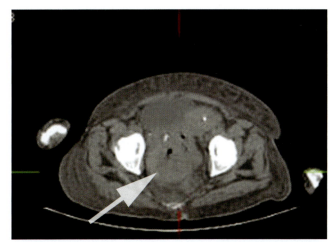

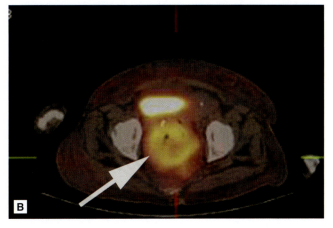

3. A. Axial, contrast-enhanced CT image demonstrates a large, irregular rectal tumor (arrow). **B.** PET/CT examination performed for staging of the tumor demonstrates high fluorodeoxyglucose (FDG) avidity of the large rectal mass lesion (arrows).

CHAPTER 9

OMENTUM, MESENTRY, ABDOMINAL WALL, AND PERITONEUM

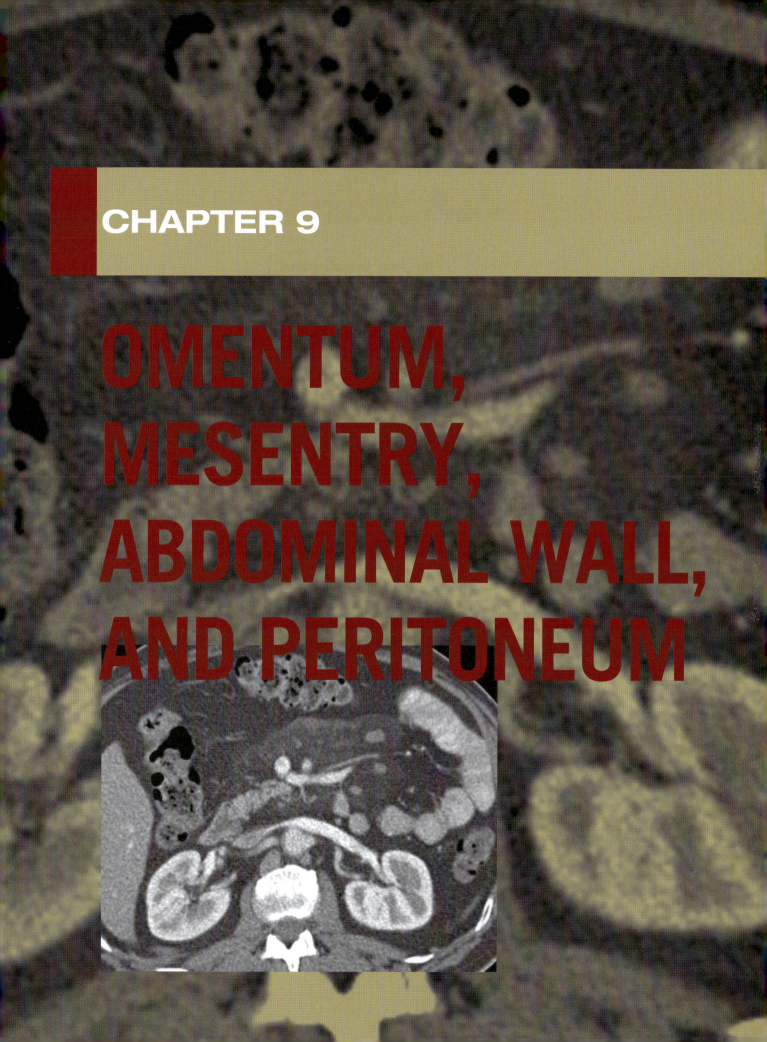

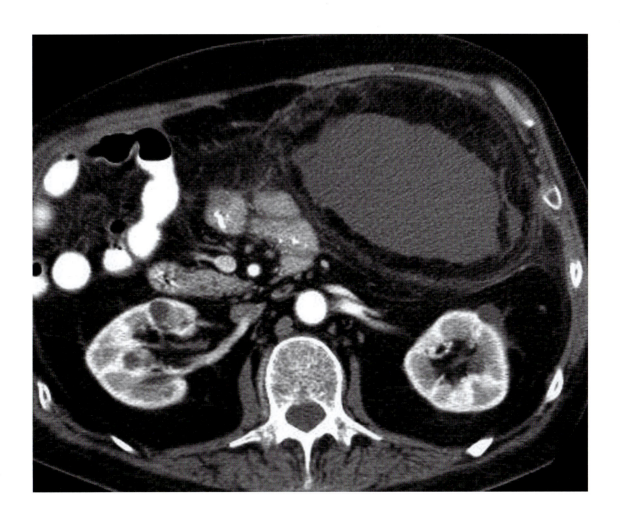

PRESENTATION

Acute abdominal pain, typically located in right upper or lower quadrants. Also, nausea, vomiting, diarrhea, fever, and leukocytosis have been reported.

FINDINGS

Omental infarctions are seen as relatively focal areas of ill-defined, heterogeneous, fat attenuation which are located between the anterior abdominal wall and the colon.

DIFFERENTIAL DIAGNOSIS

- Epiploic appendagitis
- Appendicitis
- Diverticulitis

COMMENTS

Omental infarction is an uncommon cause of acute abdominal pain which affects patients of virtually any age and is often related to abdominal surgery but is commonly idiopathic. Omental infarction may be secondary to omental torsion which may be primary and postulated to occur secondary to developmental abnormalities of the omentum such as abnormality of attachments predisposing to torsion. Secondary omental torsion is related to an inciting abnormality such as the presence of scar or a mass lesion predisposing to torsion. In cases unrelated to torsion, etiologies such as prior surgery, obesity, superior mesenteric artery thrombosis, among others have been reported.

In cases of idiopathic infarction, the location is typically in the right lower quadrant and in those cases related to surgery, the infarction is either within or in close proximity to the surgical bed.

Omental infractions are typically diagnosed by CT though ultrasound (US) and magnetic resonance imaging (MRI) findings have been reported. On computed tomography (CT), omental infarctions are seen as relatively focal areas of ill-defined, heterogeneous, fat attenuation which may or may not directly abut the adjacent colon and are located between the anterior abdominal wall and the colon. Over time, omental infarctions are seen to decrease in size, become increasingly well defined, and form a hyperdense periphery. However, progression to a frank intraperitoneal abscess has been described. In primary (idiopathic) omental infarcts, the size of omental infarcts has been reported to range from 5 to 7.5 cm in the majority of patients and exceeds 7.5 cm in those patients with infarction related to surgery.

PEARLS

- Omental infarction is an uncommon cause of acute abdominal pain which affects patients of virtually any age and is often related to abdominal surgery but is commonly idiopathic.

- In cases of idiopathic infarction, the location is typically in the right lower quadrant and in those cases related to surgery, the infarction is either within or in close proximity to the surgical bed.

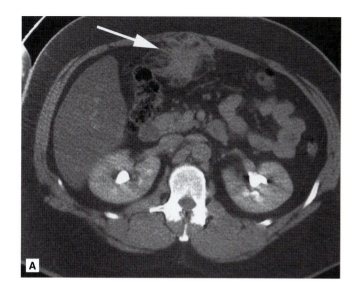

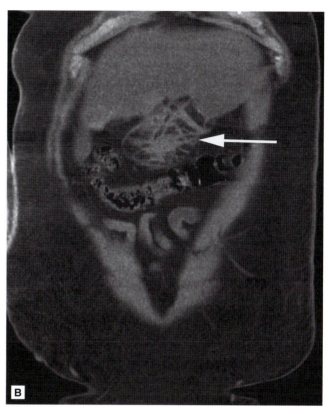

1. **A.** Axial, contrast-enhanced CT image reveals an ill-defined omental infarction within the midline (arrow). **B.** Coronal, contrast-enhanced CT image reveals an ill-defined omental infarction within the midline (arrow).

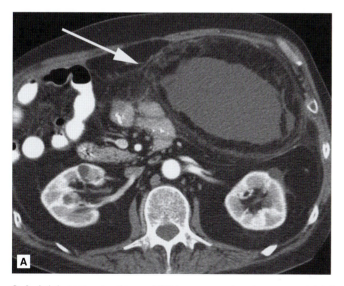

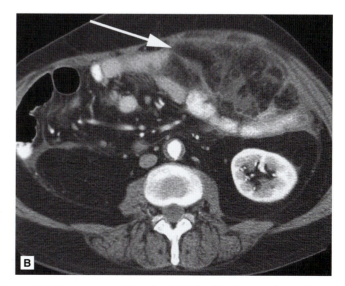

2. **A.** Axial, contrast-enhanced CT image reveals a large omental infarction which has progressed to a frank fluid collection, worrisome for an abscess in the appropriate clinical setting (arrow). **B.** Axial, contrast-enhanced CT image reveals the ill-defined inflammatory components along the inferior aspect of a large omental infarction (arrow).

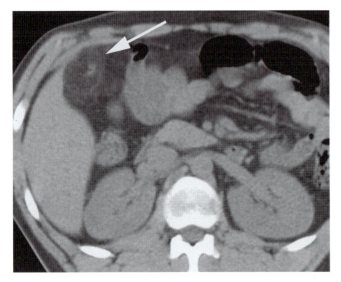

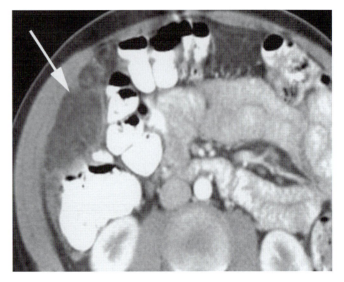

3. Axial, unenhanced CT image reveals a small, right-sided omental infarction (arrow).

4. Axial, enhanced CT image reveals a right-sided omental infarction (arrow).

PRESENTATION

When symptomatic, patients may present with abdominal pain, weight loss, and palpable abdominal mass.

FINDINGS

In cases of mesenteric panniculitis, increased attenuation of the mesenteric fat is typically noted which may be associated with a hypoattenuating halo surrounding mesenteric vessels and prominent to frankly enlarged lymph nodes.

DIFFERENTIAL DIAGNOSIS

- Desmoid tumor
- Carcinoid tumor
- Peritoneal carcinomatosis

COMMENTS

Mesenteric panniculitis is a rare, chronic inflammation of the adipose tissue of the mesentery. While the specific etiology of this disorder remains unclear, proposed pathophysiologic mechanisms include autoimmune disease, prior trauma or surgery, and ischemia. In addition, mesenteric panniculitis has been associated with other conditions including malignancy (lymphoma, lung, breast, among others), vasculitis, rheumatic diseases, granulomatous diseases, tobacco consumption, and pancreatitis, among many others. Myriad terms have been applied to mesenteric panniculitis, leading to some confusion, including mesenteric lipodystrophy, sclerosing mesenteritis, liposclerotic mesenteritis, among others. While often asymptomatic, the clinical signs and symptoms may include abdominal pain, anorexia, weight loss, as well as palpable abdominal mass lesions.

The progression of mesenteric panniculitis has been characterized by three histologic stages: (1) mesenteric lipodystrophy, (2) mesenteric panniculitis, and (3) retractile mesenteritis. In the first stage, foamy macrophages infiltrate the mesenteric fat. In the second stage, mesenteric panniculitis, additional cells are seen to infiltrate the mesenteric adipose tissue including polymorphonuclear leukocytes and foreign body giant cells. In the third stage, fibrosis, inflammation, and collagen deposition are seen, leading to tethering and retraction of the mesentery.

The imaging findings of mesenteric panniculitis depend on the histologic stage of the disease but the finding of *misty mesentery* is often identified on CT. The term *misty mesentery* refers to increased attenuation of the mesenteric fat owing to the deposition of inflammatory cell, fluid, fibrosis, or tumor. Thus, while an appearance of misty mesentery may be seen in cases of mesenteric panniculitis, this imaging finding is nonspecific and may be seen in cases of mesenteric edema related to vascular disorders, direct infiltration of tumor into the mesenteric fat, lymphedema, among various other causes. Often, the underlying cause of this nonspecific imaging finding of *misty mesentery* is idiopathic. In cases of mesenteric panniculitis, a hypoattenuating halo is often seen surrounding the mesenteric vasculature, termed the *fat-ring sign*. In addition, soft tissue nodularity within the area of increased attenuation may be seen; these nodules may also be surrounded by a peripheral area of hypoattenuation. These nodules vary in size and mesenteric mass lesions may be seen which may develop calcification or display cystic components. A pseudocapsule surrounding the involved area of mesenteric adipose tissue has also been described, sharply marginating the area of involvement. Most commonly, the involved segment of mesentery is directed toward the leftward aspect of the abdomen, extending toward the root of the jejunum. Additionally, the abnormal portion of the mesentery may exert mass effect on the surrounding bowel loops.

PEARLS

- In mesenteric panniculitis, hyperattenuation of the involved mesentery, termed misty mesentery; this imaging finding is nonspecific and is related to myriad etiologies.

- A hypoattenuating halo surrounding mesenteric vessels and associated mesenteric soft tissue nodules, termed the fat-ring sign, may be seen in cases of mesenteric panniculitis.

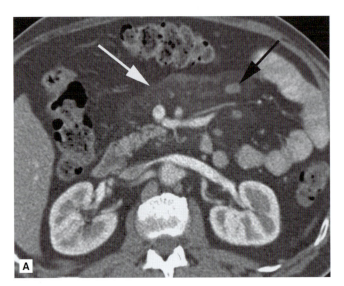

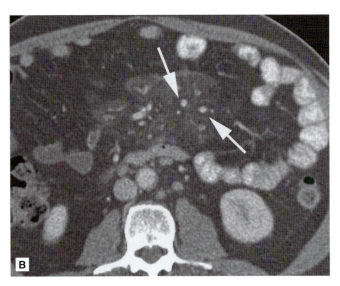

1. A. Axial CT image reveals a segmental area of mesenteric infiltration (white arrow) which contains several soft tissue nodules (black arrow) in this case of mesenteric panniculitis. **B.** Axial CT image reveals relative hypoattenuation surrounding several mesenteric vessels (arrows), termed the fat-ring sign, in this case of mesenteric panniculitis.

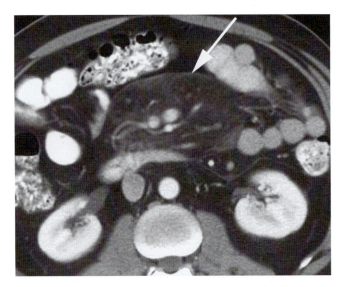

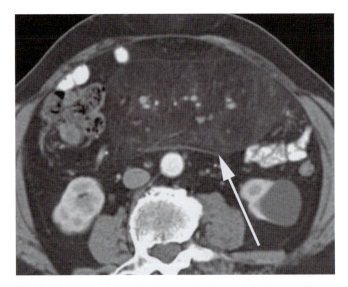

2. Axial CT image reveals a well-circumscribed peripheral pseudocapsule (arrow) surrounding an area of mesenteric panniculitis.

3. Axial CT image demonstrates a well-circumscribed area of relative hyperattenuation (arrow) within the mesenteric adipose tissue, in this case of mesenteric panniculitis.

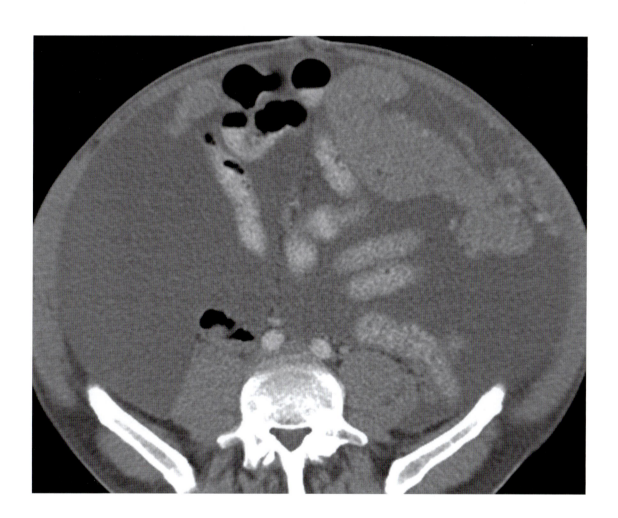

PRESENTATION

Many cases are asymptomatic but patients may report palpable mass, abdominal pain, nausea, vomiting, gastrointestinal hemorrhage depending on the location of the tumor.

FINDINGS

The imaging appearance of desmoid tumors varies depending on the composition and relative amounts of various constituent components such as collagen or vascularity. Thus, desmoid tumors may appear ill defined and infiltrative and others well circumscribed; they typically demonstrate a degree of enhancement after contrast administration.

DIFFERENTIAL DIAGNOSIS

- Fibrosarcoma
- Malignant fibrous histiocytoma
- Carcinoid tumor
- Lymphoma

COMMENTS

Desmoid tumors, also known as deep fibromatoses, originate from the connective tissue of muscle, fascia, or aponeuroses and are characterized by fibroblastic proliferation in a collagenous stroma. Desmoid tumors typically affect young adults aged 25 to 35 years with a slight female predominance and may be classified into their intra-abdominal, abdominal, or extra-abdominal location. Though benign at histology, desmoid tumors often exhibit aggressive behavior locally and may recur after surgery with rates reported to be 25% to 65%. The intra-abdominal desmoid tumors include those arising in the mesentery, a minority of which are associated with Gardner syndrome and typically occur after abdominal surgery. Desmoid tumors represent the most common primary tumor of the mesentery and they may compress the bowel and cause obstruction. Abdominal desmoid tumors which most commonly occur in association with the rectus or internal oblique musculature, are described in women with oral contraceptive use as well as during pregnancy or within 1 year of delivery suggesting a possible etiologic role of hormonal stimulation. Finally, extra-abdominal desmoid tumors are reported in relation to the muscles and fascia of the chest, back, thighs, and knees but have been reported in the mediastinum and are typically aggressive with high recurrence rates after surgery.

The imaging appearance of desmoid tumors varies depending on the composition and relative amounts of various constituent components such as collagen or vascularity. On US, desmoid tumor may have variable echogenicity but tend to exhibit smooth, well-circumscribed margins. On CT, desmoid tumors may appear ill defined and infiltrative and others well circumscribed. They are typically isoattenuating or hyperattenuating with respect to skeletal muscle. Desmoid tumors typically demonstrate a degree of enhancement after contrast administration. MR imaging affords superior soft tissue characterization in cases of desmoid tumors, which are typically T2 hyperintense in their early stages, gradually evolves to T2 isointensity found in more chronic lesions. The majority of desmoid tumors, T2 hyperintense bands corresponding to dense collagenous bands may be identified. After intravenous contrast administration, desmoid tumors demonstrate enhancement on MRI, save for the collagenous bands that typically remain hypointense.

PEARLS

- **Desmoid tumors represent the most common primary tumor of the mesentery.**

- **Desmoid tumors originate from the connective tissue of muscle, fascia, or aponeuroses and are characterized by fibroblastic proliferation in a collagenous stroma.**

- **Though benign at histology, desmoid tumors often exhibit aggressive behavior locally and may recur after surgery with rates reported to be 25% to 65%.**

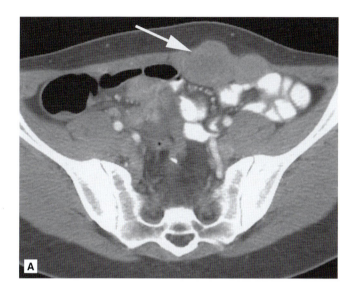

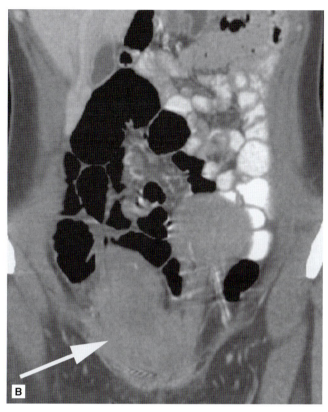

1. A. Axial, contrast-enhanced CT image reveals a lobulated desmoid tumor in the left rectus muscle (arrow). **B.** Coronal, contrast-enhanced CT image reveals a lobulated desmoid tumor in the left rectus muscle (arrow).

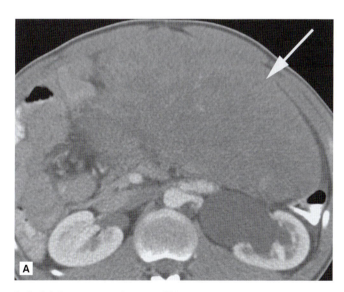

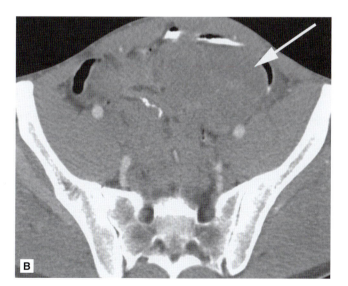

2. A. Axial, contrast-enhanced CT image reveals a large, well-circumscribed intra-abdominal desmoid tumor (arrow). **B.** Axial, contrast-enhanced CT image reveals a large, well-circumscribed intra-abdominal desmoid tumor extending into the pelvis (arrow).

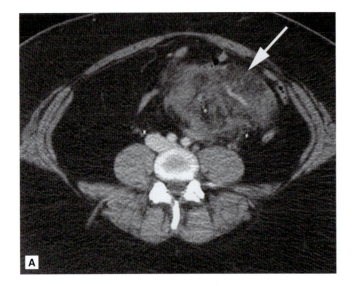

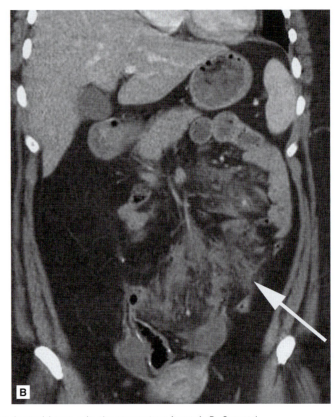

3. A. Axial, contrast-enhanced CT image reveals an infiltrative-appearing desmoid tumor in the mesentery (arrow). **B.** Coronal, contrast-enhanced CT image reveals an infiltrative-appearing desmoid tumor in the mesentery (arrow).

PRESENTATION

Many cases are asymptomatic and incidentally detected on imaging. When present, symptoms include vague abdominal pain and distention which may simulate ascites. Mesenteric cysts may lead to bowel, biliary, or urinary obstruction.

FINDINGS

The imaging findings of a mesenteric cyst typically include a well-circumscribed cyst which is typically fluid attenuating and simple, located within the mesentery and, less commonly, in the omentum.

DIFFERENTIAL DIAGNOSIS

- Splenic, renal, pancreatic, or ovarian cyst
- Hydatid cyst
- Cystic teratoma
- Duplication cysts
- Choledochal cyst

COMMENTS

The terms mesenteric and omental cysts are descriptive terms which encompass a range of histologic diagnoses. Included in the descriptive term mesenteric cyst are lymphangiomas, enteric duplication cysts, enteric cysts, mesothelial cysts, as well as nonpancreatic pseudocysts; the most common is a lymphangioma. The lining of these cysts varies depending on histologic type; lymphangiomas have an endothelial lining, enteric duplication cysts have an enteric lining, enteric cysts have an enteric lining with no muscular layer as opposed to the enteric lining of duplication cysts, mesothelial cysts have a mesothelial lining, and nonpancreatic pseudocysts do not have a lining and are circumscribed by fibrous tissue. In addition to differences in their lining, the contents of these mesenteric cysts are somewhat variable and, while typically serous, may include chylous contents in cases of communication with lymphatics, hemorrhagic fluid which may be related to trauma, or purulent fluid in cases in which the cysts become infected.

While the majority of cysts originate in the small bowel mesentery, these benign cysts may originate anywhere in the mesentery of the gastrointestinal tract and may be seen from the base of the mesentery to the retroperitoneum. Less common than mesenteric cysts, omental cysts may be seen anywhere within the lesser or greater omentum. While often asymptomatic, patients may present with vague abdominal pain or distention and complications of mesenteric cysts include secondary bowel, biliary or urinary obstruction, volvulus, as well as hemorrhage or infection. Mesenteric cysts are often seen in children; up to one-third of cases are seen in patients less than 15 years old.

The imaging findings in mesenteric and omental cysts depend on the histologic type. Typically mesenteric and omental cysts appear as simple, unilocular cysts of variable size ranging up to greater than 40 cm in dimension, however, this appearance may vary widely. Plain radiographs or barium studies are reported to reveal noncalcified masses that are seen to displace the bowel. On cross-sectional imaging, the cysts may have a variety of imaging appearances based on the contents of the cyst which include hemorrhage, serous fluid, or chyle as well as the presence of infection. On US, the most common finding is that of a simple, anechoic cyst though internal septations and solid echogenicity with a honeycomb pattern have been described. Similarly, On CT, uni- and multilocular cystic lesions have been described with attenuation ranging from fat to a more complex, hyperattenuating appearance related to variable contents ranging from chylous to hemorrhagic, respectively. Finally, while the imaging appearance of the various histologic types often overlaps, enteric duplication cysts and nonpancreatic pseudocysts have been described to have demonstrate a relatively thick, enhancing wall on CT.

PEARLS

- Mesenteric and omental cysts are descriptive terms which include a variety of histologically distinct entities, the most common of which are lymphangiomas.

- The imaging appearance of mesenteric and omental cysts depend on the histologic type as well as the contents of the cyst which may be serous, hemorrhagic, chylous, or purulent.

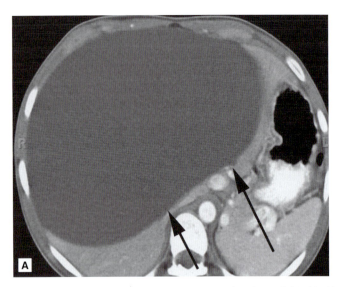 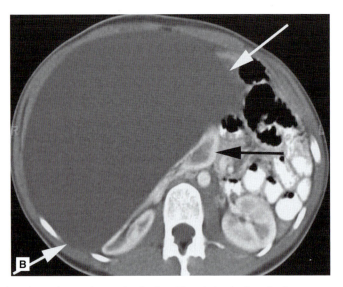

1. A. Axial, contrast-enhanced CT image reveals a large right-sided lymphangioma (arrows) seen to displace the abdominal contents leftward. **B.** Axial, contrast-enhanced CT image reveals a large right-sided lymphangioma (white arrows) seen to exert significant mass effect on the right kidney (black arrow).

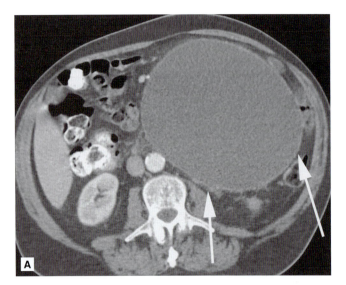 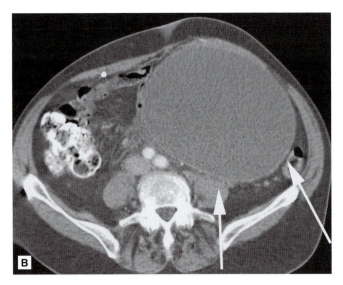

2. A. Axial, contrast-enhanced CT image reveals a large left-sided lymphangioma (arrows) displacing the bowel. **B.** Axial, contrast-enhanced CT image reveals a large left-sided lymphangioma (arrows) displacing the bowel.

PRESENTATION

Abdominal pain, distention, ascites, and weight loss

FINDINGS

Peritoneal mesotheliomas are typically seen as solid, enhancing intraperitoneal soft tissue mass lesions.

DIFFERENTIAL DIAGNOSIS

- Desmoid tumor
- Peritoneal carcinomatosis, not otherwise specified (nos)
- Tuberculosis

COMMENTS

Malignant peritoneal mesotheliomas are rare, rapidly fatal neoplasms which account for approximately 30% of all malignant mesotheliomas, the majority of which affect the pleura. As with all mesotheliomas, asbestos exposure is a risk factor for peritoneal mesothelioma with 50% of patients reporting a history of exposure. Peritoneal mesothelioma is typically confined to the peritoneal cavity though metastases to lung bone, and liver as well as thoracic and retroperitoneal lymph nodes have been reported, among others. Peritoneal mesotheliomas are aggressive with 5-year mortality of approximately 50%.

The imaging findings of peritoneal mesotheliomas are nonspecific; on CT, peritoneal mesotheliomas are typically seen as solid, enhancing intraperitoneal soft tissue mass lesions. The CT imaging findings have been categorized into three types: the "dry" appearance with absence of ascites with a single large or several smaller masses in a single abdominal quadrant, the "wet" appearance with the absence of a dominant mass with ascites and diffuse soft tissue nodules and plaques, or a combination of these two types. Mass effect with scalloping of adjacent abdominal organs may be seen. In contradistinction to pleural mesothelioma, calcification is an uncommon finding in malignant peritoneal mesothelioma. Peritoneal mesotheliomas tend to spread along serosal surfaces and often infiltrate solid or hollow visceral organs, most commonly the liver and colon. Though nonspecific from a diagnostic standpoint, imaging and in particular CT is useful in planning biopsy as well as surgical management as cytoreductive surgery is often indicated and its success impacts prognosis.

PEARLS

- Malignant peritoneal mesotheliomas are rare, rapidly fatal neoplasms which account for approximately 30% of all malignant mesotheliomas.

- Asbestos exposure is a risk factor for peritoneal mesothelioma with 50% of patients reporting a history of exposure.

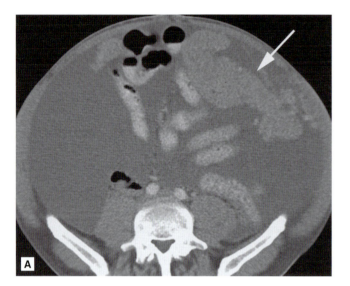
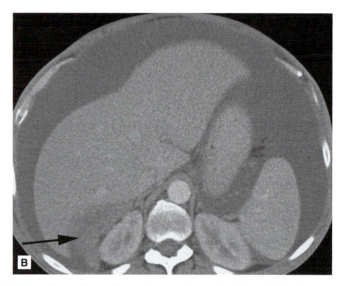

1. A. Axial, contrast-enhanced CT image reveals a large peritoneal mesothelioma (arrow) as well as a large volume of ascites. **B.** Axial, contrast-enhanced CT image reveals a large peritoneal mesothelioma extending posterior to the liver (arrow) well as a large volume of ascites.

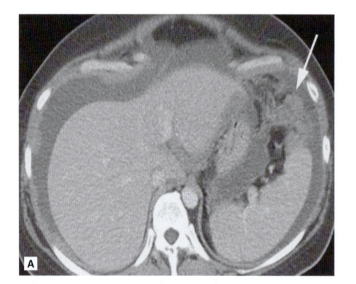
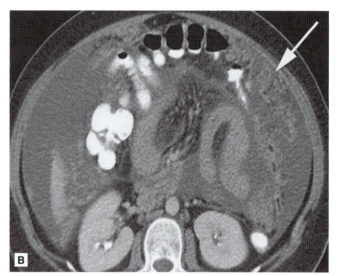

2. A. Axial, contrast-enhanced CT image reveals a peritoneal mesothelioma (arrow) as well as a large volume of ascites. **B.** Axial, contrast-enhanced CT image reveals a large peritoneal mesothelioma (arrow) as well as a large volume of ascites.

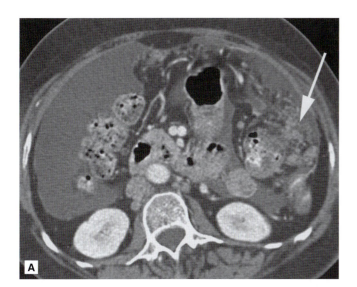

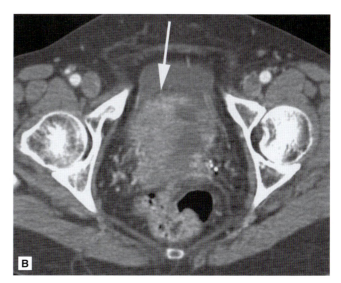

3. A. Axial, contrast-enhanced CT image reveals the presence of a peritoneal mesothelioma (arrow) as well as a large volume of ascites.
B. Axial, contrast-enhanced CT image reveals the presence of a peritoneal mesothelioma extending into the pelvis (arrow) as well as a large volume of ascites.

PRESENTATION

Abdominal pain, distention, and weight loss

FINDINGS

On CT, the gelatinous material is typically hypoattenuating though soft tissue nodularity representing tumor, compressed mesentery, or focal fibrosis may be present. Unlike simple ascites, scalloping of surface of the liver and spleen may be identified in cases of pseudomyxoma peritonei resulting from mass effect exerted by the mucinous implants.

DIFFERENTIAL DIAGNOSIS

- Ascites, not otherwise specified
- Multicystic mesothelioma

COMMENTS

Pseudomyxoma peritonei is a rare condition which refers to the finding of mucinous or gelatinous material within the peritoneal cavity. Pseudomyxoma may be classified into two categories based on the histologic characteristics of the etiology such that the classic pseudomyxoma peritonei refers to cases in which the epithelial cells are benign or borderline appearing or cells which originate from a well-differentiated mucinous tumor. The second category, referred to as peritoneal mucinous carcinomatosis originates from invasive high-grade mucinous carcinomas of the gastrointestinal tract, ovaries, or pancreas of gallbladder. The most common form of pseudomyxoma peritonei is the former which typically arises from low-grade mucinous tumors of the appendix that extend or rupture into the peritoneal cavity. The prognosis and management of the two forms of pseudomyxoma reflect the underlying histology such that the former has an indolent course amenable to surgical debulking while the latter is aggressive resulting in fatality. The relative degree of gelatinous material is larger in those patients with classic pseudomyxoma peritonei versus peritoneal mucinous carcinomatosis. In some patients with pseudomyxoma, synchronous appendiceal and ovarian mucinous tumors are diagnosed. Whether the ovarian tumor represents a synchronous primary or a site of metastasis from the appendix remains a point of controversy.

Pseudomyxoma peritonei is more common in female patients with mean age of approximately 50 years. Symptomatology is related to the large gelatinous material within the abdomen and includes abdominal distention and weight loss. As the common etiology is mucinous appendiceal tumors, right-sided symptoms are often reported.

On imaging, the gelatinous material in pseudomyxoma peritonei may appear echogenic on US, a distinguishing characteristic from simple ascites. In contradistinction to the internal echoes seen in complex ascitic fluid due to hemorrhage, for example, the internal echoes associated with pseudomyxoma are immobile. Echogenic septations may also be visible on US. With large degrees of intraperitoneal mucin, the bowel may be displaced centrally and posteriorly leading to a typical appearance of pseudomyxoma, the starburst pattern in which the echogenic, centrally displaced bowel is surrounded by relatively hypoattenuating gelatinous material. On CT, the gelatinous material is typically hypoattenuating though soft tissue nodularity representing tumor, compressed mesentery, or focal fibrosis may be present. In addition, calcification may be readily identified on CT. Unlike simple ascites, scalloping of surface of the liver and spleen may be identified in cases of pseudomyxoma peritonei resulting from mass effect exerted by the mucinous implants. On MRI, the gelatinous material exhibits T1 hypointensity and T2 hyperintensity with internal septations and soft tissue findings readily identified. Finally, differentiating classic pseudomyxoma peritonei from peritoneal mucinous carcinomatosis may be challenging on imaging but the latter often demonstrates less volume of gelatinous material, more soft tissue nodularity and lymphadenopathy, and more frequently involves the thorax with effusions of pleural masses.

PEARLS

- **Pseudomyxoma peritonei is a rare condition which refers to the finding of mucinous or gelatinous material within the peritoneal cavity.**

- **Pseudomyxoma may be classified into two categories based on the histologic characteristics of the etiology: classic pseudomyxoma peritonei from benign, borderline, or well-differentiated mucinous tumors versus peritoneal mucinous carcinomatosis related to invasive high-grade mucinous carcinomas.**

- **Unlike simple ascites, scalloping of surface of the liver and spleen may be identified in cases of pseudomyxoma peritonei.**

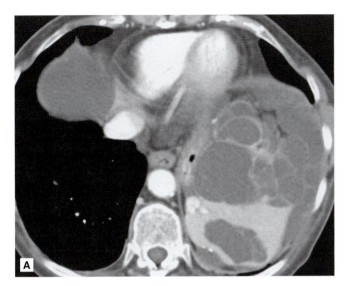

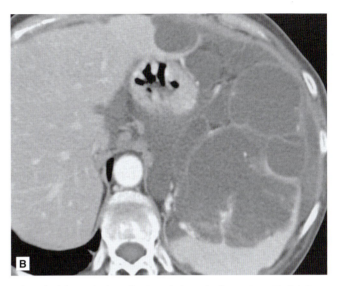

1. A. Axial, contrast-enhanced CT image reveals diffuse pseudomyxoma peritonei with marked scalloping of the splenic contour. **B.** Axial, contrast-enhanced CT image reveals diffuse pseudomyxoma peritonei with marked scalloping of the splenic and hepatic contours.

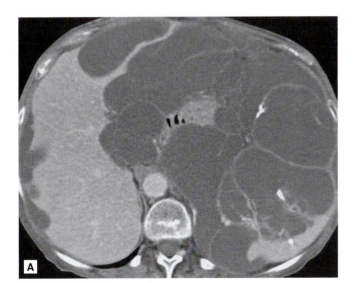

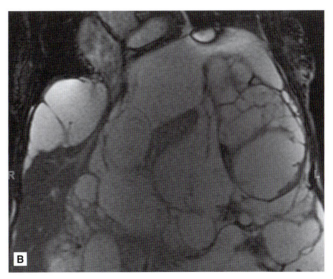

2. A. Axial, contrast-enhanced CT image reveals diffuse pseudomyxoma peritonei with marked scalloping of the splenic and hepatic contours. Areas of calcification along the septations are noted. **B.** Coronal T2-weighted MRI image reveals diffuse pseudomyxoma peritonei throughout the peritoneal cavity.

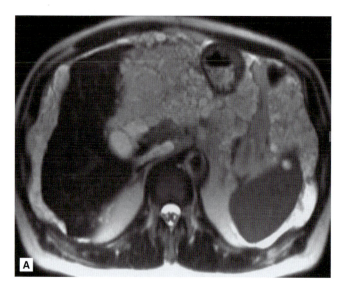

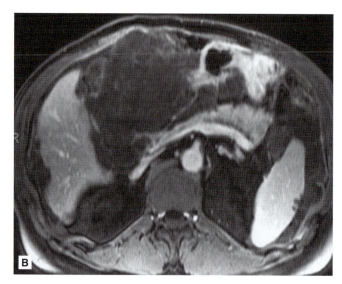

3. A. Axial T2-weighted MRI image reveals diffuse pseudomyxoma peritonei with scalloping of the liver well seen on this image. **B.** Axial, enhanced T1-weighted MRI image reveals diffuse pseudomyxoma peritonei with scalloping of the liver and spleen seen on this image.

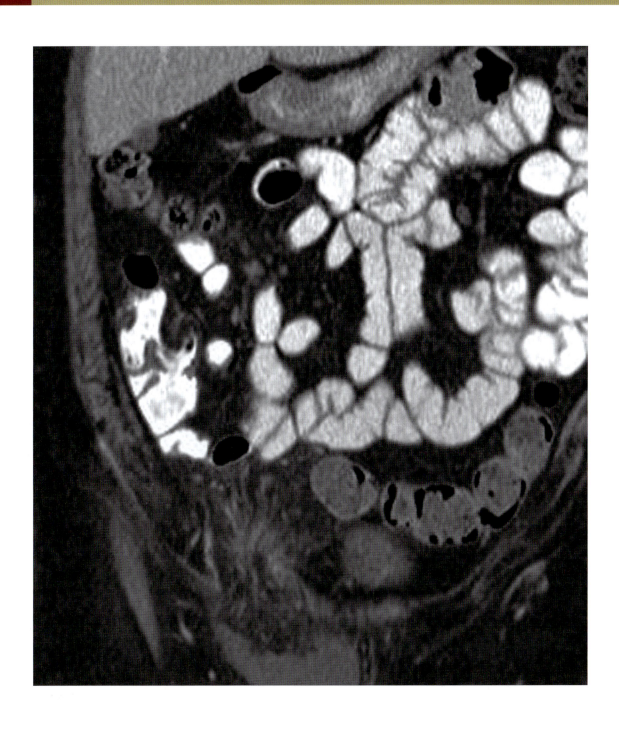

PRESENTATION

Palpable mass, groin pain and swelling, incarceration of bowel with pain, and possible bowel obstruction.

FINDINGS

Direct inguinal hernias originate medial to the inferior epigastric vessels while indirect inguinal hernias originate lateral to the inferior epigastric vessels.

DIFFERENTIAL DIAGNOSIS

• Femoral hernia

COMMENTS

Inguinal hernias may be subdivided into direct and indirect subtypes. The indirect hernias originate at the deep inguinal ring, lateral to the inferior epigastric vessels, and extend along the inguinal canal inferomedially. In contradistinction, the direct inguinal hernias pass medial to the inferior epigastric vessels through a defect of the Hesselbach triangle. The Hesselbach triangle is composed of the inferior epigastric artery superolaterally, the conjoint tendon medially, and the inguinal ligament inferiorly. Approximately 80% of abdominal wall hernias are inguinal hernias and these more commonly affect the men. When compared to femoral hernia, the likelihood of incarceration of bowel and subsequent complications is less in cases of inguinal hernia. Of the two inguinal hernias, indirect hernias are more likely to incarcerate.

On imaging, femoral hernias may be differentiated into indirect or direct subtypes based on their relationship with the inferior epigastric vessels. In addition to the relationship with the inferior epigastric vessels, the relationship of the hernia with the pubic tubercle may be used to differentiate the subtypes of inguinal hernias. The extension of the hernia sac medial to the pubic tubercle has been reported to be specific for indirect inguinal hernias. Though typically associated with femoral hernias, compression of the femoral vein may rarely occur with inguinal hernias and in these cases the relationship of the hernia to the pubic tubercle may be useful in differentiation. Finally, complications of inguinal hernias which should be evaluated on imaging include bowel incarceration which may lead to strangulation and/or obstruction.

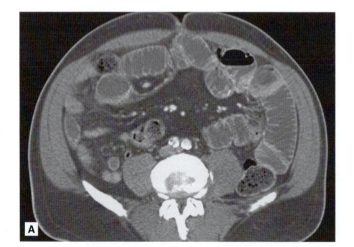 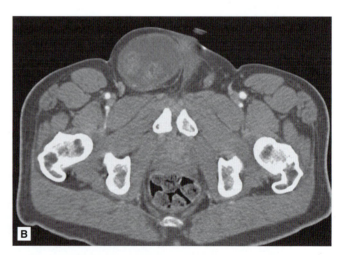

1. A. Axial CT image centered in the mid abdomen demonstrates several dilated, fluid filled small intestinal loops with relatively decompressed loops in the right abdomen. **B.** Axial image centered low in the pelvis shows the obstructing right inguinal hernia sac containing bowel and fluid.

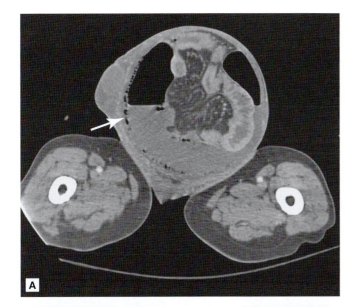

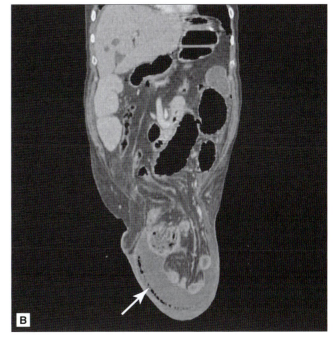

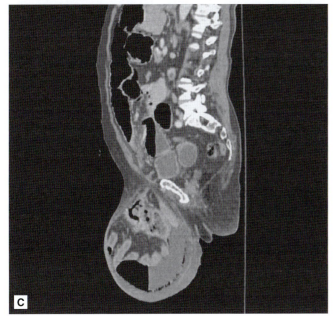

2. A, B, and **C.** Axial, coronal and sagittal images in the region of the pelvis demonstrates an obstructing right inguinal hernia with several dilated small bowel loops herniated through the right inguinal canal. The dilated herniated featureless small bowel also shows evidence of pneumatosis (arrows in A,B).

PRESENTATION

Intermittently palpable mass or abdominal pain, which may be vague

FINDINGS

Spigelian hernias may be diagnosed based on their location, along the lateral aspects of the rectus abdominus muscles on either side of the abdomen, medial to the semilunar line.

DIFFERENTIAL DIAGNOSIS

• Incisional hernia

COMMENTS

Spigelian hernia, named after a Belgian anatomist, Adriaan van den Spieghel (1578-1625), is an acquired ventral hernia along the spigelian fascia or transversus abdominis aponeurosis, a tendinous line along the lateral aspects of the rectus abdominus muscles on either side of the abdomen, medial to the semilunar line. Spigelian hernias typically occur at the level of the semicircular line which is the point at which the fascia of the transversus and oblique muscles begin to split and present a weak point. Below this point, hernias occur less likely as the aponeurosis is formed by a single layer. The hernias typically penetrate the transversus and internal oblique fascial layers and rarely extend through the external oblique fascia. The "spigelian hernia belt" is a paramedian region approximately 0 to 6 cm above an imaginary line running between anterior superior iliac spines in which the majority of hernias occur. In spigelian hernias, the incarceration rate is quite high with reported rates approaching 20%; the hernia sac often contains omentum and less commonly, small bowel or colon.

US and CT are often employed in diagnosing spigelian hernias. On US, examination may begin lateral to the rectus muscles at the approximate level of the umbilicus. Inferior to this level, the inferior epigastric artery may be located on US and it is superior to this landmark that spigelian hernias typically occur. The hernia, depending on its content, is often heterogeneously hyperechoic and loops of bowel may be identified, when present. The advantage of US over CT, in which the patients are supine which may reduce the prominence of the hernia, is the fact that the patient can attain various positions and Valsalva maneuver can be employed. On CT, spigelian hernias may be diagnosed based on their location. These hernias are interparietal, extending between layers of the abdominal wall musculature and rarely extend into the superficial fascia or deep subcutaneous fat of the abdominal wall, findings readily appreciated at CT. CT may also be useful for evaluating the possibility of strangulation or incarceration of the components of the hernia sac. On CT, as with US, Valsalva should be considered to increase sensitivity and to evaluate the full extent of the hernia.

PEARLS

• Spigelian hernias typically occur at the level of the semicircular line, the point at which the fascia of the transversus and oblique muscles begin to split and present a weak point.

• In spigelian hernias, the incarceration rate approaches 20%.

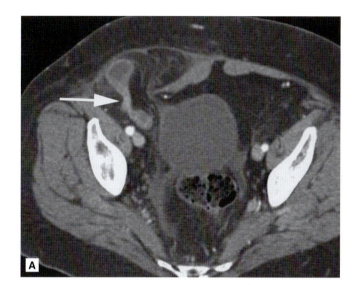

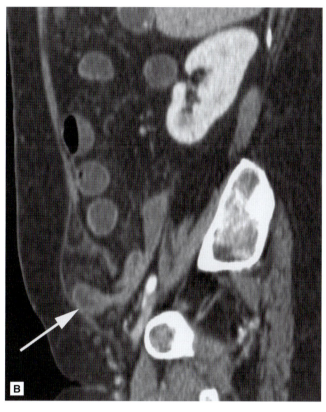

1. A. Axial, contrast-enhanced CT image reveals the presence of an incarcerated loop of small bowel within a spigelian hernia (arrow).
B. Sagittal, contrast-enhanced CT image reveals the presence of an incarcerated loop of small bowel within a spigelian hernia (arrow).

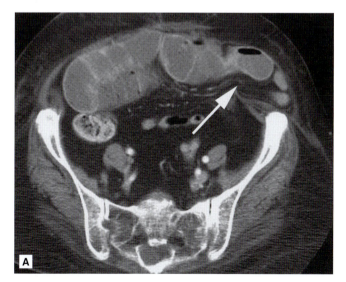

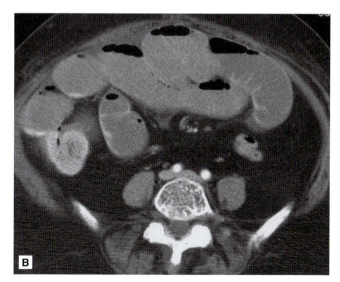

2. A. Axial, contrast-enhanced CT image demonstrates an incarcerated loop of small bowel within a left-sided spigelian hernia (arrow).
B. Axial, contrast-enhanced CT image reveals diffusely distended bowel proximal to the obstruction caused by the spigelian hernia.

547

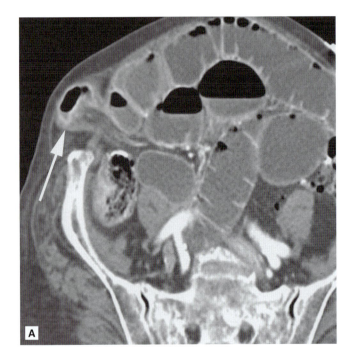

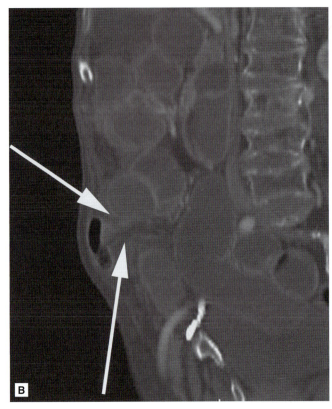

3. A. Axial, contrast-enhanced CT image reveals the presence of an incarcerated loop of small bowel within a spigelian hernia (arrow) causing small bowel obstruction. **B.** Coronal, contrast-enhanced CT image reveals the presence of an incarcerated loop of small bowel within a spigelian hernia (arrows) causing small bowel obstruction.

PRESENTATION

Palpable mass below the inguinal ligament, incarceration of bowel with pain, and possible bowel obstruction.

FINDINGS

A femoral hernia is seen to extend into the femoral canal, possibly causing compression of the adjacent femoral vein located immediately lateral to the hernia.

DIFFERENTIAL DIAGNOSIS

- Inguinal hernia

COMMENTS

Femoral hernias are postulated to result from a congenital abnormality in the attachment of the transverse fascia to the pubis. Femoral hernias are less common than inguinal hernias, accounting for approximately 5% of abdominal wall hernias, and are more commonly affect the women. Given the nature of the femoral canal, which is narrow and rigid, a potential complication of femoral hernias is bowel incarceration that may lead to strangulation or bowel obstruction. In fact, up to 40% of patients with femoral hernias are reported to present with incarceration or strangulation of bowel loops.

On imaging, the femoral hernia is seen to extend into the femoral canal, medial to the femoral vein and posterior to the inguinal ligament. These hernias are more common on the right side. A useful imaging finding to distinguish femoral hernias from inguinal hernias is compression of the femoral vein which is seen in the majority of femoral hernias and rarely seen in inguinal hernias. Thus, when a groin hernia is seen lateral to the pubic tubercle (medial extension is specific for inguinal hernia), the presence of femoral vein compression suggests the presence of a femoral hernia.

PEARLS

- **Forty percent of femoral hernias may result in incarceration or strangulation of bowel loops.**

- **A femoral hernia may cause compression of the adjacent femoral vein and do not extend medial to the pubic tubercle, a specific finding for inguinal hernias.**

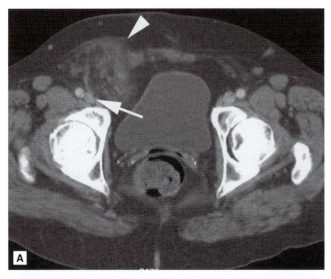

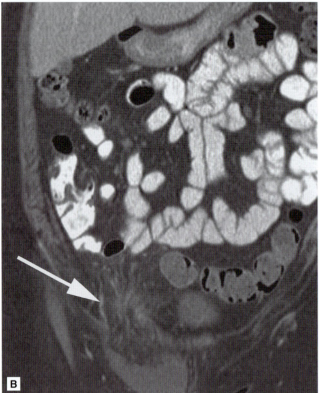

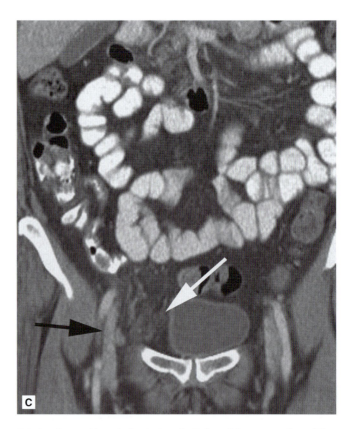

1. A. Axial, contrast-enhanced CT image reveals strangulation of a fat-containing femoral hernia (arrowhead). Note mild compression of the adjacent femoral vein (arrow). **B.** Coronal, contrast-enhanced CT image reveals strangulation of a fat-containing femoral hernia (arrow) with inflammation and fluid within the hernia noted. **C.** Coronal, contrast-enhanced CT image reveals strangulation of a fat-containing femoral hernia (white arrow) with mild compression of the femoral vein again noted (black arrow).

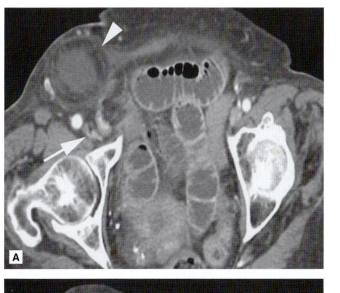

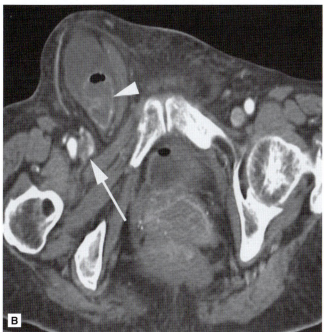

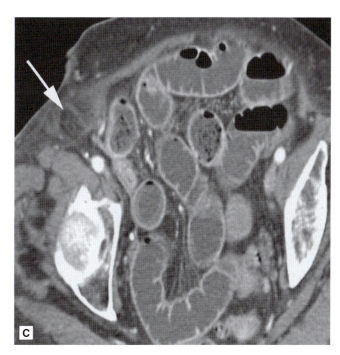

2. A. Axial, contrast-enhanced CT image reveals a femoral hernia (arrowhead) causing compression of the adjacent femoral vein (arrow).
B. Axial, contrast-enhanced CT image reveals a femoral hernia with incarcerated small bowel (arrowhead) causing compression of the adjacent femoral vein (arrow). **C.** Axial, contrast-enhanced CT image reveals diffuse distention of the small bowel related to the obstruction caused by the incarcerated loop within the femoral hernia, the superior most aspect of which is seen on this image (arrow).

PRESENTATION

Often vague, nonspecific signs and symptoms with dull abdominal pain, nausea, and vomiting.

FINDINGS

Obturator hernias may be confidently diagnosed by the presence of a portion of small bowel extending into the obturator foramen; the majority of patients also exhibit findings of secondary small bowel obstruction.

DIFFERENTIAL DIAGNOSIS

• Femoral hernia

• Inguinal hernia

COMMENTS

Obturator hernias are a rare variety of abdominal hernia which occurs through the obturator canal. The boundaries of the obturator canal include the pubic bone laterally and superiorly and the obturator membrane inferiorly. Obturator hernias are more common in women than men (up to ratio 9:1) given the anatomy of the obturator canal which is larger in women. Obturator hernias are also known as "little old lady's hernia" given their propensity to occur in elderly women. Weight loss and emaciation are also known to be predisposing factors related to the loss of preperitoneal fat about the obturator nerves and vasculature, allowing for hernia formation. While the signs and symptoms are typically nonspecific, a common clinical finding is the presence of the Howship-Romberg sign that includes pain and possibly parasthesias along the anteromedial thigh with movement of the ipsilateral hip or thigh. A more specific sign of an obturator hernia, which has been described, is the Hannington-Kiff sign that refers to an absent adductor

reflex in the thigh. In addition, a clinical clue to the diagnosis may be the presence of intermittent obstruction. Often in the case of obturator hernias, there is Richter herniation of small bowel into the obturator canal resulting in partial obstruction.

CT scan is the imaging modality of choice in confidently diagnosing an obturator hernia. Typically, in cases of obturator hernias, a portion of small bowel is visualized in the obturator foramen with the majority of patients also exhibiting findings of secondary small bowel obstruction. However, herniation of large bowel, omentum, appendix as well as fallopian tube has been described. On imaging, one of three described types of obturator hernia may be visualized: (1) herniation of bowel extending between the pectineus and obturator externus muscles, (2) herniation of bowel between the superior and middle fasciculi of the obturator externus muscle, and (3) herniation of bowel between the internal and external obturator membrane, which is a fibrous sheet, that nearly closes the obturator foramen. Given a relatively high incidence of strangulation, complications of obturator hernia such as frank ischemia as evidenced by decreased mucosal enhancement as well as bowel perforation should be considered when reviewing CT images in cases of obturator hernia.

PEARLS

• Obturator hernias often occur in elderly women and are associated with weight loss, hence the nickname is little old lady's hernia.

• Obturator hernias are diagnosed by the presence of small bowel within the obturator foramen that may extend between the pelvic musculature including pectineus and obturator externus muscles.

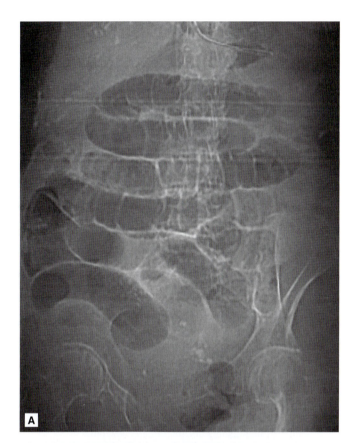

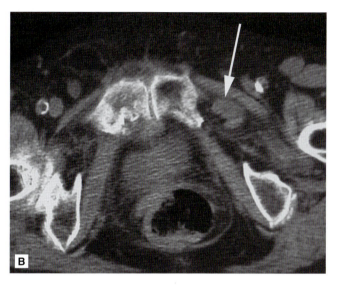

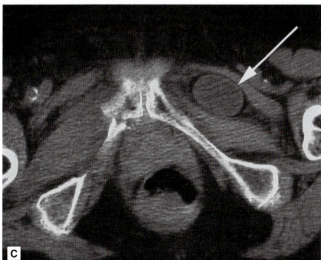

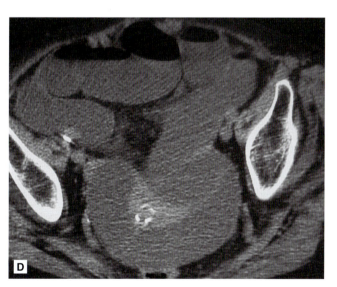

1. A. Abdominal radiograph demonstrates numerous dilated loops of small bowel suggesting a mechanical small bowel obstruction. **B.** Axial CT image reveals a small portion of small bowel (arrow) extending immediately posterior to the pectineus muscle. **C.** Axial CT image reveals a small portion of small bowel (arrow) herniating between the pectineus muscle anteriorly and the obturator externus muscle posteriorly. **D.** Axial CT image demonstrates dilated, fluid-filled loops of small bowel consistent with a mechanical small bowel obstruction related to the obturator hernia.

PRESENTATION

Typically asymptomatic but patients can present with right lower quadrant pain, nausea, and vomiting if the appendix is inflamed.

FINDINGS

The typical imaging findings in cases of Amyand hernia (AH) are the presence of a normal-appearing appendix extending into a right inguinal hernia.

DIFFERENTIAL DIAGNOSIS

- Littre hernia
- Incarcerated or strangled inguinal hernia

COMMENTS

AH is defined as the presence of a vermiform appendix within an inguinal hernia. In fact, Claudius Amyand (1660-1740) was the first surgeon to perform an appendectomy when he removed a perforated appendix from the inguinal canal of an 11-year-old boy. Thus, though typically normal, the appendix may be acutely inflamed and display complications commonly associated with appendicitis such as perforation. The complication of appendicitis is postulated to results from compression due to the inguinal ring resulting in inflammation, ischemia, and bacterial overgrowth. AHs are reported to be more common in men, occur in 1% of inguinal hernias, and have a bimodal age distribution with the majority of cases have been reported in premature neonates, infants, or postmenopausal women.

Though there is significant overlap in the clinical presentation of an AH with an incarcerated inguinal hernia, imaging is typically not employed unless the patient is also presenting with signs and symptoms to suggest an acute appendicitis. The typical imaging findings in cases of AH are the presence of a normal-appearing appendix extending into a right inguinal hernia. Though typically right sided given the location of the appendix, left-sided AH may be seen in cases of malrotation, situs inversus, or mobile cecum. When inflamed, typical imaging findings of acute appendicitis may be seen including appendiceal distention, mucosal hyperemia, periappendiceal inflammation and fluid, as well as frank perforation with abscess formation. In addition to CT, US has been reported to visualize the presence of appendicitis within an AH.

PEARLS

- AH is defined as the presence of the appendix within an inguinal hernia.

- Though typically normal, the appendix may be acutely inflamed and display complications commonly associated with appendicitis such as perforation.

- When inflamed, typical imaging findings of acute appendicitis may be seen including appendiceal distention, mucosal hyperemia, periappendiceal inflammation and fluid, as well as frank perforation with abscess formation.

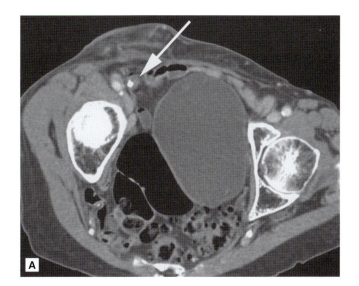

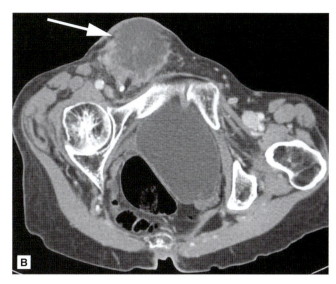

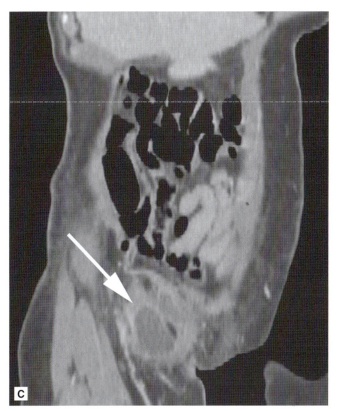

1. A. Axial, contrast-enhanced CT image reveals an appendicolith within the base of the appendix seen to extend into the right inguinal canal (arrow). **B.** Axial, contrast-enhanced CT image reveals an abscess related to a perforated appendicitis in the right inguinal canal (arrow). **C.** Coronal, contrast-enhanced CT image reveals an abscess related to a perforated appendicitis in the right inguinal canal (arrow).

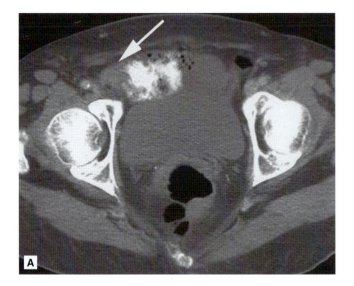

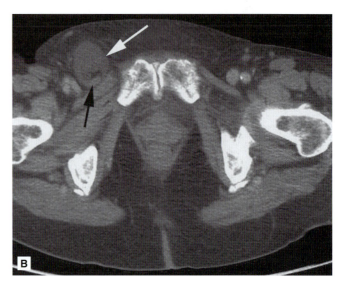

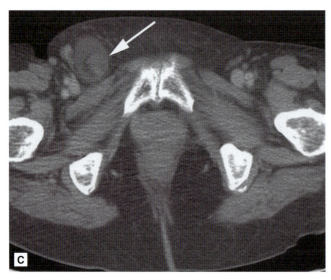

2. A. Axial, contrast-enhanced CT image reveals an abnormally thickened cecum and base of the appendix extending into the right inguinal canal (arrow). **B.** Axial, contrast-enhanced CT image reveals a fluid-filled appendix with mild mucosal hyperemia (black arrow) with surrounding fluid (white arrow) in the right inguinal canal. **C.** Axial, contrast-enhanced CT image reveals thickening of the appendiceal tip with surrounding fluid in the right inguinal canal (arrow).

VASCULAR

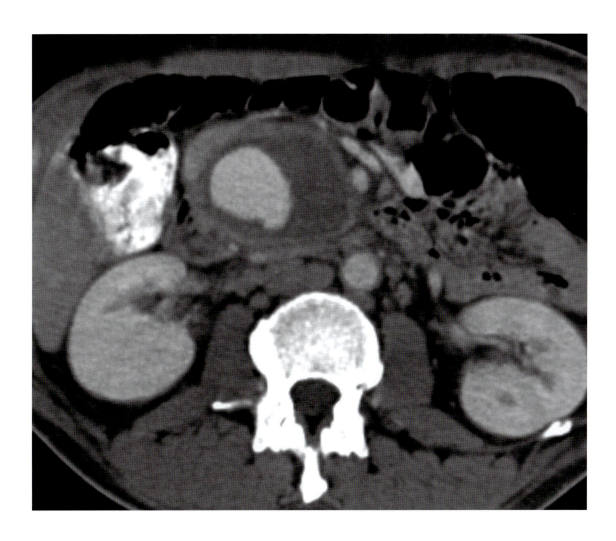

PRESENTATION

While visceral artery aneurysms (VAAs) are typically incidentally detected and asymptomatic, patients may present with abdominal pain, a palpable pulsating abdominal mass, an abdominal bruit, or signs and symptoms related to hemorrhage.

FINDINGS

Color Doppler typically demonstrates internal vascularity with an arterial flow pattern while CT angiography (CTA), the preferred modality for both diagnosis and treatment planning purposes, readily demonstrates the aneurysm as a saccular or fusiform dilation of the involved artery.

DIFFERENTIAL DIAGNOSIS

- Tortuosity of a normal artery (commonly splenic artery)
- Hypervascular pancreatic mass (neuroendocrine tumor, etc)

COMMENTS

While previously thought to be rare, VAAs are increasingly identified incidentally on imaging studies. VAAs are those that affect the hepatic, splenic, superior and inferior mesenteric, celiac, gastroduodenal, or pancreaticoduodenal, gastric and gastroepiploic, jejunal, and ileocolic arteries. In many cases, renal artery aneurysms are also considered VAAs. VAAs include both true as well as false aneurysms. The majority of VAAs are composed of splenic artery aneurysms followed by hepatic arterial aneurysms. However, over the past two decades, hepatic artery pseudoaneurysms have been the most frequently reported VAAs given the increase in invasive hepatobiliary procedures. While the underlying pathophysiology resulting in the formation of VAAs remains uncertain, most VAAs are secondary to vessel wall degeneration. Atherosclerosis, congenital syndromes, fibromuscular dysplasia, and collagen vascular disorders are other possible etiologies of VAAs. Pseudoaneurysms of the visceral arteries may develop as a result of trauma, inflammation (pancreatitis, etc), infection, vasculitides, and iatrogenic injuries. The incidence of rupture of VAAs is high, reportedly up to 25% resulting in high mortality rates. Thus, prompt diagnosis and subsequent therapy are critical in patients presenting with clinical signs and symptoms of rupture including abdominal pain or frank gastrointestinal (GI) bleeding.

On imaging, VAAs may be solitary or multiple (in up to one-third of patients), fusiform or saccular, and occur throughout any portion of a given visceral artery though certain portions of a given artery are favored. Thus, splenic artery aneurysms, which are typically solitary and saccular usually occur along the middle or distal aspects of the splenic artery and hepatic artery aneurysms, which are typically solitary and saccular, usually occur in an extrahepatic location. US examinations performed for the evaluation of unrelated clinical indications or related signs and symptoms such as abdominal pain may demonstrate a hypoechoic or anechoic round, pulsatile abdominal mass. Color Doppler typically demonstrates internal vascularity with an arterial flow pattern and a peripheral hypoechoic rim may be seen indicative of intraluminal thrombus. CTA is the preferred modality for both diagnosis and treatment planning purposes. CTA readily demonstrates the aneurysm as a saccular or fusiform dilation of the artery of origin. Peripheral intraluminal hypoattenuation is indicative of thrombus or atherosclerotic plaque. Surrounding hematoma is concerning for leak or frank rupture of VAAs.

PEARLS

- The majority of VAAs are composed of splenic artery aneurysms followed by hepatic arterial aneurysms.
- While previously thought to be rare, VAAs are increasingly identified incidentally on imaging studies.
- CTA readily demonstrates the aneurysm as a saccular or fusiform dilation of the artery of origin; surrounding hematoma is concerning for leak or frank rupture.

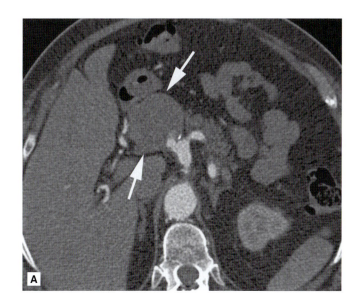

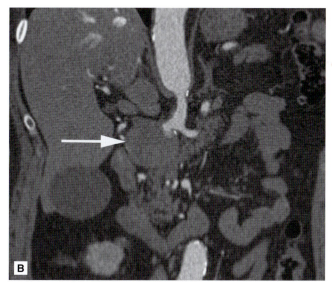

1. A. Axial CTA image demonstrates a large saccular outpouching arising from the common hepatic artery (arrows), the lack of filling of which is consistent with near-complete thrombosis. **B.** Coronal CTA image demonstrates a large, nearly completely thrombosed hepatic arterial aneurysm (arrow).

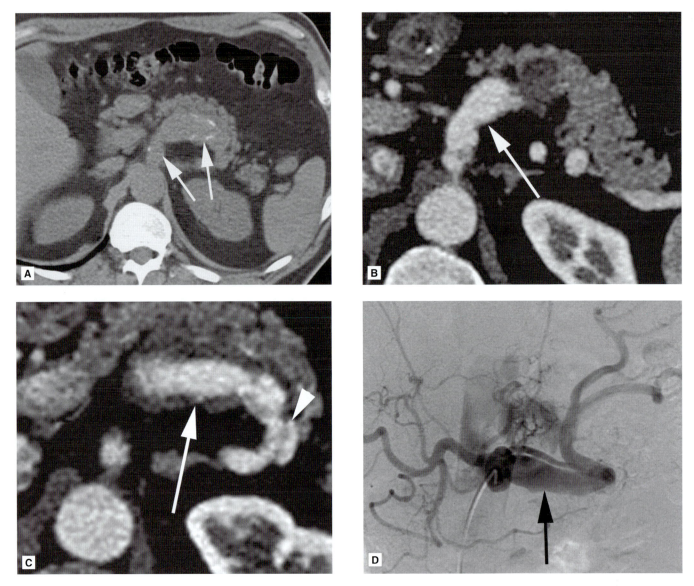

2. A. Axial, unenhanced CT image demonstrates fusiform dilatation of the celiac axis and splenic artery (arrows). **B.** Axial CTA image demonstrates fusiform dilatation of the celiac axis extending into the splenic artery (arrow). **C.** Axial CTA image demonstrates fusiform dilatation of the splenic artery (arrow) in which a dissection is seen (arrowhead). **D.** Selective celiac angiogram reveals a fusiform aneurysm of the celiac axis and proximal splenic artery (arrow) in which a dissection is seen.

PRESENTATION

While typically clinically silent, patients may present with abdominal pain or gastrointestinal hemorrhage related to complications from splenic vein (SV) thrombosis.

FINDINGS

Acute splenic thrombosis classically causes a partially occlusive, hypoattenuating filling defect within the SV on contrast-enhanced CT and, over time, results in a lack of visualization of the SV, isolated left-sided (perigastric) collaterals, as well as upstream SV dilatation.

DIFFERENTIAL DIAGNOSIS

- Mixing or streaming artifact of contrast bolus
- External SV compression
- Portal hypertension

COMMENTS

SV thrombosis is diagnosed by the presence of clot within an enlarged SV. SV thrombosis equally affects men and women of any age and is most often associated with hypercoaguable states, trauma, adjacent inflammation (chronic pancreatitis causes 10%-40% of SV thromboses), local stasis (cirrhosis), or neoplastic invasion. Feared complications of SV thrombosis and resultant left-sided portal hypertension (also referred to as sinistral hypertension) include the formation of left-sided collateral veins which may result in gastrointestinal hemorrhage.

US is employed as the initial imaging modality for patients presenting with nonspecific abdominal pain. On US, in acute cases of portal venous thrombosis, the thrombus is usually made apparent by the lack color Doppler flow; noting that the presence of flow within hilar branches does not exclude SV thrombosis. The thrombus itself varies in appearance from anechoic to hyperechoic, depending on its age. Chronic thrombosis within the splenic vein is evidenced by nonvisualization of part or the entirety of the scarred splenic vein and often also by the presence of splenogastric or splenorenal collaterals without other evidence of portal hypertension.

Acute splenic thrombosis classically causes a partially occlusive, hypoattenuating filling defect within the SV on contrast-enhanced CT. A common pitfall in diagnosing SV thrombosis is related to a mixing artifact from the administration of intravenous contrast. Thus, recognizing the sequela from SV thrombosis is useful in mitigating this imaging pitfall and increasing diagnostic confidence. SV thrombosis may result in lack of visualization of the SV, isolated left-sided (perigastric) collaterals, upstream SV dilatation and splenic parenchymal congestion leading to splenomegaly. Rarely, acute SV thrombosis can cause sever congestion leading to frank splenic infarction.

PEARLS

- SV thrombosis is most often associated with hypercoaguable states, trauma, adjacent inflammation with a large number of cases caused by pancreatis, local stasis such as related to cirrhosis, or neoplastic invasion.

- As mixing artifact is a common pitfall for SV thrombosis on CT, recognizing sequela such as isolated left-sided collaterals, upstream splenic vein dilatation, and splenic parenchymal congestion is useful in improving diagnostic confidence.

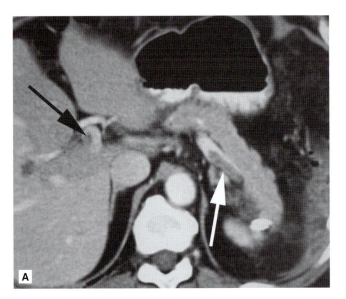

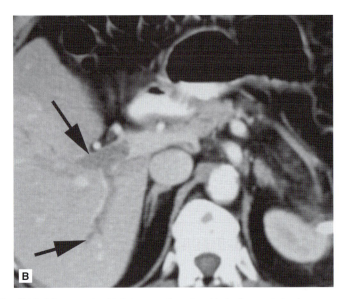

1. A. Axial, contrast-enhanced examination reveals a thrombus within the SV (white arrow) which is seen to extend into the portal vein (black arrow) in a patient with recent splenectomy. **B.** Axial, contrast-enhanced examination reveals extension of the thrombus into the main and right-sided portal venous system (arrows).

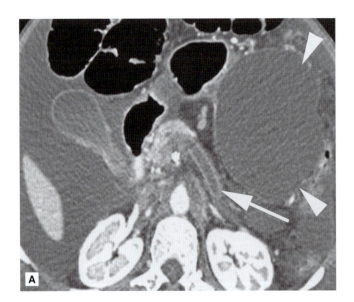

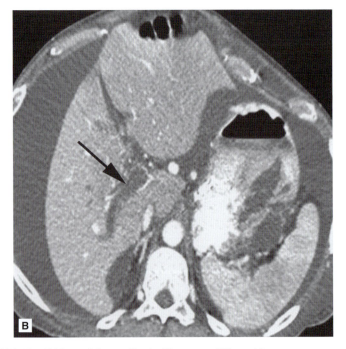

2. A. Axial, contrast-enhanced examination reveals a large thrombus within the SV (arrow) in a patient with pancreatitis and large pseudocyst formation (arrowheads). **B.** Axial, contrast-enhanced examination reveals extension of the SV thrombosis into the portal venous system (arrow) in a patient with pancreatitis.

PRESENTATION

Patients may present with abdominal pain and abnormal liver function tests.

FINDINGS

Portal vein thrombosis (PVT), directly identified as intraluminal filling defects within the portal vein may result in relative hyperattenuation of the affected segments on early-phase CT image along with enhancement of the portal vein walls.

DIFFERENTIAL DIAGNOSIS

• Mixing or streaming artifact of contrast bolus

• External compression

• Budd-Chiari syndrome

COMMENTS

PVT may cause abnormal liver function and abdominal pain. It is an uncommon finding that affects men and women of any age equally and is most often associated with hypercoagulable states, intraluminal nidus or seeding (such as in the case of appendicitis), adjacent inflammation (pancreatitis or local infection), local stasis (cirrhosis), or neoplastic invasion. Portal venous thrombi can be acute or chronic, form within the intra- or extrahepatic portal veins, propagate up- or downstream, partially or totally occlude the portal vein, and result in a spectrum of findings on virtually all imaging modalities.

US is most often the first-line evaluation of right upper quadrant pain or abnormal liver function testing. US features of PVT include absent flow or nonvisualization of the portal vein or its tributaries. The thrombus itself varies in appearance from anechoic to hyperechoic, depending on its age. In cases of chronic, completely occlusive thrombi, portal vein nonvisualization or recognition of cavernous transformation or collateral vessel formation are typical imaging findings. While acute thrombus can be occlusive, it can also cause partial occlusion resulting in upstream portal venous dilation. Care must be taken during Doppler and spectral analysis to rule out other causes of slow or near-absent portal venous blood flow, namely, portal hypertension related to conditions such as cirrhosis, external compression from adjacent lymph nodes or mass lesions, or Budd-Chiari syndrome. In suspected cases of PVT, contrast-enhanced CT may be used to confirm the diagnosis if there is suspicion of possible slow portal venous blood flow causing a false-positive diagnosis on US.

Acute portal venous thrombus classically causes a partially occlusive, hypoattenuating filling defect within the portal vein on contrast-enhanced CT and visual identification of this filling defect is the most direct method of detection. A common pitfall in making this diagnosis on CT is a mixing or streaming artifact from intravenous contrast. When a low-attenuating filling defect within the portal vein does not certainly represent a thrombus and mixing artifact is considered as a possible explanation, recognizing the indirect sequela portal venous thrombosis is useful in increasing confidence and correctly making the appropriate diagnosis. In cases of relatively acute portal venous thrombus, abnormally high attenuation within the affected hepatic segments of the liver from increased arterial blood flow may be identified on both arterial and portal venous phase imaging though this may be more evident on earlier-phase (arterial or early portal venous) imaging. In addition, enhancement of the walls of the portal vein secondary to hyperemic vasa vasorum blood flow, also known as a "rim sign" may be identified on CT. Differentiating chronic from acute PVT can be deduced by indentifying periportal collaterals or varices, splenic enlargement, hepatic artery dilatation, or atrophy/nodular regeneration of affected hepatic segments, findings seen in cases of chronic thrombosis. More distant imaging findings in cases of PVT which may be readily identified on CT include bowel wall edema and congestion, ileus, and, rarely, venous infarction or ascites. On contrast-enhanced MRI, similar findings to CT are often identified including direct visualization of the thrombus as a filling defect on portal venous phase images and increased enhancement of the affected segments during the arterial phase of image acquisition. In addition, MRI of subacute and chronic PVT typically reveals increased signal on both T1 and T2-weighted images.

While neoplastic invasion of the portal vein by adjacent tumor can also cause indistinguishable sequela on US, the

---

PEARLS

• **PVT may result in relative hyperattenuation of the affected segments on early-phase CT image acquisition related to an increase in hepatic arterial blood supply.**

• **Enhancement of the portal vein walls may be seen in cases of PVT related to hyperemia of the vasa vasorum.**

• **The presence of vascularity or contrast enhancement may be useful in distinguishing tumor from bland portal venous thrombi.**

primary tumor is typically readily identified by contrast-enhanced CT or MR. In addition, in many cases, blood flow in tumor thrombi may be identified on US (Doppler analysis) as well as contrast-enhanced CT and MRI as evidence by enhancement of the tumor thrombus itself or direct visualization of the tumoral neovascularity.

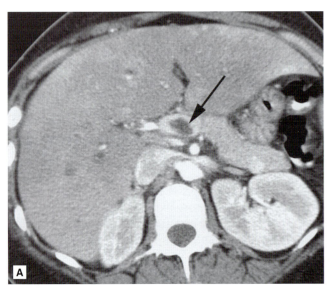

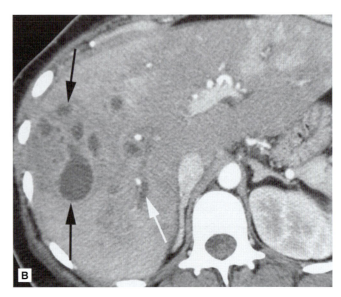

1. A. Axial, contrast-enhanced CT examination reveals a large thrombus within the portal vein (arrow) and resultant heterogeneous enhancement of the hepatic parenchyma. **B.** Axial, contrast-enhanced CT examination reveals a large hepatic abscess (black arrows) causing thrombosis of the portal veins (white arrow).

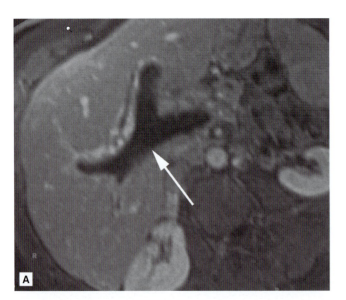

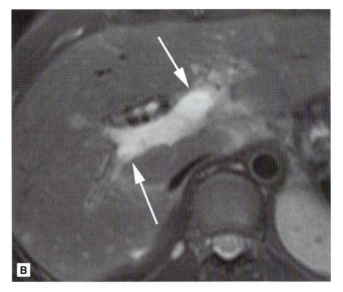

2. A. Axial, contrast-enhanced MRI examination demonstrates extensive PVT (arrow) as evidenced by a lack of contrast opacification in a patient with pancreatitis. **B.** T2-weighted MRI image reveals hyperintensity of the portal venous thrombus (arrows), suggesting liquefaction of the clot. **C.** Magnetic resonance cholangiopancreatography (MRCP) images demonstrate hyperintensity of the portal venous thrombus (arrows), suggesting liquefaction of the clot. Adjacent normal-appearing bile ducts are also seen (arrowhead).

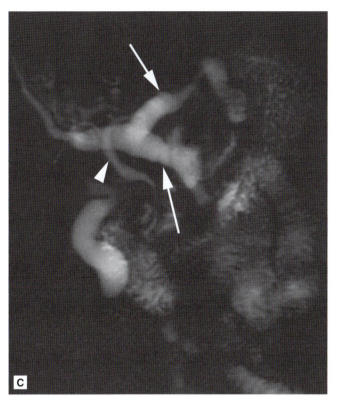

2. (*Continued*)

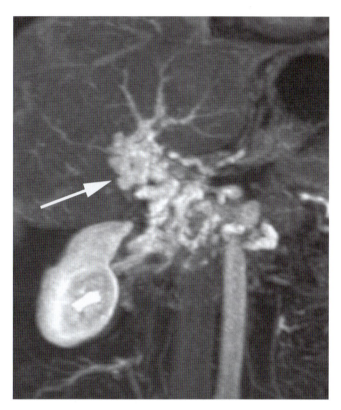

3. Contrast-enhanced MRI image demonstrates cavernous transformation of the portal vein as evidence by the presence of numerous small collateral veins in the hepatic hilum (arrow) in the expected location of the main and central portal veins, which are not visualized in this case.

PRESENTATION

While gastroduodenal artery (GDA) pseudoaneurysms may be asymptomatic, patients may present with abdominal pain, a palpable epigastric mass, melena, hematemesis, hematochezia, or obstructive jaundice.

FINDINGS

On CT angiography, opacification of pseudoaneurysm sac with direct communication with the GDA can be seen.

DIFFERENTIAL DIAGNOSIS

- True visceral arterial aneurysm
- Arteriovenous malformation
- Hypervascular pancreatic mass (neuroendocrine tumor, etc)

COMMENTS

Pseudoaneuryms occur in 3.5% to 10% of the cases of pancreatitis. Of these, approximately 30% occur in GDAs. In pancreatitis, which is the most common etiology of GDA pseudoaneurysm, pancreatic enzymes erode the peripancreatic vessels, resulting in pseudoaneurysm formation. Less common etiologies include trauma and iatrogenic causes. Similar to splenic artery pseudoaneurysms, GDA pseudoaneurysms are rarely asymptomatic and usually present with melena, hematochezia, hematemesis, or hemodynamic instability. Other presenting symptoms include abdominal pain, pulsating epigastric mass, obstructive jaundice, and, rarely, gastric outlet obstruction. GDA pseudoaneurysms have been reported to rupture into pseudocysts, the gastrointestinal (GI) tract, the peritoneal cavity, as well as the pancreatic parenchyma. Also, rupture of a GDA pseudoaneurysm into the main pancreatic duct can result in chronic or massive GI bleeding and is known as hemosuccus pancreaticus.

Initial US examination of the abdomen obtained for workup of abdominal pain may reveal a GDA pseudoaneurysm. On grayscale US imaging, an unruptured pseudoaneurysm demonstrates an anechoic "cystic" mass, often with a hypoechoic rind indicative of thrombus. Color Doppler images of the pseudoaneurysm sac may reveal the well known "yin yang" sign of swirling blood. At the neck of the pseudoaneurysm, the so-called "to and fro" appearance as blood enters the pseudoaneurysm sac may be seen. An adjacent avascular cyst indicative of a pancreatic pseudocyst may also be seen. A noncontrast CT may demonstrate high density adjacent to the pseudoaneurysm indicative of a hematoma, which could be due to hemorrhage into a pseudocyst, pancreatic parenchyma, or the peritoneal cavity. On CT angiography, opacification of pseudoaneurysm sac with visualization of its origin from the GDA can be seen. Delayed-phase CT may reveal retention of contrast within the pseudoaneurysm. In case of a ruptured GDA pseudoaneurysm, CT angiography often demonstrates extraluminal leakage of hyperattenuating contrast into a surrounding hematoma or adjacent anatomic compartment. In a patient presenting with chronic GI bleeding, a GDA pseudoaneurysm may be seen communicating with pancreatic duct, establishing a diagnosis of hemosuccus pancreaticus.

PEARLS

- Pancreatitis is the most common etiology of gastroduodenal pseudoaneurysms; less common etiologies include trauma and iatrogenic causes.

- Color Doppler images of the pseudoaneurysm sac may reveal the "yin yang" sign of swirling blood and the "to and fro" appearance of blood entering the pseudoaneurysm sac may be seen in the neck of the pseudoaneurysm.

- In case of a ruptured GDA pseudoaneurysm, computed tomographic angiography (CTA) often demonstrates extraluminal leakage of contrast into a surrounding hematoma or adjacent anatomic compartment.

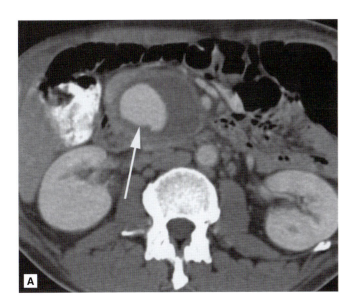

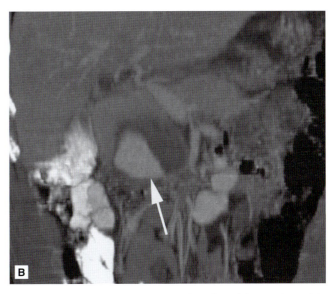

1. A. Axial, contrast-enhanced CT image demonstrates a large GDA pseudoaneurysm (arrow) which is partially thrombosed in a patient with a history of pancreatitis. **B.** Coronal, contrast-enhanced CT image demonstrates a large GDA pseudoaneurysm (arrow).

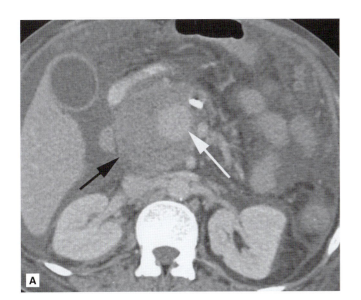

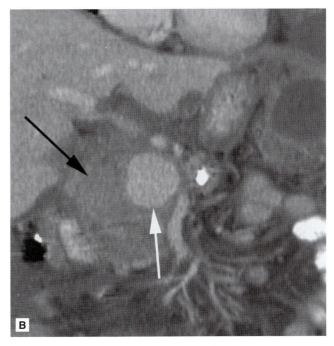

2. A. Axial, contrast-enhanced CT image demonstrates a GDA pseudoaneurysm (white arrow) with evidence of surrounding hemorrhage (black arrow) concerning for rupture. **B.** Coronal, contrast-enhanced CT image demonstrates a GDA pseudoaneurysm (white arrow) with evidence of surrounding hemorrhage (black arrow) in a patient with a history of pancreatitis.

PRESENTATION

Patients typically present with abdominal pain and clinical signs and symptoms related to rupture and hemorrhage.

FINDINGS

Splenic artery pseudoaneurysms are seen as focal out-pouchings of the splenic artery on CT angiography.

DIFFERENTIAL DIAGNOSIS

- True splenic artery aneurysm
- Arteriovenous fistula
- Hypervascular pancreatic mass (neuroendocrine tumor, etc)

COMMENTS

Splenic artery pseudoaneurysms are sequelae of an insult of the splenic arterial wall with injury to one or more layers of arterial wall, resulting in contained rupture with perfused sac that communicates with the artery. The most common causes of splenic artery pseudoaneurysms include pancreatitis, trauma, iatrogenic injury, and rarely, peptic ulcer disease. In pancreatitis, pancreatic enzymes cause a necrotizing arteritis with destruction of vessel wall architecture and fragmentation of elastic tissues, leading to pseudoaneurysm formation. Additionally, a long-standing pseudocyst may induce a pseudoaneurysm, caused by vascular erosion from enzymes within the pseudocyst, direct compression, or ischemia.

Splenic artery pseudoaneurysms nearly always present with symptoms, with only the minority of the cases presenting incidentally. The most common presentations include abdominal pain, hematochezia or melena, and hemateme-sis. The hemorrhage from splenic artery pseudoaneurysms may involve the pancreatic duct, peritoneum, retroperitoneum, adjacent organs (stomach, colon), as well as pancreatic pseudocysts. The risk of rupture of splenic arterial pseudoaneurysms, which is independent of its size, is reported to approach 40% with mortality rate approaching 90% when left untreated. The mean size of splenic artery pseudoaneurysms is nearly 5.0 cm. A coexisting pseudocyst can be seen in up to 40% of cases.

CT angiography (CTA) is the diagnostic modality of choice on which splenic artery pseudoaneurysms are seen as focal outpouchings with direct communication with the splenic artery. Splenic artery pseudoaneurysms are often identified adjacent to or within pancreatic pseudocysts, appearing as focal regions of enhancement in the low-density intracystic fluid. The enhancing component of a splenic artery pseudoaneurysm may be surrounded by thrombus or hematoma. A potential pitfall on axial imaging includes misinterpreting a splenic arterial aneurysm or pseudoaneurysm as a solid pancreatic mass.

PEARLS

- The most common causes of splenic artery pseudoaneurysms include pancreatitis, trauma, iatrogenic injury, and rarely, peptic ulcer disease.

- The risk of rupture of splenic arterial pseudoaneurysms is independent of size and is reported to approach 40% with a mortality rate approaching 90% when left untreated.

- Splenic artery pseudoaneurysms are seen as focal outpouchings with direct communication with the splenic artery which may be surrounded by thrombus or hematoma.

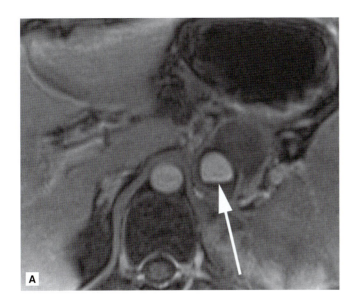

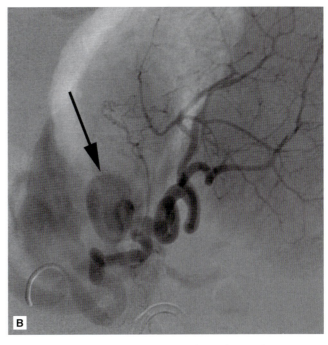

1. A. Axial, contrast-enhanced MRI image demonstrates a splenic arterial pseudoaneurysm (arrow) in a patient with a history of acute pancreatitis. **B.** Conventional angiographic image demonstrates the presence of a large splenic arterial pseudoaneurysm (arrow) in a patient with a history of acute pancreatitis.

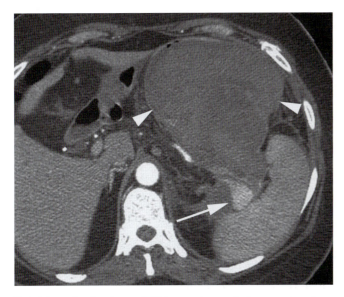

2. Axial, contrast-enhanced CT image demonstrates a ruptured splenic arterial pseudoaneurysm (arrow) as evidenced by the presence of a large perisplenic hematoma (arrowheads).

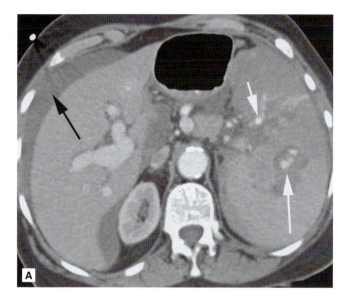 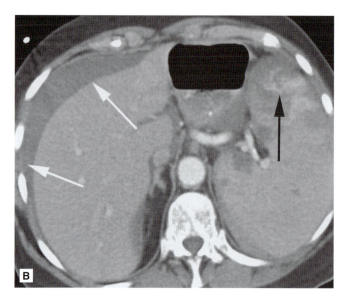

3. A. Axial, contrast-enhanced CT image demonstrates splenomegaly in a patient with polycythemia vera with resultant splenic rupture and pseudoaneurysm formation (white arrows) with large hemoperitoneum (black arrow). **B.** Axial, contrast-enhanced CT image demonstrates active hemorrhage related to splenic artery pseudoaneurysm rupture (black arrow) with resultant large hemoperitoneum (white arrows).

PRESENTATION

While rare, the classic clinical presentation of patients with aortoenteric fistula is gastrointestinal bleeding (upper and lower), pulsatile abdominal mass, and abdominal pain. More often, the diagnosis is made incidentally or after massive gastrointestinal hemorrhage.

FINDINGS

Periaortic or perigraft soft tissue edema, intramural gas, periaortic gas, pseudoaneurysm formation, or loss of the fat plane between the aorta and overlying bowel should raise the suspicion of an aortoenteric fistula.

DIFFERENTIAL DIAGNOSIS

- Peptic ulcer disease
- Infectious aortitis
- Retroperitoneal fibrosis
- Infected aneurysm
- Varices
- Vascular malformations
- Mallory-Weiss tears
- Malignancy

COMMENTS

Aortoenteric fistulas are direct communication between the aorta and any portion of the bowel which are typically found between the distal duodenum and the aorta though they may involve the jejunum or ileum. Aortoenteric fistulas are usually characterized as primary aortoenteric fistulas when they occur between the native aorta and adjacent bowel in a patient with no history of prior intervention. Primary aortoenteric fistulas are most commonly seen in patients with a history of an abdominal aortic aneurysm. In the absence of a history of an abdominal aortic aneurysm, primary aortoenteric fistulas are also found in patients with underlying infectious or inflammatory aortitis as well as in patients with a history of collagen vascular disorders.

Secondary aortoenteric fistulas are encountered more commonly than primary aortoenteric fistulas and occur as a result of aortic repair with or without the use of a graft. It is thought that the underlying reason for fistula formation is due to a chronic infection at the repair site which, in combination with the aortic pulsations, eventually leads to intestinal erosion and subsequent fistula formation.

In the absence of a history of aortic intervention, it is often difficult to make the diagnosis of aortoenteric fistula prospectively. When suspected, CT is often the first-line imaging tool employed given its speed and widespread availability. Primary aortoenteric fistulas should be suspected when there is obliteration of the fat plane between the aorta and adjacent bowel as well as gas surrounding the aorta or within the wall of the aorta. Surrounding periaortic fluid or hematoma and aortic wall disruption are additional findings suggestive of fistula formation. Secondary aortoenteric fistulas more readily prospectively suspected based on the clinical and surgical history. It should be noted that it may be difficult to distinguish graft infection from possible aortoenteric fistula formation. On imaging, outside of the immediate postsurgical period, periaortic or perigraft soft tissue edema, intramural gas, periaortic gas, pseudoaneurysm formation, or loss of the fat plane between the aorta and overlying bowel should raise the suspicion of an aortoenteric fistula formation. Both primary and secondary aortoenteric fistulas should be suspected when intravenous contrast is seen to extravasate into the lumen of the bowel.

PEARLS

- Aortoenteric fistulas are usually characterized as primary when they occur between the native aorta and adjacent bowel in a patient with no history of prior intervention.

- The more commonly encountered secondary aortoenteric fistulas occur as a result of aortic repair with or without the use of a graft.

- Currently, CT is often the first-line imaging tool in patients with suspected aortoenteric fistulas given its speed and widespread availability.

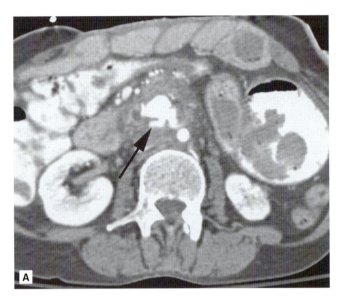

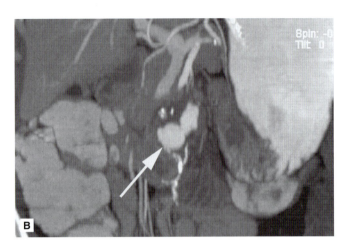

1. **A.** Axial, contrast-enhanced CT image demonstrates irregular pseudoaneurysm formation in the abdominal aorta (arrow) in a patient with massive gastrointestinal hemorrhage, highly suspicious for an aortoenteric fistula. **B.** Coronal, maximum-intensity projection image demonstrates a large, irregular pseudoaneurysm of the abdominal aorta in a patient presenting with gastrointestinal hemorrhage and found to have a secondary aortoenteric fistula.

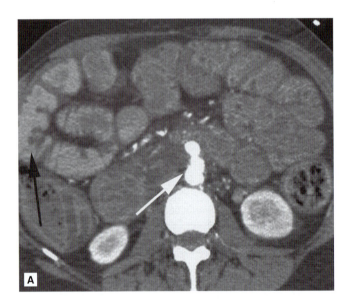

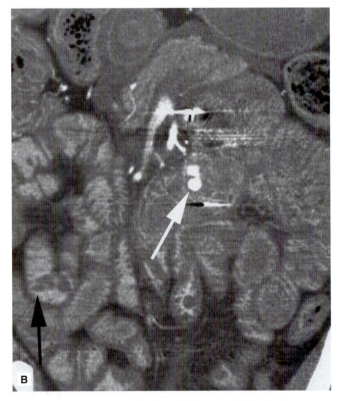

2. **A.** Axial, contrast-enhanced CT image demonstrates an abdominal aortic pseudoaneurysm extending into the lumen of the duodenum (white arrow). Note that this examination was performed without the administration of positive oral contrast agents; hyperattenuation within the small bowel lumen (black arrow) is consistent with gastrointestinal hemorrhage. **B.** Coronal, contrast-enhanced CT image demonstrates an abdominal aortic pseudoaneurysm (white arrow) as well as evidence of gastrointestinal hemorrhage (black arrow) in this patient with aortoenteric fistula.

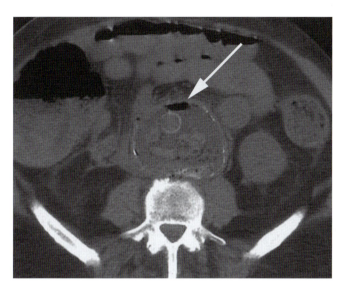

3. Axial, unenhanced CT image demonstrates the presence of air within an abdominal aortic aneurysm (arrow) as well as periaortic stranding. Outside of the immediate postsurgical period, these findings are concerning for an aortoenteric fistula, in the appropriate clinical setting.

INDEX